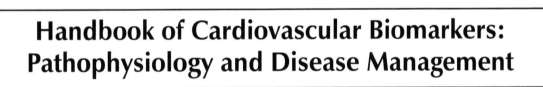

Handbook of Cardiovascular Biomarkers:
Pathophysiology and Disease Management

Handbook of Cardiovascular Biomarkers: Pathophysiology and Disease Management

Editor: John Freeman

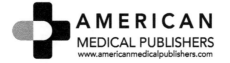

AMERICAN
MEDICAL PUBLISHERS
www.americanmedicalpublishers.com

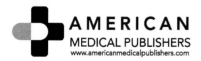

AMERICAN
MEDICAL PUBLISHERS
www.americanmedicalpublishers.com

Cataloging-in-Publication Data

Handbook of cardiovascular biomarkers : pathophysiology and disease management / edited by John Freeman.
     p. cm.
Includes bibliographical references and index.
ISBN 978-1-63927-961-6
1. Cardiovascular system--Diseases. 2. Biochemical markers. 3. Cardiovascular system--Diseases--Pathophysiology.
4. Cardiovascular system--Diseases--Diagnosis. 5. Cardiovascular system--Diseases--Treatment. I. Freeman, John.
RC667 .H36 2023
616.1--dc23

American Medical Publishers,
41 Flatbush Avenue,
1st Floor, New York,
NY 11217, USA

ISBN 978-1-63927-961-6 (Hardback)

Contents

Preface

Cardiovascular diseases (CVD) are a group of diseases that affect the heart and its functions. Biomarkers or biological markers are measurable and quantifiable biological indicators of health and some diseases. They play a crucial role in the implication of assessments related to health and physiology that cover a plethora of parameters, including disease progression and risk, psychiatric disorders, disease diagnosis, and metabolic processes. A CVD biomarker is used to improve the optimal clinical management and treatment of the patient. Various cardiac enzymes act as cardiac biomarkers, which comprise myoglobin, troponin and creatine kinase. The heart releases cardiac biomarkers into the bloodstream when it experiences damage or stress due to lack of oxygen. These biomarkers assist in determining if symptoms are due to a myocardial infarction, angina, heart failure or some other health problems. Enzyme marker test is utilized to measure specific biomarkers in the blood. This book elucidates the role of cardiovascular biomarkers in pathophysiology and disease management. It consists of contributions made by international experts. This book will serve as a valuable source of reference for scholars and researchers.

The information shared in this book is based on empirical researches made by veterans in this field of study. The elaborative information provided in this book will help the readers further their scope of knowledge leading to advancements in this field.

Finally, I would like to thank my fellow researchers who gave constructive feedback and my family members who supported me at every step of my research.

Editor

Carbohydrate Antigen 125 is a Biomarker of the Severity and Prognosis of Pulmonary Hypertension

Yi Zhang[1†], Qi Jin[1,2†], Zhihui Zhao[1], Qing Zhao[1], Xue Yu[1,3], Lu Yan[1], Xin Li[1], Anqi Duan[1], Chenhong An[1], Xiuping Ma[1], Changming Xiong[1], Qin Luo[1] and Zhihong Liu[1*]*

[1] Center for Pulmonary Vascular Diseases, Fuwai Hospital, National Center for Cardiovascular Diseases, Chinese Academy of Medical Sciences and Peking Union Medical College, Beijing, China, [2] Department of Cardiology, Shanghai Institute of Cardiovascular Diseases, Zhongshan Hospital, Fudan University, Shanghai, China, [3] Department of Cardiology, Qingdao Municipal Hospital, Qingdao, China

Correspondence:
Qin Luo
luoqin2009@163.com
Zhihong Liu
zhihongliufuwai@163.com

[†] These authors have contributed equally to this work

Background: Emerging evidence has showed that serum carbohydrate antigen 125 (CA 125) levels are associated with the severity and prognosis of heart failure. However, its role in pulmonary hypertension remains unclear. This study aimed to investigate the clinical, echocardiographic, hemodynamic, and prognostic associations of CA 125 in pulmonary hypertension.

Methods and Results: We conducted a retrospective cohort study of all idiopathic pulmonary arterial hypertension and chronic thromboembolic pulmonary hypertension patients receiving CA 125 measurement in Fuwai Hospital (January 1, 2014–December 31, 2018). The primary end-point was cumulative 1-year clinical worsening-free survival rate. Linear regression was performed to assess the association between CA 125 and clinical, echocardiographic, and hemodynamic parameters. Cox proportional hazards models were used to assess the association between CA 125 and clinical worsening events. Receiver operating characteristic (ROC) curve analysis was performed to determine the predictive performance of CA 125. A total of 231 patients were included. After adjustment, CA 125 still positively correlated with World Health Organization functional class, NT-proBNP, right ventricular end-diastolic diameter, pericardial effusion, mean right atrial pressure and pulmonary arterial wedge pressure; negatively correlated with 6-min walk distance, left ventricular end-diastolic diameter, mixed venous oxygen saturation, and cardiac index. After adjustment, CA 125 > 35 U/ml was associated with over 2 folds increased risk of 1-year clinical worsening. Further, ROC analysis showed that CA 125 provided additional predictive value in addition to the established pulmonary hypertension biomarker NT-proBNP.

Conclusion: CA 125 was associated with functional status, echocardiography, hemodynamics and prognosis of pulmonary hypertension.

Keywords: pulmonary hypertension, carbohydrate antigen 125, biomarkers, prognosis, severity

INTRODUCTION

Carbohydrate antigen 125 (CA 125), also known as mucin 16, is a glycoprotein synthesized by serosal cells in response to mechanical stress (congestion) or inflammatory stimuli (1–3). High serum CA 125 levels have been identified in malignancies such as ovarian, lung and gastrointestinal cancer (4). Currently, CA 125 is a widely used biomarker for the screening (5), monitoring (6) and risk stratification (7) of ovarian cancer. In addition, emerging evidence has linked serum CA 125 levels to non-malignant conditions such as cardiovascular disease (e.g., heart failure, pericardial diseases, and coronary artery disease) (8). More specifically, serum CA 125 levels were found to be associated with functional class (9), echocardiography (10), and hemodynamics (11) in heart failure. Furthermore, some studies have demonstrated the diagnostic and prognostic value of CA 125 in heart failure (12, 13). The capability of CA 125 to serve as a therapeutic target for heart failure has also been investigated, and the results were promising (14, 15).

As the release of CA 125 is irrelevant to the etiology of cardiac aggression, it should be considered a final organ damage marker (8). Thus, it may also play a role in pulmonary hypertension (PH). Unfortunately, there is still limited knowledge on this topic. Rahimi-Rad et al. reported that patients with PH had higher serum CA 125 levels than those without PH in chronic obstructive pulmonary disease (16). A similar phenomenon was also observed in congenital heart disease (17). Whether serum CA 125 levels are correlated with the severity and prognosis of PH remains unclear. In the present study, we aimed to investigate the correlations between CA125 and the functional status, echocardiography, hemodynamics, and prognosis of PH in a retrospective cohort.

MATERIALS AND METHODS

Study Design and Participants

This observational retrospective cohort study was conducted at Fuwai Hospital, Chinese Academy of Medical Sciences (Beijing, China). We screened all patients with idiopathic pulmonary arterial hypertension (IPAH) and chronic thromboembolic pulmonary hypertension (CTEPH) who underwent right heart catheterization (RHC) from January 1, 2014, to December 31, 2018. Patients with CA 125 data and multiple clinical visit/hospitalization records were enrolled as long as they had a minimum of 1 year of follow-up data for outcomes. In addition, echocardiography-suspected PH patients with normal invasive pulmonary arterial pressure and CA 125 data were also recruited as the control group. The establishment of IPAH and CTEPH was based on the 2009 (before January 2016) or 2015 European Society of Cardiology/European Respiratory Society (ERS) guidelines (18, 19). Normal pulmonary arterial pressure was defined as the mean pulmonary arterial pressure (mPAP) <25 mm Hg (18, 19). By design, patients were excluded if they had (1) any malignancy, (2) inflammatory diseases, or (3) active infection. The following clinical data were collected via an electronic medical record system by two independent reviewers: demographics, etiology of PH, 6-minute walk distance (6MWD), N-terminal pro-brain natriuretic peptide (NT-proBNP) levels, smoking history, alcohol consumption, World Health Organization functional class (WHO-FC), PH-specific medication, history of balloon pulmonary angioplasty/pulmonary endarterectomy, comorbidities, parameters derived from echocardiography and RHC, serum CA 125 levels, and follow-up data. The study protocol was approved by the Ethics Committee of Fuwai Hospital. Written informed consent was obtained from each patient.

CA 125 Measurement

Fasting venous blood samples were collected for CA 125 measurement on the first day of admission. Serum levels of CA125 were measured using a chemiluminescent microparticle immunoassay (product name: Access OV Monitor; Cat. No. 386357; Beckman Coulter Inc., Brea, CA, USA). Please refer to the manufacturer's website for the detailed methodology of the Access OV Monitor (https://mms.mckesson.com/product/586335/Beckman-Coulter-386357). The upper limit of normal for CA 125 was 35 U/ml with the Access OV Monitor. Accordingly, the included patients were divided into either the CA 125 > 35 U/ml group or the CA 125 $\leq$ 35 U/ml group.

RHC and Echocardiographic Examination

The detailed protocol for RHC has been provided in our previous publications (20–23). Briefly, with local anesthesia under continuous electrocardiographic monitoring, a 6 French pigtail catheter or 7 French Swan-Ganz catheter (Edwards Lifesciences World Trade Co., Ltd, Irvine, CA, USA) was advanced into the pulmonary artery through the right femoral vein or right internal jugular vein by placement of a 6 or 7 French vascular sheath. Correct catheter positioning was verified by fluoroscopy. Transducers were positioned at the midaxillary line and zeroed at atmospheric pressure. Transthoracic echocardiography was performed by experienced ultrasonologists in the Department of Echocardiography under the current guidelines (24).

Outcome

We considered the cumulative 1-year clinical worsening-free survival rate as the primary endpoint. Clinical worsening was defined as the occurrence of any of the following events: deteriorated WHO-FC, escalation of PH-specific therapy and rehospitalization due to heart failure or progression of PH. End-point events were adjudicated by two senior clinicians. Any discordance was resolved by the supervisors (QL and ZHL).

Statistical Analysis

Continuous variables are presented as the mean $\pm$ standard deviation. Categorical variables are given as counts. Comparisons between two groups were performed using an independent-sample t-test, the Mann–Whitney U-test or the chi-square test, as appropriate. Correlations between CA 125 and other variables were examined using the Spearman correlation coefficient. To adjust for potential confounding factors, associations with $P < 0.100$ were further assessed using multivariate linear regression analysis (enter method).

The Kaplan–Meier method was used to assess differences in the rate of 1-year clinical worsening events between patients with values above or below 35 U/ml; curves were compared with the log-rank test. The association between serum CA 125 levels and clinical worsening events was evaluated by a Cox proportional hazards model. Univariate Cox analysis was first performed to screen all prognostic factors. Variables with clinical significance or $P < 0.100$ in univariate analysis were selected for multivariate Cox analysis (enter method). We tested the Cox proportional hazards assumption for each covariate using Schoenfeld residuals. The linearity assumption for CA 125 was evaluated by restricted cubic splines with four knots. Collinearity diagnostics were examined for the potential presence of collinearity between independent variables in multivariate linear regression analysis and multivariate Cox analysis. Receiver operating characteristic (ROC) curve analysis was performed to assess the predictive performance of CA 125. Internal validation was performed using 500 bootstrap resamples (25, 26).

Values of CA 125 and NT-proBNP were logarithmically transformed (ln) and then used in correlation analysis, linear regression and the Cox proportional hazards model. No single missing value was replaced. A two-sided $P < 0.05$ was considered indicative of statistical significance. Data analysis was performed using SPSS (version 23.0), R-studio (version 1.4.1106), R (version 4.0.5), and MedCalc (version 19.7.2).

RESULTS

Patient Enrolment
We identified 231 (45.9%) eligible records for IPAH/CTEPH patients from the 503 records assessed; of the patients, 164 were IPAH and 67 were CTEPH. Furthermore, 84 patients with normal invasive pulmonary arterial pressure and CA 125 data were included as controls. A flow chart displaying the enrolment process is shown in **Figure 1**.

Baseline Characteristics
The baseline characteristics of all included patients are presented in **Table 1**. Among 231 patients with PH, 191 were categorized into the CA 125 ≤ 35 U/ml group and 40 into the CA 125 > 35 U/ml group. At baseline, 111 (48.1%) of 231 patients presented with WHO-FC III/IV, and 40 (17.3%) patients did not receive PH-specific medication. During the follow-up period, 73 (31.6%) patients experienced clinical worsening events. More specifically, 20 patients had deteriorated WHO-FC, 16 patients escalated their PH-specific therapy, and 37 patients were rehospitalized due to heart failure or progression of pulmonary hypertension. Among patients who experienced clinical worsening, 23 were in the CA 125>35 U/ml group, and 50 were in the CA 125 ≤ 35 U/ml group.

Patients With PH vs. Control Group
Compared to those in the control group, patients with PH were younger (40.0 ± 15.3 vs. 50.4 ± 16.2 years, $P < 0.001$), had worse WHO-FC, 6MWD, echocardiographic and haemodynamic parameters, and had higher serum levels of

NT-proBNP and CA 125 [17.3 (11.3, 25.8) vs. 9.5 (6.1, 18.2) U/ml, $P < 0.001$].

PH Patients With CA 125 > 35 U/ml vs. Those With CA 125 ≤ 35 U/ml
Compared to those with CA 125 ≤ 35 U/ml, patients with CA 125 > 35 U/ml had lower mixed venous oxygen saturation (S_vO_2), lower cardiac index (CI) values, a larger right ventricular end-diastolic diameter (RVED), higher prevalence rates of hyperlipidaemia and pericardial effusion, higher mean right atrial pressure (mRAP), and higher serum levels of NT-proBNP and CA 125 [55.9 (43.7, 83.0) vs. 14.5 (10.6, 21.1) U/ml, $P < 0.001$]. In addition, patients with CA 125 > 35 U/ml tended to have a smaller left ventricular end-diastolic diameter (LVED) (36.2 ± 6.6 vs. 38.2 ± 6.2 mm, $P = 0.064$).

CA 125 Is Weakly Associated With Established Markers of PH Severity
As shown in **Table 2**, ln(CA 125) was weakly correlated with 6MWD, WHO-FC, ln(NT-proBNP), echocardiographic parameters (LVED, RVED, and pericardial effusion), and haemodynamic parameters [S_vO_2, mRAP, CI and pulmonary vascular resistance (PVR)]. In addition, ln(CA 125) tended to correlate with pulmonary arterial wedge pressure (PAWP) ($r = 0.123$, $P = 0.062$). However, no correlations were observed between ln(CA 125) and left atrial dimension ($r = -0.066$, $P = 0.318$), left ventricular ejection fraction ($r = 0.034$, $P = 0.605$), systolic pulmonary arterial pressure ($r = -0.037$, $P = 0.585$), or mPAP ($r = 0.106$, $P = 0.109$). Similar results were observed in the CTEPH and IPAH subgroups (**Supplementary Tables 1, 2**).

In multivariate linear regression analysis (enter method), we further assessed correlations between CA 125 and functional status (6MWD, WHO-FC, and NT-proBNP) and echocardiographic (LVED, RVED and pericardial effusion) and haemodynamic (S_vO_2, mRAP, CI, PVR, and PAWP) parameters by adjusting for age, sex, and body mass index. The results showed that ln(CA 125) was still positively correlated with WHO-FC, ln(NT-proBNP), RVED, pericardial effusion, mRAP, and PAWP and negatively correlated with 6MWD, LVED, S_vO_2, and CI (**Table 2**). Similar results were observed in the CTEPH and IPAH subgroups (**Supplementary Tables 1, 2**). No problems with collinearity were detected in multivariate linear regression analysis (variance inflation factor < 5).

CA 125 Is Associated With Prognosis of PH
Kaplan–Meier analysis showed that IPAH/CTEPH patients with CA 125 > 35 U/ml had a lower cumulative one-year clinical worsening-free survival rate than those with CA 125 ≤ 35 U/ml (42.5 vs. 73.8%, $P < 0.0001$; **Figure 2**).

In univariate Cox analysis, 6MWD, ln(NT-proBNP), S_vO_2, mRAP, PAWP, and CA 125 > 35 U/ml had a $P < 0.100$ (**Table 3**). Considering their clinical importance, age, WHO-FC and pericardial effusion were also selected for multivariate Cox analysis (enter method). Events per variable are often used to estimate the sample size needed in multiple Cox analyses, and the lowest acceptable number of events per

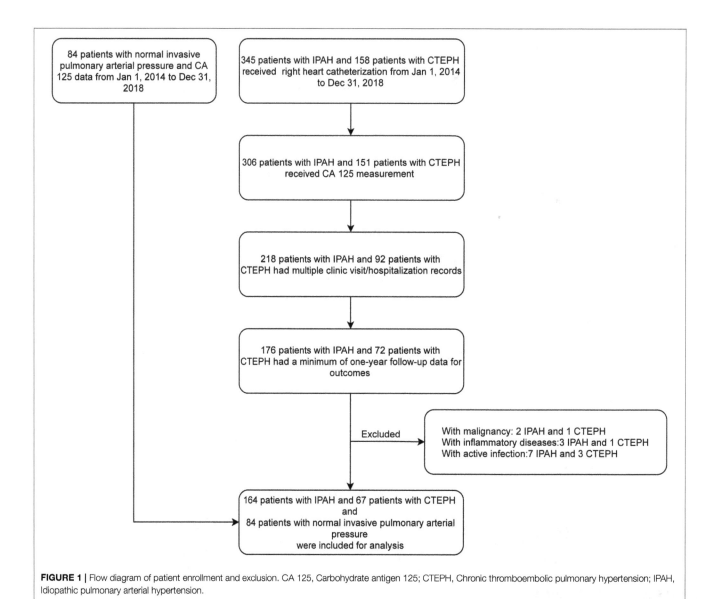

FIGURE 1 | Flow diagram of patient enrollment and exclusion. CA 125, Carbohydrate antigen 125; CTEPH, Chronic thromboembolic pulmonary hypertension; IPAH, Idiopathic pulmonary arterial hypertension.

variable is usually considered to be 10 (27). Given that 73 patients reached the primary endpoint in the present study, it was relatively safe for us to include a maximum of 7 independent variables into multivariate Cox analysis. Model 1 was adjusted for S_vO_2, 6MWD, ln(NT-proBNP), mRAP, and PAWP. Model 2 was adjusted for the variables in model 1 plus age. Model 3 was adjusted for the variables in model 1 plus hyperlipidemia. Model 4 was adjusted for the variables in model 1 plus WHO-FC. Model 5 was adjusted for the variables in model 1 plus pericardial effusion. In all 5 Cox models, CA 125 was found to be an independent predictor of clinical worsening (**Table 4**). The C statistic was 0.648 [95% CI: 0.577–0.718] for model 1, 0.652 [95% CI: 0.582–0.722] for model 2, 0.649 [95% CI: 0.578–0.720] for model 3, 0.649 [95% CI: 0.579–0.720] for model 4 and 0.647 [95% CI: 0.576–0.718] for model 5. Using bootstrap validation, the optimism-corrected C statistic was 0.609 for model 1,

0.606 for model 2, 0.603 for model 3, 0.604 for model 4 and 0.602 for model 5, indicating that the predictive ability of the models is relatively stable in future patients. We did not observe statistically significant deviations from the proportional hazards assumption in any of the Cox models (**Supplementary Table 3**). When modeled as restricted cubic splines, CA 125 showed a linear association with the HR for clinical worsening (**Supplementary Figure 1**). No problems with collinearity were detected in multivariate Cox analysis (variance inflation factor < 5). Subgroup analysis also showed that CA 125 was an independent predictor of clinical worsening in CTEPH and IPAH (**Supplementary Tables 4–7**).

CA 125 Provided Additional Predictive Value in Combination With NT-proBNP

To provide better insight into the predictive value of CA 125 for clinical worsening, we benchmarked it against the established

TABLE 1 | Basic characteristics of control group and patients with PH.

Variables	Control (n = 84)	IPAH/CTEPH			P-value*
		Total (n = 231)	CA 125 ≤ 35 U/ml (n = 191)	CA 125 > 35 U/ml (n = 40)	
Age, years	50.4 ± 16.2	40.0 ± 15.30‡	40.2 ± 15.2‡	38.9 ± 16.0‡	0.500
Female gender, no.	62 (73.8%)	158 (68.4%)	131 (68.6%)	27 (67.5%)	0.893
BMI, kg/m²	23.0 ± 3.9	23.2 ± 3.5	23.3 ± 3.5	22.8 ± 3.4	0.354
IPAH/CTEPH, no.	–	164/67	136/55	28/12	0.879
6 MWD, m	454.4 ± 96.2	420.4 ± 100.4†	424.0 ± 101.0	398.3 ± 95.2‡	0.259
NT-proBNP, pg/ml	135.0 (53.3, 314.9)	880.0 (170.3, 1908.0)‡	712.9 (151.5, 1705.0)‡	1,375.0 (888.7, 3206.5)‡	**0.002**
Smoking, no.	12 (14.3%)	29 (12.6%)	21 (11.0%)	8 (20.0%)	0.118
Alcohol intake, no.	13 (15.5%)	22 (9.5%)	16 (8.4%)	6 (15.0%)	0.194
WHO-FC		‡	‡	‡	**0.007**
I or II, no.	71 (84.5%)	120 (51.9%)	107 (56.0%)	13 (32.5%)	
III or IV, no.	13 (15.5%)	111 (48.1%)	84 (44.0%)	27 (67.5%)	
PH specific medication					0.376
None, no.	–	40 (17.3%)	35 (18.3%)	5 (12.5%)	
Mono or combination therapy, no.	–	191 (82.7%)	156 (81.7%)	35 (87.5%)	
PEA or BPA#, no.	–	24 (10.4%)	23 (12.0%)	1 (2.5%)	**0.044**
Co-morbidities					
Systemic hypertension, no.	25 (29.8%)	45 (19.5%)	40 (20.9%)	5 (12.5%)†	0.220
Diabetes mellitus, no.	4 (4.8%)	11 (4.8%)	9 (4.7%)	2 (5.0%)	1.000
Hyperlipidemia, no.	15 (17.9%)	22 (9.5%)†	22 (11.5%)	0†	**0.017**
Echocardiography					
LVEF, %	63.4 ± 6.4	63.3 ± 5.8	63.3 ± 5.8	63.0 ± 5.7	0.785
LA, mm	34.3 ± 5.9	31.0 ± 5.5‡	30.8 ± 5.0‡	31.8 ± 7.5‡	0.722
LVED, mm	44.5 ± 4.7	37.8 ± 6.3‡	38.2 ± 6.2‡	36.2 ± 6.6‡	**0.064**
RVED, mm	25.6 ± 6.6	32.2 ± 6.6‡	31.2 ± 6.4‡	33.7 ± 6.5‡	**<0.001**
sPAP, mm Hg	47.0 ± 10.0	86.7 ± 26.0‡	87.85 ± 27.2‡	81.1 ± 18.9‡	**0.096**
Pericardial effusion, no.	7 (8.3%)	32 (13.9%)	18 (9.4%)	14 (35.0%)‡	**<0.001**
Hemodynamics					
S_VO_2, %	76.0 ± 5.8	67.1 ± 6.5‡	67.8 ± 6.2‡	63.9 ± 7.4‡	**<0.001**
mRAP, mm Hg	3.0 (1.0, 5.0)	5.0 (2.0, 8.0)‡	4.0 (2.0, 7.0)‡	7.0 (3.3, 13.8)‡	**0.001**
mPAP, mm Hg	15.2 ± 3.2	51.2 ± 13.4‡	51.3 ± 13.5‡	50.9 ± 13.3‡	0.791
CI, L/min/m²	3.7 ± 0.8	3.0 ± 1.0‡	3.1 ± 1.0‡	2.7 ± 0.9‡	**0.018**
PVR, Wood units	1.2 ± 0.8	10.7 ± 5.1‡	10.6 ± 5.2‡	11.3 ± 4.4‡	0.227
PAWP, mm Hg	8.3 ± 3.3	7.7 ± 3.4	7.6 ± 3.2	8.5 ± 4.2	0.138
CA125, U/ml	9.5 (6.1, 18.2)	17.3 (11.3, 25.8)‡	14.5 (10.6, 21.1)‡	55.9 (43.7, 83.0)‡	**<0.001**

*Data are presented as mean ± standard deviation, median (range) or number (percentage). BMI, Body mass index; BPA, balloon pulmonary angioplasty; CA 125, Carbohydrate antigen 125; CI, Cardiac index; CTEPH, Chronic thromboembolic pulmonary hypertension; IPAH, Idiopathic pulmonary arterial hypertension; LA, Left atrium dimension; LVED, Left ventricular end-diastolic diameter; LVEF, Left ventricular ejection fraction; mPAP, Mean pulmonary arterial pressure; mRAP, Mean right atrial pressure; NT-proBNP, N-terminal pro-brain natriuretic peptide; PAWP, Pulmonary arterial wedge pressure; PAH, Pulmonary arterial hypertension; PEA, Pulmonary endarterectomy; PH, Pulmonary hypertension; PVR, Pulmonary vascular resistance; RVED, Right ventricular end-diastolic diameter; 6MWD, 6-min walk distance; sPAP, Systolic pulmonary arterial pressure; S_VO_2, Mixed venous oxygen saturation; WHO-FC, World Health Organization functional class. #Only for patients with CTEPH. *CA 125 > 35 U/ml compared with CA 125 ≤ 35 U/ml. †P < 0.05, compared with control group. ‡P <0.001, compared with control group. Bold values means their P value < 0.100.*

PH biomarker NT-proBNP (18). The areas under the curve for CA 125, NT-proBNP, and combined CA 125 and NT-proBNP were 0.604 (95% CI 0.537–0.667), 0.573 (95% CI 0.507–0.638), and 0.637 (0.571–0.699), respectively. The area under the curve of CA 125 + NT-proBNP was significantly higher than that of NT-proBNP alone (P = 0.0233), as shown in **Figure 3**. No significant differences were observed between CA 125 and NT-proBNP (P = 0.5108) or CA 125 and CA 125 + NT-proBNP (P = 0.2710).

DISCUSSION

In the present study, we found that serum CA 125 levels were weakly correlated with functional status (6MWD, WHO-FC, and NT-proBNP) and echocardiographic (LVED, RVED, and pericardial effusion) and haemodynamic (S_VO_2, mRAP, and CI) parameters of PH after adjustment. Moreover, CA 125>35 U/ml was found to be an independent predictor of 1-year clinical worsening in PH.

TABLE 2 | Correlations between carbohydrate antigen 125 and established markers of PH severity.

Variables	Coefficient (r)	P-value	Adjusted coefficient (r)*	P-value
6MWD	−0.168	**0.018**	−0.208	**0.004**
WHO-FC	0.277	**<0.001**	0.293	**<0.001**
ln (NT-proBNP)	0.309	**<0.001**	0.284	**<0.001**
Echocardiography				
LVEF	0.034	0.605		
LA	−0.066	0.318		
LVED	0.215	**0.001**	−0.173	**0.017**
RVED	0.306	**<0.001**	0.382	**<0.001**
sPAP	−0.037	0.585		
Pericardial effusion	0.251	**<0.001**	0.290	**<0.001**
Hemodynamics				
S$_V$O$_2$	−0.230	**<0.001**	−0.312	**<0.001**
mRAP	0.244	**0.001**	0.372	**<0.001**
mPAP	0.106	0.109		
Cardiac index	−0.243	**<0.001**	−0.208	**0.002**
PVR	0.198	**0.003**	0.127	**0.068**
PAWP	0.123	**0.062**	0.157	**0.018**

*ln, Logarithmically transformed; LA, Left atrium dimension; LVED, Left ventricular end-diastolic diameter; LVEF, Left ventricular ejection fraction; mRAP, Mean right atrial pressure; NT-proBNP, N-terminal pro-brain natriuretic peptide; PAWP, Pulmonary arterial wedge pressure; PH, Pulmonary hypertension; PVR, Pulmonary vascular resistance; RVED, Right ventricular end-diastolic diameter; 6MWD, 6-min walk distance; S$_V$O$_2$, Mixed venous oxygen saturation; WHO-FC, World Health Organization functional class. *Each variable is adjusted for age, gender, body mass index by multivariate linear regression analysis. Bold values means their P value < 0.100.*

CA 125 Is Weakly Associated With Established Markers of PH Severity

Compared to patients with normal invasive pulmonary arterial pressure, patients with PH had higher serum CA 125 levels, which was consistent with the results seen in chronic obstructive pulmonary disease (16) and congenital heart disease (17).

WHO-FC, 6MWD, NT-proBNP, pericardial effusion, mRAP, CI, and S$_V$O$_2$ are well-established prognostic markers of IPAH (18). We demonstrated that CA 125 was positively correlated with WHO-FC (9), NT-proBNP (28), RVED (10), pericardial effusion (10), mRAP (9, 11), and PAWP (9, 11) in PH, which was consistent with the results seen in heart failure. Additionally, we also found that CA 125 was negatively correlated with 6MWD, LVED, S$_V$O$_2$, and CI in PH. Therefore, CA 125 may serve as a novel biomarker of severity in PH.

To date, it remains unclear what leads to CA125 overproduction in heart failure (29, 30). It has been hypothesized to correlate with so-called "stressed" mesothelial cells: (1) mesothelial cells are stimulated by tissue stretching/mechanical stress induced by fluid overload due to heart failure. (2) mesothelial cells are stimulated by inflammatory cytokine network activation (interleukin-1, tumor necrosis factor-α, lipopolysaccharides) (29, 31). PH is characterized by increased mPAP and high PVR, which cause right ventricular hypertrophy, and finally result in right-sided heart failure. Based on our results, we hereby offered a hypothesis to explain the relationship between CA 125 elevation and right heart failure. Elevated PVR increased the afterload of right ventricle, which would further cause right ventricular dilation and elevation of right atrial filling pressure, leading to elevated hydrostatic pressure and congestion, which would further cause both serosal mechanical stretch and third space fluid retention with resultant inflammation and cytokines release (8), ultimately resulting in the elevation of CA 125 (29).

CA 125 Is Associated With Prognosis of PH

Compared to those with CA 125 ≤ 35 U/ml, patients with CA 125 > 35 U/ml had higher serum levels of NT-proBNP and worse echocardiographic and haemodynamic parameters at baseline. In all 5 Cox models we constructed, CA125 > 35 U/ml was associated with an over 2-fold increased risk of 1-year clinical worsening, which was similar to the results seen in heart failure (32, 33). Furthermore, ROC analysis showed that CA 125 provided additional predictive value in addition to the established PH biomarker NT-proBNP (18). Due to its close relationship with congestion (8), CA 125 should be considered a final organ damage marker in cardiovascular diseases. This may explain why we found that CA 125 was a severe and prognostic marker in PH.

Clinical Implications

Based on the current knowledge, CA 125 has several merits for use as a biomarker in clinical practice: (1) it is inexpensive, widely available, and measurable with standard methods and has a relatively long half-life (5–7 days) (34–36). (2) It correlates with the severity and prognosis of PH, providing additional information in combination with established risk factors. Therefore, CA 125 may become a valuable tool in the management of PH in the near future. Further studies are needed to evaluate its capacity to monitor response to treatment, serving as a therapeutic target and predicting hard outcomes (such as mortality).

Limitations

As a retrospective cohort study, follow-up bias is our biggest concern. Two hundred nine patients with CA 125 data were excluded for not having a minimum of 1 year of follow-up data for outcomes (**Figure 1**). Among these 209 patients, 29 had CA 125 > 35 U/ml, and 180 had CA 125 ≤ 35 U/ml. In other words, these two groups had similar rates of loss to follow-up [29/(40 + 29), 42.0% for CA 125 > 35 U/ml; 180/(191 + 180), 48.5% for CA 125 ≤ 35 U/ml]. Moreover, the percentage of patients who reached the endpoint was higher in the CA 125 > 35 U/ml group (57.5 vs. 26.2%). Taken together, these results indicate that the effect size (e.g., hazard ratio) in the present study would be underestimated rather than exaggerated. Follow-up bias should not undermine our conclusion. The present study included only patients with IPAH/CTEPH, which may limit its generalizability to other etiologies of PH. We planned to conduct a comprehensive retrospective study to investigate the correlations between CA 125 and functional status and echocardiographic and hemodynamic parameters in all five groups of PH patients.

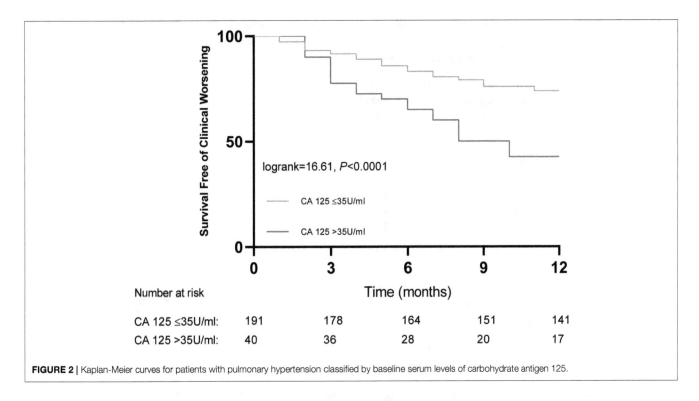

FIGURE 2 | Kaplan-Meier curves for patients with pulmonary hypertension classified by baseline serum levels of carbohydrate antigen 125.

TABLE 3 | Univariate cox analysis of proportional risks for 1-year clinical worsening.

Variable	β	Standard error	HR (95% CI)	Wald	P-value
Age	0.009	0.007	1.009 (0.994–1.024)	1.470	0.225
Female gender	−0.094	0.249	0.910 (0.559–1.484)	0.811	0.707
6MWD	−0.002	0.001	0.998 (0.995–1.000)	3.840	**0.050**
ln (NT-proBNP)	0.146	0.085	1.157 (0.979–1.368)	2.918	**0.088**
WHO-FC	0.177	0.234	1.193 (0.754–1.888)	0.568	0.451
Smoking	0.289	0.327	1.335 (0.703–2.535)	0.778	0.378
Alcohol intake	0.048	0.398	1.105 (0.482–2.288)	0.015	0.903
Systemic hypertension	−0.123	0.306	0.884 (0.485–1.611)	0.162	0.687
Diabetes mellitus	−0.662	0.717	0.516 (0.127–2.104)	0.852	0.356
Hyperlipidemia	−0.380	0.463	0.684 (0.276–1.695)	0.674	0.412
LVEF	0.000	0.020	0.982 (0.961–1.041)	0.001	0.982
LA	0.004	0.021	1.004 (0.963–1.047)	0.034	0.854
LVED	−0.016	0.019	0.985 (0.949–1.021)	0.695	0.404
RVED	0.016	0.017	1.017 (0.983–1.051)	0.949	0.330
sPAP	0.005	0.004	1.005 (0.998–1.013)	1.829	0.176
Pericardial effusion	0.410	0.306	1.507 (0.827–2.746)	1.797	0.180
S_VO_2	−0.061	0.018	0.941 (0.909–0.974)	12.023	**0.001**
mRAP	0.090	0.023	1.095 (1.047–1.145)	15.558	**<0.001**
mPAP	0.004	0.008	1.004 (0.988–1.020)	0.218	0.641
CI	−0.145	0.135	0.865 (0.664–1.127)	1.156	0.282
PVR	0.016	0.022	1.016 (0.974–1.061)	0.568	0.451
PAWP	0.064	0.035	1.067 (0.996–1.142)	3.411	**0.065**
CA 125 (category#)	0.975	0.253	2.650 (1.615–4.349)	14.866	**<0.001**

CA 125, Carbohydrate antigen 125; CI, Cardiac index; HR, Hazard ratio; LA, Left atrium dimension; LVED, Left ventricular end-diastolic diameter; LVEF, Left ventricular ejection fraction; ln, Logarithmically transformed; mPAP, Mean pulmonary arterial pressure; mRAP, Mean right atrial pressure; NT-proBNP, N-terminal pro-brain natriuretic peptide; PAWP, Pulmonary arterial wedge pressure; PVR, Pulmonary vascular resistance; RVED, Right ventricular end-diastolic diameter; 6MWD, 6-min walk distance; sPAP, Systolic pulmonary arterial pressure; S_VO_2, Mixed venous oxygen saturation; WHO-FC, World Health Organization functional class. #CA 125 is classified into two groups, namely CA 125 ≤35 U/ml and CA 125 >35 U/ml. Bold values means their P value < 0.100.

TABLE 4 | Multivariate cox analysis of proportional risks for 1-year clinical worsening.

Model	Variable	β	HR (95% CI)	P-value
1	CA 125 (category#)	0.860	2.362 (1.286–4.340)	**0.006**
	S_vO_2	−0.052	0.949 (0.904–0.996)	**0.035**
	6MWD	−0.001	0.999 (0.996–1.002)	0.576
	ln (NT-proBNP)	−0.042	0.959 (0.800–1.150)	0.650
	mRAP	0.009	1.009 (0.942–1.080)	0.802
	PAWP	0.040	1.041 (0.967–1.120)	0.282
2	CA 125 (category#)	0.876	2.401 (1.303–4.422)	**0.005**
	S_vO_2	−0.049	0.952 (0.906–1.000)	**0.050**
	6MWD	−0.001	0.999 (0.997–1.002)	0.691
	ln (NT-proBNP)	−0.037	0.964 (0.802–1.158)	0.692
	mRAP	0.011	1.011 (0.944–1.083)	0.759
	PAWP	0.037	1.037 (0.965–1.115)	0.323
	Age	0.007	1.007 (0.990–1.024)	0.424
3	CA 125 (category#)	1.474	4.366 (1.306–14.590)	**0.017**
	S_vO_2	−0.028	0.972 (0.883–1.071)	0.570
	6MWD	−0.003	0.997 (0.991–1.002)	0.225
	ln (NT-proBNP)	−0.153	0.858 (0.603–1.221)	0.396
	mRAP	−0.013	0.987 (0.878–1.110)	0.826
	PAWP	0.003	1.003 (0.883–1.138)	0.969
	Hyperlipidemia	−0.856	0.425 (0.088–2.043)	0.285
4	CA 125 (category#)	0.914	2.494 (1.339–4.645)	**0.004**
	S_vO_2	−0.054	0.948 (0.902–0.995)	**0.031**
	6MWD	−0.001	0.999 (0.996–1.002)	0.526
	ln (NT-proBNP)	−0.020	0.980 (0.810–1.186)	0.835
	mRAP	0.012	1.012 (0.944–1.084)	0.741
	PAWP	0.037	1.038 (0.963–1.118)	0.331
	WHO-FC	−0.244	0.784 (0.441–1.393)	0.406
5	CA 125 (category#)	0.843	2.323 (1.245–4.333)	**0.008**
	S_vO_2	−0.053	0.949 (0.904–0.996)	**0.034**
	6MWD	−0.001	0.999 (0.996–1.002)	0.607
	ln (NT-proBNP)	−0.048	0.953 (0.789–1.151)	0.616
	mRAP	0.010	1.010 (0.943–1.081)	0.783
	PAWP	0.040	1.040 (0.967–1.120)	0.289
	Pericardial effusion	0.095	1.100 (0.516–2.342)	0.806

CA 125, Carbohydrate antigen 125; HR, Hazard ratio; ln, logarithmically transformed; mRAP, Mean right atrial pressure; NT-proBNP, N-terminal pro-brain natriuretic peptide; PAWP, Pulmonary arterial wedge pressure; 6MWD, 6-min walk distance; S_vO_2, Mixed venous oxygen saturation; WHO-FC, World Health Organization functional class. #CA 125 is classified into two groups, namely CA 125 ≤35 U/ml and CA 125 >35 U/ml. Bold values means their P value < 0.100.

CONCLUSION

CA 125 was associated with the functional status, echocardiography and hemodynamics of PH. It was found to be an independent predictor of 1-year clinical worsening in PH. Moreover, it provided additional predictive value in combination with the established PH biomarker NT-proBNP. Given that the number of patients with elevated CA 125 levels

was low, our results, despite being promising, need to be confirmed in a large prospective study.

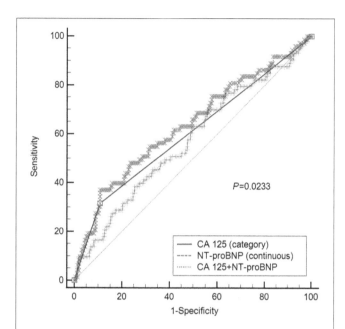

FIGURE 3 | ROC curve for CA 125, NT-proBNP, and CA 125+ NT-proBNP in predicting clinical worsening. P-value refers to the comparison between NT-proBNP and NT-proBNP + CA 125. No statistical significances were observed between CA 125 and NT-proBNP (P = 0.5108), or CA 125 and CA 125 + NT-proBNP (P = 0.2710). CA 125 is classified into two groups, namely CA 125 ≤ 35 U/ml and CA 125 > 35 U/ml; CA 125, Carbohydrate antigen 125; NT-proBNP, N-terminal pro-brain natriuretic peptide.

AUTHOR CONTRIBUTIONS

ZL and QL contributed to the conception of the study. YZ and QJ performed the data analyses and wrote the manuscript. ZZ, QZ, and CX contributed significantly to analysis and manuscript preparation. XY, LY, XL, AD, CA, and XM contributed to data collection. All authors critically reviewed the manuscript for intellectual content and had final responsibility for the decision to submit for publication.

ACKNOWLEDGMENTS

We are especially thankful to Dr. Yang Wang and Yanyan Zhao (Department of Statistics, National Center for Cardiovascular Diseases, Beijing, China) for their invaluable and dedicated assistance with the statistics.

REFERENCES

1. O'Brien TJ, Tanimoto H, Konishi I, Gee M. More than 15 years of CA 125: what is known about the antigen, its structure and its function. *Int J Biol Markers.* (1998) 13:188–95. doi: 10.1177/172460089801300403

2. Barbieri RL, Niloff JM, Bast RC Jr, Scaetzl E, Kistner RW, Knapp RC. Elevated serum concentrations of CA-125 in patients with advanced endometriosis. *Fertil Steril.* (1986) 45:630–4. doi: 10.1016/S0015-0282(16)49333-7

3. Halila H, Stenman UH, Seppälä M. Ovarian cancer antigen CA 125 levels in pelvic inflammatory disease and pregnancy. *Cancer.* (1986) 57:1327–9. doi: 10.1002/1097-0142(19860401)57:7<1327::AID-CNCR2820570713>3.0.CO;2-Z

4. Lee G, Ge B, Huang TK, Zheng G, Duan J, Wang IH. Positive identification of CA215 pan cancer biomarker from serum specimens of cancer patients. *Cancer Biomark.* (2010) 6:111–7. doi: 10.3233/CBM-2009-0134

5. Clarke-Pearson DL. Clinical practice. Screening for ovarian cancer. *N Engl J Med.* (2009) 361:170–7. doi: 10.1056/NEJMcp0901926

6. Bouanène H, Miled A. [Tumor marker CA125: biochemical and molecular properties]. *Bull Cancer.* (2009) 96:597–601. doi: 10.1684/bdc.2009.0859

7. Burger RA, Darcy KM, DiSaia PJ, Monk BJ, Grosen EA, Gatanaga T, et al. Association between serum levels of soluble tumor necrosis factor receptors/CA 125 and disease progression in patients with epithelial ovarian malignancy: a gynecologic oncology group study. *Cancer.* (2004) 101:106–15. doi: 10.1002/cncr.20314

8. Falcão F, de Oliveira FRA, da Silva M, Sobral Filho DC. Carbohydrate antigen 125: a promising tool for risk stratification in heart diseases. *Biomark Med.* (2018) 12:367–81. doi: 10.2217/bmm-2017-0452

9. D'Aloia A, Faggiano P, Aurigemma G, Bontempi L, Ruggeri G, Metra M, et al. Serum levels of carbohydrate antigen 125 in patients with chronic heart failure: relation to clinical severity, hemodynamic and doppler echocardiographic abnormalities, short-term prognosis. *J Am Coll Cardiol.* (2003) 41:1805–11. doi: 10.1016/S0735-1097(03)00311-5

10. Yilmaz MB, Zorlu A, Tandogan I. Plasma CA-125 level is related to both sides of the heart: a retrospective analysis. *Int J Cardiol.* (2011) 149:80–2. doi: 10.1016/j.ijcard.2009.12.003

11. Nägele H, Bahlo M, Klapdor R, Schaeperkoetter D, Rödiger W. CA 125 and its relation to cardiac function. *Am Heart J.* (1999) 137:1044–9. doi: 10.1016/S0002-8703(99)70360-1

12. Núñez J, Núñez E, Bayés-Genís A, Fonarow GC, Miñana G, Bodí V, et al. Long-term serial kinetics of N-terminal pro B-type natriuretic peptide and carbohydrate antigen 125 for mortality risk prediction following acute heart failure. *Euro Heart J Acute Cardiovasc Care.* (2017) 6:685–96. doi: 10.1177/2048872616649757

13. Hung CL, Hung TC, Liu CC, Wu YJ, Kuo JY, Hou CJ, et al. Relation of carbohydrate antigen-125 to left atrial remodeling and its prognostic usefulness in patients with heart failure and preserved left ventricular ejection fraction in women. *Am J Cardiol.* (2012) 110:993–1000. doi: 10.1016/j.amjcard.2012.05.030

14. Núñez J, Sanchis J, Núñez E, Fonarow GC, Bodí V, Bertomeu-González V, et al. [Benefits of statin therapy based on plasma carbohydrate antigen 125 values following an admission for acute heart failure]. *Rev Esp Cardiol.* (2011) 64:1100–8. doi: 10.1016/j.rec.2011.05.033

15. Núñez J, Llàcer P, Bertomeu-González V, Bosch MJ, Merlos P, García-Blas S, et al. Carbohydrate antigen-125-Guided therapy in acute heart failure: CHANCE-HF: a randomized study. *JACC Heart Failure.* (2016) 4:833–43. doi: 10.1016/j.jchf.2016.06.007

16. Rahimi-Rad MH, Rahimi P, Rahimi B, Gholamnaghad M. Serum CA-125 level in patients with chronic obstructive pulmonary disease with and without pulmonary hypertension. *Pneumologia.* (2014) 63:164–6.

17. Pektaş A, Olguntürk R, Kula S, Çilsal E, Oguz AD, Tunaoglu FS. Biomarker and shear stress in secondary pediatric pulmonary hypertension. *Turk J Med Sci.* (2017) 47:1854–60. doi: 10.3906/sag-1609-13

18. Galiè N, Humbert M, Vachiery JL, Gibbs S, Lang I, Torbicki A, et al. 2015 ESC/ERS guidelines for the diagnosis and treatment of pulmonary hypertension: the joint task force for the diagnosis and treatment of pulmonary hypertension of the European society of cardiology (ESC) and the European respiratory society (ERS): endorsed by: association for European paediatric and congenital cardiology (AEPC), international society

19. Galiè N, Hoeper MM, Humbert M, Torbicki A, Vachiery JL, Barbera JA, et al. Guidelines for the diagnosis and treatment of pulmonary hypertension: the task force for the diagnosis and treatment of pulmonary hypertension of the European society of cardiology (ESC) and the European respiratory society (ERS), endorsed by the international society of heart and lung transplantation (ISHLT). *Eur Heart J.* (2009) 30:2493–537. doi: 10.1093/eurheartj/ehp297

20. Tang Y, Luo Q, Liu Z, Ma X, Zhao Z, Huang Z, et al. Oxygen uptake efficiency slope predicts poor outcome in patients with idiopathic pulmonary arterial hypertension. *J Am Heart Assoc.* (2017) 6:e005037. doi: 10.1161/JAHA.116.005037

21. Zhang HL, Liu ZH, Wang Y, Xiong CM, Ni XH, He JG, et al. Acute responses to inhalation of iloprost in patients with pulmonary hypertension. *Chin Med J.* (2012) 125:2826–31. doi: 10.3760/cma.j.issn.0366-6999.2012.16.005

22. Yu X, Luo Q, Liu Z, Zhao Z, Zhao Q, An C, et al. Prevalence of iron deficiency in different subtypes of pulmonary hypertension. *Heart Lung.* (2018) 47:308–13. doi: 10.1016/j.hrtlng.2018.05.002

23. Jin Q, Luo Q, Yang T, Zeng Q, Yu X, Yan L, et al. Improved hemodynamics and cardiopulmonary function in patients with inoperable chronic thromboembolic pulmonary hypertension after balloon pulmonary angioplasty. *Respir Res.* (2019) 20:250. doi: 10.1186/s12931-019-1211-y

24. Rudski LG, Lai WW, Afilalo J, Hua L, Handschumacher MD, Chandrasekaran K, et al. Guidelines for the echocardiographic assessment of the right heart in adults: a report from the American society of echocardiography endorsed by the European association of echocardiography, a registered branch of the European society of cardiology, and the Canadian society of echocardiography. *J Am Soc Echocardiogr.* (2010) 23:685–713; quiz 786–688. doi: 10.1016/j.echo.2010.05.010

25. Harrell FE, Jr., Califf RM, Pryor DB, Lee KL, Rosati RA. Evaluating the yield of medical tests. *JAMA.* (1982) 247:2543–6. doi: 10.1001/jama.1982.03320430047030

26. Harrell FE, Jr., Lee KL, Mark DB. Multivariable prognostic models: issues in developing models, evaluating assumptions and adequacy, and measuring and reducing errors. *Stat Med.* (1996) 15:361–87. doi: 10.1002/(SICI)1097-0258(19960229)15:4<361::AID-SIM168>3.0.CO;2-4

27. Pavlou M, Ambler G, Seaman SR, Guttmann O, Elliott P, King M, et al. How to develop a more accurate risk prediction model when there are few events. *BMJ.* (2015) 351:h3868. doi: 10.1136/bmj.h3868

28. Duman D, Palit F, Simsek E, Bilgehan K. Serum carbohydrate antigen 125 levels in advanced heart failure: relation to B-type natriuretic peptide and left atrial volume. *Eur J Heart Fail.* (2008) 10:556–9. doi: 10.1016/j.ejheart.2008.04.012

29. Hung CL, Hung TC, Lai YH, Lu CS, Wu YJ, Yeh HI. Beyond malignancy: the role of carbohydrate antigen 125 in heart failure. *Biomark Res.* (2013) 1:25. doi: 10.1186/2050-7771-1-25

30. Núñez J, Miñana G, Núñez E, Chorro FJ, Bodí V, Sanchis J. Clinical utility of antigen carbohydrate 125 in heart failure. *Heart Fail Rev.* (2014) 19:575–584. doi: 10.1007/s10741-013-9402-y

31. Frigy A, Belényi B, Kirchmaier Á, Fekete N, Szabó IA. Elevated CA-125 as humoral biomarker of congestive heart failure: illustrative cases and a short review of literature. *Case Rep Cardiol.* (2020) 2020:1642914. doi: 10.1155/2020/1642914

32. Shi C, van der Wal HH, Silljé HHW, Dokter MM, van den Berg F, Huizinga L, et al. Tumour biomarkers: association with heart failure outcomes. *J Intern Med.* (2020) 288:207–18. doi: 10.1111/joim.13053

33. Chen YX, Wang XQ, Fang CF, Wang JF, Tang LJ. Value of BNP and tumour marker CA125 in patients with heart failure. *Acta Cardiol.* (2008) 63:501–6. doi: 10.2143/AC.63.4.2033050

34. Schmidt T, Rein DT, Foth D, Eibach HW, Kurbacher CM, Mallmann P, et al. Prognostic value of repeated serum CA 125 measurements in first trimester pregnancy. *Eur J Obstet Gynecol Reprod Biol.* (2001) 97:168–73. doi: 10.1016/S0301-2115(00)00533-9

35. Colaković S, Lukiç V, Mitroviç L, Jeliç S, Susnjar S, Marinkoviç J. Prognostic value of CA125 kinetics and half-life in advanced ovarian cancer. *Int J Biol Markers.* (2000) 15:147–52. doi: 10.1177/172460080001500204

2

Diagnostic and Prognostic Value of Neutrophil Extracellular Trap Levels in Patients with Acute Aortic Dissection

Shuofei Yang[1†], Yongsheng Xiao[2†], Yuanfeng Du[3], Jiaquan Chen[1], Qihong Ni[1], Xiangjiang Guo[1], Guanhua Xue[1*] and Xupin Xie[4*]

[1] Department of Vascular Surgery, Renji Hospital, School of Medicine, Shanghai Jiaotong University, Shanghai, China, [2] Department of Vascular Surgery, Tianjin 4th Centre Hospital, The Fourth Central Hospital Affiliated to Nankai University, The Fourth Center Clinical College of Tianjin Medical University, Tianjin, China, [3] Department of Neurosurgery, School of Medicine, Affiliated Hangzhou First People's Hospital, Zhejiang University, Hangzhou, China, [4] Department of Vascular Surgery, School of Medicine, Affiliated Hangzhou First People's Hospital, Zhejiang University, Hangzhou, China

*Correspondence:
Guanhua Xue
xueguanhua2018@163.com
Xupin Xie
xiexupin@163.com

†These authors have contributed equally to this work and share first authorship

Background: Acute aortic dissection (AAD) is a fatal disease demanding prompt diagnosis and proper treatment. There is a lack of serum markers that can effectively assist diagnosis and predict prognosis of AAD patients.

Methods: Ninety-six AAD patients were enrolled in this study, and 249 patients with chest pain due to acute myocardial infarction, pulmonary embolism, intramural hematoma, angina or other causes and 80 healthy controls were included as control group and healthy control group. Demographics, biochemical and hematological data and risk factors were recorded as baseline characteristics. The 1-year follow-up data were collected and analyzed. The diagnostic performance and ability to predict disease severity and prognosis of NET components in serum and aortic tissue were evaluated.

Results: Circulating NET markers, citH3 (citrullination of histone 3), cell-free DNA (cfDNA) and nucleosomes, had good diagnostic value for AAD, with superior diagnostic performance to D-dimer in discriminating patients with chest pain due to other reasons in the emergency department. Circulating NET marker levels (i.e., citH3, cfDNA and nucleosomes) of AAD patients were significantly higher than that of control group and healthy control group. In addition, circulating NET markers levels were closely associated with the disease severity, in-hospital death and 1-year survival of AAD patients. Systolic blood pressure < 90 mmHg and serum citH3 levels were identified as independent risk factors for 1-year survival of AAD patients. Excessive NET components (i.e., neutrophil elastase and citH3) in the aortic tissue of AAD patient were significantly higher than that of healthy donor aortic tissue. The expression levels of granules and nuclear NET components were significantly higher in aortic tissue from AAD patients than controls.

Conclusions: Circulating NET markers, citH3, cfDNA and nucleosomes, have significant diagnostic value and predictive value of disease severity and prognosis of AAD patients. The NETs components may constitute a useful diagnostic and prognostic marker in AAD patients.

Keywords: neutrophil extracellular trap, acute aortic dissection, serum biomarker, diagnostic marker, prognostic marker

INTRODUCTION

Acute aortic dissection (AAD) is a fatal aortic disease with high mortality and morbidity that demands prompt diagnosis and proper treatment (1). Despite recent advances in diagnostic imaging methods, AAD remains a challenge to diagnose. A widely available and cost-effective measure such as a blood test that can rule in and/or rule out the disease would indeed aid in quick diagnosis, benefiting patients and caregivers. Several major diseases that cause chest pain, such as acute myocardial infarction (AMI), pulmonary embolism (PE), intramural hematoma and angina, require differential diagnosis with AAD. Moreover, there is still a lack of effective markers to accurately predict the in-hospital and long-term outcomes of patients with AAD after surgical repair.

Neutrophils are the most abundant cell type in leukocytes and play a crucial role in the innate immune system (2). Neutrophils are also involved in the pathological mechanism of aortic dissection (AD) (3). AAD is initiated by neutrophil infiltration of the aortic intima, and local neutrophil recruitment and activation in response to AAD can lead to aortic rupture (4, 5). In patients with AAD receiving surgical repair, the neutrophil to lymphocyte ratio may be used to predict worse outcomes and hospital mortality (6). In the inflammatory response, neutrophils play critical roles through the release of neutrophil extracellular traps (NETs), which are extracellular neutrophil-derived web-like structures that constitute a DNA backbone containing histones and neutrophil granule proteins. A critical step in NET release is the citrullination of histone 3 (citH3), a process mediated by protein deiminase 4, and citH3 is considered one of the most specific markers for NET formation assessment (7). Initially, NETs were thought to provide defense against pathogens (8). In recent years, NETs have been implicated in a number of cardiovascular diseases (9). By immunophenotypic analysis, NETs were found to participate in the tissue repair of AD (10).

NETs could be used as a new circulating marker for several cardiovascular diseases, such as acute coronary syndrome, acute ischemic stroke, myocardial infarction, and deep venous thrombosis (11–13). Data on NET presence in the serum and tissue of AAD patients and the association between NET levels and clinical outcomes are scarce. Hence, this study sought to determine whether NETs may serve as disease biomarkers in AAD patients. Specifically, our aims were to examine the diagnostic value of NETs for AAD and the predictive significance of NETs for disease severity, in-hospital mortality and 1-year survival in AAD patients receiving surgical repair.

Abbreviations: AAD, acute aortic dissection; AMI, acute myocardial infarction; AD, aortic dissection; PE, pulmonary embolism; NETs, neutrophil extracellular traps; citH3, citrullination of histone 3; CTA, computed tomography angiography; MRA, magnetic resonance angiography; TAAD, type A aortic dissection; TABD, type B aortic dissection; APACHE II, the Acute Physiology, Age, Chronic Health Evaluation II; cfDNA, cell-free DNA; NE, neutrophil elastase; ROC, receiver operating characteristic curve; AUR, area under the ROC; NET, neutrophil extracellular trap; SBP, systolic blood pressure; TF, tissue factor.

PATIENTS AND METHODS

Patients

The study was approved by the ethical committee of Renji Hospital, School of Medicine, Shanghai Jiaotong University (No. RA2020-253). All patients or their proxies provided written informed consent. Ninety-six consecutive patients with AAD hospitalized in Renji Hospital between May 01, 2016, and April 04, 2019, were enrolled in this study. Diagnoses were made based on computed tomography angiography (CTA), digital subtraction angiography and, when appropriate, magnetic resonance angiography (MRA). The Stanford classifications of AAD were evaluated at the time of diagnosis. Stanford type A aortic dissection (TAAD) involves the ascending aorta, whereas type B aortic dissection (TABD) involves the descending aorta only. The severity of disease was measured by the Acute Physiology, Age, Chronic Health Evaluation II (APACHE II) score at hospital entrance and discharge. The detection risk score of AD was calculated at admission to the emergency department according to the guidelines (14). During the same time period, 249 patients admitted to the emergency chest pain center with a diagnosis of AMI, PE, angina or others were included in the control group. In addition, 80 healthy controls were included in this study. Demographics, biochemical and hematological data, clinical history, and risk factors were recorded as baseline patient characteristics. Clinical follow-up was performed 1 year after hospital discharge in all AAD patients. This was conducted by reviewing the electronic records in clinics or by telephone contact. Follow-up records included reoperation information, CTA or MRA follow-up information, mortality, and cause and date of death.

Citrated-anticoagulated venous blood was obtained from all the patients within 3 h of diagnosis and on the last morning before discharge. Platelet-poor plasma was prepared by centrifugation of the blood ($2,500 \times g$) for 10 min at 22°C, and the plasma was stored at −80°C until analysis. Aortic tissue samples were obtained from 45 AAD patients included in this study who received open surgery. Twenty normal aortic tissues were obtained from organ donors (crash victims or brain-dead patients). Tissue samples were stored at −80°C until analysis.

NET Markers

We evaluated three different markers of NETs [i.e., cfDNA (cell-free DNA), nucleosomes and citH3]. citH3 is currently considered to be the most specific marker, as H3 citrullination is required for chromatin decondensation in neutrophils. Detection of cfDNA and nucleosomes was performed as described previously (13). For cfDNA determination, plasma was diluted 1:10 with phosphate-buffered saline and mixed with an equal volume of 1 mM SytoxGreen (Invitrogen, Carlsbad, CA, USA; No. S7020) in PBS. Fluorescence was determined in a fluorescence microplate reader (Gemini XPS; Molecular Devices, Sunnyvale, CA, USA). A calibration curve was generated with calf thymus DNA (Invitrogen; No. 15633019) in PBS. Nucleosomes were measured with the Cell Death Detection ELISAPLUS kit (Roche Diagnostics, Madrid, Spain; No. 11774425001) according to the manufacturer's instructions. Determination of citH3 was

TABLE 1 | Baseline characteristics of chest pain patients included in this study.

Characteristics	AAD (n = 96)	Controls (n = 249)	P-value
Age, mean (range)	59.1 (35–85)	60.3 (40–92)	0.45
Male sex, n (%)	53 (55.2)	128 (51.4)	0.53
Medical history and risk factors, n (%)			
Hypertension	72 (75.0)	129 (51.8)	<0.05
Diabetes	44 (45.8)	109 (43.8)	0.62
Stroke	28 (29.2)	80 (32.1)	0.60
Hyperlipidemia	48 (50.0)	135 (54.2)	0.48
Smoking	55 (57.3)	125 (50.2)	0.24
Marfan syndrome	12 (12.5)	1 (0.4)	<0.01
Atrial fibrillation	28 (29.2)	63 (25.3)	0.47
Valvulopathy	20 (20.8)	42 (16.9)	0.39
Diagnosis, n (%)			
TAAD	42 (43.8)	/	/
TBAD	54 (56.3)	/	/
IH	/	10 (4.0)	/
AMI	/	63 (25.3)	/
PE	/	42 (16.9)	/
Angina	/	66 (26.5)	/
Others	/	68 (27.3)	/
Biochemical and hematological data, mean ± SD			
Glucose, mg/dL	130.3 ± 52.4	125.4 ± 44.2	0.42
Creatinine, μmol/L	148.7 ± 33.6	142.9 ± 40.7	0.36
Uric acid, mg/dL	6.1 ± 2.4	5.9 ± 2.9	0.37
Cholesterol, mg/dL	178.3 ± 39.2	183.2 ± 29.9	0.72
Triglycerides, mg/dL	182.1 ± 88.4	189.1 ± 79.2	0.60
AST, U/L	28.2 ± 13.4	30.2 ± 20.2	0.13
ALT, U/L	38.3 ± 16.7	39.6 ± 26.3	0.22
Bilirubin, mg/dL	1.9 ± 1.6	1.8 ± 0.8	0.82
Hematocrit, %	41.3 ± 6.3	39.4 ± 5.6	0.63
Platelets, 10^3/μL	248.3 ± 56.4	256.6 ± 47.2	0.20
Leukocytes, 10^3/μL	6.4 ± 3.4	6.8 ± 3.9	0.74
Lymphocytes, %	26.3 ± 9.2	27.5 ± 8.4	0.20
Neutrophils, %	74.4 ± 18.3	73.9 ± 19.8	0.48
Monocytes, %	8.8 ± 4.2	9.0 ± 7.3	0.33
D-dimer, ng/ml	2080.5 ± 1131.9	1867.3 ± 2007.3	<0.05

AAD, acute aortic dissection; TAAD, type A aortic dissection; TBAD, type B aortic dissection; IH, intramural hematoma; AMI, acute myocardial infarction; PE, pulmonary embolism; SD, standard deviation; AST, aspartate transaminase; ALT, alanine aminotransferase.

performed as previously described (15). Briefly, plasma samples were mixed with a monoclonal mouse anti-histone biotinylated antibody in a streptavidin-coated plate. A rabbit polyclonal anti-histone-H3 (citrullinated R17 + R2 + R8) (Abcam Inc., MA, USA; No. ab81797) antibody was used in the second step. Detection was performed with a peroxidase-linked antibody (GE Biosciences, Barcelona, Spain; No. A1783). Values were normalized to a pool of samples from normal subjects. Values are expressed as individual absorption values. The neutrophil elastase (NE) concentration was measured using commercially available ELISA kits.

Proteomics Analysis

In this study, we built a custom pathway of NET-associated proteins as described previously (16). To build a custom "NETosis" pathway, twenty-three proteins that belonged to five subcellular compartments (nucleus, granules, cytoplasm/cytoskeleton, enzymes, and plasma membrane) were identified by a literature screen for detailed characterization of NET proteins (17, 18). According to a Gene Set Enrichment Analysis heat map, the custom NETosis pathway was enriched in aortic tissue from AAD patients vs. normal controls. Samples were reduced, alkylated and trypsin-digested according to the iTRAQ manufacturer's instructions (AB Sciex Inc., MA, USA). To diminish any potential variation introduced by the labeling reaction, samples from AAD patients and normal controls were split into two aliquots of 60 μg to perform two technical replicates with tag swapping. Each peptide solution was labeled at room temperature for 1 h with one iTRAQ reagent vial. To verify the labeling efficiency, 1 μg of each labeled sample was individually analyzed by liquid chromatography-tandem mass spectrometry (LC-MS/MS) as specified below. Acquired data were searched against the Mascot database, setting iTRAQ labeling as the variable modification. No unmodified peptides were identified from the search, and all the peptides were correctly modified at the N-terminus and at each lysine residue. Finally, the four iTRAQ-labeled samples were combined in a 1:1:1:1 ratio, and the pool was vacuum dried in a SpeedVac system.

Immunofluorescence

NET identification in tissue samples was performed by immunofluorescence staining. The NE/citH3 pair was researched in paraffin-embedded, 3-μm-thick sections. The slides were incubated with the primary antibodies (anti-NE antibody, MAB91671, R&D Systems, Minneapolis, USA; anti-H3Cit antibody, ab5103, Abcam, Cambridge, UK; both 1:50 dilution) at 4°C overnight after blocking with goat serum. Then, the sections were incubated with secondary antibodies (Alexa Fluor 488, green, ab150077; Alexa Fluor 647, red, ab150075; both from Abcam, Cambridge, UK) for 1 h at room temperature. DAPI was used for nuclear staining (ZSGB Biotech, Beijing, China; No. ZLI-9577). The slides were analyzed with a confocal laser scanning microscope (TCS-SP5; Leica, Wetzlar, Germany). The average numbers of NE and H3Cit double-positive cells were calculated by two independent researchers counting five random microscopic fields.

Statistics

Data are expressed as the means ± SEM of absolute values or as percentages. Continuous variables were analyzed with the Mann-Whitney test. Discrete variables were evaluated with a contingency χ^2 test. By the Shapiro-Wilk test, the value of citH3, cfDNA and nucleosomes were found to be normally distributed. The Spearman coefficient (r) was used to quantify the correlations between variables. Compared with D-dimer, the diagnostic performance of NET markers for distinguishing AAD from all other diseases, AMI, PE, or angina was assessed using receiver operating characteristic curve (ROC) analysis. The area under the ROC (AUR),

TABLE 2 | NETs and risk factors before the onset of the acute event.

Characteristics		citH3 (ng/ml)	P	cfDNA (AU)	P	Nucleosomes (AU)	P
Hypertension	Yes	0.46 ± 0.23	0.73	698.82 ± 306.28	0.11	1.56 ± 0.82	0.82
	No	0.47 ± 0.26		788.13 ± 438.75		1.58 ± 0.88	
Diabetes	Yes	0.46 ± 0.23	0.56	692.48 ± 317.45	0.31	1.53 ± 0.85	0.75
	No	0.47 ± 0.25		745.40 ± 365.98		1.59 ± 0.83	
Smoking	Yes	0.48 ± 0.24	0.12	749.98 ± 355.40	0.21	1.61 ± 0.85	0.32
	No	0.44 ± 0.24		682.46 ± 328.01		1.50 ± 0.82	
Marfan syndrome	Yes	0.47 ± 0.21	0.52	664.25 ± 210.41	0.04	1.52 ± 0.74	0.21
	No	0.47 ± 0.24		729.27 ± 359.05		1.57 ± 0.85	
Atrial fibrillation	Yes	0.49 ± 0.25	0.44	757.68 ± 359.99	0.09	1.57 ± 0.80	0.71
	No	0.45 ± 0.24		706.10 ± 338.55		1.56 ± 0.85	

citH3, citrullination of histone 3; cfDNA, cell-free DNA; AU, arbitrary units.

sensitivity, specificity, accuracy, positive predictive value, and negative predictive value were calculated. The Wald test was used to assess the significance of the difference between areas under the ROC curve. The optimal cutoff point from the study was the threshold leading to the maximum summation of sensitivity and specificity. Univariate logistic regression analysis was used to assess the association between risk factors and in-hospital death or 1-year survival, and a multivariate Cox regression analysis was performed using variables with $P \leq 0.20$ in univariate analysis. A two-sided P-value <0.05 was considered statistically significant. Statistical analyses were performed with SPSS 20 (SPSS, Inc., Chicago, IL, USA).

RESULTS

Baseline Demographic Information and Hematological Parameters

A total of 96 patients, 42 TAADs and 54 TBADs, were enrolled in the AAD group. Another 249 patients were enrolled in the control group, including 10 IH cases, 63 AMI cases, 42 PE cases, 66 angina cases and 68 cases with other causes. The baseline demographic information, medical history, risk factors, and biochemical and hematological data are shown in **Table 1**. The demographic information, biochemical and hematological data of 80 healthy controls are shown in **Supplementary Table 1**. The rates of hypertension and Marfan syndrome were significantly higher in the AAD group than in the control group. Moreover, AAD patients had significantly higher levels of D-dimer than patients in the control group. There was no significant difference between the two groups regarding other parameters. The AAD patients were stratified according to classical risk factors. No significant differences among any of the three NET markers were observed between patients with or without hypertension, diabetes, smoking history and atrial fibrillation. The cfDNA levels in patients with Marfan syndrome were significantly higher than those in patients without Marfan syndrome. However, the levels of citH3 and nucleosomes were comparable between patients with or without Marfan syndrome (**Table 2**).

Diagnostic Performance of Circulating NET Markers for Discriminating AAD

The values of citH3, cfDNA and nucleosomes in patients with AAD were significantly higher than those in the control group or healthy controls (**Figure 1A**) Circulating levels of citH3, cfDNA, and nucleosomes were positively correlated with the detection risk score of AD (**Figure 1B**). In the ROC curve, the AURs in patients with AAD vs. all control patients were 0.87 for citH3, 0.95 for cfDNA, 0.92 for nucleosomes, and 0.64 for D-dimer (**Figure 1C**). Thus, circulating NET markers showed superior overall diagnostic performance compared with D-dimer when sudden-onset chest pain was present in the emergency department. cfDNA at cutoff levels of 403.5 ng/ml and D-dimer at 2015 ng/ml were the thresholds leading to the maximum summation of sensitivity and specificity in discriminating AAD from all other diagnoses. The corresponding sensitivities were 77.08% for cfDNA and 57.29% for D-dimer, and the specificities were 100% for cfDNA and 84.74% for D-dimer, resulting in 93.62% of patients for cfDNA and 55.61% of patients for D-dimer being correctly classified (**Supplementary Table 2**).

The time course was also examined in the AAD group using box plot analysis according to the admission time from symptom onset. The peak NET marker levels occurred within 12–24 h after symptom onset (**Figure 1D**). In addition, no significant difference in circulating NET markers was found between patients with TAAD and TBAD or among different subsets of the control group. There was no correlation between age and circulating levels of NET markers (**Supplementary Figure 1**).

Association Between Circulating NET Markers and Disease Severity of AAD at Onset and Discharge

There was a positive correlation between the APACHE II score and the levels of all three NET markers at disease onset (**Figure 2A**). When patients were classified according to the APACHE II score into four groups, those with higher scores had significantly higher levels of all three NET markers (**Figure 2B**). At discharge, the levels of all three NET markers were also positively correlated with the APACHE II score (**Figure 2C**). Classified by APACHE II score into three groups, patients with

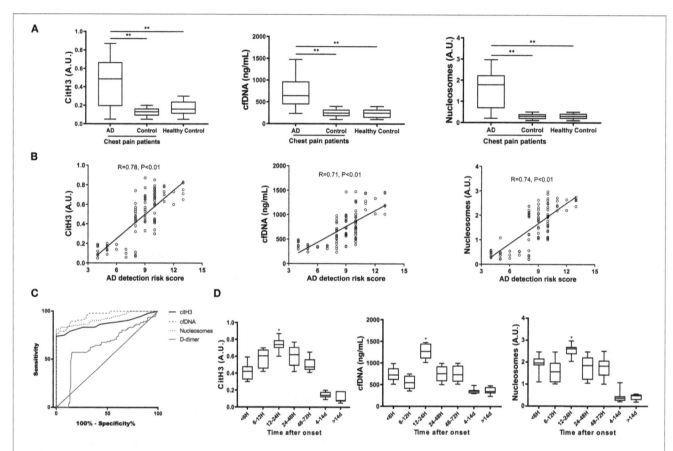

FIGURE 1 | The diagnostic performance of circulating NET markers for discriminating AAD. **(A)** Serum levels of citrullinated H3 (citH3), cell-free DNA (cfDNA), and nucleosomes were evaluated in 96 patients with AAD and 249 patients in the control group. CitH3 and nucleosomes are expressed in arbitrary units (AU). The cfDNA concentration (ng/mL) was determined based on a calibration curve of calf thymus DNA. All three markers were significantly higher in the AAD group than in the control group. **(B)** Serum levels of citH3, cfDNA and nucleosomes were positively correlated with the detection risk score of AD. **(C)** ROC curve for the diagnosis of AAD. Circulating NET markers showed superior overall diagnostic performance compared with D-dimer when sudden-onset chest pain was present in the emergency department. **(D)** The time course of NET markers was examined in patients with AAD according to the admission time from symptom onset. The peak NET marker levels occurred within 12–24 h of symptom onset. *$P < 0.05$, **$P < 0.01$.

greater disease severity showed significantly higher levels of the three NET markers (**Figure 2D**). These results demonstrated the association between circulating levels of NET markers and disease severity at both admission and discharge.

Prognostic Significance of Circulating NET Markers for Predicting In-hospital Death and 1-year Survival of Patients With AAD

The results in **Figure 3A** show that the levels of NET markers in patients with in-hospital death were significantly higher than those in patients without in-hospital death. AAD patients with the highest quartiles of citH3, cfDNA, or nucleosome levels presented significantly lower survival rates by 1 year than patients with the lower three quartiles of citH3 (**Figure 3B**). Based on the ROC curve, three circulating NET markers showed superior predictive ability for 1-year survival compared with D-dimer (**Figure 3C**). The AURs were 0.72 for citH3, 0.76 for cfDNA, 0.73 for nucleosomes, and 0.51 for D-dimer. The cfDNA at cutoff levels of 1,052 ng/ml and D-dimer at 915 ng/ml were threshold values. The corresponding sensitivities were 46.15% for cfDNA

and 26.92% for D-dimer, and the specificities were 94.29% for cfDNA and 82.86% for D-dimer (**Supplementary Table 3**).

Risk Factor Analysis of 1-year Survival in AAD Patients

We next examined whether NET markers were independently associated with the 1-year survival of AAD patients. By univariate and multivariate risk factor analysis, systolic blood pressure (SBP) < 90 mmHg and citH3 levels were identified as independent risk factors for 1-year survival ($p < 0.05$) (**Figure 4A** and **Supplementary Table 4**). AAD patients with SBP < 90 mmHg had significantly increased circulating NET markers compared with patients with SBP > 90 mmHg (**Figure 4B**).

Excess NET Components in Aortic Tissue and Their Association With Disease Severity and Prognosis in Patients With AAD

The expression levels of granule and nuclear NET components were significantly higher, and non-granular enzymes and

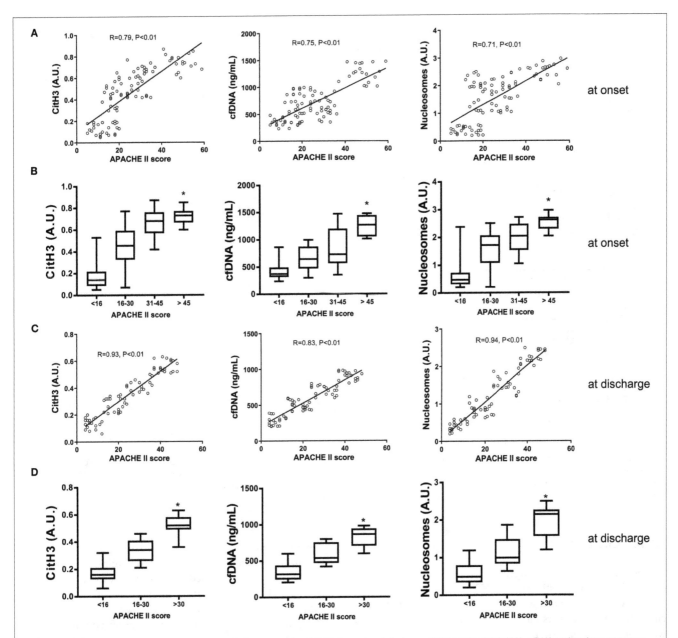

FIGURE 2 | The association between NET markers and disease severity of AAD at onset and discharge. **(A)** Serum levels of citH3, cfDNA and nucleosomes were positively correlated with the APACHE II score at disease onset. **(B)** AAD patients were classified into four groups according to APACHE II score. Patients with higher scores had significantly higher levels of all three NET markers. **(C)** The levels of all three NET markers were positively correlated with the APACHE II score at discharge. **(D)** AAD patients with greater disease severity showed significantly higher levels of NET markers. *$P < 0.05$.

membrane components were mildly enriched in aortic tissue from AAD patients compared with normal controls (**Figures 5A,B**). The expression of neutrophil elastase, the prototypical NET marker, was significantly higher in aortic tissue from the AAD group than in aortic tissue from the control group (**Figure 5C**). Additionally, the elastase level in patients with in-hospital death or without 1-year survival was significantly higher than that in patients without in-hospital death or with 1-year survival (**Figures 5D,E**).

Local NETosis was detected in the aortic samples from AAD patients, as colocalization of NE with citH3 was observed by confocal microscopy (**Figure 6A**). Compared with healthy donor aortic tissue, the numbers of NETs formed per field in the tissue samples from AAD patients were significantly increased (**Figure 6B**). Moreover, the number of NETs formed per field was positively correlated with the detection risk score of AD and the APACHE II score (**Figures 6C,D**). The number of NETs formed per field in patients with in-hospital death or death within 1-year was significantly higher than that in patients without in-hospital death or death within 1-year (**Figures 6E,F**). These results indicated that excess NET components in aortic tissue samples are associated with the disease severity and prognosis of AAD.

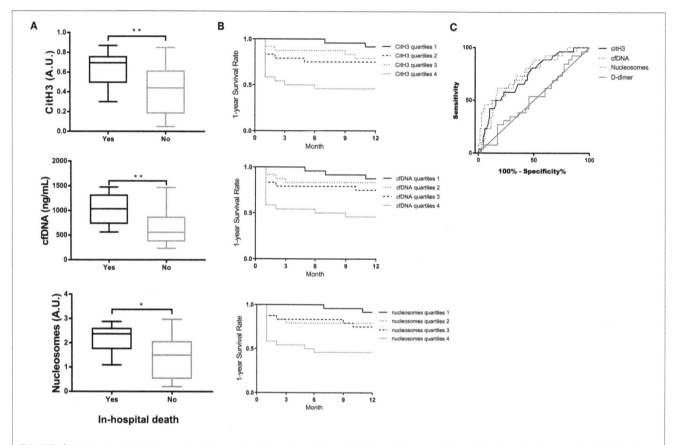

FIGURE 3 | Prognostic significance of circulating NET markers for predicting in-hospital death and 1-year survival of AAD patients. **(A)** Serum levels of citH3, cfDNA and nucleosomes in patients with in-hospital death were significantly higher than those in patients without in-hospital death. **(B)** AAD patients with the highest quartiles of citH3, cfDNA or nucleosome levels presented significantly lower survival rates by 1 year than patients with the lower three quartiles of citH3. **(C)** Based on the ROC curve, three circulating NET markers showed superior prediction ability of 1-year survival compared with D-dimer. $*P < 0.05$, $**P < 0.01$.

DISCUSSION

To the best of our knowledge, this is the first time that the diagnostic and prognostic value of NETs has been evaluated in patients with AAD. In this study, the major findings were that: (a) circulating NET markers had reliable diagnostic value of AAD, with superior diagnostic performance to discriminate patients with chest pain from other reasons in the emergency department compared with D-dimer; (b) circulating NET markers were independently associated with the disease severity, in-hospital death and 1-year survival of patients with AAD; and (c) excessive NET components in the aortic tissue were associated with the disease severity and prognosis of AAD patients.

It is well-known that neutrophils are the first line of defense against infections by pathogens. Neutrophils are also pivotal as primary effector cells at sites of inflammation, but through regulation of their survival by means of regulated cell death, these cells are also involved in the resolution of inflammation (19). Significant neutrophilic infiltration was found not only in early but also in later stages of organizing dissections and not only in the clot but also in adventitial fat (10, 20). This could reflect an upregulation of neutrophil survival to maintain the intense

tissue remodeling required for the repair of the arterial wall. In both surgical and autopsy cases of AAD, immunohistochemical staining for citH3 revealed a massive presence of NETs in the clot and in the adventitia in the subacute stage and less abundantly in early organizing stage dissections (10). It is worth noting that aortic tissue samples were collected during surgery in this study. However, in surgical cases, awareness of the pattern of margination, transmigration and extravasation around microvessels that may occur due to robust handling during surgery should be considered to avoid overinterpration of the more diffuse patterns of neutrophil infiltration and NET release related to dissection.

Our results elucidated that the three markers of NETs are significantly elevated in patients with AAD compared with the corresponding levels in subjects from the control group. Recent reports have documented the association of NETs with the severity of stroke evaluated by clinical indexes (21, 22). Our study showed for the first time that the three markers of NETs were in line with the disease severity score of AAD at onset and discharge. However, the APAHE II scoring system is predictive of disease severity only when specific baseline and wound characteristics are accounted for. A plasma marker that can be easily and quickly

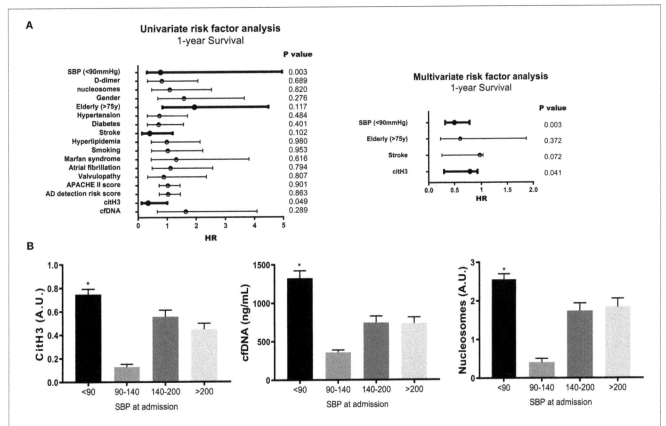

FIGURE 4 | Risk factor analysis of 1-year survival in AAD patients. (A) By univariate and multivariate risk factor analysis, systolic blood pressure (SBP) < 90 mmHg and citH3 levels were identified as independent risk factors for 1-year survival. (B) AAD patients with SBP < 90 mmHg had significantly increased circulating NET markers compared with patients with SBP > 90 mmHg. *P < 0.05.

tested to stratify patients with different risks of mortality is of great prognostic significance.

In this study, a time course study of NET markers was performed in AAD patients according to the admission time from symptom onset. The levels of all three NET markers peaked within 12–24 h after symptom onset. However, the concentrations of NET markers were measured using leftover samples of the patients from initial presentation. However, strictly speaking, the time after the actual onset of disease might be different for each patient. It would be beneficial to study the changes in concentrations according to time course or disease progression intraindividually. In addition, the time window for NET concentrations returning to the baseline level after surgery also needs to be determined. This will provide a stable time horizon for the testing of NET markers to predict the outcome of treatment for patients with AAD.

The mechanism underlying the increased NET formation in AAD remains unknown. AAD is considered an active inflammatory process that occurs in response to endothelial damage through high shear stress. Neutrophils and NETs are emerging as important mediators of pathogenic inflammation in the aorta (23). When aortic dissection occurs, disruption of the aortic media immediately changes aorta hemodynamics, with intramural hemorrhage leading to propagation and tracking of

blood within the media, which will overactivate the coagulation system. Currently, there is increasing awareness that NETs are linked to thrombosis since they may shift the hemostatic balance toward excessive coagulation (24). AAD exhibits high concentrations of tissue factor (TF) in serum, and the ability of neutrophils to expose functional TF on NETs is considered a link between inflammation and coagulation (25, 26).

In the last two decades, much progress has been made to make effective biochemical diagnoses of AAD, which is an unmet need with lifesaving value. Several promising biomarkers have emerged. Vinculin, lumican, MMP-12 and high levels of ischemia-modified albumin have been considered potential AAD-related serum markers that may assist in the diagnosis and prediction of the in-hospital mortality of patients with AAD (27–30). However, most of these biomarkers are still clinically unavailable. In real-world clinical practice, in patients with acute chest pain and elevated D-dimer, a diagnosis of AAD should be considered. D-dimer might be a useful complementary tool to the current diagnostic work-up of patients with suspected AAD (31, 32). D-dimer levels may be useful in risk-stratifying patients with potential AD to rule out AD if used within the first 24 h after symptom onset (33). Nevertheless, D-dimers are not always elevated in patients with AAD (34). The results of this study demonstrated that circulating NET markers showed

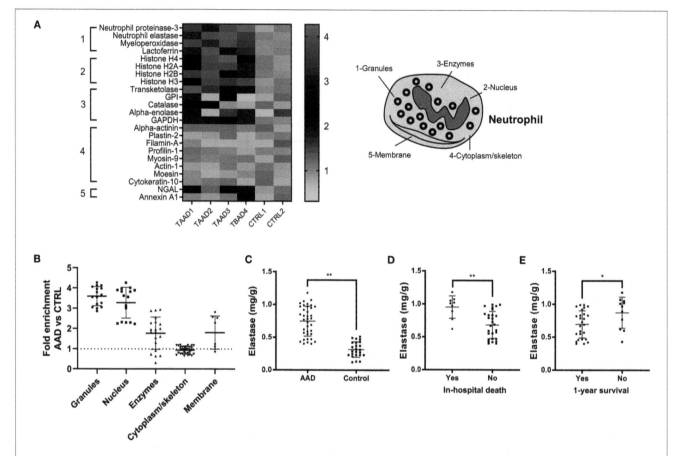

FIGURE 5 | Custom proteomic analysis of aortic tissue lysates from AAD patients. **(A)** Twenty-three proteins that belonged to five subcellular compartments (nucleus, granules, cytoplasm/cytoskeleton, enzymes, and plasma membrane) were identified to build a custom "NETosis" pathway. Profile plot from the Gene Set Enrichment Analysis (GSEA) showing highly significant enrichment of most proteins in the custom NETosis pathway in the 4 replicates (TAAD1-3, TBAD 4) compared with negative control subjects (CTRL1-2). The false discovery rate–adjusted P value for this analysis, according to GSEA output, was < 0.01. **(B)** The expression of granules and nuclear NET components was significantly higher, and non-granular enzymes and membrane components were mildly enriched in aortic tissue from AAD patients. **(C)** Neutrophil elastase was significantly higher in aortic tissue from the AAD group than in aortic tissue from the control group. **(D,E)** The elastase level in patients with in-hospital death or without 1-year survival was significantly higher than that in patients without in-hospital death or with 1-year survival. *P < 0.05, **P < 0.01.

significantly superior diagnostic performance compared with D-dimer to discriminate AAD patients with chest pain due to other reasons.

Despite acceptable reproducibility, as indicated by interassay cutoff values, the variability of the data makes clinically relevant cutoffs infeasible, and causality cannot be addressed. Although we used methods in line with current standards, the observed results highlight the need for improved methods when quantifying circulating NET markers (35). However, the inconsistent findings among the levels of cfDNA, citH3 and nucleosomes call into question their specificity in terms of reflecting NETosis. Previous studies have used various methods for evaluating the suitability of NETs as biomarkers in different clinical conditions, in which the main analytical targets were cfDNA, histones, and other components of NETs, such as neutrophil elastase or myeloperoxidase in plasma (36). cfDNA has repeatedly been described as a NET marker due to the objectivity of DNA quantification methods, yet its source is ambiguous, as non-neutrophil cells also release chromatin through cell death processes (35). The citrullination of histone

3 is a necessary step in the formation of NETs, as demonstrated by genetic and pharmacological approaches (37). Thus, citH3 appears to be the most specific marker of NETs, and it has been used to test for the presence of NETs in plasma. Importantly, citH3 has been reported to be independently associated with all-cause mortality during the 1-year follow-up in patients with acute ischemic stroke (21). In this study, citH3 was also identified as an independent risk factor for 1-year survival in patients with AAD.

Some limitations should be considered in the interpretation of our results. First, this is a single-center study with a relatively small number of subjects. Potential selection biases are not negligible. Future research on this topic should aim to include a larger study population. Secondly, a long-term follow-up period would be necessary to obtain statistically significant results in the prediction of disease prognoses. In this study, we reported major outcomes observed during the 1-year follow-up. Analysis of the changes in circulating levels of NETs during the follow-up period is also meaningful. Thirdly, our study was mostly descriptive, whereas the specific mechanism of NETs in circulation or aortic tissue promoting the occurrence and progression of AAD was not

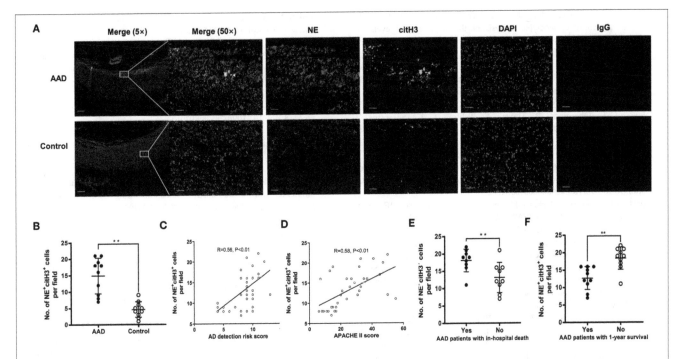

FIGURE 6 | The association between excess NETs in aortic tissue and disease severity or prognosis of patients with AAD. **(A)** Local NETosis was detected in aortic samples from AAD patients, as colocalization of NE with citH3 was observed by confocal microscopy. NE was stained green (Alexa Fluor 488) and citH3 was stained red (Alexa Fluor 647). DAPI staining was used to mark nucleus (blue fluorescence). **(B)** Compared with normal controls, the number of NETs formed per field in the tissue samples from AAD patients was significantly increased. **(C,D)** The number of NETs formed per field was positively correlated with the detection risk score of AD and the APACHE II score. **(E)** The number of NETs formed per field in patients with in-hospital death was significantly higher than that in patients without in-hospital death. **(F)** The number of NETs formed per field in patients with 1-year survival was significantly lower than that in patients without 1-year survival. $^{**}P < 0.01$.

addressed in this study. Further research is needed to determine whether NET components could be used as potential therapeutic targets for AAD.

In conclusion, the present study demonstrates that circulating NET markers have significant diagnostic value for AAD with good diagnostic performance to discriminate patients with chest pain from other causes. NET markers, in both the serum and aortic tissue, are associated with disease severity and the prognosis of AAD patients at the 1-year follow-up. Our results suggest that NETs may constitute a useful diagnostic and prognostic marker in patients with AAD and open new avenues for future drug therapy for AAD.

AUTHOR CONTRIBUTIONS

Study conception and design and drafting of article were performed by SY and YX. Data collection was performed by JC and QN. Analysis and interpretation of data was performed by SY, YD, and XG. Critical revision was performed by GX and XX. All authors contributed to the article and approved the submitted version.

REFERENCES

1. Bossone E, LaBounty TM, Eagle KA. Acute aortic syndromes: diagnosis and management, an update. *Eur Heart J.* (2018) 39:739–49d. doi: 10.1093/eurheartj/ehx319

2. Nathan C. Neutrophils and immunity: challenges and opportunities. *Nat Rev Immunol.* (2006) 6:173–82. doi: 10.1038/nri1785

3. Yoshida S, Yamamoto M, Aoki H, Fukuda H, Akasu K, Takagi K, et al. STAT3 activation correlates with adventitial neutrophil infiltration in human aortic dissection. *Ann Vasc Dis.* (2019) 12:187–93. doi: 10.3400/avd.oa.19-00007

4. Anzai A, Shimoda M, Endo J, Kohno T, Katsumata Y, Matsuhashi T, et al. Adventitial CXCL1/G-CSF expression in response to acute aortic dissection triggers local neutrophil recruitment and activation leading to aortic rupture. *Circ Res.* (2015) 116:612–23. doi: 10.1161/CIRCRESAHA.116.304918

5. Kurihara T, Shimizu-Hirota R, Shimoda M, Adachi T, Shimizu H, Weiss SJ, et al. Neutrophil-derived matrix metalloproteinase

9 triggers acute aortic dissection. *Circulation.* (2012) 126:3070–80. doi: 10.1161/CIRCULATIONAHA.112.097097

6. Kalkan ME, Kalkan AK, Gündeş A, Yanartaş M, Oztürk S, Gurbuz AS, et al. Neutrophil to lymphocyte ratio: a novel marker for predicting hospital mortality of patients with acute type A aortic dissection. *Perfusion.* (2017) 32:321–7. doi: 10.1177/0267659115590625

7. Li P, Li M, Lindberg MR, Kennett MJ, Xiong N, Wang Y. PAD4 is essential for antibacterial innate immunity mediated by neutrophil extracellular traps. *J Exp Med.* (2010) 207:1853–62. doi: 10.1084/jem.20100239

8. Brinkmann V, Reichard U, Goosmann C, Fauler B, Uhlemann Y, Weiss DS, et al. Neutrophil extracellular traps kill bacteria. *Science.* (2004) 303:1532–5. doi: 10.1126/science.1092385

9. Döring Y, Libby P, Soehnlein O. Neutrophil extracellular traps participate in cardiovascular diseases: recent experimental and clinical insights. *Circ Res.* (2020) 126:1228–41. doi: 10.1161/CIRCRESAHA.120.315931

10. Visonà SD, de Boer OJ, Mackaaij C, de Boer HH, Pertiwi KR, de Winter RW, et al. Immunophenotypic analysis of the chronological events of tissue repair in aortic medial dissections. *Cardiovasc Pathol.* (2018) 34:9–14. doi: 10.1016/j.carpath.2018.01.009

11. Lim HH, Jeong IH, An GD, Woo KS, Kim KH, Kim JM, et al. Evaluation of neutrophil extracellular traps as the circulating marker for patients with acute coronary syndrome and acute ischemic stroke. *J Clin Lab Anal.* (2020) 34:e23190. doi: 10.1002/jcla.23190

12. Novotny J, Oberdieck P, Titova A, Pelisek J, Chandraratne S, Nicol P, et al. Thrombus NET content is associated with clinical outcome in stroke and myocardial infarction. *Neurology.* (2020) 94:e2346–60. doi: 10.1212/WNL.0000000000009532

13. Yang S, Qi H, Kan K, Chen J, Xie H, Guo X, et al. Neutrophil extracellular traps promote hypercoagulability in patients with sepsis. *Shock.* (2017) 47:132–9. doi: 10.1097/SHK.0000000000000741

14. Hiratzka LF, Bakris GL, Beckman JA, Bersin RM, Carr VF, Casey DE Jr, et al. 2010 ACCF/AHA/AATS/ACR/ASA/SCA/SCAI/SIR/STS/SVM Guidelines for the diagnosis and management of patients with thoracic aortic disease. A Report of the American College of Cardiology Foundation/American Heart Association Task Force on Practice Guidelines, American Association for Thoracic Surgery, American College of Radiology, American Stroke Association, Society of Cardiovascular Anesthesiologists, Society for Cardiovascular Angiography and Interventions, Society of Interventional Radiology, Society of Thoracic Surgeons, and Society for Vascular Medicine. *J Am Coll Cardiol.* (2010) 55:e27–129. doi: 10.1016/j.jacc.2010.02.010

15. Borissoff JI, Joosen IA, Versteylen MO, Brill A, Fuchs TA, Savchenko AS, et al. Elevated levels of circulating DNA and chromatin are independently associated with severe coronary atherosclerosis and a prothrombotic state. *Arterioscler Thromb Vasc Biol.* (2013) 33:2032–40. doi: 10.1161/ATVBAHA.113.301627

16. Fadini GP, Menegazzo L, Rigato M, Scattolini V, Poncina N, Bruttocao A, et al. NETosis delays diabetic wound healing in mice and humans. *Diabetes.* (2016) 65:1061–71. doi: 10.2337/db15-0863

17. Ravindran M, Khan MA, Palaniyar N. neutrophil extracellular trap formation: physiology, pathology, and pharmacology. *Biomolecules.* (2019) 9:365. doi: 10.3390/biom9080365

18. Papayannopoulos V. Neutrophil extracellular traps in immunity and disease. *Nat Rev Immunol.* (2018) 18:134–47. doi: 10.1038/nri.2017.105

19. Witko-Sarsat V, Mocek J, Bouayad D, Tamassia N, Ribeil J-A, Candalh C, et al. Proliferating cell nuclear antigen acts as a cytoplasmic platform controlling human neutrophil survival. *J Exp Med.* (2010) 207:2631–45. doi: 10.1084/jem.20092241

20. del Porto F, Proietta M, Tritapepe L, Miraldi F, Koverech A, Cardelli P, et al. Inflammation and immune response in acute aortic dissection. *Ann Med.* (2010) 42:622–9. doi: 10.3109/07853890.2010.518156

21. Valles J, Lago A, Santos MT, Latorre AM, Tembl JI, Salom JB, et al. Neutrophil extracellular traps are increased in patients with acute ischemic stroke: prognostic significance. *Thromb Haemost.* (2017) 117:1919–29. doi: 10.1160/TH17-02-0130

22. Tsai NW, Lin TK, Chen SD, Chang WN, Wang HC, Yang TM, et al. The value of serial plasma nuclear and mitochondrial DNA levels in patients with acute ischemic stroke. *Clin Chim Acta.* (2011) 412:476–9. doi: 10.1016/j.cca.2010.11.036

23. Liu Y, Carmona-Rivera C, Moore E, Seto NL, Knight JS, Pryor M, et al. Myeloid-specific deletion of peptidylarginine deiminase 4 mitigates atherosclerosis. *Front Immunol.* (2018) 9:1680. doi: 10.3389/fimmu.2018.01680

24. Gould TJ, Lysov Z, Liaw PC. Extracellular DNA and histones: double-edged swords in immunothrombosis. *J Thromb Haemost.* (2015) 13(Suppl. 1):S82–91. doi: 10.1111/jth.12977

25. Kambas K, Chrysanthopoulou A, Vassilopoulos D, Apostolidou E, Skendros P, Girod A, et al. Tissue factor expression in neutrophil extracellular traps and neutrophil derived microparticles in antineutrophil cytoplasmic antibody associated vasculitis may promote thromboinflammation and the thrombophilic state associated with the disease. *Ann Rheum Dis.* (2014) 73:1854–63. doi: 10.1136/annrheumdis-2013-203430

26. Gao Z, Pei X, He C, Wang Y, Lu J, Jin M, et al. Oxygenation impairment in patients with acute aortic dissection is associated with disorders of coagulation and fibrinolysis: a prospective observational study. *J Thorac Dis.* (2019) 11:1190–201. doi: 10.21037/jtd.2019.04.32

27. Gu G, Cheng W, Yao C, Yin J, Tong C, Rao A, et al. Quantitative proteomics analysis by isobaric tags for relative and absolute quantitation identified Lumican as a potential marker for acute aortic dissection. *J Biomed Biotechnol.* (2011) 2011:920763. doi: 10.1155/2011/920763

28. Proietta M, Tritapepe L, Cifani N, Ferri L, Taurino M, Del Porto F. MMP-12 as a new marker of Stanford-A acute aortic dissection. *Ann Med.* (2014) 46:44–8. doi: 10.3109/07853890.2013.876728

29. Yang G, Zhou Y, He H, Pan X, Chai X. Ischemia-modified albumin, a novel predictive marker of in-hospital mortality in acute aortic dissection patients. *Front Physiol.* (2019) 10:1253. doi: 10.3389/fphys.2019.01253

30. Wang HQ, Yang H, Tang Q, Gong YC, Fu YH, Wan F, et al. Identification of vinculin as a potential diagnostic biomarker for acute aortic dissection using label-free proteomics. *Biomed Res Int.* (2020) 2020:7806409. doi: 10.1155/2020/7806409

31. Ohlmann P, Faure A, Morel O, Petit H, Kabbaj H, Meyer N, et al. Diagnostic and prognostic value of circulating D-Dimers in patients with acute aortic dissection. *Crit Care Med.* (2006) 34:1358–64. doi: 10.1097/01.CCM.0000216686.72457.EC

32. Marill KA. Serum D-dimer is a sensitive test for the detection of acute aortic dissection: a pooled meta-analysis. *J Emerg Med.* (2008) 34:367–76. doi: 10.1016/j.jemermed.2007.06.030

33. Suzuki T, Distante A, Zizza A, Trimarchi S, Villani M, Salerno Uriarte JA, et al. Diagnosis of acute aortic dissection by D-dimer: the International Registry of Acute Aortic Dissection Substudy on Biomarkers (IRAD-Bio) experience. *Circulation.* (2009) 119:2702–7. doi: 10.1161/CIRCULATIONAHA.108.833004

34. Paparella D, Malvindi PG, Scrascia G, de Ceglia D, Rotunno C, Tunzi F, et al. D-dimers are not always elevated in patients with acute aortic dissection. *J Cardiovasc Med.* (2009) 10:212–4. doi: 10.2459/JCM.0b013e32831c849e

35. Masuda S, Nakazawa D, Shida H, Miyoshi A, Kusunoki Y, Tomaru U, et al. NETosis markers: quest for specific, objective, and quantitative markers. *Clin Chim Acta.* (2016) 459:89–93. doi: 10.1016/j.cca.2016.05.029

36. Jorch SK, Kubes P. An emerging role for neutrophil extracellular traps in noninfectious disease. *Nat Med.* (2017) 23:279–87. doi: 10.1038/nm.4294

37. Martinod K, Demers M, Fuchs TA, Wong SL, Brill A, Gallant M, et al. Neutrophil histone modification by peptidylarginine deiminase 4 is critical for deep vein thrombosis in mice. *Proc Natl Acad Sci USA.* (2013) 110:8674–9. doi: 10.1073/pnas.1301059110

3

The Association Between Plasma Osmolarity and In-Hospital Mortality in Cardiac Intensive Care Unit Patients

Guangyao Zhai, Jianlong Wang, Yuyang Liu and Yujie Zhou*

Beijing Anzhen Hospital, Capital Medical University, Beijing, China

*Correspondence:
Yujie Zhou
azzyj12@163.com

Objectives: Plasma osmolarity is a common marker used for evaluating the balance of fluid and electrolyte in clinical practice, and it has been proven to be related to prognosis of many diseases. The purpose of this study was to identify the association between plasma osmolarity and in-hospital mortality in cardiac intensive care unit (CICU) patients.

Method: All of the patients were divided into seven groups stratified by plasma osmolarity, and the group with 290–300 mmol/L osmolarity was used as a reference group. Primary outcome was in-hospital mortality. The local weighted regression (Lowess) smoothing curve was drawn to determine the "U"-shaped relationship between plasma osmolarity and in-hospital mortality. Binary logistic regression analysis was performed to determine the effect of plasma osmolarity on the risk of in-hospital mortality.

Result: Overall, 7,060 CICU patients were enrolled. A "U"-shaped relationship between plasma osmolarity and in-hospital mortality was observed using the Lowess smoothing curve. The lowest in-hospital mortality (7.2%) was observed in the reference group. whereas hyposmolarity (<280 mmol/L vs. 290–300 mmol/L: 13.0 vs. 7.2%) and hyperosmolarity (≥330 mmol/L vs. 290–300 mmol/L: 31.6 vs. 7.2%) had higher in-hospital mortality. After adjusting for possible confounding variables with binary logistic regression analysis, both hyposmolarity (<280 mmol/L vs. 290–300 mmol/L: OR, 95% CI: 1.76, 1.08–2.85, $P = 0.023$) and hyperosmolarity (≥330 mmol/L vs. 290–300 mmol/L: OR, 95% CI: 1.65, 1.08–2.52, $P = 0.021$) were independently associated with an increased risk of in-hospital mortality. Moreover, lengths of CICU and hospital stays were prolonged in patients with hyposmolarity or hyperosmolarity.

Conclusion: A "U"-shaped relationship between plasma osmolarity and in-hospital mortality was observed. Both hyposmolarity and hyperosmolarity were independently associated with the increased risk of in-hospital mortality.

Keywords: cardiac care intensive unit, cardiovascular, in-hospital mortality, "U"-shaped, plasma osmolarity

INTRODUCTION

Although the prognosis of cardiovascular diseases has greatly improved due to technological advances and innovative drug use, cardiovascular diseases still remain the leading cause of death and disability worldwide (1). Much research is still needed in the field of cardiovascular diseases, especially for severe cardiovascular diseases with high mortality (2). Cardiac intensive care unit (CICU) has been established to manage severe cardiovascular diseases, and patients admitted to the CICU are usually at great risk of adverse outcomes (3). For CICU patients, readily available risk factors are always welcomed by clinicians, which will help doctors in assessment of the patients' condition and prognosis.

As a common marker used for evaluating the balance of fluid and electrolyte in clinical practice (4–7), plasma osmolarity can be calculated easily from serum sodium, potassium, glucose, and blood nitrogen urea (8). Previous clinical studies have shown that plasma osmolarity is associated with prognosis of many diseases, such as stroke (9), intracerebral hemorrhage (10), and gastrointestinal diseases (11). Plasma osmolarity is also tightly related to a higher rate of mortality and adverse cardiac events in patients with heart failure (12, 13). Likewise, in patients with coronary artery disease undergoing percutaneous coronary intervention (PCI), higher plasma osmolarity was shown to be associated with higher mortality and acute kidney injury (14, 15). Plasma osmolarity is also closely associated with the severity of disease, in-hospital mortality, and other adverse outcomes in critically ill patients (11). However, no research has been done to explore the influence of plasma osmolarity on the prognosis of CICU patients. Therefore, the purpose of this study was to identify the association between plasma osmolarity and in-hospital mortality in CICU patients.

METHOD

Population Selection Criteria and Definition of Plasma Osmolarity

As shown in **Figure 1**, all adult CICU patients at their first admission were eligible. Patients meeting the following criteria were excluded: (1) age under 18 years; (2) hospital admission for non-heart disease; (3) insufficient data to calculate plasma osmolarity; and (4) Acute Physiology and Chronic Health Evaluation IV (APACHE IV) data missing. A total of 7,060 CICU patients were included.

Plasma osmolarity was calculated as follows: 2 × [serum sodium concentration (mmol/L)] + 2 × [serum potassium concentration (mmol/L)] + [blood glucose (mmol/L)] + [blood nitrogen urea (mmol/L)] (8). Initial plasma osmolarity referred to the plasma osmolarity obtained from the first blood test after admission, while maximum osmolarity referred to the maximum plasma osmolarity during hospitalization. Plasma osmolarity was calculated from the serum sodium, potassium, glucose, and blood nitrogen urea levels measured at the same time.

Data Extraction

The data used in this study were taken from eICU Collaborative Research Database (16), which collected information on 200,859

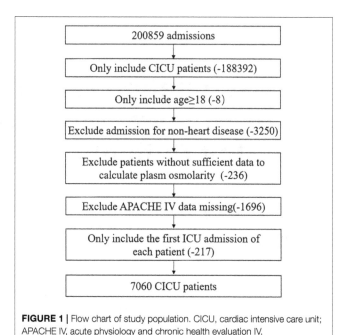

FIGURE 1 | Flow chart of study population. CICU, cardiac intensive care unit; APACHE IV, acute physiology and chronic health evaluation IV.

admissions from 208 hospitals in the United States between 2014 and 2015. This database is available at: https://doi.org/10.13026/C2WM1R, and the author was granted access to the database through Protecting Human Research Participants exam (certificate number: 9,728,458).

The following data were collected: demographics (age, gender, and race), vital signs (blood pressure, heart rate, respiration rate, oxygen saturation), body mass index, diagnoses and comorbidities [coronary artery disease, acute coronary syndrome, ST-elevation myocardial infarction (STEMI), non-ST-elevation myocardial infarction (NSTEMI), congestive heart failure, arrhythmias, cardiac arrest, atrial fibrillation, ventricular arrhythmias, atrioventricular block, cardiomyopathy, valve disease, shock, pulmonary embolism, pulmonary hypertension, hypertension, diabetes, chronic obstructive pulmonary disease (COPD), respiratory failure, chronic kidney disease, acute kidney injury, malignancy, stroke, sepsis], laboratory parameters (white blood cells, red blood cells, platelets, hemoglobin, hematocrit, glucose, creatinine, blood nitrogen urea, sodium, potassium), medication use [antiplatelet, oral anticoagulants, beta-blockers, angiotensin-converting enzyme inhibitor/angiotensin receptor blocker (ACEI/ARB), statins], acute physiology score (APS), and Acute Physiology and Chronic Health Evaluation IV (APACHE IV) (17).

Grouping and Outcomes

In clinical practice, we usually consider 285–307 mmol/L as a normal range of plasma osmolarity (8); however, according to the Lowess smoothing curve (**Figure 2**), we found that in-hospital mortality was the lowest when plasma osmolarity ranged from 290 to 300 mmol/L. Therefore, we decided to use osmolarity of 290–300 mmol/L as the reference group in binary logistic regression analysis. In order to better explore the association

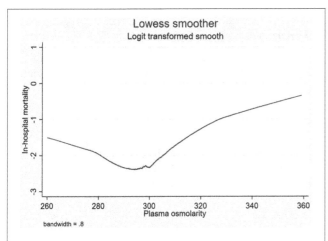

FIGURE 2 | Association between plasma osmolarity and in-hospital mortality presented through Lowess smoothing. Lowess, local weighted regression.

between plasma osmolarity and in-hospital mortality of CICU patients, all of the enrolled patients were divided into seven groups according to their initial plasma osmolarity: group 1 (< 280 mmol/L), group 2 (280–290 mmol/L), group 3 (290–300 mmol/L), group 4 (300–310 mmol/L), group 5 (310–320 mmol/L), group 6 (320–330 mmol/L), and group 7 (≥ 330 mmol/L).

The primary outcome was in-hospital mortality. Secondary outcomes were length of CICU stay and length of hospital stay.

Statistical Analysis

Normally distributed continuous variables were expressed as mean ± standard deviation (SD) and compared between the groups using Student's t-test. Skewed data were expressed as median and interquartile range (IQR) and were compared using the Kruskal–Wallis test or the Mann–Whitney U-test. Categorical variables were expressed as a number (percentage) and compared between the groups using the chi-square test.

The relationship between plasma osmolarity and in-hospital mortality was identified by binary logistic regression analysis, and the results were expressed as odds ratio (OR) with 95% confidence interval (CI). Covariates were selected on basis of statistical analysis and clinical suspicion that the factors may modulate the result. The curve in line with overall trend was drawn by local weighted regression (Lowess). All the tests were two-sided, and P < 0.05 was considered statistically significant. All of the data analyses were performed in Stata V.15.1.

RESULTS

Subjects and Baseline Characteristics

As shown in **Figure 1**, a total of 7,060 CICU patients were enrolled after screening step by step; most of them were White and male. Baseline characteristics of survivors and non-survivors are shown in **Table 1**. Initial plasma osmolarity and maximum plasma osmolarity of all the patients were 302.2 ± 14.4 and 308.4 ± 15.6 mmol/L, respectively. Non-survivors had higher

initial plasma osmolarity (308.1 ± 18.1 vs. 301.4 ± 13.7, P < 0.001) and maximum plasma osmolarity (321.0 ± 19.9 vs. 306.7 ± 14.1, P < 0.001) than survivors. Non-survivors were more likely to have lower blood pressure, oxygen saturation, and body mass index, but higher heart rate and respiration rate. Moreover, non-survivors more often presented congestive heart failure, cardiac arrest, atrial fibrillation, ventricular arrhythmias, shock, COPD, respiratory failure, chronic kidney disease, acute kidney injury, malignancy, stroke, and sepsis, but less commonly coronary artery disease, acute coronary syndrome, STEMI, and hypertension. Non-survivors also had higher white blood cell count, glucose, creatinine, blood nitrogen urea, sodium, and potassium levels, but lower red blood cell and platelet counts, hemoglobin, and hematocrit. Non-survivors less often received oral anticoagulant, antiplatelet, beta-blocker, ACEI/ARB, and statin therapy. APS and APACHE IV of non-survivors were significantly higher than those of survivors.

Association Between Osmolarity and Outcomes

The primary outcome was in-hospital mortality. Through the Lowess smoothing curve shown in **Figure 2**, a "U"-shaped relationship between in-hospital mortality and plasma osmolarity was found. When plasma osmolarity ranged from 290 to 300 mmol/L, in-hospital mortality of CICU patients was the lowest. Therefore, we decided to use osmolarity of 290–300 mmol/L as the reference group in binary logistic regression analysis.

Table 2 shows crude outcomes by plasma osmolarity categories. The lowest in-hospital mortality (7.2%) was observed in the group with 290–300 mmol/L osmolarity. When plasma osmolarity was >290 mmol/L, as plasma osmolarity increased, in-hospital mortality increased significantly (≥330 vs. 290–300 mmol/L: 31.6 vs. 7.2%, respectively). When plasma osmolarity was below 300 mmol/L, as plasma osmolarity decreased, in-hospital mortality increased significantly (<280 vs. 290–300 mmol/L: 13.0 vs. 7.2%, respectively). Higher in-hospital mortality was confirmed in both lower and higher plasma osmolarity group, which was similar with the conclusion drawn by Lowess smoothing shown in **Figure 2**. Moreover, the lengths of CICU and hospital stays were the lowest in the 290–300 mmol/L group; in contrast, the lengths of CICU and hospital stays were prolonged in both hyposmolarity and hyperosmolarity groups (**Table 2**).

As shown in **Table 3**, in unadjusted logistic regression model, with the 290–300 mmol/L group serving as the reference group, both hyposmolarity (<280 vs. 290–300 mmol/L: OR, 95% CI: 1.92, 1.27–2.90, P = 0.002) and hyperosmolarity (≥330 mmol/L vs. 290–300 mmol/L: OR, 95% CI: 5.92, 4.33–8.09, P < 0.001) were related to the increased risk of in-hospital mortality. When plasma osmolarity was >290 mmol/L, the risk of in-hospital mortality increased gradually as plasma osmolarity increased. When plasma osmolarity was below 300 mmol/L, the risk of in-hospital mortality increased gradually as plasma osmolarity decreased. After adjusting for age, gender, and ethnicity in the model 1, the conclusion was basically consistent with that

TABLE 1 | Baseline characteristics between survivors and non-survivors.

Characteristics	Total (n = 7,060)	Survivors (n = 6,207)	Non-survivors (n = 853)	P-value
Age (years)	65.6 ± 15.2	65.1 ± 15.3	69.4 ± 13.7	<0.001
Gender, n (%)				0.701
Male	3,958 (56.1)	3,485 (56.2)	473 (55.5)	
Female	3,102 (43.9)	2,722 (43.9)	380 (44.6)	
Ethnicity, n (%)				<0.001
Caucasian	4,989 (70.7)	4,366 (70.3)	623 (73.0)	
African American	1,185 (16.8)	1,022 (16.5)	163 (19.1)	
Other	886 (12.6)	819 (13.2)	67 (7.9)	
Vital signs				
Systolic blood pressure (mmHg)	122.3 ± 19.7	123.7 ± 19.3	111.7 ± 19.4	<0.001
Diastolic blood pressure (mmHg)	66.1 ± 11.3	66.7 ± 11.2	61.3 ± 10.8	<0.001
Mean blood pressure (mmHg)	82.3 ± 13.0	83.1 ± 12.9	76.0 ± 12.3	<0.001
Heart rate (beats/min)	87.4 ± 22.4	86.4 ± 21.9	95.0 ± 24.1	<0.001
Respiration rate (beats/min)	21.0 ± 6.7	20.7 ± 6.5	22.9 ± 7.7	<0.001
Oxygen saturation (%)	96.3 ± 5.3	96.5 ± 4.4	94.4 ± 9.5	<0.001
Body mass index (kg/m^2)	29.1 ± 7.5	29.2 ± 7.4	28.4 ± 8.1	0.006
Diagnoses and comorbidities, n (%)				
Congestive heart failure	1,396 (19.8)	1,200 (19.3)	196 (23.0)	0.012
Coronary artery disease	2,619 (37.1)	2,417 (38.9)	202 (23.7)	<0.001
Acute coronary syndrome	1,646 (23.3)	1,518 (24.5)	128 (15.0)	<0.001
STEMI	688 (9.8)	641 (10.3)	47 (5.5)	<0.001
NSTEMI	499 (7.1)	441 (7.1)	58 (6.8)	0.774
Arrhythmias	2,205 (31.2)	1,935 (31.2)	270(32.7)	0.777
Cardiac arrest	577 (8.2)	270 (4.4)	307 (36.0)	<0.001
Atrial fibrillation	1,260 (17.9)	1,077 (17.4)	183 (21.5)	0.003
Ventricular arrhythmias	114 (1.6)	83 (1.3)	31 (3.6)	<0.001
Atrioventricular block	176 (2.5)	161 (2.6)	15 (1.8)	0.142
Cardiomyopathy	419 (5.9)	370 (6.0)	49 (5.7)	0.802
Valve disease	182 (2.6)	157 (2.5)	25 (2.9)	0.488
Shock	1,951 (27.6)	1,534 (24.7)	417 (48.9)	<0.001
Pulmonary embolism	143 (2.0)	122 (2.0)	21 (2.5)	0.335
Pulmonary hypertension	76 (1.1)	65 (1.1)	11 (1.3)	0.520
Hypertension	2,019 (28.6)	1,868 (30.1)	151 (17.7)	<0.001
Diabetes	1,306 (18.5)	1,146 (18.5)	160 (18.8)	0.836
COPD	717 (10.2)	610 (9.8)	107 (12.5)	0.014
Respiratory failure	1,894 (26.8)	1,416 (22.8)	478 (56.0)	<0.001
Chronic kidney disease	982 (13.9)	821 (13.2)	161 (18.9)	<0.001
Acute kidney injury	1,178 (16.7)	895 (14.4)	283 (33.2)	<0.001
Malignancy	371 (5.3)	294 (4.7)	77 (9.0)	<0.001
Stroke	262 (3.7)	212 (3.4)	50 (5.9)	<0.001
Sepsis	1,396 (19.8)	1,113 (17.9)	283 (33.2)	<0.001
Laboratory parameters				
White blood cell (10^9/L)	11.7 ± 8.4	11.3 ± 7.9	14.6 ± 11.1	<0.001
Red blood cell (10^9/L)	4.1 ± 0.8	4.1 ± 0.8	3.9 ± 0.8	<0.001
Platelet (10^9/L)	226.6	227.8 ± 96.4	217.4 ± 108.3	0.004
Hemoglobin (g/dL)	12.1 ± 2.5	12.2 ± 2.5	11.5 ± 2.5	<0.001
Hematocrit (%)	36.7 ± 7.0	36.9 ± 7.0	35.4 ± 7.4	<0.001
Glucose (mmol/L)	8.9 ± 5.1	8.7 ± 5.0	10.2 ± 6.0	<0.001
Creatinine (mg/dL)	1.69 ± 1.48	1.64 ± 1.48	2.02 ± 1.47	<0.001

(Continued)

TABLE 1 | Continued

Characteristics	Total (n = 7,060)	Survivors (n = 6,207)	Non-survivors (n = 853)	P-value
Blood nitrogen urea (mmol/L)	28.7 ± 21.7	27.4 ± 20.6	38.1 ± 26.3	<0.001
Sodium (mmol/L)	137.2 ± 5.3	137.2 ± 5.2	137.6 ± 6.4	0.043
Potassium (mmol/L)	4.2 ± 0.8	4.2 ± 0.7	4.4 ± 0.9	<0.001
Medication use, n (%)				
Antiplatelet	3,396 (48.1)	3,078 (49.6)	318 (37.3)	<0.001
Oral anticoagulants	767 (10.9)	710 (11.4)	57 (6.7)	<0.001
Beta-blockers	3,034 (43.0)	2,795 (45.0)	239 (28.0)	<0.001
ACEI/ARB	1,914 (27.1)	1,805 (29.1)	109 (12.8)	<0.001
Statin	2,150 (30.5)	1,999 (32.2)	151(17.7)	<0.001
APS	38 (27–55)	36 (25–49)	76 (52–106)	<0.001
APACHE IV	52 (38–70)	49 (36–64)	92 (67–121)	<0.001
Initial osmolarity (mmol/L)	302.2 ± 14.4	301.4 ± 13.7	308.1 ± 18.1	<0.001
Maximum osmolarity (mmol/L)	308.4 ± 15.6	306.7 ± 14.1	321.0 ± 19.9	<0.001

Normally distributed continuous variables were presented as mean ± SD or median (IQR). Categorical variables were presented as number (percentage). STEMI, ST-elevation myocardial infarction; NSTEMI, non-ST-elevation myocardial infarction; COPD, chronic obstructive pulmonary disease; ACEI, angiotensin-converting enzyme inhibitor; ARB, angiotensin receptor blocker; APS, acute physiology score; APACHE IV, acute physiology and chronic health evaluation IV.

TABLE 2 | Outcomes by osmolarity categories in CICU patients.

Outcome	Osmolarity (mmol/L)							
	<280 (n = 231)	280–290 (n = 732)	290–300 (n = 2,283)	300–310 (n = 2290)	310–320 (n = 917)	320–330 (n = 363)	≥330 (n = 244)	P-value
In-hospital mortality, n (%)	30 (13.0)	71 (9.7)	165 (7.2)	243 (10.6)	173 (18.9)	94 (25.9)	77 (31.6)	<0.001
Length of CICU stay (days)	2.2 (1.4–4.6)	2.0 (1.1–3.9)	1.8 (1.0–3.1)	1.9 (1.1–3.4)	2.2 (1.2–4.1)	2.7 (1.5–5.0)	3.3 (1.6–6.0)	<0.001
Length of hospital stay (days)	5.7 (3.0–10.7)	5.2 (2.9–9.9)	4.6 (2.5–8.9)	5.0 (2.8–9.2)	5.9 (3.1–10.3)	7.4 (3.6–12.2)	7.9 (4.3–14.9)	<0.001

Lengths of CICU and hospital stays were skewed. Therefore, they were presented as median (IQR). Categorical variables were presented as number (percentage). CICU, cardiac intensive care unit.

of the unadjusted model. After adjusting for more possible confounding variables in the model 2, the association between osmolarity and in-hospital mortality was attenuated but still remained statistically significant. Both hyposmolarity (<280 vs. 290–300 mmol/L: OR, 95% CI: 1.76, 1.08–2.85, $P = 0.023$) and hyperosmolarity (≥330 mmol/L vs. 290–300 mmol/L: OR, 95% CI: 1.65, 1.08–2.52, $P = 0.021$) were independently associated with the increased risk of in-hospital mortality. OR values increased gradually as plasma osmolarity increased when plasma osmolarity was >290 mmol/L; when plasma osmolarity was below 300 mmol/L, OR values increased gradually as plasma osmolarity decreased. **Figure 3** vividly presents the change of OR with the change of osmolarity groups in the unadjusted model, model 1, and model 2.

DISCUSSION

This study identified the association between plasma osmolarity and in-hospital mortality in CICU patients. A "U"-shaped relationship between plasma osmolarity and in-hospital mortality was observed. With the group of 290–300 mmol/L serving as the reference group, both hyposmolarity and hyperosmolarity were associated with the increased risk of in-hospital mortality, even after adjusting for possible confounding variables. The lengths of CICU and hospital stays were prolonged in both hyposmolarity and hyperosmolarity groups.

As a common clinical marker to evaluate the balance of fluid and electrolytes (4–7), plasma osmolarity can be easily calculated from the concentrations of serum sodium, potassium, glucose, and blood nitrogen urea (8). Plasma osmolarity is the most commonly used indicator of hydration (18), which can influence cell size and function (19). Therefore, changes in plasma osmolarity can reflect changes in cell function. A great number of studies have been done on plasma osmolarity, and there is sufficient evidence that plasma osmolarity is associated with the prognosis of many diseases, such as stroke (9), intracerebral hemorrhage (10), and acute pulmonary embolism (20). Moreover, recent studies have shown a correlation between

TABLE 3 | The association between in-hospital mortality and osmolarity (mmol/L).

	Unadjusted		Model 1		Model 2	
	OR(95% CIs)	P-value	OR(95% CIs)	P-value	OR(95% CIs)	P-value
Osmolarity (<280)	1.92 (1.27–2.90)	0.002	1.85 (1.22–2.80)	0.004	1.76 (1.08–2.85)	0.023
Osmolarity (280–290)	1.38 (1.03–1.85)	0.031	1.39 (1.04–1.87)	0.027	1.20 (0.85–1.69)	0.289
Osmolarity (290–300)	1.0 (reference)		1.0 (reference)		1.0 (reference)	
Osmolarity (300–310)	1.52 (1.24–1.87)	<0.001	1.45 (1.18–1.78)	<0.001	1.13(0.88–1.45)	0.351
Osmolarity (310–320)	2.98 (2.37–3.75)	<0.001	2.80 (2.22–3.53)	<0.001	1.46 (1.09–1.96)	0.012
Osmolarity (320–330)	4.49 (3.38–5.95)	<0.001	4.16 (3.13–5.53)	<0.001	1.46 (1.00–2.13)	0.052
Osmolarity (≥330)	5.92 (4.33–8.09)	<0.001	5.58 (4.07–7.65)	<0.001	1.65 (1.08–2.52)	0.021

Models were derived from binary logistic regression analysis. Unadjusted model: unadjusted. Model 1: adjusted for age, gender, ethnicity. Model 2: adjusted for age, gender, ethnicity, systolic blood pressure, diastolic blood pressure, mean blood pressure, heart rate, respiration rate, congestive heart failure, coronary artery disease, acute coronary syndrome, STEMI, NSTEMI, cardiac arrest, ventricular arrhythmias, shock, hypertension, diabetes, respiratory failure, acute kidney injury, sepsis, stroke, malignancy, white blood cell, red blood cell, hemoglobin, creatinine, ACEI/ARB, beta-blockers, statin, and oral anticoagulants, APS, APACHE IV. OR, odds ratio; CI, confidence interval.

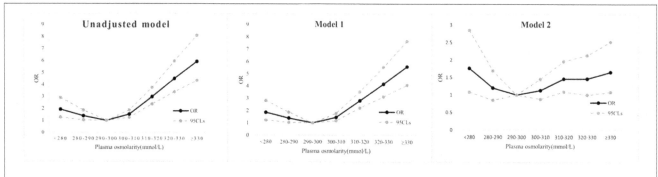

FIGURE 3 | Line graphs reflecting the trend of change in OR of in-hospital mortality in unadjusted model, model 1, and model 2. OR, odds ratio; CI, confidence interval.

plasma osmolarity and cardiovascular diseases. A single-center retrospective study with 1,927 patients after PCI showed that the rate of acute kidney injury and 1-year mortality increased significantly as plasma osmolarity increased (14). Another study, which enrolled 985 patients with acute coronary syndrome undergoing PCI, confirmed higher mortality in the higher osmolarity group (15). In patients with STEMI, higher rates of all-cause mortality, recurrent myocardial infarction, and revascularization were found in those with higher plasma osmolarity (21). Previous studies also showed that both low and high plasma osmolarity were related to more cardiovascular deaths, deterioration of cardiac function, and rehospitalization in patients with heart failure (12, 13). In this study exploring the relationship between plasma osmolarity and in-hospital mortality in CICU patients, we came to a similar conclusion that plasma osmolarity was closely associated with in-hospital mortality. Moreover, through Lowess smoothing, we found a "U"-relationship between in-hospital mortality and osmolarity, which provided a more graphic description of the overall trend.

Plasma osmolarity is mainly determined by serum sodium, chloride, potassium, blood glucose, and blood nitrogen urea. Hypernatremia, hyperchloremia, hyperkalemia, hyperglycemia, and high urea contribute to high plasma osmolarity.

Hypernatremia was shown to be associated with higher mortality and more cardiovascular diseases in older men (22). Another study confirmed that increased hypernatremia was associated with higher perioperative 30-day mortality (23). For patients with intracranial hemorrhage, hypernatremia was associated with more adverse cardiac events (24). Patel et al. found that hyperchloremia was independently associated with acute kidney injury in patients with STEMI undergoing PCI (25). Hyperkalemia can lead to malignant arrhythmia and increase mortality (26). Hyperglycemia is very common in clinical practice and it is related to higher mortality and more adverse cardiac events in patients with or without diabetes (27). A prospective study with 1,667 patients diagnosed with acute coronary syndrome showed that high blood nitrogen was associated with more adverse cardiac events and higher mortality (28). These studies can explain why high plasma osmolarity leads to high mortality, which can also explain the results of our study. The lengths of CICU and hospital stays were prolonged in both the hyposmolarity and the hyperosmolarity groups, indicating that patients with hyposmolarity or hyperosmolarity had a more complex condition and therefore required a longer treatment. The increased lengths of CICU and hospital stays imposed not only the financial but also mental burden on patients. In exceptional cases, some patients may abandon treatment because of financial problems. Therefore, more attention to plasma osmolarity of CICU patients is needed.

Changes in plasma osmolarity can provide guidance for clinical practice. Usually, the clinicians tend to pay more attention to the outliers, but when all the variables are within the normal range but close to the upper limit of the normal value, plasma osmolarity will increase significantly. At this time, plasma osmolarity can better reflect the patient's condition and give the clinician a hit. The independent association between in-hospital mortality and plasma osmolarity was confirmed in this study. As a readily accessible and inexpensive prognostic marker, plasma osmolarity is clinically valuable for critically ill patients admitted to CICU, especially in some cases that more complex prognostic score can't be calculated, for example, the patient is unable to undergo complex examination or the patient is in a remote area without the means to do so, plasma osmolarity may alert the clinicians.

We confirmed the association between plasma osmolarity and in-hospital mortality in CICU patients in this study, which is convenient for clinical use. The multicenter and large sample size makes the conclusion more reliable. However, some limitations in this study should be noted. First, bias was inevitable due to the retrospective nature of the study. Second, some important information, such as left ventricular ejection fraction and information about smoking and alcohol, could not be collected.

In general, the variables included in the model determine the accuracy of the model; thus, the accuracy of the model was likely affected by the missing variables. Third, we were not able to dynamically observe plasma osmolarity. Fourth, although the optimal equation was used, the calculated plasma osmolarity cannot be the exactly the same as the real plasma osmolarity.

CONCLUSION

A "U"-shaped relationship between plasma osmolarity and in-hospital mortality was observed. The lowest in-hospital mortality was shown in the group with 290–300 mmol/L osmolarity; patients with hyposmolarity or hyperosmolarity had higher in-hospital mortality. With the group with 290–300 mmol/L osmolarity serving as the reference group, both hyposmolarity and hyperosmolarity were shown to be independently associated with the increased risk of in-hospital mortality.

AUTHOR CONTRIBUTIONS

GZ and YZ contributed to study design, data analysis, and article writing. JW and YL contributed to data collection. All authors contributed to the article and approved the submitted version.

REFERENCES

1. GBD 2017 DALYs and HALE Collaborators. Global, regional, and national disability-adjusted life-years (DALYs) for 359 diseases and injuries and healthy life expectancy (HALE) for 195 countries and territories, 1990–2017: a systematic analysis for the Global Burden of Disease Study 2017. *Lancet.* (2018) 392:1859–922. doi: 10.1016/S0140-6736(18)32335-3

2. Vervoort D. Global cardiac surgery: a wake-up call. *Eur J Cardio Thoracic Surg.* (2019) 55:1022–3. doi: 10.1093/ejcts/ezy319

3. Katz JN, Shah BR, Volz EM, Horton JR, Shaw LK, Newby LK, et al. Evolution of the coronary care unit: clinical characteristics and temporal trends in healthcare delivery and outcomes. *Crit Care Med.* (2010) 38:375–81. doi: 10.1097/CCM.0b013e3181cb0a63

4. Earley LE, Sanders CA. The effect of changing serum osmolality on the release of antidiuretic hormone in certain patients with decompensated cirrhosis of the liver and low serum osmolality. *J Clin Invest.* (1959) 38:545–50. doi: 10.1172/JCI103832

5. Rasouli M. Basic concepts and practical equations on osmolality: biochemical approach. *Clin Biochem.* (2016) 49:936–41. doi: 10.1016/j.clinbiochem.2016.06.001

6. Gennari FJ. Current concepts. Serum osmolality. Uses and limitations. *N Engl J Med.* (1984) 310:102–5. doi: 10.1056/NEJM198401123100207

7. Cheuvront SN, Kenefick RW, Sollanek KJ, Ely BR, Sawka MN. Water-deficit equation: systematic analysis and improvement. *Am J Clin Nutr.* (2013) 97:79–85. doi: 10.3945/ajcn.112.046839

8. Heavens KR, Kenefick RW, Caruso EM, Spitz MG, Cheuvront SN. Validation of equations used to predict plasma osmolality in a healthy adult cohort. *Am J Clin Nutr.* (2014) 100:1252–6. doi: 10.3945/ajcn.114.091009

9. Bhalla A, Sankaralingam S, Dundas R, Swaminathan R, Wolfe CD, Rudd AG. Influence of raised plasma osmolality on clinical outcome after acute stroke. *Stroke.* (2000) 31:2043–8. doi: 10.1161/01.STR.31.9.2043

10. Nag C, Das K, Ghosh M, Khandakar MR. Plasma osmolality in acute spontanious intra-cerebral hemorrhage: does it influence hematoma volume and clinical outcome? *J Res Med Sci.* (2012) 17:548–51.

11. Shen Y, Cheng X, Ying M, Chang HT, Zhang W. Association between serum osmolarity and mortality in patients who are critically ill: a retrospective cohort study. *BMJ Open.* (2017) 7:e015729. doi: 10.1136/bmjopen-2016-015729

12. Vaduganathan M, Marti CN, Mentz RJ, Greene SJ, Ambrosy AP, Subacius HP, et al. Serum osmolality and postdischarge outcomes after hospitalization for heart failure. *Am J Cardiol.* (2016) 117:1144–50. doi: 10.1016/j.amjcard.2015.12.059

13. Kaya H, Yücel O, Ege MR, Zorlu A, Yücel H, Güneş H, et al. Plasma osmolality predicts mortality in patients with heart failure with reduced ejection fraction. *Kardiologia polska.* (2017) 75:316–22. doi: 10.5603/KP.a2016.0168

14. Farhan S, Vogel B, Baber U, Sartori S, Aquino M, Chandrasekhar J, et al. Calculated serum osmolality, acute kidney injury, and relationship to mortality after percutaneous coronary intervention. *Cardiorenal Med.* (2019) 9:160–7. doi: 10.1159/000494807

15. Rohla M, Freynhofer MK, Tentzeris I, et al. Plasma osmolality predicts clinical outcome in patients with acute coronary syndrome undergoing percutaneous coronary intervention. *Eur Heart J Acute Cardiovasc Care.* (2014) 3:84–92. doi: 10.1177/2048872613516018

16. Pollard TJ, Johnson AEW, Raffa JD, Celi LA, Mark RG, Badawi O. The eICU collaborative research database, a freely available multi-center database for critical care research. *Sci Data.* (2018) 5:180178. doi: 10.1038/sdata.2018.178

17. Zimmerman JE, Kramer AA, McNair DS, Malila FM. Acute physiology and chronic health evaluation (APACHE IV) IV: hospital mortality assessment for today's critically ill patients. *Crit Care Med.* (2006) 34:1297–310. doi: 10.1097/01.CCM.0000215112.84523.F0

18. Francesconi RP, Hubbard RW, Szlyk PC, Schnakenberg D, Carlson D, Leva N, et al. Urinary and hematologic indexes of hypohydration. *J Appl Physiol.* (1987) 62:1271–6. doi: 10.1152/jappl.1987.62.3.1271

19. Danziger J, Zeidel ML. Osmotic homeostasis. *Clin J Am Soc Nephrol.* (2015) 10:852–62. doi: 10.2215/CJN.10741013

20. Öz A, Çinar T, Hayiroglu M, Avşar S, Keskin M, Orhan AL. The predictive value of plasma osmolality for in-hospital mortality in patients with acute pulmonary embolism. *Clin Respir J.* (2019) 13:174–83. doi: 10.1111/crj.13001

21. Tatlisu MA, Kaya A, Keskin M, Uzman O, Borklu EB, Cinier G, et al. Can we use plasma hyperosmolality as a predictor of mortality for ST-segment elevation myocardial infarction? *Coron Artery Dis.* (2017) 28:70–6. doi: 10.1097/MCA.0000000000000426

22. Wannamethee SG, Shaper AG, Lennon L, Papacosta O, Whincup P. Mild hyponatremia, hypernatremia and incident cardiovascular disease and mortality in older men: a population-based cohort study. *Nutr Metab Cardiovasc Dis.* (2016) 26:12–9. doi: 10.1016/j.numecd.2015.07.008

23. Leung AA, McAlister FA, Finlayson SR, Bates DW. Preoperative hypernatremia predicts increased perioperative morbidity and mortality. *Am J Med.* (2013) 126:877–6. doi: 10.1016/j.amjmed.2013.02.039

24. Fisher LA, Ko N, Miss J, Tung PP, Kopelnik A, Banki NM, et al. Hypernatremia predicts adverse cardiovascular and neurological outcomes after SAH. *Neurocrit Care.* (2006) 5:180–5. doi: 10.1385/NCC:5:3:180

25. Patel N, Baker SM, Walters RW, Kaja A, Kandasamy V, Abuzaid A, et al. Serum hyperchloremia as a risk factor for acute kidney injury in patients with ST-segment elevation myocardial infarction undergoing percutaneous coronary intervention. Proc (Bayl Univ Med Cent). (2016) 29:7–11. doi: 10.1080/08998280.2016.11929341

26. Dunn JD, Benton WW, Orozco-Torrentera E, Adamson RT. The burden of hyperkalemia in patients with cardiovascular and renal disease. *Am J Manag Care.* (2015) 21(15 Suppl):s307–15.

27. Capes SE, Hunt D, Malmberg K, Gerstein HC. Stress hyperglycaemia and increased risk of death after myocardial infarction in patients with and without diabetes: a systematic overview. *Lancet.* (2000) 355:773–8. doi: 10.1016/S0140-6736(99)08415-9

28. Saygitov RT, Glezer MG, Semakina SV. Blood urea nitrogen and creatinine levels at admission for mortality risk assessment in patients with acute coronary syndromes. *Emerg Med J.* (2010) 27:105–9. doi: 10.1136/emj.2008.068155

4

Aortic Stiffness: Epidemiology, Risk Factors and Relevant Biomarkers

Rebecca Angoff[1], Ramya C. Mosarla[2] and Connie W. Tsao[1]*

[1] Cardiovascular Division, Department of Medicine, Beth Israel Deaconess Medical Center, Boston, MA, United States,
[2] Division of Cardiology, Department of Medicine, New York University Langone Health, New York, NY, United States

*Correspondence:
Connie W. Tsao
ctsao1@bidmc.harvard.edu

Aortic stiffness (AoS) is a maladaptive response to hemodynamic stress and both modifiable and non-modifiable risk factors, and elevated AoS increases afterload for the heart. AoS is a non-invasive marker of cardiovascular health and metabolic dysfunction. Implementing AoS as a diagnostic tool is challenging as it increases with age and varies amongst races. AoS is associated with lifestyle factors such as alcohol and smoking, as well as hypertension and comorbid conditions including metabolic syndrome and its components. Multiple studies have investigated various biomarkers associated with increased AoS, and this area is of particular interest given that these markers can highlight pathophysiologic pathways and specific therapeutic targets in the future. These biomarkers include those involved in the inflammatory cascade, anti-aging genes, and the renin-angiotensin aldosterone system. In the future, targeting AoS rather than blood pressure itself may be the key to improving vascular health and outcomes. In this review, we will discuss the current understanding of AoS, measurement of AoS and the challenges in interpretation, associated biomarkers, and possible therapeutic avenues for modulation of AoS.

Keywords: aortic stiffness, pulse wave velocity, cardiovascular health, risk factors, biomarkers

INTRODUCTION

Aortic stiffness (AoS) is a measure of the elasticity of the blood vessel wall, and elevated AoS may result from and contribute to increased stress on the vessel walls. It is a non-invasive method of measuring maladaptive change and remodeling to aortic properties and is a promising marker of subclinical disease. Its measurement is based on principles of physics. The arterial tree has varying mechanical properties along its length, primarily determined by different contributions of collagen and elastin to its structure, in addition to varying degrees of modulation by smooth muscle. Pulse waves generated from pulsatile hemodynamics of the cardiac cycle travel down the large conduit arteries to the mid-sized arteries where they incur increased resistance due to branch points and increased arterial tone. The incident waves are then reflected back toward the central arteries from the periphery. The stiffness of the central conduit arteries determines the velocity with which the reflected waves return, with increased AoS resulting in more rapid propagation of reflected waves, determining the measured pulse wave velocity (PWV) (1). Pathologically increased AoS allows waves reflected from the periphery to return in phase with cardiac systole, augmenting central systolic pressure and increasing hemodynamic load on the left ventricle. AoS is able to capture a unique measure of central hemodynamics not reflected by simply the blood pressure alone, likely explaining the ability of carotid-femoral PWV (cfPWV) to serve as an independent predictor of cardiovascular outcomes. Further, the processes implicated in AoS, which include activation of oxidative stress pathways and inflammation may be reflective of underlying vascular risk (2).

The purpose of this review is to discuss the clinical implications of AoS, its measurements including PWV and augmentation index (AI), and the factors that contribute to and alter AoS. We will also review AoS involvement in disease processes as well as biomarkers involved in AoS. The goal is to gain a better understanding of AoS as a subclinical marker of chronic disease.

CLINICAL SIGNIFICANCE

Stiffening of the aorta is a marker of subclinical disease and has been demonstrated to precede the onset of hypertension in a longitudinally followed cohort (3). Earlier studies first implicated elevated PWV to be associated with atherosclerosis (4) and as a predictor of worse cardiovascular outcomes and mortality in high-risk conditions such as diabetes mellitus (DM), chronic kidney disease, and hypertension, as well as coronary artery disease post-myocardial infarction (5–7). AoS was later demonstrated in healthy community dwelling individuals to predict incident events including coronary disease, heart failure, stroke, and cardiovascular mortality independently of adjustment for cardiovascular risk factors (8–11). Further, there is evidence that AoS reflects the presence of composite end-organ damage and has been shown to have superior prognostic value to measurements of office and ambulatory systolic blood pressures in patients with advanced kidney disease (12).

The adverse outcomes related to elevated AoS suggested by the prior studies have been corroborated and further evaluated through meta-analyses. In such a 2010 study by Vlachopoulos et al. an increase in PWV of 1 m/s conferred an increased risk of cardiovascular events, cardiovascular mortality, and all-cause mortality (13). Moreover, a meta-analysis of over 17,000 participants showed that a 1-standard deviation difference in log-transformed cfPWV was associated with an increased risk of future cardiovascular events over 5 years even after adjusting for more traditional risk factors; furthermore, this same meta-analysis showed that using cfPWV in addition to traditional risk factors was able to reclassify patient risk for cardiovascular disease (CVD) for those who had an intermediate 10 year CVD risk (14). Therefore, by measuring AoS in patients, practitioners may be able to detect patients at risk for CVD at an early, subclinical stage. This early detection may provide the opportunity for early intervention, patient education on risk factors, and potentially help to decrease the incidence of overt disease.

MEASUREMENT

Several modalities are available to measure AoS by PWV including recording the pulse waves by a tonometer transducer, standard blood pressure cuff, doppler ultrasound, and magnetic resonance imaging (MRI) (15). The transducer methods consist of placing a tonometer over the carotid and femoral arteries and monitoring an ECG signal for timing of the pressure waveforms. These methods have historically been the gold standard but can be a challenging learning curve for the operator. Thus, there has been increased interest in comparing the various AoS measurement methods to determine which is most accurate and easiest to implement. Pulse wave doppler ultrasound allows measurement of AoS without the need for a specific measurement device, is quicker, and has been shown to be comparable to transducer methods (16, 17). While blood pressure cuff measured cfPWV may be easier to acquire than the doppler approach, it often requires correction (18). MRI based techniques also offer promise due to their ability to directly and accurately visualize path-length and ability to quantify AoS in more proximal aortic segments but lack practicality (19).

cfPWV is the gold standard measure of aortic wall stiffness (2). cfPWV is obtained via transcutaneous measurement of the pressure waveform at the common carotid artery and at the femoral artery by either probes or blood pressure cuffs; alternatively, this can be measured from Doppler or MRI flow waveforms (20). The distance between the two surface sites and the time delay between the waveforms is used to determine the velocity component (2). **Figure 1** depicts how the cfPWV is calculated. It is important to note that blood pressure and PWV are closely intertwined with higher mean arterial pressures correlated with increased AoS (15, 22).

However, there are additional challenges to measuring cfPWV. The surface distance between carotid and femoral sites of measurement may not represent true arterial path-length, especially in patients with obesity. Therefore, proposed correction factor equations account for these systematic inaccuracies such as multiplying the distance from the carotid artery to the femoral artery by 0.8 (23). In addition, there are challenges with measuring pressure waveforms in obese patients and in controlling for existing atherosclerotic disease in vessels. Furthermore, conditions during time of measurements such as patient positioning, temperature in the room, and white coat hypertension can all confound the results (2). Brachial PWV methods also exist, but because of PWV amplification in peripheral arteries, it is considered a less reliable measure of central artery stiffness (24).

Augmentation index (AI) is another measurement of AoS (**Figure 1**). It is measured by dividing the augmentation pressure by the pulse pressure and multiplying by 100 to provide a number (percentage). AI is a stronger predictor of left ventricular mass reduction in response to lowering the blood pressure compared to other more conventional measures such as brachial blood pressure (25), and increased AI is independently associated with increased cardiovascular events in those undergoing percutaneous coronary interventions (26). Furthermore, more recent data has shown that higher augmentation index is associated with poor exercise capacity after heart transplant (27). However, AI is impacted by other factors such as age, systolic blood pressure, heart rate, left ventricular ejection time, and height to a greater extent than PWV (28, 29). Therefore, PWV, and in particular cfPWV, is used more often in trials.

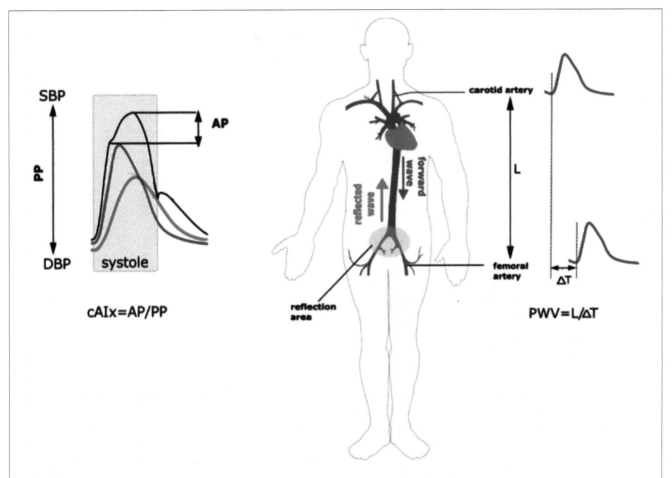

FIGURE 1 | Measurement of augmentation index and cfPWV. On the left panel, the central augmentation index is calculated as the ratio of the augmentation pressure over the pulse pressure. On the right panel, the cfPWV is measured by evaluating waveforms at the common carotid and femoral artery. This is the foot-to-foot method as it measures the beginning of the waveform at each site. The velocity component is then calculated by measuring the distance between the two sites divided by the time it takes for the waveform to travel from site to site. AP, augmentation pressure; PP, pulse pressure; cAIx, central augmentation index; PWV, pulse wave velocity; SBP, systolic blood pressure; DBP, diastolic blood pressure. Reproduced from (21).

NORMATIVE VALUES AND IMPACT OF DEMOGRAPHICS

Despite having known prognostic implications distinct from traditional cardiovascular risk factors, the clinical use of cfPWV has been limited due to lack of widespread use of population specific reference ranges. The 2007 ESC/ESH guidelines proposed a cut-off value of 12 m/s for elevated AoS based on clinical outcome data (30). Furthermore, multiple studies have sought to establish reference ranges for PWV. The Reference Values for Arterial Stiffness Collaboration Database was one of the first large-scale efforts to establish reference ranges for cfPWV in 16,867 European individuals across 13 centers (31). A subset of 11,092 individuals without prevalent CVD or use of anti-hypertensive or lipid-lowering medications were used to draw reference values presented in **Table 1**. However, a challenge with creating normative values is that experienced laboratories are needed for cfPWV measurement, and disparate measurement devices and methodologies can

produce a variance in PWV affecting generalizability even within the same patient (32).

AGE, SEX, AND RACE

Age

A rise in AoS with age has been well-described in large, diverse groups free of clinical CVD (31, 33–35). Central artery stiffness results in a reduced arterial reservoir effect, augmenting pressure during systole and diminishing it during diastole (36). This is thought to be one mechanism for the observed age-related increase in systolic blood pressure and decline in diastolic blood pressure, which lead to adverse ventricular and vascular hemodynamics, poor cardiac perfusion, and cardiac remodeling (37, 38).

Several mechanisms may contribute to age-related arteriosclerosis. Intrinsic remodeling of arteries has been demonstrated with increasing intima media thickness with age (39). Changes in the mechanical properties of the vascular

TABLE 1 | Distribution of pulse wave velocity (PWV) values (m/s) in the reference value population (11,092 subject) according to age and blood pressure category.

Age category (years)	Blood pressure category				
	Optimal	Normal	High Normal	Grade I HTN	Grade II/III HTN
PWV as mean					
(±2SD)					
<30	6.1 (4.6–7.5)	6.6 (4.9–8.2)	6.8 (5.1–8.5)	7.4 (4.6–10.1)	7.7 (4.4–11.0)
30–39	6.6 (4.4–8.9)	6.8 (4.2–9.4)	7.1 (4.5–9.7)	7.3 (4.0–10.7)	8.2 (3.3–13.0)
40–49	7.0 (4.5–9.6)	7.5 (5.1–10.0)	7.9 (5.2–10.7)	8.6 (5.1–12.0)	9.8 (3.8–15.7)
50–59	7.6 (4.8–10.5)	8.4 (5.1–11.7)	8.8 (4.8–12.8)	9.6 (4.9–14.3)	10.5 (4.1–16.8)
60–69	9.1 (5.2–12.9)	9.7 (5.7–13.6)	10.3 (5.5–15.1)	11.1 (6.1–16.2)	12.2 (5.7–18.6)
≥70	10.4 (5.2–15.6)	11.7 (6.0–17.5)	11.8 (5.7–17.9)	12.9 (6.9–18.9)	14.0 (7.4–20.6)
PWV as median					
(10th–90th percentile)					
<30	6.0 (5.2–7.0)	6.4 (5.7–7.5)	6.7 (5.8–7.9)	7.2 (5.7–9.3)	7.6 (5.9–9.9)
30–39	6.5 (5.4–7.9)	6.7 (5.3–8.2)	7.0 (5.5–8.8)	7.2 (5.5–9.3)	7.6 (5.8–11.2)
40–49	6.8 (5.8–8.5)	7.4 (5.3–8.2)	7.7 (6.5–9.5)	8.1 (6.8–10.8)	9.2 (7.1–13.2)
50–59	7.5 (6.2–9.2)	8.1 (6.7–10.4)	8.4 (7.0–11.3)	9.2 (7.2–12.5)	9.7 (7.4–14.9)
60–69	8.7 (7.0–11.4)	9.3 (7.6–12.2)	9.8 (7.9–13.2)	10.7 (8.4–14.1)	12.0 (8.5–16.5)
≥70	10.1 (7.6–13.8)	11.1 (8.6–15.5)	11.2 (8.6–15.8)	12.7 (9.3–16.7)	13.5 (10.3–18.2)

Modified from Reference Values for Arterial Stiffness (31).
HTN, hypertension; SD, standard deviation.

media are also observed, with maladaptive remodeling with increased deposition of collagen (40). Age related arteriosclerosis that is independent of atherosclerosis is supported by the strong independent association between age and cfPWV that persists in those without aortic calcifications (41). The cumulative exposure to vascular risk factors including DM also contributes to increases in AoS with age (42).

Sex

The relationship between sex and AoS is complex and varies with age. Whereas pre-pubescent females have higher PWV than pre-pubescent males, this difference is abrogated post-puberty as the average PWV in females decreases but PWV in males increases (43). In the Jackson Heart Study, while adult men were more likely to have elevated cfPWV in the overall cohort, women had steeper rise in both cfPWV and forward wave amplitude with age >60 (35). Brachial-ankle PWV (baPWV) has been shown to be similar in males and females until about age 50–60 years old, at which point there is a greater proportional increase in female baPWV (44). This accelerated increase in the baPWV around age 50–60, when females are post-menopausal, provides further evidence that there is a hormonal component to the sex differences in AoS. Furthermore, when corrected for age and blood pressure, middle aged females with metabolic syndrome had higher aortic PWV as compared to males, again supporting the role of sex the relationship of age with PWV (45).

The mechanism behind sex differences in AoS may be related to downstream effects of sex hormones. Men with acquired hypogonadism have higher PWV compared to normal men, and treatment with testosterone therapy helps to lower PWV,

supporting a possible role for testosterone in lowering AoS (46). Indeed, in animal models, testosterone induces endothelium-independent vasodilation of arterial beds (47). Sex hormones in women also seem to play roles in modulating AoS. Decreases in estradiol with menopause are associated with a proinflammatory state, which may be a cause of elevated AoS in women after menopause (48). Furthermore, female sex steroids such as 17 beta estradiol and progesterone promote elastin deposition, and thus withdrawal following menopause may also contribute to increased AoS during this time period (49).

Race

African Americans (AA) suffer a disproportionately increased risk of CVD, hypertension, and microvascular dysfunction compared to whites, highlighting the disparities in vascular morbidity and mortality (50–52). Data suggests that these differences may be driven by a difference in risk factor burden, sociodemographic factors including income, as well as intrinsic differences in mechanical properties of blood vessels and baseline AoS (53).

Differences in AoS between AA and whites have been observed in childhood. AA boys as young as 6–8 years old have elevated mean arterial pressure (MAP), intimal media thickness, and cfPWV compared to white boys (54). Sociodemographic factors including education, lower family income, and lower socioeconomic status were all associated with higher PWV (55). However, higher aortic PWV is seen in AA children compared to whites even after adjusting for age, sex, body mass index, mean arterial pressure, and socioeconomic status (56). This difference in AoS among children persists in adults. In the Multi-Ethnic Study of Atherosclerosis of multiple community cohorts, AA had a higher prevalence of hypertension and lower aortic distensibility (57). In the Dallas Heart Study, both AA and Hispanic individuals had greater aortic arch PWV independent of cardiovascular risk factors including mean arterial pressure, heart rate, DM, and smoking (58).

However, other studies suggest that there may be confounding variables that account for the differences in AoS among races. In the ELSA-Brasil study, investigators noted that AAs had a higher burden of hypertension, DM, and obesity compared to the other racial groups and had higher unadjusted cfPWV compared to browns and whites who were similar. However, after adjusting for characteristics including mean arterial pressure, age, waist circumference, heart rate, and fasting glucose, the inter-group differences were abrogated. The results of this study indicate that ~40% of the difference between cfPWV values could be explained by age and mean arterial pressure, suggesting less contribution by race itself to AoS. Though there may be a race-sex interaction in women, with AA and brown women having higher cfPWV than whites particularly in the highest quartiles of cfPWV, the strength of that relationship was much weaker than the effects of MAP and age (59).

Several mechanisms have been proposed to contribute to the differences of AoS among racial/ethnic groups. First, risk factor sensitivity may vary among different racial groups. For example, cfPWV progression is affected by risk factors such as diastolic blood pressure, glucose, and low-density lipoprotein cholesterol in AA women, while it was not in Caucasian women (60). Furthermore, it has been demonstrated that AAs living in the northern hemisphere likely suffer a greater burden of Vitamin D deficiency relative to white counterparts (61). Vitamin D has been proposed to improve vascular health by suppressing oxidative pathways and the sensitivity to renin-angiotensin-aldosterone system (RAAS) mediated remodeling. Vitamin D supplementation has been shown to decrease PWV in AAs with vitamin D deficiency (62). While the paucity of large-scale studies suggests the need for further research to determine the clinical utility of improving Vitamin D to improve vascular health, this modifiable risk factor creates a targetable treatment regimen for AAs.

Generalized endothelial dysfunction has also been posited as a mediator of progressive AoS in AAs compared to whites. Studies have demonstrated that AAs tend to have impaired nitric oxide signaling and thus more endothelial cell dysfunction at baseline and when compared to whites (63, 64). This impaired nitric oxide signaling in AAs compared to white Americans has been shown to be present even after adjusting for CVD risk factors, suggesting that impaired vascular function precedes incident disease (65). Whether additional intrinsic differences in the properties of vessels or unmeasured risk factors exist between racial/ethnic groups remains to be determined.

COMORBIDITIES ASSOCIATED WITH AoS

Hypertension

Hypertension demonstrates a very strong association with AoS compared to other cardiometabolic risk factors studied. A major shift has occurred regarding the understanding of

directionality between hypertension on AoS and vice versa. The initial paradigm posited that arterial stress induced by elevated pressure and pulsatility-mediated breaks in elastin led to maladaptive remodeling by inducing inflammation (1, 66, 67). Both baseline blood pressure and blood pressure variability have been linked to increased vascular stiffness (68). Higher blood pressure variability is thought to promote vascular smooth muscle cell proliferation and atherosclerosis as well as increase oscillatory wall stress (69, 70). This increased variability may lead to increased AoS which in turn, with stiffer arteries, may increase blood pressure (71).

Clinical and experimental studies have demonstrated that the relationship between hypertension and AoS is interdependent (72–74). Elevated AoS preceding the development of overt hypertension has been demonstrated in population-based studies (3, 75). Additionally, Weisbrod et al. evaluated the temporal relationship between AoS and hypertension in a mouse model of diet induced obesity, demonstrating that AoS increased within 1 month while hypertension evolved in 5 months (76). Increased AoS and blood pressure were reversed with weight loss. Understanding this temporal relationship is of particular clinical significance, as AoS can be used as a marker for patients that are high risk to develop hypertension, prompting earlier risk factor modification and potential treatment.

Metabolic Syndrome

While hypertension alone can increase AoS, metabolic syndrome is also associated with increased AoS. Metabolic syndrome is a constellation of disorders consisting of obesity, insulin resistance, hypertension, and dyslipidemia. Investigators from the Bogalusa Heart Study showed that even in asymptomatic, young (ages 24–44) subjects, baPWV rose with increasing number of components of the metabolic syndrome (77). Multiple other studies have shown that metabolic syndrome components were associated with elevated PWV (78–80). Investigators of the CRAVE study also showed that patients with both hypertension and dyslipidemia had a four-fold increase in the annual progression of cfPWV compared to controls (80). There is also evidence to suggest that resolving metabolic syndrome is associated with lower PWV compared to those with current metabolic syndrome (81).

Diabetes Mellitus

Patients with DM are at a high risk for CVD (82, 83). Aortic PWV serves as an additional tool to help risk stratify patients as increased PWV has been shown to be associated with CVD in those with DM (84). An interesting dose dependent relationship between level of glucose dysregulation and elevation of cfPWV has also been described (85).

The pathogenesis of AoS in DM is likely to be mediated by the pro-inflammatory milieu generated by metabolic dysregulation and direct damage to the vascular wall. For example, high intake of advanced end glycation products, such as carboxy-methyl-lysine, have been associated with higher PWVs among those with DM (86). Furthermore, a trial of ALT-711, a non-enzymatic breaker of these products, decreased PWV in the elderly (87). Different genotypes of advanced end glycation products and their

TABLE 2 | Association of lifestyle risk factors with aortic stiffness.

	Population studied	Exposure	Effect
Diet	Adults 20–59 years of age	Salt consumption (varied)	An increase in urinary sodium excretion by >100 mmol over a 24-h period is associated with increased systolic pressures by 3–6 mm Hg and increased diastolic pressures by 0–3 mm Hg (90)
	11 adults aged 60 ± 2 years with elevated BP (139 ± 2 over 83±2 mmHg)	Low sodium (77 ± 2 mmol/d) vs. normal sodium (144 ± 7 mmol/d)	Low sodium group with 17% reduction in aortic PWV compared to normal sodium (7 ± 0.40 vs. 8.43 ± 0.36 m/s, $p = 0.001$) (91)
Exercise	Endurance trained males age 69 ± 2.5 years	Fitness level: VO2 max at least 1 SD above age matched sedentary counterparts	26% decrease in Aortic PWV relative to peers their age (92)
	Pre-menopausal women aged 31 ± 1 years and post-menopausal women age 59±2 years	6 ± 1 hour/week of endurance exercise	No significant difference in aortic PWV or AI between pre and post-menopausal women with exercise (suggesting age related increase in AoS is halted by exercise) (93)
	Systematic review/meta-analysis of 14 RCTs of adults with pre-hypertension and hypertension	Exercise types: aerobic/endurance, dynamic resistance, isometric resistance, combined exercise	Exercise significantly reduced PWV by 0.76 m/s (CI 1.05–0.47) (94)
Smoking	Healthy adults 33 ± 6 years of age	Acute: 5 min after smoking 1 cigarette	FMD % decreased from 13.5 ± 5 to 6.9 ± 4% (95)
	Adults 15–57 years of age	Chronic: 1–75 pack years	FMD 10±3.3% (4–22%) in controls vs. 4 ± 3.9% (0–17%) in smokers; FMD is inversely related to the duration of smoking (96)
	Males 30–64 years of age	Non-smokers, former smokers, and current smokers	Men who quit smoking <1 year prior had elevated AI (β 3.94, SE 1.54, $p = 0.011$) similar to current smokers (β 4.39, SE 0.74, $p < 0.001$) compared to non-smokers; those that quit 1– <10 years prior with AI similar to non-smokers (β 1.87, SE 0.94, $p < 0.047$) (97)
E-cigarettes	Adults 30 ± 8 years of age	5 min of usage and 30 min of usage	Smoking over 5 min increased cfPWV by 0.19 m/s after 15 min; over 30 min increased cfPWV by 0.36 m/s (98)
Alcohol	Males 40–80 years of age	4–10, 11–21, and 22–58 drinks/week	Compared to those consuming 0–3 drinks per week; decreased cfPWV by 0.77 m/s (4–10 drinks), 0.57 m/s (11–21 drinks), 0.14 m/s (22–58 drinks) (99)
	Post-menopausal women 50–74 years of age	1–3, 4–9, 10–14, and 15–35 drinks/week	Compared to non-drinkers: those consuming 1–3, 4–9, 10–14, and 15–35 drinks/week had the following difference in mean cfPWV 0.044 (95% CI −0.47–0.56), −0.085 (95% CI −0.59–0.43), −0.869 (95% CI −1.44–0.29), and −0.225 (95% CI −0.98–0.53) m/s (100)

AI, augmentation index; AoS, aortic stiffness; β, beta; BP, blood pressure; cfPWV, carotid-femoral pulse wave velocity; FMD, flow-mediated dilation; PWV, pulse wave velocity; RCT, randomized control trial; SD, standard deviation; SE, standard error.

receptors have also been associated with increased blood pressure and AoS in patients with DM (88). Therefore, modulation of advanced end glycation products remains an interesting target to halt disease progression. Furthermore, increased glucose may lead to increased activity of RAAS and thus the detrimental consequences as described in the section on RAAS below (89).

LIFESTYLE RISK FACTORS

The association of lifestyle risk factors with AoS detailed below are summarized in **Table 2**.

Alcohol

Much of the evidence for the association of alcohol with AoS is data derived from self-reported alcohol consumption in cross-sectional epidemiology studies. Interestingly, evidence

suggests there may be a J shaped relationship of alcohol use to central aortic hemodynamics, with more favorable measures among those with light to moderate consumption compared with negligible and heavy drinkers. In young individuals, those who reported light alcohol consumption, 2–6 drinks per week, had lower central blood pressure than those who drank lower or greater amounts (101). Similar findings have been reported in middle aged to older adults. In men aged 40–80 years old, those who drank moderate to large amounts of 4–10 and 11–21 drinks per week had lower PWV than those who drank more or less than these groups (99). Additionally, in post-menopausal women aged 50–74 years, moderate alcohol intake was inversely related to PWV (100). Furthermore, in controlled experiments, alcohol ingestion appears to acutely decrease AoS. Even drinking 200 or 350 cc of beer leads to decreased baPWV and cfPWV compared to controls (102). There are many proposed mechanisms as to why low doses of alcohol can be beneficial to the heart such as by increasing HDL, insulin sensitivity, and decreasing oxidative stress (103). More acutely, small amounts of alcohol may decrease PWV through alcohol induced increases in nitric oxide (104). Ultimately, future prospective studies will shed light on the ideal alcohol consumption with respect to long-term outcomes and recommended exposure for vascular health.

Smoking

Smoking is a major modifiable risk factor for CVD (105). One cigarette causes acute increases in brachial and aortic blood pressure, arterial wave reflection, and AoS (106). Even passive smoking has been shown to worsen the elasticity of the aorta (107). Cigarette smoking has been shown to have a dose-response relationship to elevated PWV, which is only reversed after prolonged smoking cessation >10 years (108). There is also evidence to suggest that e-cigarettes are detrimental to AoS (98). The effect of cigarettes on AoS may be due to endothelial cell damage and subsequent impaired vasodilatory capacity (95, 96). Additional mechanisms appear to be an increase in cholesterol, increased vascular remodeling and arterial calcification, increased vascular tone, and oxidative stress/inflammation (109).

Diet and Physical Activity

There is a growing body of evidence that lifestyle habits including smoking cessation, diet modification, and exercise/weight loss can reverse AoS (110). It is well-supported that high salt intake leads to higher blood pressures (90) and that reduction in salt intake leads to lower blood pressures (111). Low salt diets similarly have been associated with lower PWV independent of blood pressure (112). Furthermore, in men, over a period of 17.8 years, higher consumption of saturated fatty acids was associated with higher cfPWV and higher consumption of poly-unsaturated fatty acids was associated with lower cfPWV (113). Greater dairy consumption, particularly in those with DM, as well as increased intake of vegetables has also been associated with lower AoS (114–116).

Physical activity leads to lower central PWV and age-related increases in PWV can be mitigated by exercise in both men and women (92, 93). The Baltimore Longitudinal Study of Aging rigorously phenotyped adults and measured VO2 max in adults aged 21–96 years of age. These investigators demonstrated that with greater age in the entire cohort, augmentation index and aortic PWV increased out of proportion to the blood pressure increase. However, these measures of AoS were lower in endurance trained male athletes (defined by a VO2 max 1 standard deviation above their age matched non-trained controls), compared with sedentary individuals (defined as less than at least 20 min of aerobic exercise three times weekly) of similar age (92). Similarly, while sedentary post-menopausal women have higher augmentation index and PWV than comparable pre-menopausal women, these measures of AoS were similar in both pre- and post-menopausal active women who were physically active (performed endurance training, actively competing in running races, with average exercise of 6 +/- 1 hour of activity per week) (93). The effect of exercise on reducing AoS

is thought to relate to exercise induced changes in vessel wall stress, a reduction in vasoconstrictors and ultimately vasodilation via increased nitric oxide activity (117, 118). These studies add to the growing body of evidence that improved lifestyle modifications could make a large impact on the development and progression of disease.

BIOMARKERS ILLUMINATING PATHOPHYSIOLOGY AND THERAPEUTICS

Given the association of AoS with adverse outcomes, serum biomarkers that correlate with AoS allow further insight into mechanisms of AoS, non-invasive detection and monitoring of AoS, and may highlight therapeutic targets. In this section, we will discuss key serum biomarkers that modulate AoS, and the associated evidence for therapies targeting these pathways.

Inflammatory Biomarkers

The presence of chronic inflammatory and infectious conditions is associated with elevated AoS. In patients with systemic lupus erythematosus, cfPWV was shown to be elevated even when traditional risk stratification categorized patients into low risk for CVD (119). Furthermore, higher aortic PWV has been seen in patients with inflammatory bowel disease and has been associated with disease duration (120). Many other inflammatory conditions have been associated with increased AoS such as rheumatoid arthritis (121, 122), psoriatic arthritis (123, 124), and Sjogren's syndrome (125, 126). The increase in AoS in those with autoimmune disorders and chronic inflammatory diseases is independent of more traditional risk factors and related to disease duration and the elevation in inflammatory markers, suggesting inflammation as a key player in this pathology (127).

Multiple inflammatory biomarkers have been associated with AoS. A prospective study that followed middle-aged Japanese men without hypertension for 9 years demonstrated that sustained elevations in serum C-reactive protein (CRP) were associated with a longitudinal increase in baPWV. Higher baPWV was in turn associated with higher blood pressures during follow-up (128). The accelerated vascular disease in this cohort at relatively low vascular risk suggests that chronic inflammation may contribute to progressive vascular stiffness and dysfunction. Though CRP is associated with several cardiovascular risk factors, models adjusting for these demonstrated a persistent linear association between CRP and AoS in the population-based Rotterdam Study (129). A potential mechanism may lie in endothelial dysfunction: in men with coronary artery disease with forearm blood flow response studied with venous occlusion plethysmography, CRP levels were associated with blunted endothelial vasodilator capacity in models including risk factors (130). Additionally, normalization of CRP levels was associated with improved blood flow response in these individuals. IL-6 is another inflammatory cytokine that has been shown to be associated with cfPWV in individuals with hypertension (131). Furthermore, there is research establishing a link between polymorphisms on IL-6 with increased cfPWV (132). These studies suggest that inflammation is associated with AoS but more studies are needed to fully elucidate the mechanistic relationships.

The relationship between inflammatory states and CVD has been further elucidated by studies that have examined the effect of treatment of inflammatory diseases. Patients with rheumatoid arthritis treated with anti-tumor necrosis factor-a agents have shown significant declines in cfPWV after treatment (133). Furthermore, statins have been shown to decrease AoS in patients with inflammatory joint diseases, suggesting that controlling inflammation and possibly lowering lipids is beneficial in this population (134).

Klotho and Sirtuin-1

Klotho is predominantly expressed in the kidney and has been described as an anti-aging gene (135). When mice are deficient in Klotho, they have decreased lifespan and calcifications of multiple organs. Haplodeficiency of Klotho in mice leads to increased PWV and hypertension (136, 137). The association of Klotho levels with AoS has also been demonstrated in patients with chronic kidney disease (CKD) (138). Klotho appears to directly regulate SIRT1, a gene encoding a NAD+ dependent-deacetylase with anti-inflammatory and anti-oxidant effects and importance in endothelial cell function (139, 140). Klotho

---

TABLE 3 | Association of serum biomarkers with aortic stiffness.

Biomarker	Clinical relevance	Association with aortic stiffness
Key biomarkers with independent association with AoS		
Inflammatory biomarkers	• The presence of conditions like SLE (155), IBD (156), psoriasis (157), and HIV (158) are linked with high higher risk of CVD	• Elevated PWV in IBD patients (120) • Elevated carotid AI and PWV in SLE patients (159)
CRP	• Associated with insulin resistance (160), carotid intima-media thickness and markers of atherosclerosis (161)	• Sustained elevation in serum CRP correlated with increased baPWV and BP in middle aged Japanese men (128) • In Chinese general population baseline hs-CRP associated with baPWV (162)
Klotho	• Klotho levels lower in those with renovascular hypertension and essential hypertension compared to healthy controls (163) • Klotho levels lower in those with significant coronary artery disease (164)	• Haplodeficiency in Klotho in mice led to increased AoS (136, 137)
Aldosterone	• Increases insulin resistance, oxidative stress, inflammation (89) • Promotes vascular calcification (165)	• Associated with increased PWV (143) • Fibronectin accumulation (166)
Other biomarkers associated with AoS		
Adipocyte-Fatty-Acid-Binding protein (A-FABP)	• Elevated levels have been associated with endothelial dysfunction in patients with type 2 diabetes (167) • Elevated levels associated with diastolic dysfunction (168) and cardiovascular death (169)	• In patients with hypertension and metabolic syndrome, increased levels of A-FABP associated with increased cfPWV (170) • A-FABP levels positively correlated with cfPWV in patients with type 2 diabetes (171)
Leptin	• Leptin levels predicted ischemic heart disease in patients with type 2 diabetes (172) • Patients with coronary artery disease have higher levels of serum leptin (173)	• Higher leptin levels associated with increased cfPWV in patients with kidney transplants (174) and in geriatric patients on dialysis (175) • Meta-analysis demonstrated leptin is positively associated with cfPWV (176)
Natriuretic peptides	• Released in response to ventricular hypertrophy, inflammation, and fibrosis (177) • Predictor for heart failure or death in patients with an acute MI (178, 179)	• AoS is associated with NT-proBNP level and MR-proANP months after MI (180, 181)
Parathyroid hormone	• Parathyroid hormone is associated with atherosclerosis (182)	• Patients with mild hyperparathyroidism had increased cfPWV which then decreased after a thyroidectomy (183) • cfPWV increased independently with parathyroid hormone in Chinese patients with untreated hypertension (184)
Resistin	• Increased resistin associated with increased risk of heart failure, coronary heart disease, CVD (185)	• High levels of resistin associated with increased cfPWV in sample with high prevalence of untreated hypertension/obesity (186) • Serum resistin is an independent predictor of cfPWV in patients with coronary artery disease (187)
Uric Acid	• High levels of uric acid associated with acute myocardial infarction (188) cardiovascular events (189, 190) stroke (190)	• Association between higher uric acid and cfPWV in men after adjustment for confounders (191) • Overall positive association between uric acid and cfPWV at adjusted analysis in both males and females (192) • Serum uric acid is independently associated with cfPWV in post-menopausal women (193) • Significant association between uric acid cf PWV and carotid radial PWV in young Caucasian population (194)

AI, augmentation index; AoS, aortic stiffness; ba-PWV, brachial-ankle pulse wave velocity; CVD, cardiovascular disease; HIV, human immunodeficiency virus; hs-CRP, high sensitivity CRP; IBD, Inflammatory Bowel Disease; MI, myocardial infarction; PWV, pulse wave velocity; SLE, Systemic lupus erythematosus.

haplodeficiency downregulates SIRT1 in arterial endothelial and smooth muscle cells, with associated increased arterial wall collagen deposition and elastin fragmentation, both of which explain the association with AoS (137). Zhou et al. demonstrated that CYP11B2, a rate-limiting enzyme in aldosterone synthesis, is up-regulated in Klotho deficiency, and that treatment with eplerenone reversed increased AoS (141). Thus, another mechanism by which Klotho deficiency may mediate increased AoS is through the aldosterone pathway.

The interaction between Klotho and SIRT1 has illuminated a number of possible targets for therapies that modulate pro-oxidant and pro-inflammatory pathways. Further, improved calcium and phosphate homeostasis may be of increased importance in CKD patients where impaired calcium homeostasis and a pro-inflammatory milieu may accelerate vascular dysfunction. Thus, understanding these mechanisms provides opportunities for possible therapeutic interventions.

RAAS

The role of RAAS in the progression of AoS is supported by observational studies, clinical studies relating to modulation with therapeutics, biochemical studies demonstrating involvement in vascular remodeling, and mapping of related gene loci.

RAAS-associated AoS is proposed to be due to aldosterone and angiotensin II increased inflammation as well as vasoconstriction from activation of angiotensin I receptors and mineralocorticoid receptors (142). Aldosterone has been shown to be involved in many pathologic processes such as increased insulin resistance, increased oxidative stress, and increased inflammation (89). In multivariable adjusted models, serum aldosterone is linearly associated with PWV in hypertensive patients (143). The importance of RAAS is further highlighted by multiple studies that demonstrate a positive association between cfPWV and polymorphisms in the angiotensin II type 1 receptor (144, 145), angiotensin converting enzyme gene (146, 147) as well as in the aldosterone gene (148). Polymorphisms in RAAS may thus contribute to the highly heritable traits of AoS and blood pressure (149). Additional future work may determine the appropriate application of genetic testing to guide detection and management of AoS.

With respect to therapies, inhibiting aldosterone with spironolactone has been shown to decrease collagen density and thus AoS (150). London et al. demonstrated that central systolic blood pressure was decreased to a greater extent with perindopril/indapamide treatment compared to treatment with atenolol, implying a distinct role of RAAS modulation in central hemodynamics (151). This data on the role of RAAS inhibition in AoS may be useful to consider for physicians choosing an anti-hypertensive medication. When compared with atenolol, eplerenone has been shown to decrease AoS, decrease the collagen to elastin ratio, and decrease concentrations of inflammatory markers including MCP-1, basic fibroblast growth factor, and interleukin-10 (152). Furthermore, when comparing atenolol, nebivolol, aliskiren, and quinapril, the RAAS modulating agents demonstrated continued reductions of cfPWV, possibly implicating arterial remodeling rather than modulation of hemodynamics alone

(153). Lastly, non-pharmacologic augmentation to the RAAS system is also important to consider. Decreased salt intake has been shown to decrease AoS independent of blood pressure reductions that may be mediated through RAAS modulation (154).

In addition to the above, other general biomarkers associated with AoS are presented in **Table 3**.

GENERALIZABILITY AND FUTURE DIRECTIONS

Despite data illuminating pathways important in AoS pathophysiology and the promising data for their modulation, there has been a paucity of data in this field. Controlled trials thus far have been of relatively small size with short duration, with possibly insufficient follow up time to adequately assess for aortic remodeling and change in AoS (195). However, encouraging data on the prognostic impact of PWV continues to emerge. In the past 2 years, a *post-hoc* analysis of 8,450 patients in the Systolic Blood Pressure Intervention Trial (SPRINT) demonstrated that reductions in PWV after 1 year of anti-hypertensive therapy were associated with 42% lower risk of death compared to individuals who did not have reductions in PWV, independent of Framingham Risk Score and blood pressure (196). Additionally, an innovative experiment performed on mice aortas *ex vivo* used a synthetic peptide targeted to a cytoskeletal protein known to be associated with AoS in human genome wide association studies (197). This study illustrated the proof of concept that such decoy peptides decreased cfPWV, illustrating that approaches targeted to AoS rather than blood pressure *per se*, may be able to be applied in the future. Ultimately, larger therapeutic trials that target AoS and demonstrate improved outcomes are needed to establish widespread clinical utility of AoS assessment and treatment.

CONCLUSION

AoS is a precursor to hypertension and an accepted risk factor for CVD independent of blood pressure. Despite its demonstrated prognostic value, thus far broad clinical applicability has been limited by measurement variation in multiple methodologies illustrated, lack of age and blood pressure specific reference values applicable to all populations, and effective therapeutics targeting AoS. AoS may be addressed indirectly through treating several lifestyle risk factors and associated comorbidities. Continued research will help to add to the illustrated biologic pathways of AoS. In the future, novel approaches and applications of existing drugs to specifically target pathways involved in modulating AoS may provide further support to its broader assessment and treatment to improve cardiovascular outcomes.

AUTHOR CONTRIBUTIONS

RA: drafted manuscript, manuscript editing, and figure copyright permissions. RM: drafted manuscript. CT: manuscript concept and editing. All authors contributed to the article and approved the submitted version.

ACKNOWLEDGMENTS

We would like to thank Matthew Borinshteyn for his assistance in drafting the tables.

REFERENCES

1. O'Rourke MF, Mancia G. Arterial stiffness. *J Hypertens.* (1999) 17:1065–72. doi: 10.1097/00004872-199917010-00001
2. Laurent S, Cockcroft J, Van Bortel L, Boutouyrie P, Giannattasio C, Hayoz D, et al. Expert consensus document on arterial stiffness: methodological issues and clinical applications. *Eur Heart J.* (2006) 27:2588–605. doi: 10.1093/eurheartj/ehl254
3. Kaess BM, Rong J, Larson MG, Hamburg NM, Vita JA, Levy D, et al. Aortic stiffness, blood pressure progression, incident hypertension. *JAMA.* (2012) 308:875–81. doi: 10.1001/2012.jama.10503
4. van Popele NM, Grobbee DE, Bots ML, Asmar R, Topouchian J, Reneman RS, et al. Association between arterial stiffness and atherosclerosis: the rotterdam study. *Stroke.* (2001) 32:454–60. doi: 10.1161/01.STR.32.2.454
5. Baumann M, Wassertheurer S, Suttmann Y, Burkhardt K, Heemann U. Aortic pulse wave velocity predicts mortality in chronic kidney disease stages 2-4. *J Hypertens.* (2014) 32:899–903. doi: 10.1097/HJH.0000000000000113
6. Feistritzer HJ, Klug G, Reinstadler SJ, Reindl M, Niess L, Nalbach T, et al. prognostic value of aortic stiffness in patients after st-elevation myocardial infarction. *J Am Heart Assoc.* (2017) 6:e005590. doi: 10.1161/JAHA.117.005590
7. Laurent S, Boutouyrie P, Asmar R, Gautier I, Laloux B, Guize L, et al. Aortic stiffness is an independent predictor of all-cause and cardiovascular mortality in hypertensive patients. *Hypertension.* (2001) 37:1236–41. doi: 10.1161/01.HYP.37.5.1236
8. Mitchell GF, Hwang SJ, Vasan RS, Larson MG, Pencina MJ, Hamburg NM, et al. Arterial stiffness and cardiovascular events: the framingham heart study. *Circulation.* (2010) 121:505–11. doi: 10.1161/CIRCULATIONAHA.109.886655
9. Mattace-Raso FU, van der Cammen TJ, Hofman A, van Popele NM, Bos ML, Schalekamp MA, et al. Arterial stiffness and risk of coronary heart disease and stroke: the rotterdam study. *Circulation.* (2006) 113:657–63. doi: 10.1161/CIRCULATIONAHA.105.555235
10. Sutton-Tyrrell K, Najjar SS, Boudreau RM, Venkitachalam L, Kupelian V, Simonsick EM, et al. Elevated aortic pulse wave velocity, a marker of arterial stiffness, predicts cardiovascular events in well-functioning older adults. *Circulation.* (2005) 111:3384–90. doi: 10.1161/CIRCULATIONAHA.104.483628
11. Willum-Hansen T, Staessen JA, Torp-Pedersen C, Rasmussen S, Thijs L, Ibsen H, et al. Prognostic value of aortic pulse wave velocity as index of arterial stiffness in the general population. *Circulation.* (2006) 113:664–70. doi: 10.1161/CIRCULATIONAHA.105.579342
12. Sarafidis PA, Loutradis C, Karpetas A, Tzanis G, Piperidou A, Koutroumpas G, et al. Ambulatory pulse wave velocity is a stronger predictor of cardiovascular events and all-cause mortality than office and ambulatory blood pressure in hemodialysis patients. *Hypertension.* (2017) 70:148–57. doi: 10.1161/HYPERTENSIONAHA.117.09023
13. Vlachopoulos C, Aznaouridis K, Stefanadis C. Prediction of cardiovascular events and all-cause mortality with arterial stiffness: a systematic review and meta-analysis. *J Am Coll Cardiol.* (2010) 55:1318–27. doi: 10.1016/j.jacc.2009.10.061
14. Ben-Shlomo Y, Spears M, Boustred C, May M, Anderson SG, Benjamin EJ, et al. Aortic pulse wave velocity improves cardiovascular event prediction: an individual participant meta-analysis of prospective observational data from 17,635 subjects. *J Am Coll Cardiol.* (2014) 63:636–46. doi: 10.1016/j.jacc.2013.09.063
15. Townsend RR, Wilkinson IB, Schiffrin EL, Avolio AP, Chirinos JA, Cockcroft JR, et al. Recommendations for improving and standardizing vascular research on arterial stiffness: a scientific statement from the American heart association. *Hypertension.* (2015) 66:698–722. doi: 10.1161/HYP.0000000000000033
16. Calabia J, Torguet P, Garcia M, Garcia I, Martin N, Guasch B, et al. Doppler ultrasound in the measurement of pulse wave velocity: agreement with the complior method. *Cardiovasc Ultrasound.* (2011) 9:13. doi: 10.1186/1476-7120-9-13
17. Jiang B, Liu B, McNeill KL, Chowienczyk PJ. Measurement of pulse wave velocity using pulse wave doppler ultrasound: comparison with arterial tonometry. *Ultrasound Med Biol.* (2008) 34:509–12. doi: 10.1016/j.ultrasmedbio.2007.09.008
18. Hickson SS, Butlin M, Broad J, Avolio AP, Wilkinson IB, McEniery CM. Validity and repeatability of the vicorder apparatus: a comparison with the SphygmoCor device. *Hypertens Res.* (2009) 32:1079–85. doi: 10.1038/hr.2009.154
19. Laurent S, Marais L, Boutouyrie P. The noninvasive assessment of vascular AGING. *Can J Cardiol.* (2016) 32:669–79. doi: 10.1016/j.cjca.2016.01.039
20. Wilkinson IB, Mäki-Petäjä KM, Mitchell GF. Uses of arterial stiffness in clinical practice. *Arterioscler Thromb Vasc Biol.* (2020) 40:1063–7. doi: 10.1161/ATVBAHA.120.313130
21. Jeroncic A, Gunjaca G, Mrsic DB, Mudnic I, Brizic I, Polasek O, et al. Normative equations for central augmentation index: assessment of inter-population applicability and how it could be improved. *Sci Rep.* (2016) 6:27016. doi: 10.1038/srep27016
22. Kim EJ, Park CG, Park JS, Suh SY, Choi CU, Kim JW, et al. Relationship between blood pressure parameters and pulse wave velocity in normotensive and hypertensive subjects: invasive study. *J Hum Hypertens.* (2007) 21:141–8. doi: 10.1038/sj.jhh.1002120
23. Van Bortel LM, Laurent S, Boutouyrie P, Chowienczyk P, Cruickshank JK, De Backer T, et al. Expert consensus document on the measurement of aortic stiffness in daily practice using carotid-femoral pulse wave velocity. *J Hypertens.* (2012) 30:445–8. doi: 10.1097/HJH.0b013e32834fa8b0
24. Cavalcante JL, Lima JA, Redheuil A, Al-Mallah MH. Aortic stiffness: current understanding and future directions. *J Am Coll Cardiol.* (2011) 57:1511–22. doi: 10.1016/j.jacc.2010.12.017
25. Hashimoto J, Imai Y, O'Rourke MF. Indices of pulse wave analysis are better predictors of left ventricular mass reduction than cuff pressure. *Am J Hypertens.* (2007) 20:378–84. doi: 10.1016/j.amjhyper.2006.09.019
26. Weber T, Auer J, O'Rourke M F, Kvas E, Lassnig E, Lamm G, et al. Increased arterial wave reflections predict severe cardiovascular events in patients undergoing percutaneous coronary interventions. *Eur Heart J.* (2005) 26:2657–63. doi: 10.1093/eurheartj/ehi504
27. Chun KH, Lee CJ, Oh J, Won C, Lee T, Park S, et al. Increased aortic augmentation index is associated with reduced exercise capacity after heart transplantation. *J Hypertens.* (2020) 38:1777–85. doi: 10.1097/HJH.0000000000002455
28. Sakurai M, Yamakado T, Kurachi H, Kato T, Kuroda K, Ishisu R, et al. The relationship between aortic augmentation index and pulse wave velocity: an invasive study. *J Hypertens.* (2007) 25:391–7. doi: 10.1097/HJH.0b013e3280115b7c
29. Yasmin, Brown MJ. Similarities and differences between augmentation index and pulse wave velocity in the assessment of arterial stiffness. *QJM.* (1999) 92:595–600. doi: 10.1093/qjmed/92.10.595
30. Mancia G, De Backer G, Dominiczak A, Cifkova R, Fagard R, Germano G, et al. 2007 guidelines for the management of arterial hypertension: the task force for the management of arterial hypertension of the European society of hypertension (ESH) and of the European society of cardiology (ESC). *J Hypertens.* (2007) 25:1105–87. doi: 10.1097/HJH.0b013e3281fc975a

31. Reference Values for Arterial Stiffness Collaboration. Determinants of pulse wave velocity in healthy people and in the presence of cardiovascular risk factors: 'establishing normal and reference values'. *Eur Heart J.* (2010) 31:2338–50. doi: 10.1093/eurheartj/ehq165

32. Rajzer MW, Wojciechowska W, Klocek M, Palka I, Brzozowska-Kiszka M, Kawecka-Jaszcz K. Comparison of aortic pulse wave velocity measured by three techniques: complior, SphygmoCor and arteriograph. *J Hypertens.* (2008) 26:2001–7. doi: 10.1097/HJH.0b013e32830a4a25

33. Khoshdel AR, Thakkinstian A, Carney SL, Attia J. Estimation of an age-specific reference interval for pulse wave velocity: a meta-analysis. *J Hypertens.* (2006) 24:1231–7. doi: 10.1097/01.hjh.0000234098.85497.31

34. Mitchell GF, Parise H, Benjamin EJ, Larson MG, Keyes MJ, Vita JA, et al. Changes in arterial stiffness and wave reflection with advancing age in healthy men and women: the framingham heart study. *Hypertension.* (2004) 43:1239–45. doi: 10.1161/01.HYP.0000128420.01881.aa

35. Tsao CW, Washington F, Musani SK, Cooper LL, Tripathi A, Hamburg NM, et al. Clinical correlates of aortic stiffness and wave amplitude in black men and women in the community. *J Am Heart Assoc.* (2018) 7:e008431. doi: 10.1161/JAHA.117.008431

36. Franklin SS, Gustin Wt, Wong ND, Larson MG, Weber MA, Kannel WB, et al. Hemodynamic patterns of age-related changes in blood pressure. The framingham heart study. *Circulation.* (1997) 96:308–15. doi: 10.1161/01.CIR.96.1.308

37. Saba PS, Roman MJ, Pini R, Spitzer M, Ganau A, Devereux RB. Relation of arterial pressure waveform to left ventricular and carotid anatomy in normotensive subjects. *J Am Coll Cardiol.* (1993) 22:1873–80. doi: 10.1016/0735-1097(93)90772-S

38. Cruickshank JM. The role of coronary perfusion pressure. *Euro Heart J.* (1992) 13:39–43. doi: 10.1093/eurheartj/13.suppl_D.39

39. Madhuri V, Chandra S, Jabbar A. Age associated increase in intima media thickness in adults. *Indian J Physiol Pharmacol.* (2010) 54:371–5.

40. Lakatta EG, Levy D. Arterial and cardiac aging: major shareholders in cardiovascular disease enterprises. *Circulation.* (2003) 107:139–46. doi: 10.1161/01.CIR.0000048892.83521.58

41. Tsao CW, Pencina KM, Massaro JM, Benjamin EJ, Levy D, Vasan RS, et al. Cross-sectional relations of arterial stiffness, pressure pulsatility, wave reflection, arterial calcification. *Arterioscler Thromb Vasc Biol.* (2014) 34:2495–500. doi: 10.1161/ATVBAHA.114.303916

42. Loboz-Rudnicka M, Jaroch J, Bociaga Z, Kruszynska E, Ciecierzynska B, Dziuba M, et al. Relationship between vascular age and classic cardiovascular risk factors and arterial stiffness. *Cardiol J.* (2013) 20:394–401. doi: 10.5603/CJ.2013.0098

43. Rossi P, Francès Y, Kingwell BA, Ahimastos AA. Gender differences in artery wall biomechanical properties throughout life. *J Hypertens.* (2011) 29:1023–33. doi: 10.1097/HJH.0b013e328344da5e

44. Tomiyama H, Yamashina A, Arai T, Hirose K, Koji Y, Chikamori T, et al. Influences of age and gender on results of noninvasive brachial-ankle pulse wave velocity measurement–a survey of 12517 subjects. *Atherosclerosis.* (2003) 166:303–9. doi: 10.1016/S0021-9150(02)00332-5

45. Protogerou AD, Blacher J, Aslangul E, Le Jeunne C, Lekakis J, Mavrikakis M, et al. Gender influence on metabolic syndrome's effects on arterial stiffness and pressure wave reflections in treated hypertensive subjects. *Atherosclerosis.* (2007) 193:151–8. doi: 10.1016/j.atherosclerosis.2006.05.046

46. Yaron M, Greenman Y, Rosenfeld JB, Izkhakov E, Limor R, Osher E, et al. Effect of testosterone replacement therapy on arterial stiffness in older hypogonadal men. *Eur J Endocrinol.* (2009) 160:839–46. doi: 10.1530/EJE-09-0052

47. Yue P, Chatterjee K, Beale C, Poole-Wilson PA, Collins P. Testosterone relaxes rabbit coronary arteries and aorta. *Circulation.* (1995) 91:1154–60. doi: 10.1161/01.CIR.91.4.1154

48. Pfeilschifter J, Köditz R, Pfohl M, Schatz H. Changes in proinflammatory cytokine activity after menopause. *Endocr Rev.* (2002) 23:90–119. doi: 10.1210/edrv.23.1.0456

49. Natoli AK, Medley TL, Ahimastos AA, Drew BG, Thearle DJ, Dilley RJ, et al. Sex steroids modulate human aortic smooth muscle cell matrix protein deposition and matrix metalloproteinase expression. *Hypertension.* (2005) 46:1129–34. doi: 10.1161/01.HYP.0000187016.06549.96

50. Muntner P, Lewis CE, Diaz KM, Carson AP, Kim Y, Calhoun D, et al. Racial differences in abnormal ambulatory blood pressure monitoring measures: results from the coronary artery risk development in young adults (CARDIA) study. *Am J Hypertens.* (2015) 28:640–8. doi: 10.1093/ajh/hpu193

51. Heffernan KS, Jae SY, Wilund KR, Woods JA, Fernhall B. Racial differences in central blood pressure and vascular function in young men. *Am J Physiol Heart Circul Physiol.* (2008) 295:H2380–7. doi: 10.1152/ajpheart.00902.2008

52. Hozawa A, Folsom AR, Sharrett AR, Chambless LE. Absolute and attributable risks of cardiovascular disease incidence in relation to optimal and borderline risk factors: comparison of African American with white subjects–atherosclerosis risk in communities study. *Arch Intern Med.* (2007) 167:573–9. doi: 10.1001/archinte.167.6.573

53. Din-Dzietham R, Couper D, Evans G, Arnett DK, Jones DW. Arterial stiffness is greater in African Americans than in whites: evidence from the forsyth county, north carolina, ARIC cohort. *Am J Hypertens.* (2004) 17:304–13. doi: 10.1016/j.amjhyper.2003.12.004

54. Mokwatsi GG, Schutte AE, Kruger R. Ethnic differences regarding arterial stiffness of 6-8-year-old black and white boys. *J Hypertens.* (2017) 35:960–7. doi: 10.1097/HJH.0000000000001267

55. Thurston RC, Matthews KA. Racial and socioeconomic disparities in arterial stiffness and intima media thickness among adolescents. *Soc Sci Med.* (2009) 68:807–13. doi: 10.1016/j.socscimed.2008.12.029

56. Lefferts WK, Augustine JA, Spartano NL, Atallah-Yunes NH, Heffernan KS, Gump BB. Racial differences in aortic stiffness in children. *J Pediatr.* (2017) 180:62–7. doi: 10.1016/j.jpeds.2016.09.071

57. Malayeri AA, Natori S, Bahrami H, Bertoni AG, Kronmal R, Lima JA, et al. Relation of aortic wall thickness and distensibility to cardiovascular risk factors [from the multi-ethnic study of atherosclerosis (MESA)]. *Am J Cardiol.* (2008) 102:491–6. doi: 10.1016/j.amjcard.2008.04.010

58. Goel A, Maroules CD, Mitchell GF, Peshock R, Ayers C, McColl R, et al. Ethnic difference in proximal aortic stiffness: an observation from the dallas heart study. *JACC Cardiovasc Imaging.* (2017) 10:54–61. doi: 10.1016/j.jcmg.2016.07.012

59. Baldo MP, Cunha RS, Ribeiro ALP, Lotufo PA, Chor D, Barreto SM, et al. Racial differences in arterial stiffness are mainly determined by blood pressure levels: results from the ELSA-Brasil study. *J Am Heart Assoc.* (2017) 6:e005477. doi: 10.1161/JAHA.117.005477

60. Birru MS, Matthews KA, Thurston RC, Brooks MM, Ibrahim S, Barinas-Mitchell E, et al. African-American ethnicity and cardiovascular risk factors are related to aortic pulse-wave velocity progression. *Am J Hypertens.* (2011) 24:809–15. doi: 10.1038/ajh.2011.57

61. Dong Y, Pollock N, Stallmann-Jorgensen IS, Gutin B, Lan L, Chen TC, et al. Low 25-hydroxyvitamin D levels in adolescents: race, season, adiposity, physical activity, and fitness. *Pediatrics.* (2010) 125:1104–11. doi: 10.1542/peds.2009-2055

62. Raed A, Bhagatwala J, Zhu H, Pollock NK, Parikh SJ, Huang Y, et al. Dose responses of vitamin D3 supplementation on arterial stiffness in overweight African Americans with vitamin D deficiency: a placebo controlled randomized trial. *PLoS ONE.* (2017) 12:e0188424. doi: 10.1371/journal.pone.0188424

63. Kalinowski L, Dobrucki IT, Malinski T. Race-specific differences in endothelial function: predisposition of African Americans to vascular diseases. *Circulation.* (2004) 109:2511–7. doi: 10.1161/01.CIR.0000129087.81352.7A

64. Campia U, Choucair WK, Bryant MB, Waclawiw MA, Cardillo C, Panza JA. Reduced endothelium-dependent and -independent dilation of conductance arteries in African Americans. *J Am Coll Cardiol.* (2002) 40:754–60. doi: 10.1016/S0735-1097(02)02015-6

65. Morris AA, Patel RS, Binongo JN, Poole J, Al Mheid I, Ahmed Y, et al. Racial differences in arterial stiffness and microcirculatory function between black and white Americans. *J Am Heart Assoc.* (2013) 2:e002154. doi: 10.1161/JAHA.112.002154

66. McEniery CM, Spratt M, Munnery M, Yarnell J, Lowe GD, Rumley A, et al. An analysis of prospective risk factors for aortic stiffness in men: 20-year follow-up from the caerphilly prospective study. *Hypertension.* (2010) 56:36–43. doi: 10.1161/HYPERTENSIONAHA.110.150896

67. Zieman SJ, Melenovsky V, Kass DA. Mechanisms, pathophysiology, and therapy of arterial stiffness. *Arterioscler Thromb Vasc Biol.* (2005) 25:932–43. doi: 10.1161/01.ATV.0000160548.78317.29

68. Tedla YG, Yano Y, Carnethon M, Greenland P. Association between long-term blood pressure variability and 10-year progression in arterial stiffness: the multiethnic study of atherosclerosis. *Hypertension.* (2017) 69:118–27. doi: 10.1161/HYPERTENSIONAHA.116.08427

69. Aoki Y, Kai H, Kajimoto H, Kudo H, Takayama N, Yasuoka S, et al. Large blood pressure variability aggravates arteriolosclerosis and cortical sclerotic changes in the kidney in hypertensive rats. *Circ J.* (2014) 78:2284–91. doi: 10.1253/circj.CJ-14-0027

70. Chappell DC, Varner SE, Nerem RM, Medford RM, Alexander RW. Oscillatory shear stress stimulates adhesion molecule expression in cultured human endothelium. *Circ Res.* (1998) 82:532–9. doi: 10.1161/01.RES.82.5.532

71. Shimbo D, Shea S, McClelland RL, Viera AJ, Mann D, Newman J, et al. Associations of aortic distensibility and arterial elasticity with long-term visit-to-visit blood pressure variability: the multi-ethnic study of atherosclerosis (MESA). *Am J Hypertens.* (2013) 26:896–902. doi: 10.1093/ajh/hpt040

72. Dernellis J, Panaretou M. Aortic stiffness is an independent predictor of progression to hypertension in nonhypertensive subjects. *Hypertension.* (2005) 45:426–31. doi: 10.1161/01.HYP.0000157818.58878.93

73. Franklin SS. Arterial stiffness and hypertension: a two-way street? *Hypertension.* (2005) 45:349–51. doi: 10.1161/01.HYP.0000157819.31611.87

74. Mitchell GF. Arterial stiffness and hypertension: chicken or egg? *Hypertension.* (2014) 64:210–4. doi: 10.1161/HYPERTENSIONAHA.114.03449

75. Najjar SS, Scuteri A, Shetty V, Wright JG, Muller DC, Fleg JL, et al. Pulse wave velocity is an independent predictor of the longitudinal increase in systolic blood pressure and of incident hypertension in the Baltimore longitudinal study of aging. *J Am Coll Cardiol.* (2008) 51:1377–83. doi: 10.1016/j.jacc.2007.10.065

76. Weisbrod RM, Shiang T, Al Sayah L, Fry JL, Bajpai S, Reinhart-King CA, et al. Arterial stiffening precedes systolic hypertension in diet-induced obesity. *Hypertension.* (2013) 62:1105–10. doi: 10.1161/HYPERTENSIONAHA.113.01744

77. Li S, Chen W, Srinivasan SR, Berenson GS. Influence of metabolic syndrome on arterial stiffness and its age-related change in young adults: the bogalusa heart study. *Atherosclerosis.* (2005) 180:349–54. doi: 10.1016/j.atherosclerosis.2004.12.016

78. Gomez-Sanchez L, Garcia-Ortiz L, Patino-Alonso MC, Recio-Rodriguez JI, Fernando R, Marti R, et al. Association of metabolic syndrome and its components with arterial stiffness in caucasian subjects of the MARK study: a cross-sectional trial. *Cardiovasc Diabetol.* (2016) 15:148. doi: 10.1186/s12933-016-0465-7

79. Safar ME, Thomas F, Blacher J, Nzietchueng R, Bureau JM, Pannier B, et al. Metabolic syndrome and age-related progression of aortic stiffness. *J Am Coll Cardiol.* (2006) 47:72–5. doi: 10.1016/j.jacc.2005.08.052

80. Terentes-Printzios D, Vlachopoulos C, Xaplanteris P, Ioakeimidis N, Aznaouridis K, Baou K, et al. Cardiovascular risk factors accelerate progression of vascular aging in the general population: results from the CRAVE Study (cardiovascular risk factors affecting vascular age). *Hypertension.* (2017) 70:1057–64. doi: 10.1161/HYPERTENSIONAHA.117.09633

81. Tomiyama H, Hirayama Y, Hashimoto H, Yambe M, Yamada J, Koji Y, et al. The effects of changes in the metabolic syndrome detection status on arterial stiffening: a prospective study. *Hypertens Res.* (2006) 29:673–8. doi: 10.1291/hypres.29.673

82. Haffner SM, Lehto S, Ronnemaa T, Pyorala K, Laakso M. Mortality from coronary heart disease in subjects with type 2 diabetes and in nondiabetic subjects with and without prior myocardial infarction. *N Engl J Med.* (1998) 339:229–34. doi: 10.1056/NEJM199807233390404

83. Kannel WB, McGee DL. Diabetes and glucose tolerance as risk factors for cardiovascular disease: the framingham study. *Diabetes Care.* (1979) 2:120–6. doi: 10.2337/diacare.2.2.120

84. Mansour AS, Yannoutsos A, Majahalme N, Agnoletti D, Safar ME, Ouerdane S, et al. Aortic stiffness and cardiovascular risk in type 2 diabetes. *J Hypertens.* (2013) 31:1584–92. doi: 10.1097/HJH.0b013e32836 13074

85. Pietri P, Vlachopoulos C, Vyssoulis G, Ioakeimidis N, Stefanadis C. Macro- and microvascular alterations in patients with metabolic syndrome: sugar makes the difference. *Hypertens Res.* (2014) 37:452–6. doi: 10.1038/hr.2013.148

86. Di Pino A, Currenti W, Urbano F, Scicali R, Piro S, Purrello F, et al. High intake of dietary advanced glycation end-products is associated with increased arterial stiffness and inflammation in subjects with type 2 diabetes. *Nutr Metab Cardiovasc Dis.* (2017) 27:978–84. doi: 10.1016/j.numecd.2017.06.014

87. Kass DA, Shapiro EP, Kawaguchi M, Capriotti AR, Scuteri A, deGroof RC, et al. Improved arterial compliance by a novel advanced glycation end-product crosslink breaker. *Circulation.* (2001) 104:1464–70. doi: 10.1161/hc3801.097806

88. Engelen L, Ferreira I, Gaens KH, Henry RM, Dekker JM, Nijpels G, et al. The association between the−374T/A polymorphism of the receptor for advanced glycation endproducts gene and blood pressure and arterial stiffness is modified by glucose metabolism status: the hoorn and CoDAM studies. *J Hypertens.* (2010) 28:285–93. doi: 10.1097/HJH.0b013e3283 330931

89. Lastra-Lastra G, Sowers JR, Restrepo-Erazo K, Manrique-Acevedo C, Lastra-Gonzalez G. Role of aldosterone and angiotensin II in insulin resistance: an update. *Clin Endocrinol.* (2009) 71:1–6. doi: 10.1111/j.1365-2265.2008.03498.x

90. Elliott P, Stamler J, Nichols R, Dyer AR, Stamler R, Kesteloot H, et al. Intersalt revisited: further analyses of 24 hour sodium excretion and blood pressure within and across populations. Intersalt cooperative research group. *BMJ.* (1996) 312:1249–53. doi: 10.1136/bmj.312.7041.1249

91. Jablonski KL, Fedorova OV, Racine ML, Geolfos CJ, Gates PE, Chonchol M, et al. Dietary sodium restriction and association with urinary marinobufagenin, blood pressure, aortic stiffness. *Clin J Am Soc Nephrol.* (2013) 8:1952–9. doi: 10.2215/CJN.00900113

92. Vaitkevicius PV, Fleg JL, Engel JH, O'Connor FC, Wright JG, Lakatta LE, et al. Effects of age and aerobic capacity on arterial stiffness in healthy adults. *Circulation.* (1993) 88:1456–62. doi: 10.1161/01.CIR.88.4.1456

93. Tanaka H, DeSouza CA, Seals DR. Absence of age-related increase in central arterial stiffness in physically active women. *Arterioscler Thromb Vasc Biol.* (1998) 18:127–32. doi: 10.1161/01.ATV.18.1.127

94. Lopes S, Afreixo V, Teixeira M, Garcia C, Leitão C, Gouveia M, et al. Exercise training reduces arterial stiffness in adults with hypertension: a systematic review and meta-analysis. *J Hypertens.* (2021) 39:214–22. doi: 10.1097/HJH.0000000000002619

95. Lekakis J, Papamichael C, Vemmos C, Nanas J, Kontoyannis D, Stamatelopoulos S, et al. Effect of acute cigarette smoking on endothelium-dependent brachial artery dilatation in healthy individuals. *Am J Cardiol.* (1997) 79:529–31. doi: 10.1016/S0002-9149(96)00805-3

96. Celermajer DS, Sorensen KE, Georgakopoulos D, Bull C, Thomas O, Robinson J, et al. Cigarette smoking is associated with dose-related and potentially reversible impairment of endothelium-dependent dilation in healthy young adults. *Circulation.* (1993) 88:2149–55. doi: 10.1161/01.CIR.88.5.2149

97. Lee GB, Shim JS, Kim HC. Dose-response association between smoking cessation and arterial stiffness: the cardiovascular and metabolic diseases etiology research center (CMERC) cohort. *Korean Circ J.* (2020) 50:361–9. doi: 10.4070/kcj.2019.0270

98. Vlachopoulos C, Ioakeimidis N, Abdelrasoul M, Terentes-Printzios D, Georgakopoulos C, Pietri P, et al. Electronic cigarette smoking increases aortic stiffness and blood pressure in young smokers. *J Am Coll Cardiol.* (2016) 67:2802–3. doi: 10.1016/j.jacc.2016.03.569

99. Sierksma A, Muller M, van der Schouw YT, Grobbee DE, Hendriks HF, Bots ML. Alcohol consumption and arterial stiffness in men. *J Hypertens.* (2004) 22:357–62. doi: 10.1097/00004872-200402000-00020

100. Sierksma A, Lebrun CE, van der Schouw YT, Grobbee DE, Lamberts SW, Hendriks HF, et al. Alcohol consumption in relation to aortic stiffness and aortic wave reflections: a cross-sectional study in healthy postmenopausal women. *Arterioscler Thromb Vasc Biol.* (2004) 24:342–8. doi: 10.1161/01.ATV.0000110784.52412.8f

101. Yu A, Cooke AB, Scheffler P, Doonan RJ, Daskalopoulou SS. Alcohol exerts a shifted u-shaped effect on central blood pressure in young adults. *J Gen Intern Med.* (2021) 36:2975–81. doi: 10.1007/s11606-021-06665-0

102. Nishiwaki M, Kora N, Matsumoto N. Ingesting a small amount of beer reduces arterial stiffness in healthy humans. *Physiol Rep.* (2017) 5:e13381. doi: 10.14814/phy2.13381

103. Gardner JD, Mouton AJ. Alcohol effects on cardiac function. *Compr Physiol.* (2015) 5:791–802. doi: 10.1002/cphy.c140046

104. Kuhlmann CR, Li F, Lüdders DW, Schaefer CA, Most AK, Backenköhler U, et al. Dose-dependent activation of Ca2+-activated K+ channels by ethanol contributes to improved endothelial cell functions. *Alcohol Clin Exp Res.* (2004) 28:1005–11. doi: 10.1097/01.ALC.0000130811.92457.0D

105. Centers for Disease Control and Prevention. Cigarette smoking among adults–United States, 2000. *MMWMorb Rep.* (2002) 51:642–5.

106. Mahmud A, Feely J. Effect of smoking on arterial stiffness and pulse pressure amplification. *Hypertension.* (2003) 41:183–7. doi: 10.1161/01.HYP.0000047464.66901.60

107. Stefanadis C, Vlachopoulos C, Tsiamis E, Diamantopoulos L, Toutouzas K, Giatrakos N, et al. Unfavorable effects of passive smoking on aortic function in men. *Ann Intern Med.* (1998) 128:426–34. doi: 10.7326/0003-4819-128-6-199803150-00002

108. Jatoi NA, Jerrard-Dunne P, Feely J, Mahmud A. Impact of smoking and smoking cessation on arterial stiffness and aortic wave reflection in hypertension. *Hypertension.* (2007) 49:981–5. doi: 10.1161/HYPERTENSIONAHA.107.087338

109. Doonan RJ, Hausvater A, Scallan C, Mikhailidis DP, Pilote L, Daskalopoulou SS. The effect of smoking on arterial stiffness. *Hypertens Res.* (2010) 33:398–410. doi: 10.1038/hr.2010.25

110. Tanaka H, Safar ME. Influence of lifestyle modification on arterial stiffness and wave reflections. *Am J Hypertens.* (2005) 18:137–44. doi: 10.1016/j.amjhyper.2004.07.008

111. He FJ, Li J, Macgregor GA. Effect of longer term modest salt reduction on blood pressure: Cochrane systematic review and meta-analysis of randomised trials. *BMJ.* (2013) 346:f1325. doi: 10.1136/bmj.f1325

112. Avolio AP, Clyde KM, Beard TC, Cooke HM, Ho KK, O'Rourke MF. Improved arterial distensibility in normotensive subjects on a low salt diet. *Arteriosclerosis.* (1986) 6:166–9. doi: 10.1161/01.ATV.6.2.166

113. Livingstone KM, Givens DI, Cockcroft JR, Pickering JE, Lovegrove JA. Is fatty acid intake a predictor of arterial stiffness and blood pressure in men? Evidence from the caerphilly prospective study. *Nutr Metab Cardiovasc Dis.* (2013) 23:1079–85. doi: 10.1016/j.numecd.2012.12.002

114. Crichton GE, Elias MF, Dore GA, Abhayaratna WP, Robbins MA. Relations between dairy food intake and arterial stiffness: pulse wave velocity and pulse pressure. *Hypertension.* (2012) 59:1044–51. doi: 10.1161/HYPERTENSIONAHA.111.190017

115. Petersen KS, Keogh JB, Meikle PJ, Garg ML, Clifton PM. Dietary predictors of arterial stiffness in a cohort with type 1 and type 2 diabetes. *Atherosclerosis.* (2015) 238:175–81. doi: 10.1016/j.atherosclerosis.2014.12.012

116. Aatola H, Koivistoinen T, Hutri-Kähönen N, Juonala M, Mikkilä V, Lehtimäki T, et al. Lifetime fruit and vegetable consumption and arterial pulse wave velocity in adulthood: the cardiovascular risk in young finns study. *Circulation.* (2010) 122:2521–8. doi: 10.1161/CIRCULATIONAHA.110.969279

117. Green D, Cheetham C, Mavaddat L, Watts K, Best M, Taylor R, et al. Effect of lower limb exercise on forearm vascular function: contribution of nitric oxide. *Am J Physiol Heart Circul Physiol.* (2002) 283:H899–907. doi: 10.1152/ajpheart.00049.2002

118. Green DJ, Bilsborough W, Naylor LH, Reed C, Wright J, O'Driscoll G, et al. Comparison of forearm blood flow responses to incremental handgrip and cycle ergometer exercise: relative contribution of nitric oxide. *J Physiol.* (2005) 562:617–28. doi: 10.1113/jphysiol.2004.075929

119. Sacre K, Escoubet B, Pasquet B, Chauveheid MP, Zennaro MC, Tubach F, et al. Increased arterial stiffness in systemic lupus erythematosus (SLE) patients at low risk for cardiovascular disease: a cross-sectional controlled study. *PLoS ONE.* (2014) 9:e94511. doi: 10.1371/journal.pone.0094511

120. Zanoli L, Boutouyrie P, Fatuzzo P, Granata A, Lentini P, Ozturk K, et al. Inflammation and aortic stiffness: an individual participant data meta-analysis in patients with inflammatory bowel disease. *J Am Heart Assoc.* (2017) 6. doi: 10.1161/JAHA.117.007003

121. Anyfanti P, Triantafyllou A, Gkaliagkousi E, Koletsos N, Aslanidis S, Douma S. Association of non-invasive hemodynamics with arterial stiffness in rheumatoid arthritis. *Scand Cardiovasc J.* (2018) 52:171–6. doi: 10.1080/14017431.2018.1453943

122. Maloberti A, Riva M, Tadic M, Valena C, Villa P, Boggioni I, et al. Association between atrial, ventricular and vascular morphofunctional alterations in rheumatoid arthritis. *High Blood Press Cardiovasc Prev.* (2018) 25:97–104. doi: 10.1007/s40292-017-0246-8

123. Costa L, Caso F, D'Elia L, Atteno M, Peluso R, Del Puente A, et al. Psoriatic arthritis is associated with increased arterial stiffness in the absence of known cardiovascular risk factors: a case control study. *Clin Rheumatol.* (2012) 31:711–5. doi: 10.1007/s10067-011-1892-1

124. Shen J, Shang Q, Li EK, Leung YY, Kun EW, Kwok LW, et al. Cumulative inflammatory burden is independently associated with increased arterial stiffness in patients with psoriatic arthritis: a prospective study. *Arthritis Res Ther.* (2015) 17:75. doi: 10.1186/s13075-015-0570-0

125. Sezis Demirci M, Karabulut G, Gungor O, Celtik A, Ok E, Kabasakal Y. Is there an increased arterial stiffness in patients with primary sjögren's syndrome? *Intern Med.* (2016) 55:455–9. doi: 10.2169/internalmedicine.55.3472

126. Ozisler C, Kaplanoglu H. Evaluation of subclinical atherosclerosis by ultrasound radiofrequency data technology in patients with primary Sjögren's syndrome. *Clin Rheumatol.* (2019) 38:709–17. doi: 10.1007/s10067-018-4330-9

127. Roman MJ, Devereux RB, Schwartz JE, Lockshin MD, Paget SA, Davis A, et al. Arterial stiffness in chronic inflammatory diseases. *Hypertension.* (2005) 46:194–9. doi: 10.1161/01.HYP.0000168055.89955.db

128. Tomiyama H, Shiina K, Matsumoto-Nakano C, Ninomiya T, Komatsu S, Kimura K, et al. The contribution of inflammation to the development of hypertension mediated by increased arterial stiffness. *J Am Heart Assoc.* (2017) 6:e05729. doi: 10.1161/JAHA.117.005729

129. Mattace-Raso FU, van der Cammen TJ, van der Meer IM, Schalekamp MA, Asmar R, Hofman A, et al. C-reactive protein and arterial stiffness in older adults: the rotterdam study. *Atherosclerosis.* (2004) 176:111–6. doi: 10.1016/j.atherosclerosis.2004.04.014

130. Fichtlscherer S, Rosenberger G, Walter DH, Breuer S, Dimmeler S, Zeiher AM. Elevated C-reactive protein levels and impaired endothelial vasoreactivity in patients with coronary artery disease. *Circulation.* (2000) 102:1000–6. doi: 10.1161/01.CIR.102.9.1000

131. Mahmud A, Feely J. Arterial stiffness is related to systemic inflammation in essential hypertension. *Hypertension.* (2005) 46:1118–22. doi: 10.1161/01.HYP.0000185463.27209.b0

132. Sie MP, Mattace-Raso FU, Uitterlinden AG, Arp PP, Hofman A, Pols HA, et al. The interleukin-6-174 G/C promoter polymorphism and arterial stiffness; the rotterdam study. *Vasc Health Risk Manag.* (2008) 4:863–9. doi: 10.2147/VHRM.S1693

133. Vlachopoulos C, Gravos A, Georgiopoulos G, Terentes-Printzios D, Ioakeimidis N, Vassilopoulos D, et al. The effect of TNF-a antagonists on aortic stiffness and wave reflections: a meta-analysis. *Clin Rheumatol.* (2018) 37:515–26. doi: 10.1007/s10067-017-3657-y

134. Ikdahl E, Rollefstad S, Hisdal J, Olsen IC, Pedersen TR, Kvien TK, et al. Sustained Improvement of arterial stiffness and blood pressure after long-term rosuvastatin treatment in patients with inflammatory joint diseases: results from the RORA-AS study. *PLoS ONE.* (2016) 11:e0153440. doi: 10.1371/journal.pone.0153440

135. Wang Y, Sun Z. Current understanding of klotho. *Ageing Res Rev.* (2009) 8:43–51. doi: 10.1016/j.arr.2008.10.002

136. Chen K, Zhou X, Sun Z. Haplodeficiency of klotho gene causes arterial stiffening via upregulation of scleraxis expression and induction of autophagy. *Hypertension.* (2015) 66:1006–13. doi: 10.1161/HYPERTENSIONAHA.115.06033

137. Gao D, Zuo Z, Tian J, Ali Q, Lin Y, Lei H, et al. Activation of SIRT1 attenuates klotho deficiency-induced arterial stiffness and hypertension by enhancing AMP-activated protein kinase activity. *Hypertension.* (2016) 68:1191–9. doi: 10.1161/HYPERTENSIONAHA.116.07709

138. Kitagawa M, Sugiyama H, Morinaga H, Inoue T, Takiue K, Ogawa A, et al. A decreased level of serum soluble Klotho is an independent biomarker associated with arterial stiffness in patients with chronic kidney disease. *PLoS ONE.* (2013) 8:e56695. doi: 10.1371/journal.pone.0056695

139. Zarzuelo MJ, Lopez-Sepulveda R, Sanchez M, Romero M, Gomez-Guzman M, Ungvary Z, et al. SIRT1 inhibits NADPH oxidase activation and protects endothelial function in the rat aorta: implications for vascular aging. *Biochem Pharmacol.* (2013) 85:1288–96. doi: 10.1016/j.bcp.2013.02.015

140. Fry JL, Al Sayah L, Weisbrod RM, Van Roy I, Weng X, Cohen RA, et al. Vascular smooth muscle sirtuin-1 protects against diet-induced aortic stiffness. *Hypertension.* (2016) 68:775–84. doi: 10.1161/HYPERTENSIONAHA.116.07622

141. Zhou X, Chen K, Wang Y, Schuman M, Lei H, Sun Z. Antiaging gene klotho regulates adrenal CYP11B2 expression and aldosterone synthesis. *J Am Soc Nephrol.* (2016) 27:1765–76. doi: 10.1681/ASN.2015010093

142. Neves MF, Cunha AR, Cunha MR, Gismondi RA, Oigman W. The role of renin-angiotensin-aldosterone system and its new components in arterial stiffness and vascular aging. *High Blood Press Cardiovasc Prev.* (2018) 25:137–45. doi: 10.1007/s40292-018-0252-5

143. Park S, Kim JB, Shim CY, Ko YG, Choi D, Jang Y, et al. The influence of serum aldosterone and the aldosterone-renin ratio on pulse wave velocity in hypertensive patients. *J Hypertens.* (2007) 25:1279–83. doi: 10.1097/HJH.0b013e3280f31b6e

144. Benetos A, Topouchian J, Ricard S, Gautier S, Bonnardeaux A, Asmar R, et al. Influence of angiotensin II type 1 receptor polymorphism on aortic stiffness in never-treated hypertensive patients. *Hypertension.* (1995) 26:44–7. doi: 10.1161/01.HYP.26.1.44

145. Lajemi M, Labat C, Gautier S, Lacolley P, Safar M, Asmar R, et al. Angiotensin II type 1 receptor-153A/G and 1166A/C gene polymorphisms and increase in aortic stiffness with age in hypertensive subjects. *J Hypertens.* (2001) 19:407–13. doi: 10.1097/00004872-200103000-00008

146. Dima I, Vlachopoulos C, Alexopoulos N, Baou K, Vasiliadou C, Antoniades C, et al. Association of arterial stiffness with the angiotensin-converting enzyme gene polymorphism in healthy individuals. *Am J Hypertens.* (2008) 21:1354–8. doi: 10.1038/ajh.2008.295

147. Taniwaki H, Kawagishi T, Emoto M, Shoji T, Hosoi M, Kogawa K, et al. Association of ACE gene polymorphism with arterial stiffness in patients with type 2 diabetes. *Diabetes Care.* (1999) 22:1858–64. doi: 10.2337/diacare.22.11.1858

148. Pojoga L, Gautier S, Blanc H, Guyene TT, Poirier O, Cambien F, et al. Genetic determination of plasma aldosterone levels in essential hypertension. *Am J Hypertens.* (1998) 11:856–60. doi: 10.1016/S0895-7061(98)00048-X

149. Laurent S, Boutouyrie P, Lacolley P. Structural and genetic bases of arterial stiffness. *Hypertension.* (2005) 45:1050–5. doi: 10.1161/01.HYP.0000164580.39991.3d

150. Nehme JA, Lacolley P, Labat C, Challande P, Robidel E, Perret C, et al. Spironolactone improves carotid artery fibrosis and distensibility in rat post-ischaemic heart failure. *J Mol Cell Cardiol.* (2005) 39:511–9. doi: 10.1016/j.yjmcc.2005.05.015

151. London GM, Asmar RG, O'Rourke MF, Safar ME. Mechanism(s) of selective systolic blood pressure reduction after a low-dose combination of perindopril/indapamide in hypertensive subjects: comparison with atenolol. *J Am Coll Cardiol.* (2004) 43:92–9. doi: 10.1016/j.jacc.2003.07.039

152. Savoia C, Touyz RM, Amiri F, Schiffrin EL. Selective mineralocorticoid receptor blocker eplerenone reduces resistance artery stiffness in hypertensive patients. *Hypertension.* (2008) 51:432–9. doi: 10.1161/HYPERTENSIONAHA.107.103267

153. Koumaras C, Tziomalos K, Stavrinou E, Katsiki N, Athyros VG, Mikhailidis DP, et al. Effects of renin-angiotensin-aldosterone system inhibitors and beta-blockers on markers of arterial stiffness. *J Am Soc Hypertens.* (2014) 8:74–82. doi: 10.1016/j.jash.2013.09.001

154. D'Elia L, Galletti F, La Fata E, Sabino P, Strazzullo P. Effect of dietary sodium restriction on arterial stiffness: systematic review and meta-analysis of the randomized controlled trials. *J Hypertens.* (2018) 36:734–43. doi: 10.1097/HJH.0000000000001604

155. Zeller CB, Appenzeller S. Cardiovascular disease in systemic lupus erythematosus: the role of traditional and lupus related risk factors. *Curr Cardiol Rev.* (2008) 4:116–22. doi: 10.2174/157340308784245775

156. Yarur AJ, Deshpande AR, Pechman DM, Tamariz L, Abreu MT, Sussman DA. Inflammatory bowel disease is associated with an increased incidence of cardiovascular events. *Am J Gastroenterol.* (2011) 106:741–7. doi: 10.1038/ajg.2011.63

157. Ahlehoff O, Gislason GH, Charlot M, Jorgensen CH, Lindhardsen J, Olesen JB, et al. Psoriasis is associated with clinically significant cardiovascular risk: a Danish nationwide cohort study. *J Intern Med.* (2011) 270:147–57. doi: 10.1111/j.1365-2796.2010.02310.x

158. Holloway CJ, Ntusi N, Suttie J, Mahmod M, Wainwright E, Clutton G, et al. Comprehensive cardiac magnetic resonance imaging and spectroscopy reveal a high burden of myocardial disease in HIV patients. *Circulation.* (2013) 128:814–22. doi: 10.1161/CIRCULATIONAHA.113.001719

159. Shang Q, Tam LS, Li EK, Yip GW, Yu CM. Increased arterial stiffness correlated with disease activity in systemic lupus erythematosus. *Lupus.* (2008) 17:1096–102. doi: 10.1177/0961203308092160

160. Yudkin JS, Stehouwer CD, Emeis JJ, Coppack SW. C-reactive protein in healthy subjects: associations with obesity, insulin resistance, and endothelial dysfunction: a potential role for cytokines originating from adipose tissue? *Arterioscler Thromb Vasc Biol.* (1999) 19:972–8. doi: 10.1161/01.ATV.19.4.972

161. van der Meer IM, de Maat MP, Bots ML, Breteler MM, Meijer J, Kiliaan AJ, et al. Inflammatory mediators and cell adhesion molecules as indicators of severity of atherosclerosis: the rotterdam study. *Arterioscler Thromb Vasc Biol.* (2002) 22:838–42. doi: 10.1161/01.ATV.0000016249.96529.B8

162. Xue H, Li JJ, Wang JL, Chen SH, Gao JS, Chen YD, et al. Changes in pulse pressure × heart rate, hs-CRP, and arterial stiffness progression in the Chinese general population: a cohort study involving 3978 employees of the Kailuan company. *J Geriatr Cardiol.* (2019) 16:710–6. doi: 10.11909/j.issn.1671-5411.2019.09.010

163. Park MY, Herrmann SM, Saad A, Eirin A, Tang H, Lerman A, et al. Biomarkers of kidney injury and klotho in patients with atherosclerotic renovascular disease. *Clin J Am Soc Nephrol.* (2015) 10:443–51. doi: 10.2215/CJN.07290714

164. Navarro-González JF, Donate-Correa J, Muros de Fuentes M, Pérez-Hernández H, Martínez-Sanz R, Mora-Fernández C. Reduced KLOTHO is associated with the presence and severity of coronary artery disease. *Heart.* (2014) 100:34–40. doi: 10.1136/heartjnl-2013-304746

165. Chirinos JA, Sardana M, Syed AA, Koppula MR, Varakantam S, Vasim I, et al. Aldosterone, inactive matrix gla-protein, and large artery stiffness in hypertension. *J Am Soc Hypertens.* (2018) 12:681–9. doi: 10.1016/j.jash.2018.06.018

166. Lacolley P, Labat C, Pujol A, Delcayre C, Benetos A, Safar M. Increased carotid wall elastic modulus and fibronectin in aldosterone-salt-treated rats: effects of eplerenone. *Circulation.* (2002) 106:2848–53. doi: 10.1161/01.CIR.0000039328.33137.6C

167. Aragones G, Ferre R, Lazaro I, Cabre A, Plana N, Merino J, et al. Fatty acid-binding protein 4 is associated with endothelial dysfunction in patients with type 2 diabetes. *Atherosclerosis.* (2010) 213:329–31. doi: 10.1016/j.atherosclerosis.2010.07.026

168. Fuseya T, Furuhashi M, Yuda S, Muranaka A, Kawamukai M, Mita T, et al. Elevation of circulating fatty acid-binding protein 4 is independently associated with left ventricular diastolic dysfunction in a general population. *Cardiovasc Diabetol.* (2014) 13:126. doi: 10.1186/s12933-014-0126-7

169. von Eynatten M, Breitling LP, Roos M, Baumann M, Rothenbacher D, Brenner H. Circulating adipocyte fatty acid-binding protein levels and cardiovascular morbidity and mortality in patients with coronary heart disease: a 10-year prospective study. *Arterioscler Thromb Vasc Biol.* (2012) 32:2327–35. doi: 10.1161/ATVBAHA.112.248609

170. Chen MC, Hsu BG, Lee CJ, Yang CF, Wang JH. High serum adipocyte fatty acid binding protein level as a potential biomarker of aortic arterial stiffness in hypertensive patients with metabolic syndrome. *Clin Chim Acta.* (2017) 473:166–72. doi: 10.1016/j.cca.2017.08.030

171. Tseng PW, Hou JS, Wu DA, Hsu BG. High serum adipocyte fatty acid binding protein concentration linked with increased aortic arterial

stiffness in patients with type 2 diabetes. *Clin Chim Acta*. (2019) 495:35–9. doi: 10.1016/j.cca.2019.03.1629

172. Vavruch C, Länne T, Fredrikson M, Lindström T, Östgren CJ, Nystrom FH. Serum leptin levels are independently related to the incidence of ischemic heart disease in a prospective study of patients with type 2 diabetes. *Cardiovasc Diabetol*. (2015) 14:62. doi: 10.1186/s12933-015-0208-1

173. Montazerifar F, Bolouri A, Paghalea RS, Mahani MK, Karajibani M. Obesity. Serum resistin and leptin levels linked to coronary artery disease. *Arq Bras Cardiol*. (2016) 107:348–353. doi: 10.5935/abc.20160134

174. Tsai JP, Lee MC, Chen YC, Ho GJ, Shih MH, Hsu BG. Hyperleptinemia is a risk factor for the development of central arterial stiffness in kidney transplant patients. *Transplant Proc*. (2015) 47:1825–30. doi: 10.1016/j.transproceed.2015.06.002

175. Kuo CH, Lin YL, Wang CH, Lai YH, Syu RJ, Hsu BG. High serum leptin levels are associated with central arterial stiffness in geriatric patients on hemodialysis. *Ci Ji Yi Xue Za Zhi*. (2018) 30:227–32. doi: 10.4103/tcmj.tcmj_10_18

176. D'Elia L, Giaquinto A, De Luca F, Strazzullo P, Galletti F. Relationship between circulating leptin levels and arterial stiffness: a systematic review and meta-analysis of observational studies. *High Blood Press Cardiovasc Prev*. (2020) 27:505–13. doi: 10.1007/s40292-020-00404-y

177. Clerico A, Giannoni A, Vittorini S, Passino C. Thirty years of the heart as an endocrine organ: physiological role and clinical utility of cardiac natriuretic hormones. *Am J Physiol Heart Circul Physiol*. (2011) 301:H12–20. doi: 10.1152/ajpheart.00226.2011

178. Khan SQ, O'Brien RJ, Struck J, Quinn P, Morgenthaler N, Squire I, et al. Prognostic value of midregional pro-adrenomedullin in patients with acute myocardial infarction: the LAMP (leicester acute myocardial infarction peptide) study. *J Am Coll Cardiol*. (2007) 49:1525–32. doi: 10.1016/j.jacc.2006.12.038

179. O'Malley RG, Bonaca MP, Scirica BM, Murphy SA, Jarolim P, Sabatine MS, et al. Prognostic performance of multiple biomarkers in patients with non-ST-segment elevation acute coronary syndrome: analysis from the MERLIN-TIMI 36 trial (metabolic efficiency with ranolazine for less ischemia in non-ST-elevation acute coronary syndromes-thrombolysis in myocardial infarction 36). *J Am Coll Cardiol*. (2014) 63:1644–53. doi: 10.1016/j.jacc.2013.12.034

180. Klug G, Feistritzer HJ, Reinstadler SJ, Krauter L, Mayr A, Mair J, et al. Association of aortic stiffness with biomarkers of myocardial wall stress after myocardial infarction. *Int J Cardiol*. (2014) 173:253–8. doi: 10.1016/j.ijcard.2014.02.038

181. Reinstadler SJ, Feistritzer HJ, Klug G, Mayr A, Huybrechts L, Hammerer-Lercher A, et al. Biomarkers of hemodynamic stress and aortic stiffness after STEMI: a cross-sectional analysis. *Dis Markers*. (2015) 2015:717032. doi: 10.1155/2015/717032

182. Hagstrom E, Michaelsson K, Melhus H, Hansen T, Ahlstrom H, Johansson L, et al. Plasma-parathyroid hormone is associated with subclinical and clinical atherosclerotic disease in 2 community-based cohorts. *Arterioscler Thromb Vasc Biol*. (2014) 34:1567–73. doi: 10.1161/ATVBAHA.113.303062

183. Schillaci G, Pucci G, Pirro M, Monacelli M, Scarponi AM, Manfredelli MR, et al. Large-artery stiffness: a reversible marker of cardiovascular risk in primary hyperparathyroidism. *Atherosclerosis*. (2011) 218:96–101. doi: 10.1016/j.atherosclerosis.2011.05.010

184. Cheng YB, Li LH, Guo QH, Li FK, Huang QF, Sheng CS, et al. Independent effects of blood pressure and parathyroid hormone on aortic pulse wave velocity in untreated Chinese patients. *J Hypertens*. (2017) 35:1841–8. doi: 10.1097/HJH.0000000000001395

185. Muse ED, Feldman DI, Blaha MJ, Dardari ZA, Blumenthal RS, Budoff MJ, et al. The association of resistin with cardiovascular disease in the multi-ethnic study of atherosclerosis. *Atherosclerosis*. (2015) 239:101–8. doi: 10.1016/j.atherosclerosis.2014.12.044

186. Norman G, Norton GR, Gomes M, Michel F, Majane OH, Sareli P, et al. Circulating resistin concentrations are independently associated with aortic pulse wave velocity in a community sample. *J Hypertens*. (2016) 34:274–81. doi: 10.1097/HJH.0000000000000792

187. Wang JH, Lee CJ, Yang CF, Chen YC, Hsu BG. Serum resistin as an independent marker of aortic stiffness in patients with coronary artery disease. *PLoS ONE*. (2017) 12:e0183123. doi: 10.1371/journal.pone.0183123

188. Krishnan E, Baker JF, Furst DE, Schumacher HR. Gout and the risk of acute myocardial infarction. *Arthritis Rheum*. (2006) 54:2688–96. doi: 10.1002/art.22014

189. Verdecchia P, Schillaci G, Reboldi G, Santeusanio F, Porcellati C, Brunetti P. Relation between serum uric acid and risk of cardiovascular disease in essential hypertension. The PIUMA study. *Hypertension*. (2000) 36:1072–8. doi: 10.1161/01.HYP.36.6.1072

190. Bos MJ, Koudstaal PJ, Hofman A, Witteman JC, Breteler MM. Uric acid is a risk factor for myocardial infarction and stroke: the rotterdam study. *Stroke*. (2006) 37:1503–7. doi: 10.1161/01.STR.0000221716.55088.d4

191. Baena CP, Lotufo PA, Mill JG, Cunha Rde S, Bensenor IJ. Serum uric acid and pulse wave velocity among healthy adults: baseline data from the brazilian longitudinal study of adult health (ELSA-Brasil). *Am J Hypertens*. (2015) 28:966–70. doi: 10.1093/ajh/hpu298

192. Rebora P, Andreano A, Triglione N, Piccinelli E, Palazzini M, Occhi L, et al. Association between uric acid and pulse wave velocity in hypertensive patients and in the general population: a systematic review and meta-analysis. *Blood Press*. (2020) 29:220–31. doi: 10.1080/08037051.2020.1735929

193. Park JS, Kang S, Ahn CW, Cha BS, Kim KR, Lee HC. Relationships between serum uric acid, adiponectin and arterial stiffness in postmenopausal women. *Maturitas*. (2012) 73:344–8. doi: 10.1016/j.maturitas.2012.09.009

194. Mehta T, Nuccio E, McFann K, Madero M, Sarnak MJ, Jalal D. Association of uric acid with vascular stiffness in the framingham heart study. *Am J Hypertens*. (2015) 28:877–83. doi: 10.1093/ajh/hpu253

195. Boutouyrie P, Chowienczyk P, Humphrey JD, Mitchell GF. Arterial stiffness and cardiovascular risk in hypertension. *Circ Res*. (2021) 128:864–886. doi: 10.1161/CIRCRESAHA.121.318061

196. Vlachopoulos C, Terentes-Printzios D, Laurent S, Nilsson PM, Protogerou AD, Aznaouridis K, et al. Association of estimated pulse wave velocity with survival: a secondary analysis of SPRINT. *JAMA Netw Open*. (2019) 2:e1912831. doi: 10.1001/jamanetworkopen.2019.12831

197. Nicholson CJ, Singh K, Saphirstein RJ, Gao YZ, Li Q, Chiu JG, et al. Reversal of aging-induced increases in aortic stiffness by targeting cytoskeletal protein-protein interfaces. *J Am Heart Assoc*. (2018) 7:e008926. doi: 10.1161/JAHA.118.008926

5

Plasma Oxylipins: A Potential Risk Assessment Tool in Atherosclerotic Coronary Artery Disease

D. Elizabeth Le[1†], Manuel García-Jaramillo[2,3,4†‡], Gerd Bobe[3,5†],
Armando Alcazar Magana[3,6], Ashish Vaswani[3,6], Jessica Minnier[7], Donald B. Jump[2,3],
Diana Rinkevich[1], Nabil J. Alkayed[1,8], Claudia S. Maier[3,6*] and Sanjiv Kaul[1*]

[1] Knight Cardiovascular Institute, Oregon Health and Science University, Portland, OR, United States, [2] Nutrition Program, School of Biological and Population Health Sciences, Oregon State University, Corvallis, OR, United States, [3] Linus Pauling Institute, Oregon State University, Corvallis, OR, United States, [4] Helfgott Research Institute, National University of Natural Medicine, Portland, OR, United States, [5] Department of Animal and Rangeland Sciences, Oregon State University, Corvallis, OR, United States, [6] Department of Chemistry, Oregon State University, Corvallis, OR, United States, [7] Department of Biostatistics and Knight Cancer Institute, Oregon Health and Science University, Portland, OR, United States, [8] Department of Anesthesiology and Perioperative Medicine, Oregon Health and Science University, Portland, OR, United States

*Correspondence:
Sanjiv Kaul
kauls@ohsu.edu
Claudia S. Maier
claudia.maier@oregonstate.edu

[†] These authors have contributed equally to this work and share first authorship

[‡] Present address:
Manuel García-Jaramillo,
Department of Environmental and Molecular Toxicology, Oregon State University, Corvallis, OR, United States

Background: While oxylipins have been linked to coronary artery disease (CAD), little is known about their diagnostic and prognostic potential.

Objective: We tested whether plasma concentration of specific oxylipins may discriminate among number of diseased coronary arteries and predict median 5-year outcomes in symptomatic adults.

Methods: Using a combination of high-performance liquid chromatography (HPLC) and quantitative tandem mass spectrometry, we conducted a targeted analysis of 39 oxylipins in plasma samples of 23 asymptomatic adults with low CAD risk and 74 symptomatic adults ($\geq$70% stenosis), aged 38–87 from the Greater Portland, Oregon area. Concentrations of 22 oxylipins were above the lower limit of quantification in >98% of adults and were compared, individually and in groups based on precursors and biosynthetic pathways, in symptomatic adults to number of diseased coronary arteries [(1) $n = 31$; (2) $n = 23$; (3) $n = 20$], and outcomes during a median 5-year follow-up (no surgery: $n = 7$; coronary stent placement: $n = 24$; coronary artery bypass graft surgery: $n = 26$; death: $n = 7$).

Results: Plasma levels of six quantified oxylipins decreased with the number of diseased arteries; a panel of five oxylipins diagnosed three diseased arteries with 100% sensitivity and 70% specificity. Concentrations of five oxylipins were lower and one oxylipin was higher with survival; a panel of two oxylipins predicted survival during follow-up with 86% sensitivity and 91% specificity.

Conclusions: Quantification of plasma oxylipins may assist in CAD diagnosis and prognosis in combination with standard risk assessment tools.

Keywords: coronary artery disease, oxylipins, diagnosis, prognosis, mass spectrometry, LCMS

INTRODUCTION

Coronary artery disease (CAD) is the leading cause of death worldwide (1–3). Traditional CAD risk factors such as diabetes, smoking, hypertension, hyperlipidemia, and family history of premature cardiovascular disease (CVD), as well as nontraditional risk factors of rheumatic inflammatory disease, human immunodeficiency disease, and gestational diabetes can assist clinicians in decisions for CAD primary prevention but have limited efficacy in high CAD risk patient management (4). This is currently done using expensive invasive tests, such as exercise stress testing (without or with concomitant imaging for myocardial perfusion and/or function) or measuring the coronary calcium score on X-ray computed tomography (CT). Our objective is to develop a point-of-care blood test that could assist in decision making regarding CAD patient management.

Ruptured arterial plaques are a major reason for adverse cardiac events with resultant thrombus formation that partially or completely impairs blood flow to the heart (5). The progression from asymptomatic to ruptured arterial plaques involves lipid oxidation and inflammation (6, 7). Conventional indicators of lipid oxidation include secondary products such as 4-hydroxynonenal (4-HNE) (8), malondialdehyde (MDA) (9), and oxidized low-density lipoproteins (Ox-LDL) (10), and its associated oxidized phospholipids (11). Technological advancements in soft ionization tandem mass spectrometry (MS/MS) have allowed multiplexed quantification of oxidized lipids in one analytical run and with it the emergence of isoprostanes and oxylipins as indicators of oxidative tissue injuries, implicating oxidative tissue injuries in the pathology of a variety of chronic diseases (3, 12).

Oxylipins are oxidized long and very long chain polyunsaturated fatty acids (PUFA), which are derived from phospholipids. Oxylipins can be classified based on their fatty acid (FA) precursor (**Figure 1**). The dominant precursors of oxylipins are the more proinflammatory omega-6 PUFA linoleic acid (LA; C18:2 $n{-}6$) and arachidonic acid (ARA; C20:4 $n{-}6$) and the more anti-inflammatory omega-3 PUFA linolenic acid (LNA; C18:3 $n{-}3$), eicosapentaenoic acid (EPA; C20:5 $n{-}3$), and docosahexaenoic acid (DHA; C22:6 $n{-}3$). The dominant oxylipin biosynthesis pathways are named after the enzymes involved, as follows: lipoxygenases (LOX), cyclooxygenases (COX), cytochrome P450 (CYP450) epoxygenases and hydroxylases, and soluble epoxide hydrolases. Reactive oxygen species (ROS) can initiate the formation of a few, specific oxylipins from PUFAs (13). Prior human studies with limited sample sizes reported elevated concentrations of ARA-derived oxylipins in unstable arterial plaques (14) and ischemic heart

tissue (15). Elevated circulating concentrations were observed in individuals after cardiac surgery (16) and those experiencing adverse cardiac events on follow-up (17, 18). Furthermore, CAD patients had higher circulating concentrations of ARA-derived oxylipins than non-CAD adults (19–21).

In the present study, we evaluated whether plasma oxylipins, alone or in panels, may discriminate among number of diseased coronary arteries and predict median 5-year outcomes in high CAD risk symptomatic patients and $\geq$70% stenosis which, to our knowledge, has not been previously published. In doing so, a point-of-care plasma oxylipin test could assist in decision making regarding CAD patient management. Here, we report results of a small study confirming this hypothesis.

MATERIALS AND METHODS

Participants and Study Design

The study was approved by the Institutional Review Board of the Oregon Health and Science University (OHSU) in Portland, Oregon. We prospectively enrolled 74 individuals from the greater Portland metropolitan area from October 2012 and January 2017 (IRB00008606) who were referred to OHSU for an invasive coronary angiography because of symptoms suggestive of CAD (median age: 66 years; range: 38–87 years). Inclusion criteria were inducible myocardial ischemia during stress (either on echocardiography or single-photon computed tomography) and $\geq$70% coronary luminal narrowing of one or more major coronary artery or its major branch on subsequent coronary angiography. Exclusion criteria were <70% coronary stenosis on angiography, prior myocardial infarction, hemodynamically significant valvular heart disease, prior revascularization, or congestive heart failure. The CAD patients were classified as having one-vessel ($n = 31$), two-vessel ($n = 23$), or three-vessel ($n = 20$) CAD and were followed up until November 2019 (**Figure 2**) for a median of 60 months (range: 25–84 months) for adverse events [i.e., coronary stent placement; coronary artery bypass graft (CABG) surgery; death]. Ten CAD patients were lost to follow-up (unable to contact: $n = 8$; declined to follow-up: $n = 2$).

To establish ranges of plasma oxylipin concentrations in low CAD risk populations, we established the Astoria cohort and prospectively enrolled 220 individuals from Astoria, a rural community within the same area as the CAD patients, from July 2016 to February 2017 (IRB00011193). For the current study, we selected individuals of the same age range (range: 38–71 years) that fulfilled all the exclusion criteria ($n = 23$). Exclusion criteria were self-reported history of hyperlipidemia, diabetes, myocardial infarction, ischemia, coronary artery revascularization surgery, coronary atherosclerosis on coronary angiography, active tobacco use, and family history of CAD. Participants from the Astoria and Portland were not age-matched.

Sample Collection and Preparation for Oxylipin Analysis

All participants fasted for at least 6 h before 4.5 mL blood was collected in tubes containing 0.01 M buffered sodium citrate and immediately placed on ice. Blood samples were collected 1–4 h

---

Abbreviations: ACN, acetonitrile; ARA, arachidonic acid; CAD, coronary artery disease; COX, cyclooxygenases; CUDA, 1-cyclohexyl ureido, 3-dodecanoic acid; CVD, cardiovascular diseases; CYP450, cytochrome P450; CYPEPOX, CYP epoxide; DHA, docosahexaenoic acid; EPA, eicosapentaenoic acid; FA, fatty acid; 4-HNE, 4-hydroxynonenal; HPLC-MS/MS, high-performance liquid chromatography tandem mass spectrometry; IMS, ionization mass spectrometry; IPA, isopropanol; LA, linoleic acid; LDL, low-density lipoproteins; LNA, linolenic acid; LOD, limit of detection; LOQ, limit of quantification; LOX, lipoxygenases; MDA, malondialdehyde; MRM, multi-reaction monitoring; PUFA, polyunsaturated fatty acids; ROS, reactive oxygen species; RT, retention time; sEH, soluble epoxide hydrolases.

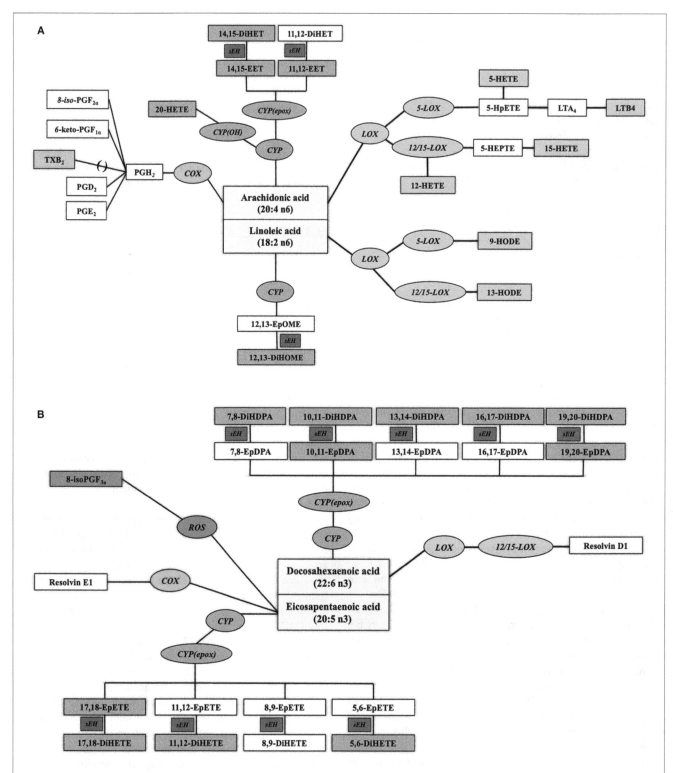

FIGURE 1 | Biosynthetic pathways of plasma oxylipins from omega-6 **(A)** and omega-3 **(B)** polyunsaturated fatty acids (PUFA). Normal text designates PUFA (yellow rectangular boxes) and oxylipins. Italic text designates enzymes involved in the metabolic transformation [blue oval boxes for cyclo-oxygenases or aspirin, orange oval boxes for lipoxygenases or CYP1B1, green oval boxes for cytochrome P450, and gray rectangular boxes for soluble epoxide hydrolase (sEH)] with their quantified oxylipins in the same color and oxylipins below the limit of quantification (LOQ) in noncolored squares. See Abbreviation Index and **Appendix** for full names description.

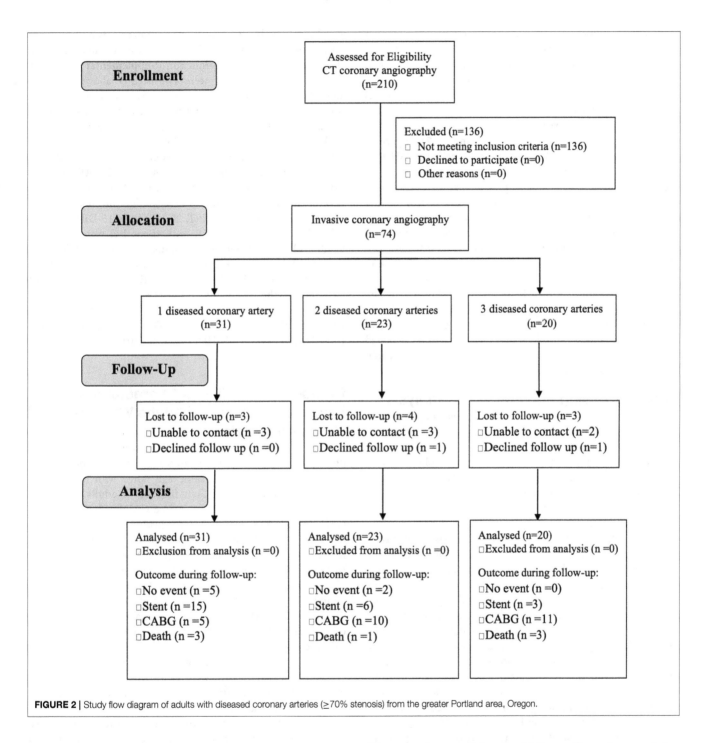

FIGURE 2 | Study flow diagram of adults with diseased coronary arteries (≥70% stenosis) from the greater Portland area, Oregon.

prior to coronary angiography of participants with CAD. Whole blood samples were then centrifuged at 3,000 rpm for 15 min in a refrigerated centrifuge at 4°C, after which the plasma was aliquoted into 1 mL Eppendorf tubes and immediately stored at −80°C until analysis.

Oxylipins from plasma were extracted as described in Pedersen et al. (22) with minor modifications. The internal oxylipin standards used during the extraction (**Supplementary Table 1**) were used to correct the recovery of the quantified oxylipins (23).

Chromatographic and Mass Spectrometric Analysis of Oxylipins

The high-performance liquid chromatography (HPLC) and mass spectrometry methods used for the analysis of plasma oxylipins was based on methods previously described for the analysis of oxylipins in liver (24). The analysis was performed using a Shimadzu Prominence HPLC system (Shimadzu, Columbia, MD) coupled to an Applied Biosystems 4000 QTRAP (AB SCIEX, Framingham, MA). Employing dynamic multireaction monitoring (dMRM), we evaluated 60 oxylipins in a targeted approach (**Supplementary Figure 1**). For each compound, optimal transitions were determined by flow injection of pure standards using the optimizer application, and transitions were compared with literature when available. A detailed list of MRM transitions and experimental conditions is provided in **Supplementary Table 2**.

Compounds were separated using a Waters Acquity UPLC CSH C18 column (100 mm length × 2.1 mm id; 1.7 μm particle size) with an additional Waters Acquity VanGuard CSH C18 pre-column (5 mm × 2.1 mm id; 1.7 μm particle size). Column oven was set to 60°C. The mobile phase consisted of (A) water containing 0.1% acetic acid and (B) acetonitrile/isopropanol (ACN/IPA) (90/10, v/v) containing 0.1% acetic acid. Gradient elution (22) was carried out for 22 min at a flow rate of 0.15 ml min^{-1}. Gradient conditions were as follows: 0–1.0 min, 0.1–25% B; 1.0–2.5 min, 25–40% B; 2.5–4.5 min, 40–42% B; 4.5–10.5 min, 42–50% B; 10.5–12.5 min, 50–65% B; 12.5–14 min, 65–75% B; 14–14.5 min, 75–85% B; 14.5–20 min, 85–95% B; 20–20.5 min, 95–95% B; 20.5–22 min, 95–25% B. A 5-μl aliquot of each sample was injected. Limits of detection (LOD) and quantification (LOQ) (**Supplementary Table 1**) were calculated based on one concentration point (0.1 ng μl^{-1}) for each oxylipin and deuterated surrogate.

Data Processing and Statistical Analysis

Raw data from targeted oxylipin analyses were imported into MultiQuant 3.0.2 software (AB SCIEX) in order to perform the alignment and integration of the peaks (obtaining peak areas). This software allows for the correction of metabolite intensity with the intensity of the internal standards. Data obtained with MultiQuant were imported into MarkerView 1.3.1 software (AB SCIEX) for initial data visualization (25).

Data were analyzed using SAS version 9.2 (SAS Ins. Inc., Cary, NC). Demographic and clinical characteristics of groups were compared using Fisher's exact test for binary data and t-test for nonbinary data. Concentrations of oxylipins were compared using Wilcoxon rank sum test. To evaluate diagnostic and predictive efficacy of oxylipins, we used logistic regression analysis and calculated receiver operating characteristic (ROC) values, including area under the curves (AUC). Our goal was to identify oxylipin panels that could achieve an ROC of 0.90 or higher. To compare diagnostic and predictive efficacy of oxylipins with current standard risk assessment tool, we compared ROC values of our best oxylipin models with those of the 10-year Framingham general CVD risk scores using the ROCCONTRAST statement in PROC LOGISTIC. We were not able to use the 10-year atherosclerotic CVD risk score of the American College of Cardiology (ACC) because 41 of 74 CAD patient scores could not be calculated. All statistical tests were two sided. Significance was declared at $P \leq 0.05$.

RESULTS

Analysis of Oxylipins

In order to achieve a representative coverage of LA-, ARA-, EPA-, and DHA-derived oxylipins and the enzymatic and nonenzymatic pathways involved in their production,

a library with 39 oxylipin standards was analyzed (**Supplementary Table 1**). Our LC-MRM method detected all 39 oxylipins in one 22-min run (**Supplementary Figure 1**). Of the 39 oxylipins, 24 were consistently above the LOD and 22 oxylipins were consistently above the LOQ. Oxylipin concentrations below the LOQ were set at 80% of the lowest quantifiable sample. The library included (i) four LA-derived oxylipins (two each from CYP450 and LOX pathways), of which three [CYP450: 12,13-DiHOME, LOX: 9(S) HODE, 13(S) HODE] were above the LOQ; (ii) 14 ARA-derived oxylipins (five from COX, five from CYP450, and four from LOX pathways), of which nine (COX: thromboxane B2; CYP450: 11,12-EET, 14,15-EET, 20-HETE, 14,15-DiHET; LOX: 5-HETE, 12-HETE, 15-HETE, leukotriene B4) were above the LOQ; (iii) 10 EPA-derived oxylipins (one from COX, eight from CYP450, and one from ROS pathways), of which three (CYP450: 11,12-DiHETE, 17,18-EpETE; ROS: 8-iso PGF3a) were above the LOQ; (iv) 11 DHA-derived oxylipins (10 CYP450 and one from LOX pathways) of which seven (CYP450: 10,11-EpDPA, 19,20 EpDPA, 7,8-DiHDPA, 10,11-DiHDPA, 13,14-DiHDPA, 16,17-DiHDPA, 19,20-DiHDPA) were above the LOQ.

Demographic, Clinical Characteristics, and Levels of Oxylipins of Adults With Diseased Coronary Arteries

Selected demographic and clinical characteristics of adults with diseased coronary arteries stratified by number of diseased arteries and adults of the same age range with a low CAD risk are listed in **Table 1**. Sixty-nine of 74 adults with CAD had multiple CVD risk factors (three CAD1 patients and one CAD2 patient had one CVD risk factor and one CAD2 patient had no CVD risk factor). Almost all adults with CAD had hypertension and hypercholesterolemia. Most adults with CAD were on aspirin, were overweight or obese, or had a history of smoking. About half adults with CAD had diabetes or a family history of CVD. Demographic and clinical characteristics of adults with CAD had a limited efficacy to diagnose number of diseased arteries. The 10-year Framingham general CVD risk score and the number of CAD risk factors increased with the number of diseased arteries; specifically, adults with multiple diseased arteries were more likely to be male, were overweight or obese, former smokers, or had lower plasma HDL cholesterol concentrations.

Ten of 22 (45%) individual oxylipin concentrations decreased with greater number of diseased arteries by at least 10%; six individual oxylipins (27%) had significantly lower concentrations in adults with three vs. one diseased artery (**Table 2**). For pattern detection, oxylipins were grouped in **Table 3** by (1) FA precursors (i.e., LA, ARA, EPA, and DHA), oxylipin groups (i.e., mid-chain HODE, EET, mid-chain HETE, EpDPA, DiHDPA), (2) enzymes involved in their synthesis [i.e., oxygenation of PUFAs by LOX followed by reduction or alternatively hydroxylation of PUFAs by CYP1B1; oxidation of PUFAs by CYP450 followed by hydroxylation of oxidized PUFAs by soluble epoxide hydrolase (sEH)], and (3) based on enzymatic product to substrate

TABLE 1 | Demographic and clinical characteristics of adults with diseased coronary arteries ($\geq$70% stenosis) and adults of the same age range with a low coronary artery disease (CAD) risk.

Characteristics	Low CAD risk (n = 23) Mean ± STD	Number of diseased arteries 1 (n = 31) Mean ± STD	2 (n = 23) Mean ± STD	3 (n = 20) Mean ± STD	Contrast CAD1/2 vs. CAD3 P-value
Age (year)	49 ± 10[b]	65 ± 9[a]	67 ± 12[a]	66 ± 1[a]	0.89
Male [n (%)]	4 (17)[c]	17 (55)[b]	19 (83)[a]	17 (85)[a]	0.15
BMI (kg/m^2)	28.3 ± 6.7[ab]	28.1 ± 4.9[b]	31.0 ± 9.3[ab]	31.7 ± 6.1[a]	0.20
Overweight	3 (13)[ab]	15 (48)[a]	9 (39)[ab]	8 (40)[ab]	0.80
Obese	9 (39)	8 (26)	10 (43)	10 (50)	0.28
Blood pressure (mmHg)					
Systolic	124 ± 9	131 ± 20	133 ± 17	129 ± 17	0.58
Diastolic	79 ± 6[a]	71 ± 13[b]	69 ± 11[b]	70 ± 11[b]	0.89
Plasma					
Triacylglycerol (mg/dl)	88 ± 38[b]	136 ± 72[a]	165 ± 106[a]	218 ± 326[ab]	0.40
Total cholesterol (mg/dl)	195 ± 32	182 ± 49[a]	156 ± 33[b]	177 ± 60[ab]	0.62
HDL cholesterol (mg/dl)	65 ± 13[a]	52 ± 16[b]	46 ± 14[b]	40 ± 12[c]	0.03
LDL cholesterol (mg/dl)	126 ± 28[a]	101 ± 35[b]	76 ± 25[b]	104 ± 48[ab]	0.28
Hba1c (mmol/mol)	5.3 ± 0.4[b]	6.1 ± 1.1[a]	6.5 ± 1.3[a]	6.3 ± 1.1[a]	0.90
Medication	0[b]	30 (97)[a]	21 (91)[a]	18 (90)[a]	0.61
Blood pressure [total, n (%)]	0[b]	24 (77)[b]	21 (91)[ab]	20 (100)[a]	0.10
ACE inhibitor [n (%)]	0[b]	10 (32)[a]	8 (35)[a]	5 (25)[a]	0.58
Angiotension receptor blocker	0[b]	5 (16)[ab]	3 (13)[ab]	5 (25)[a]	0.32
Beta blocker [n (%)]	0[b]	18 (58)[a]	19 (83)[a]	13 (65)[a]	0.79
Calcium channel blocker [n (%)]	0[b]	7 (23)[a]	4 (17)[ab]	5 (25)[a]	0.75
Diabetes [total, n (%)]	0[b]	6 (19)[a]	6 (26)[a]	6 (30)[a]	0.55
Oral hyperglycemia [n (%)]	0[b]	3 (10)[ab]	3 (13)[ab]	4 (20)[a]	0.44
Insulin [n (%)]	0	3 (10)	3 (13)	2 (10)	1
Hyperlipidemia (total)					
Statin [n (%)]	0[b]	24 (77)[a]	16 (70)[a]	13 (65)[a]	0.56
Aspirin [n (%)]	0[b]	23 (74)[a]	19 (83)[a]	15 (75)[a]	0.77
CVD risk factors					
Tobacco use [n (%)]					
Former	6 (26)	8 (26)	9 (39)	6 (30)	1
Active	0[b]	4 (13)[ab]	2 (9)[ab]	5 (25)[a]	0.15
History of [n (%)]					
Hypertension	2 (9)[b]	25 (81)[a]	22 (96)[a]	20 (100)[a]	0.18
Diabetes	0[b]	8 (26)[a]	8 (49)[a]	9 (45)[a]	0.27
Hypercholesterolemia	0[b]	30 (97)[a]	21 (91)[a]	19 (95)[a]	1
CVD in family	0[b]	14 (45)[a]	12 (52)[a]	11 (55)[a]	0.79
Total risk (1–5)	0[c]	2.6 ± 0.9[b]	2.8 ± 0.9[ab]	3.2 ± 0.8[a]	0.04
Framingham 10-year CVD risk (%)	4.0 ± 2.3[c]	21.6 ± 16.2[b]	29.4 ± 17.5[ab]	35.7 ± 19.7[a]	0.04
ACC 10-year ASCVD risk (%)	1.8 ± 1.2[b]	15.6 ± 11.7[a]	18.6 ± 7.5[a]	25.7 ± 12.3[a]	0.05

The superscripts denote whether averages of specific groups in a row differed at $P \leq 0.05$. If none of the groups differed from each other, no superscripts are shown. If two groups differed from each other, the significantly higher group got a superscript a, and the significantly lower group got a superscript b, and the group that did not significantly differ from the higher or the lower group got a superscript ab. If three groups differed from each other, the significantly highest group got a superscript a, the significantly lower group got a superscript b, and the group that was significantly lower than the group with a superscript b, got a, c. Quantitative data were compared using Student's t-test. Proportions were compared using Fisher's exact test.
ACE, angiotension converting enzyme; ACC, American College of Cardiology; ASCVD, atherosclerotic cardiovascular disease.

ratio (i.e., hydroxylation of 10,11-EpDPA to 10,11-DiHDPA, 14,15-EET to 14,15-DiHET, or 19,20-EpDPA to 19,20-DiHDPA by sEH).

Total oxylipin concentrations significantly declined with number of diseased arteries, specifically omega-3 FA-derived oxylipins and within those hydroxylated DHA-epoxide

TABLE 2 | Plasma oxylipin concentrations of adults with diseased coronary arteries (≥70% stenosis) and adults of the same age range with a low coronary artery disease (CAD) risk.

Oxylipins (nM)	Low	Number of diseased arteries			Contrast
	CAD risk (n = 23)	1 (n = 31)	2 (n = 23)	3 (n = 20)	CAD1/2 vs. CAD3
	Median (IQR)	Median (IQR)	Median (IQR)	Median (IQR)	P-value
12,13-DiHOME	8.71[a] (5.27, 11.8)	6.97[ab] (4.76, 8.85)	5.59[bc] (4.07, 8.45)	5.11[c] (4.17, 5.89)	0.07
13(S)-HODE	29.1[b] (26.7, 33.8)	37.6[a] (25.5, 49.9)	34.1[ab] (23.4, 41.7)	31.0[ab] (24.4, 43.2)	0.64
9(S)-HODE	19.0 (17.6, 21.6)	22.3 (16.8, 28.8)	20.3 (16.9, 25.0)	20.5 (14.9, 26.7)	0.64
Leukotriene B4	0.19[ab] (0.15, 0.24)	0.23[a] (0.18, 0.28)	0.24[a] (0.16, 0.27)	0.18[b] (0.15, 0.21)	0.01
Thromboxane B2	0.05 (0.03, 0.08)	0.03 (0.02, 0.05)	0.04 (0.02, 0.04)	0.04 (0.03, 0.06)	0.10
20-HETE	9.18 (7.04, 11.2)	8.60 (7.39, 10.4)	9.37 (7.35, 10.7)	8.43 (6.98, 9.52)	0.36
14,15-EET	0.27[b] (0.18, 0.34)	0.34[a] (0.28, 0.45)	0.22[b] (0.18, 0.36)	0.35[a] (0.23, 0.40)	0.70
11,12-EET	0.25[b] (0.19, 0.30)	0.32[a] (0.26, 0.41)	0.32[a] (0.27, 0.37)	0.35[a] (0.28, 0.46)	0.35
14,15-DiHET	0.98[ab] (0.78, 1.13)	1.12[a] (0.93, 1.23)	0.99[ab] (0.84, 1.17)	0.90[b] (0.78,1.09)	0.08
5-HETE	2.69[b] (2.30, 3.14)	4.63[a] (3.37, 7.29)	4.37[a] (2.87, 6.86)	3.87[ab] (2.21, 6.65)	0.38
12-HETE	2.41[b] (1.13, 4.19)	8.14[a] (5.60, 20.8)	11.2[a] (6.51, 19.6)	7.92[a] (2.78, 12.0)	0.10
15-HETE	1.18[b] (1.02,1.53)	2.41[a] (1.84, 3.29)	2.39[a] (1.73, 3.49)	2.26[a] (1.47, 3.11)	0.47
8-iso PGF3a	0.93[a] (0.49, 1.58)	0.99[a] (0.55, 1.95)	0.87[ab] (0.40, 2.70)	0.58[b] (0.37, 0.81)	0.02
17,18-EpETE	0.29 (0.23, 0.35)	0.26 (0.20, 0.35)	0.26 (0.21, 0.34)	0.29 (0.24, 0.33)	0.51
11,12-DiHETE	0.08 (0.04, 0.11)	0.06 (0.04, 0.12)	0.09 (0.06, 0.12)	0.05 (0.01, 0.09)	0.07
19,20-EpDPA	0.53 (0.32, 0.95)	0.59 (0.43, 0.91)	0.50 (0.40, 0.76)	0.60 (0.48, 0.83)	0.37
10,11-EpDPA	0.11 (0.05, 0.16)	0.11 (0.07, 0.14)	0.12 (0.09, 0.20)	0.11 (0.07, 0.15)	0.16
19,20-DiHDPA	2.22[a] (1.40, 2.83)	1.92[a] (1.19, 2.76)	1.69[ab] (1.00, 2.63)	0.60[b] (0.48, 0.83)	0.04
13,14-DiHDPA	0.14[a] (0.07, 0.20)	0.11[ab] (0.07, 0.14)	0.09[ab] (0.07, 0.19)	0.09[b] (0.06, 0.12)	0.39
16,17-DiHDPA	0.24[ab] (0.15, 0.34)	0.24[a] (0.16, 0.28)	0.19[ab] (0.14, 0.27)	0.17[b] (0.14, 0.21)	0.04
10,11-DiHDPA	0.09 (0.06, 0.15)	0.11 (0.08, 0.17)	0.09 (0.06, 0.18)	0.08 (0.05, 0.11)	0.06
7,8-DiHDPA	0.12 (0.08, 0.14)	0.13 (0.09, 0.16)	0.11 (0.09, 0.17)	0.12 (0.10, 0.18)	0.74

The superscripts denote whether averages of specific groups in a row differed at P ≤ 0.05 using Kruskal–Wallis test. If none of the groups differed from each other, no superscripts are shown. If two groups differed from each other, the significantly higher group got a superscript a, and the significantly lower group got a superscript b, and the group that did not significantly differ from the higher or the lower group got a superscript ab. If three groups differed from each other, the significantly highest group got a superscript a, the significantly lower group got a superscript b, and the group that was significantly lower than the group with a superscript b, got a, c.

DiHOME, dihydroxy-octadecenoic acid; HODE, hydroxy-octadecadienoic acid; HETE, hydroxy-eicosatetraenoic acid; EET, epoxy-eicosatrienoic acid; DiHET, dihydroxy-eicosatrienoic acid; EpDPA, epoxy-docosapentaenoic acid; DiHDPA, dihydroxy-docosapentaenoic acid.

TABLE 3 | Plasma concentrations of oxylipin groups in adults with diseased coronary arteries (≥70% stenosis) and adults of the same age range with a low coronary artery disease (CAD) risk.

Oxylipins (nM)	Low	Number of diseased arteries			Contrast
	CAD risk ($n = 23$)	1 ($n = 31$)	2 ($n = 23$)	3 ($n = 20$)	CAD1/2 vs. CAD3
	Median (IQR)	Median (IQR)	Median (IQR)	Median (IQR)	P-value
Total	80.3[b] (75.9, 102)	109[a] (85.8, 171)	97.9[ab] (82.0, 116)	85.4[b] (74.4, 108)	0.05
Fatty acid precursor					
C18:2 derived	47.7[b] (43.9, 54.7)	59.7[a] (41.7, 76.7)	54.1[ab] (47.4, 63.0)	55.5[ab] (45.0, 73.4)	0.64
C20:4 derived	18.5[b] (14.8, 21.3)	28.0[a] (22.0, 40.7)	28.6[a] (22.6, 42.8)	24.4[a] (18.5, 28.9)	0.11
C20:5 derived	1.35[a] (0.91, 2.01)	1.41[a] (0.83, 2.48)	1.14[ab] (0.76, 3.08)	0.94[b] (0.64, 1.24)	0.04
C22:6 derived	3.36[a] (2.26, 5.06)	3.36[ab] (2.16, 4.25)	3.14[ab] (2.01, 4.03)	2.59[b] (2.20, 3.19)	0.18
Oxylipin group					
Mid-chain HODE	47.7[b] (44.7, 54.7)	59.7[a] (41.7, 76.7)	54.1[ab] (47.4, 63.0)	51.2[ab] (40.1, 68.7)	0.64
EET	1.45[b] (1.28, 1.68)	1.77[a] (1.45, 2.16)	1.63[ab] (1.32, 1.87)	1.51[ab] (1.39, 1.89)	0.47
Mid-chain HETE	6.34[b] (5.06, 9.50)	17.1[a] (12.1, 27.0)	19.0[a] (10.6, 32.4)	13.2[a] (8.07, 19.8)	0.11
EpDPA	0.67 (0.36, 1.06)	0.75 (0.51, 1.13)	0.66 (0.50, 0.94)	0.74 (0.57, 0.99)	0.72
DiHDPA	2.84[a] (1.89, 3.70)	2.50[a] (1.63, 3.45)	2.34[ab] (1.37, 3.28)	1.89[b] (1.37, 2.33)	0.04
Enzyme products					
LOX/CYP1B1 products	55.8[b] (53.0, 68.0)	78.9[a] (60.7, 114)	79.1[a] (59.3, 92.3)	68.8[ab] (55.4, 89.4)	0.27
LOX12-15 products	32.9[b] (19.7, 40.4)	47.9[a] (37.2, 72.2)	53.8[a] (31.5, 62.5)	43.5[a] (31.6, 55.1)	0.26
LOX5 products	21.9[b] (20.1, 25.6)	27.2[a] (21.0, 37.3)	26.5[ab] (19.9, 30.2)	25.1[ab] (18.4, 31.4)	0.55
CYP epoxides	1.44 (1.19, 1.90)	1.70 (1.41, 2.19)	1.56 (1.22, 2.14)	1.94 (1.32, 2.11)	0.86
Hydroxylated CYP epoxides	11.8[a] (8.61, 20.8)	10.0[ab] (8.02, 14.1)	9.50[bc] (7.35, 11.9)	7.77[c] (6.40, 9.21)	0.008
sEH product to substrate ratios					
10,11-DiHDPA/10,11-EpDPA	0.90[a] (0.78, 1.30)	0.81[b] (0.63, 0.93)	0.79[b] (0.59, 1.04)	0.71[b] (0.52, 0.92)	0.21
14,15-DiHET/14,15-EET	4.03[a] (2.91, 5.34)	2.88[b] (2.39, 4.13)	3.76[a] (2.63, 5.37)	2.56[b] (2.29, 4.17)	0.08
19,20-DiHDPA/19,20-EpDPA	4.26[a] (2.48, 6.55)	2.97[a] (2.19, 3.92)	2.95[a] (2.13, 4.77)	1.91[b] (1.58, 2.98)	0.002

The superscripts denote whether averages of specific groups in a row differed at $P \leq 0.05$ using Kruskal–Wallis test. If none of the groups differed from each other, no superscripts are shown. If two groups differed from each other, the significantly higher group got a superscript a, and the significantly lower group got a superscript b, and the group that did not significantly differ from the higher or the lower group got a superscript ab. If three groups differed from each other, the significantly highest group got a superscript a, the significantly lower group got a superscript b, and the group that was significantly lower than the group with a superscript b, got a, c.
HODE, hydroxy-octadecadienoic acid; HETE, hydroxy-eicosatetraenoic acid; EET, epoxy-eicosatrienoic acid; DiHET, dihydroxy-eicosatrienoic acid; EpDPA, epoxy-docosapentaenoic acid; DiHDPA, dihydroxy-docosapentaenoic acid; LOX, lipoxygenase; CYP, cytochrome P450; sEH, soluble epoxide hydrolases.

DiHDPAs, which are generated by hydroxylation of oxidized PUFAs by sEH (**Table 3**). The strongest decline was observed for hydroxylation of 19,20-EpDPA to 19,20-DiHDPA.

Low CAD risk adults had lower total oxylipin concentrations than adults with CAD, specifically omega-6 FA-derived oxylipins and within those mid-chain HETEs (**Tables 2, 3**). These include

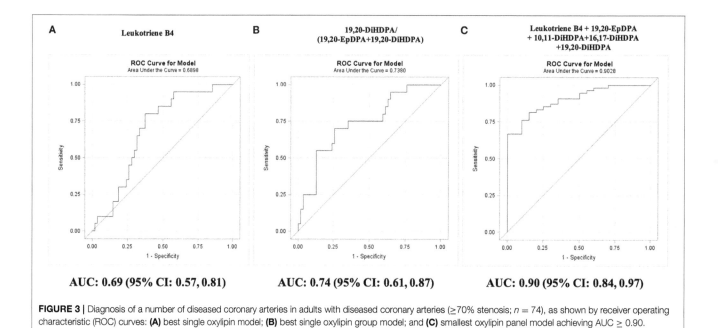

FIGURE 3 | Diagnosis of a number of diseased coronary arteries in adults with diseased coronary arteries (≥70% stenosis; n = 74), as shown by receiver operating characteristic (ROC) curves: **(A)** best single oxylipin model; **(B)** best single oxylipin group model; and **(C)** smallest oxylipin panel model achieving AUC ≥ 0.90.

the following three oxylipins that were significantly lower than in each CAD group: 11,12-EET, 12-HETE, and 15-HETE. We also observed less hydroxylation of 10,11-EpDPA to 10,11-DiHDPA, which is generated by sEH. Concentrations of LA-derived 12,13-DiHOME and DHA-derived DiHDPAs, specifically 19,20-DiHDPA and 16,17-DiHDPA, decreased gradually from adults with low CAD risk to those with three diseased arteries.

Diagnostic Efficacy of Oxylipins

Differences in plasma oxylipin concentrations were noted primarily between two and three diseased vessels. Among individual oxylipins, ARA-derived leukotriene B4 discriminated best three vs. less diseased arteries (AUC: 0.69; 95% CI: 0.57–0.81; P = 0.003; **Figure 3A**). Leukotriene B4 concentrations ≤0.21 nM diagnosed three diseased arteries in 80% of CAD3 adults and less diseased arteries in 65% CAD1 adults, 61% CAD2 adults, and 43% adults with low CAD risk.

Significant AUC values were also observed for EPA-derived 8-iso PGF3a (AUC: 0.67; 95% CI: 0.54–0.80; P = 0.009), three DHA-derived DiHDPA 19,20-DiHDPA (AUC: 0.66; 95% CI: 0.54–0.78; P = 0.01), 16,17-DiHDPA (AUC: 0.65; 95% CI: 0.52–0.79; P = 0.02), 10,11-DiHDPA (AUC: 0.64; 95% CI: 0.51–0.78; P = 0.04), and LA-derived 12,13-DiHOME (AUC: 0.64; 95% CI: 0.51–0.77; P = 0.04).

Among oxylipin groups and ratios, three diseased arteries were best diagnosed by the 19,20-DiHDPA fraction of the sum of 19,20-EpDPA and 19,20-DiHDPA (AUC: 0.74; 95% CI: 0.61–0.87; P = 0.0003; **Figure 3B**). A fraction of <72% diagnosed three diseased arteries in 70% of CAD3 adults and less diseased arteries in 74% CAD1 adults, 70% CAD2 adults, and 78% adults with low CAD risk. Adding 8-iso PGF3a to the fraction improved diagnosis of three diseased arteries to 80% but decreased diagnosis of less diseased arteries to 60% in CAD2

adults. An oxylipin panel of leukotriene B4, 19,20-EpDPA, 19,20-DiHDPA, 13,14-DiHDPA, and 10,11-DiHDPA diagnosed three diseased arteries in all CAD3 adults and less diseased arteries in 70% CAD1 and CAD2 adults (AUC: 0.90; 95% CI: 0.84–0.97; P < 0.0001; **Figure 3C**). The oxylipin panel improved (P = 0.02) diagnosis of three diseased arteries compared with the 10-year Framingham general CVD risk score (AUC: 0.68; 95% CI: 0.52–0.83; P = 0.02).

Prediction of Outcomes in Adults With Diseased Coronary Arteries

Adults with CAD were followed up until November 2019 for a median of 5 years (range: 25–84 months) and adverse events were recorded (i.e., coronary stent placement; CABG surgery; death). Ten participants (three women and seven men; median age: 61 years; range: 51–81 years) were lost to follow-up (**Figure 2**). Given the degree of stenosis, 52 of 64 adults with CAD underwent CABG surgery within 3 months of the angiography (CAD1: 19 of 28; CAD2: 16 of 19; CAD3: 17 of 17): 28 had a CABG surgery (CAD1: 5 of 19; CAD2: 10 of 16; CAD3: 13 of 17) and 26 had a coronary stent placement (CAD1: 16; CAD2: 6; CAD3: 4). Adults with multiple diseased coronary arteries were more likely to receive a CABG. Of the remaining 12 adults with CAD, seven had no further event, two adults with one diseased artery received a coronary artery stent during follow-up, and three died (CAD1: 2; CAD2: 1). In addition, four CAD adults that had undergone open-heart surgery within 3 months (two stents and two CABG) died during follow-up (CAD1: 1; CAD2: 0; CAD3: 3). Survival was not linked to the number of diseased coronary arteries.

Table 4 lists selected demographic and clinical characteristics of adults with diseased coronary arteries (≥70% stenosis) based on outcomes during follow-up. Survival was linked to lower systolic blood pressure or being a male, whereas

TABLE 4 | Demographic and clinical characteristics of adults with diseased coronary arteries (≥70% stenosis) stratified by outcome during 5-year follow-up.

Characteristics	Outcome during follow-up				Contrasts		
	No event (n = 7)	Stent (n = 24)	CABG (n = 26)	Death (n = 7)	No event vs. others	CABG/death vs. others	Death vs. Others
	Mean ± STD	Mean ± STD	Mean ± STD	Mean ± STD	P-value	P-value	P-value
Age (year)	65 ± 8	68 ± 8	67 ± 10	60 ± 17	0.71	0.52	0.31
Male [n (%)]	3 (43)[bc]	19 (79)[ab]	22 (85)[a]	2 (29)[c]	0.08	1	0.02
BMI (kg/m^2)	30.2 ± 8.5	29.9 ± 8.8	28.3 ± 3.3	29.9 ± 5.6	0.70	0.46	0.78
Overweight [n (%)]	1 (14)[b]	9 (38)[ab]	16 (62)[a]	4 (57)[ab]	0.11	0.03	0.70
Obese [n (%)]	3 (43)	9 (38)	7 (27)	2 (29)	0.67	0.43	1
Blood pressure (mmHg)							
Systolic	130 ± 16[ab]	130 ± 16[b]	130 ± 19[ab]	147 ± 15[a]	0.81	0.42	0.02
Diastolic	65 ± 12	72 ± 10	70 ± 11	67 ± 8	0.20	0.63	0.42
Plasma							
Triacylglycerol (mg/dl)	197 ± 131	167 ± 100	123 ± 59	89 ± 42	0.29	0.02	0.13
Total cholesterol (mg/dl)	174 ± 44	187 ± 50	162 ± 42	153 ± 46	0.91	0.06	0.29
HDL cholesterol (mg/dl)	48 ± 14	49 ± 12	44 ± 18	53 ± 14	0.94	0.51	0.39
LDL cholesterol (mg/dl)	92 ± 35	104 ± 37	94 ± 41	73 ± 39	0.79	0.29	0.17
Hba1c (mmol/mol)	5.9 ± 0.8	6.9 ± 0.4	6.2 ± 1.3	6.5 ± 2.5	0.61	0.74	0.95
Medication [n (%)]	7 (100)	23 (96)	25 (96)	7 (100)	1	1	1
Blood pressure (total)	6 (86)	22 (92)	22 (85)	6 (86)	1	0.71	1
ACE inhibitor	2 (29)	10 (42)	6 (23)	2 (29)	1	0.28	1
AR blocker	2 (29)	4 (17)	3 (12)	2 (29)	0.59	0.75	0.59
Beta blocker	3 (43)[b]	20 (83)[a]	17 (65)[ab]	4 (57)[ab]	0.19	0.43	0.67
Calcium channel blocker	3 (43)	4 (17)	6 (23)	1 (14)	0.17	1	1
Diabetes (total)	2 (29)	5 (21)	6 (23)	3 (43)	1	0.78	0.35
Oral hyperglycemia	2 (29)	3 (13)	3 (12)	1 (14)	0.25	0.73	1
Insulin	0	2 (8)	3 (12)	2 (29)	1	0.43	0.17
Hyperlipidemia (total)							
Statin	6 (86)	19 (79)	20 (77)	5 (71)	1	0.77	0.64
Aspirin	6 (86)	20 (83)	21 (81)	5 (71)	1	0.75	0.61
CAD risk factors							
Tobacco use [n (%)]							
Former	0	9 (40)	8 (31)	1 (14)	0.18	1	0.12
Active	1 (14)	2 (8)	4 (15)	3 (43)	1	0.30	0.07
History of [n (%)]							
Hypertension	6 (86)	22 (92)	22 (85)	7 (100)	0.57	1	1
Diabetes	3 (43)	6 (25)	8 (31)	4 (57)	0.67	0.60	0.20
Hypercholesterolemia	7 (100)	24 (100)	23 (88)	7 (100)	1	0.49	1
CVD in family	4 (57)	12 (50)	13 (50)	3 (43)	1	1	1
Total risk (1–5)	3.0 ± 0.8[ab]	2.8 ± 0.7[b]	2.7 ± 1.0[ab]	3.4 ± 1.0[a]	0.60	0.85	0.06
Framingham 10-year CVD risk (%)	23.0 ± 18.8	28.0 ± 17.9	30.1 ± 18.3	28.4 ± 22.2	0.41	0.53	0.98
ACC 10-year ASCVD risk (%)	17.5 ± 11.9	18.9 ± 10.1	20.9 ± 13.8	9.0	0.77	0.77	ND

The superscripts denote whether averages of specific groups in a row differed at P ≤ 0.05. If none of the groups differed from each other, no superscripts are shown. If two groups differed from each other, the significantly higher group got a superscript a, and the significantly lower group got a superscript b, and the group that did not significantly differ from the higher or the lower group got a superscript ab. If three groups differed from each other, the significantly highest group got a superscript a, the significantly lower group got a superscript b, and the group that was significantly lower than the group with a superscript b, got a, c. Data were compared using Student's t-test. Proportions were compared using Fisher's exact test.

CABG, coronary artery bypass grafting; ACE, angiotension converting enzyme; AR, angiotension receptor; ACC, American College of Cardiology; ASCVD, Atherosclerotic Cardiovascular Disease.

survival without CABG was linked to higher plasma triacylglycerol concentrations. Unfavorable outcomes were linked to elevated oxylipin concentrations (**Table 5**), specifically omega-6 FA-derived oxylipins and within those LA-derived mid-chain HODEs and ARA-derived mid-chain HETEs, which are either generated by oxygenation of lipoxygenases

TABLE 5 | Plasma oxylipin concentrations of adults with diseased coronary arteries (≥70% stenosis) stratified by outcome during 5-year follow-up.

Oxylipins (nM)	Outcome during follow-up				Contrasts		
	No event (n = 7)	Stent (n = 24)	CABG (n = 26)	Death (n = 7)	No event vs. others	CABG/death vs. others	Death vs. others
	Median (IQR)	Median (IQR)	Median (IQR)	Median (IQR)	P-value	P-value	P-value
12,13-DiHOME	5.05 (3.81, 6.68)	5.71 (4.25, 7.64)	5.47 (4.29, 8.56)	5.69 (5.09, 6.93)	0.38	0.66	0.82
13(S)-HODE	33.9[cb] (18.5, 37.8)	27.4[b] (17.6, 40.2)	34.1[b] (25.2, 42.2)	46.2[a] (42.6, 58.9)	0.71	0.04	0.007
9(S)-HODE	19.4[cb] (12.2, 25.8)	20.0[b] (11.5, 22.4)	20.9[b] (17.1, 25.8)	30.6[a] (21.9, 56.9)	0.65	0.03	0.01
Leukotriene B4	0.22 (0.15, 0.24)	0.24 (0.17, 0.28)	0.22 (0.17, 0.25)	0.19 (0.16, 0.22)	0.47	0.36	0.14
Thromboxane B2	0.04[ab] (0.02, 0.11)	0.03[b] (0.02, 0.04)	0.04[a] (0.02, 0.06)	0.04[a] (0.04, 0.12)	0.89	0.04	0.08
20-HETE	8.03 (7.75, 9.93)	8.57 (6.88, 10.2)	8.62 (8.11, 10.4)	8.63 (5.66, 9.20)	0.54	0.44	0.58
14,15-EET	0.31 (0.22, 0.41)	0.28 (0.20, 0.38)	0.36 (0.22, 0.46)	0.29 (0.18, 0.38)	0.89	0.20	0.67
11,12-EET	0.35[ab] (0.27, 0.41)	0.29[b] (0.23, 0.38)	0.36[a] (0.22, 0.46)	0.32[ab] (0.24, 0.39)	0.72	0.08	0.92
14,15-DiHET	1.04 (0.87, 1.23)	0.97 (0.74, 1.13)	1.05 (0.89, 1.19)	1.03 (0.86, 1.18)	0.79	0.38	0.97
5-HETE	5.87[a] (4.12, 11.08)	3.68[b] (2.28, 5.00)	4.50[ab] (2.89, 5.98)	5.00[a] (4.43, 8.63)	0.07	0.31	0.04
12-HETE	8.14 (5.42, 11.2)	7.00 (4.60, 10.0)	10.9 (5.54, 20.8)	11.1 (5.48, 25.5)	0.97	0.09	0.38
15-HETE	2.92[ab] (1.84, 2.97)	1.86[b] (1.48, 2.34)	2.52[a] (2.05, 3.19)	2.44[a] (2.13, 4.17)	0.51	0.03	0.27
8-iso PGF3a	0.60[b] (0.29, 0.99)	1.48[a] (0.60, 14.6)	0.64[ab] (0.43, 1.95)	0.39[b] (0.34, 0.72)	0.28	0.08	0.06
17,18-EpETE	0.22 (0.19, 0.33)	0.28 (0.22, 0.35)	0.29 (0.19, 0.35)	0.31 (0.24, 0.39)	0.42	0.68	0.34
11,12-DiHETE	0.06 (0.04, 0.19)	0.05 (0.03, 0.13)	0.08 (0.04,0.12)	0.06 (0.04, 0.09)	0.67	0.81	0.57
19,20-EpDPA	0.70 (0.47, 1.04)	0.51 (0.28, 0.76)	0.64 (0.46, 0.83)	0.49 (0.40-0.56)	0.33	0.54	0.38
10,11-EpDPA	0.12 (0.10, 0.38)	0.10 (0.06, 0.19)	0.13 (0.06, 0.20)	0.09 (0.08, 0.11)	0.35	0.93	0.60
19,20-DiHDPA	1.61 (1.26, 2.81)	1.63 (0.91, 2.36)	1.44 (0.97, 2.18)	1.78 (1.19, 2.73)	0.63	0.64	0.45
13,14-DiHDPA	0.07 (0.06, 0.21)	0.10 (0.06, 0.15)	0.11 (0.08, 0.15)	0.08 (0.04, 0.12)	0.97	0.91	0.20
16,17-DiHDPA	0.20 (0.15, 0.41)	0.20 (0.13, 0.28)	0.18 (0.14, 0.24)	0.20 (0.15, 0.24)	0.43	0.43	0.99
10,11-DiHDPA	0.11 (0.04, 0.33)	0.09 (0.05, 0.13)	0.09 (0.06, 0.16)	0.08 (0.06, 0.11)	0.58	0.79	0.48
7,8-DiHDPA	0.15 (0.08, 0.20)	0.12 (0.08, 0.15)	0.12 (0.09, 0.17)	0.14 (0.11, 0.18)	0.48	0.82	0.67

The superscripts denote whether averages of specific groups in a row differed at P ≤ 0.05 using Kruskal–Wallis test. If none of the groups differed from each other, no superscripts are shown. If two groups differed from each other, the significantly higher group got a superscript a, and the significantly lower group got a superscript b, and the group that did not significantly differ from the higher or the lower group got a superscript ab. If three groups differed from each other, the significantly highest group got a superscript a, the significantly lower group got a superscript b, and the group that was significantly lower than the group with a superscript b, got a, c.

CABG, coronary artery bypass grafting; DiHOME, dihydroxy-octadecenoic acid; HODE, hydroxy-octadecadienoic acid; HETE, hydroxy-eicosatetraenoic acid; EET, epoxy-eicosatrienoic acid; DiHET, dihydroxy-eicosatrienoic acid; EpDPA, epoxy-docosapentaenoic acid; DiHDPA, dihydroxy-docosapentaenoic acid.

TABLE 6 | Plasma concentrations of oxylipin groups in adults with diseased coronary arteries (≥70% stenosis) stratified by outcome during 5-year follow-up.

Oxylipins (nM)	Outcomes during follow-up				Contrasts		
	No event (n = 7)	Stent (n = 24)	CABG (n = 26)	Death (n = 7)	No event vs. others	CABG/death vs. others	Death vs. others
	Median (IQR)	Median (IQR)	Median (IQR)	Median (IQR)	P-value	P-value	P-value
Total	97.8[ab] (62.2, 112)	86.4[b] (69.4, 132)	103[ab] (81.4, 116)	119[a] (97.4, 180)	0.71	0.16	0.05
Fatty acid precursor							
C18:2 derived	59.7[b] (30.7, 62.4)	47.6[b] (28.9, 62.5)	54.9[b] (45.9, 65.8)	76.7[a] (64.5, 135)	0.76	0.04	0.004
C20:4 derived	28.0[ab] (24.9, 35.6)	23.3[b] (18.3, 30.5)	28.4[a] (23.6, 41.1)	29.0[a] (27.3, 44.9)	0.51	0.03	0.19
C20:5 derived	0.87[ab] (0.67, 1.37)	1.95[a] (0.87, 14.9)	0.97[ab] (0.74, 2.48)	0.86[b] (0.66, 1.07)	0.31	0.13	0.17
C22:6 derived	3.02 (2.25, 5.86)	2.95 (1.48, 4.21)	2.58 (2.13, 3.93)	2.96 (2.13, 3.66)	0.58	0.80	0.84
Oxylipin group							
Mid-chain HODE	59.7[b] (30.7, 62.4)	47.6[b] (28.9, 62.5)	54.9[b] (45.9, 65.8)	76.7[a] (64.5, 135)	0.76	0.04	0.004
EET	1.71 (1.45, 1.80)	1.51 (1.37, 1.83)	1.75 (1.44, 2.25)	1.46 (1.32, 1.99)	0.84	0.20	0.76
Mid-chain HETE	17.4[a] (15.2, 21.4)	12.9[b] (10.1, 18.4)	18.0[ab] (11.5, 30.8)	17.9[a] (17.1, 34.1)	0.36	0.08	0.17
EpDPA	0.82 (0.53, 1.42)	0.63 (0.33, 0.92)	0.77 (0.57, 0.97)	0.56 (0.50, 0.75)	0.32	0.59	0.35
DiHDPA	2.07 (1.72, 4.05)	2.13 (1.24, 3.01)	1.89 (1.35, 2.83)	2.26 (1.58, 3.27)	0.64	0.67	0.61
Enzyme products							
LOX/CYP1B1 products	77.7[ab] (47.2, 89.7)	62.6[b] (41.9, 89.6)	73.6[b] (61.7, 92.3)	96.4[a] (87.0, 154)	0.94	0.03	0.01
LOX12-15 products	46.2[bc] (30.3, 48.9)	37.4[c] (24.9, 58.4)	44.9[b] (38.0, 62.5)	57.1[a] (54.7, 72.2)	0.85	0.02	0.02
LOX5 products	26.7[ab] (18.3, 37.3)	23.9[b] (16.0, 28.7)	25.3[b] (21.4, 30.7)	37.1[a] (28.7, 64.8)	0.92	0.07	0.007
CYP epoxides	1.97 (1.41, 2.19)	1.57 (1.07, 1.95)	1.83 (1.34, 2.17)	1.56 (1.27, 1.97)	0.37	0.46	0.58
Hydroxylated CYP epoxides	10.0 (6.94, 10.4)	9.19 (7.50, 10.8)	9.22 (7.29, 12.0)	9.05 (7.96, 9.63)	0.89	0.91	0.94
sEH product to substrate ratios							
10,11-DiHDPA/10,11-EpDPA	0.79 (0.64, 0.94)	0.79 (0.60, 0.96)	0.79 (0.57, 1.04)	0.78 (0.58, 0.93)	0.89	0.88	0.96
14,15-DiHET/14,15-EET	2.83 (2.39, 5.27)	3.31 (2.54, 4.39)	2.79 (2.31, 4.17)	2.96 (2.51, 5.95)	0.99	0.66	0.71
19,20-DiHDPA/19,20-EpDPA	2.85[ab] (1.61, 3.11)	3.83[a] (2.13, 4.39)	2.57[b] (1.70, 3.31)	3.41[ab] (2.69, 4.86)	0.22	0.25	0.23

The superscripts denote whether averages of specific groups in a row differed at P ≤ 0.05 using Kruskal–Wallis test. If none of the groups differed from each other, no superscripts are shown. If two groups differed from each other, the significantly higher group got a superscript a, and the significantly lower group got a superscript b, and the group that did not significantly differ from the higher or the lower group got a superscript ab. If three groups differed from each other, the significantly highest group got a superscript a, the significantly lower group got a superscript b, and the group that was significantly lower than the group with a superscript b, got a, c.
CABG, coronary artery bypass grafting; HODE, hydroxy-octadecadienoic acid; HETE, hydroxy-eicosatetraenoic acid; EET, epoxy-eicosatrienoic acid; DiHET, dihydroxy-eicosatrienoic acid; EpDPA, epoxy-docosapentaenoic acid; DiHDPA, dihydroxy-docosapentaenoic acid; LOX, lipoxygenase; CYP, cytochrome P450; sEH, soluble epoxide hydrolases.

or hydroxylation of CYP1B1 (**Table 6**). Concentrations of LA-derived 9(S)-HODE and 13(S)-HODE and ARA-derived thromboxane B2, 5-HETE, and 15-HETE increased gradually from stent placement to CABG to death. In contrast, concentrations of EPA-derived 8-iso PGF3α were lower with unfavorable outcomes.

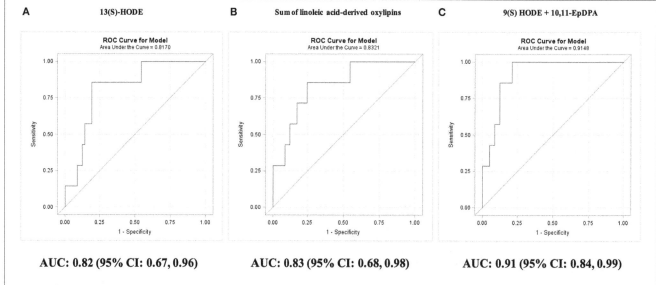

FIGURE 4 | Prediction of survival during 5-year follow-up in adults with diseased coronary arteries (≥70% stenosis; *n* = 64), as shown by receiver operating characteristic (ROC) curves: **(A)** best single oxylipin model; **(B)** best single oxylipin group model; and **(C)** smallest oxylipin panel model achieving AUC ≥ 0.90.

Predictive Efficacy of Oxylipins

Among individual oxylipins, survival was predicted best by LA-derived 13(S)-HODE (AUC: 0.82; 95% CI: 0.67–0.96; $P <$ 0.0001); concentrations of 13(S)-HODE >42.5 nM predicted mortality in 86% nonsurviving adults with CAD and predicted survival in 81% surviving adults with CAD and 91% Astoria cohort adults (**Figure 4A**).

Adding 10,11-EpDPA concentrations <0.20 nM for classification, improved survival prediction to 91% surviving adults with CAD and 96% Astoria cohort adults (AUC: 0.90; 95% CI: 0.81–0.99; $P <$ 0.0001). The two-oxylipin panel improved ($P =$ 0.02) survival prediction compared with the 10-year Framingham general CVD risk score (AUC: 0.49; 95% CI: 0.16–0.83; $P =$ 0.97).

The four remaining individual oxylipins that could significantly predict survival were ordered by P-value: EPA-derived 9(S)-HODE (AUC: 0.79; 95% CI: 0.62–0.96; $P =$ 0.0007), ARA-derived 5-HETE (AUC: 0.73; 95% CI: 0.58–0.89; $P =$ 0.01), EPA-derived 8-iso PGF3α (AUC: 0.72; 95% CI: 0.54–0.89; $P =$ 0.02), and ARA-derived thromboxane B2 (AUC: 0.72; 95% CI: 0.54–0.89; $P =$ 0.03). The best single predictor for survival was the sum of LA-derived oxylipins (AUC: 0.83; 95% CI: 0.68–0.98; $P <$ 0.0001; **Figure 4B**). The targeted AUC value of at least 0.90 was achieved with a two-oxylipin panel of 9(S)-HODE and 10,11-EpDPA (AUC: 0.91; 95% CI: 0.84–0.99; $P <$ 0.0001; **Figure 4C**).

Among individual oxylipins, survival without requiring CABG was best predicted by LA-derived 9(S)-HODE (AUC: 0.65; 95% CI: 0.52–0.79; $P =$ 0.03; **Figure 5A**). The two-remaining individual oxylipins that could significantly predict survival without requiring CABG were ordered by P-value: ARA-derived 15-HETE (AUC: 0.65; 95% CI: 0.52–0.79; $P =$ 0.03) and ARA-derived thromboxane B2 (AUC: 0.65; 95% CI: 0.51–0.79; $P =$ 0.03). The best single predictor was the sum of

LOX12/15-epoxygenated oxylipins (AUC: 0.67; 95% CI: 0.54–0.81; $P =$ 0.01; **Figure 5B**). The targeted AUC value of ≥0.85 was achieved with a linear combination of 9(S)-HODE, 5-HETE, 14,15-DiHET, thromboxane B2, 19,20-EPDPA, and 16,17-DiHDPA (AUC: 0.85; 95% CI: 0.75–0.94; $P =$ 0.0001; **Figure 5C**). The oxylipin panel improved predictive efficacy ($P =$ 0.004) compared with the 10-year Framingham general CVD risk score (AUC: 0.55; 95% CI: 0.40–0.71; $P =$ 0.51).

The only single oxylipin that could significantly predict no events in CAD adults was ARA-derived 5-HETE (AUC: 0.71; 95% CI: 0.52–0.91; $P =$ 0.03). In general, patients without follow-up events had oxylipin values similar to patients who died during follow-up or had a surgery for a full blockage. The 10-year Framingham general CVD risk score had an AUC of 0.62 (95% CI: 0.38–0.87; $P =$ 0.33).

DISCUSSION

In the current study, we provide evidence that in adults with diseased coronary arteries (>70% stenosis), plasma oxylipin panels may discriminate among the number of diseased coronary arteries and predict median 5-year outcomes, which, to our knowledge, has not been previously reported.

Analysis of Plasma Oxylipins

Novel analytical methods for extraction, detection, and data processing allow for the separation of a large number of diverse oxylipins in a short period of time (3, 12, 22, 23). In the present study, we detected and verified with standards 39 oxylipins of diverse origin and biosynthetic pathways in a 22-min LC-MS/MS run. Similar to inflammatory cytokines, low abundance, limited dynamic range, limited tissue specificity, very short half-life, significant daily fluctuation, and high inter- and intra-assay variation, limit the use of oxylipins as diagnostic biomarkers

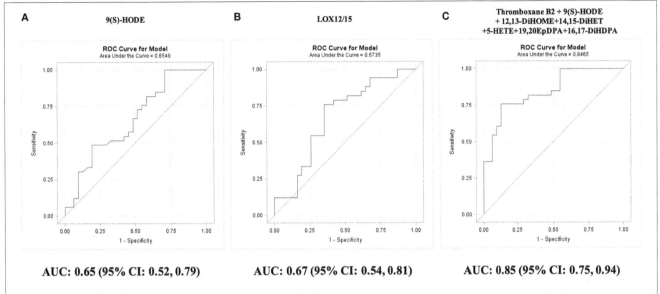

FIGURE 5 | Prediction of survival without coronary artery bypass graft (CABG) surgery during 5-year follow-up in adults with diseased coronary arteries (≥70% stenosis; *n* = 64), as shown by receiver operating characteristic (ROC) curves: **(A)** best single oxylipin model; **(B)** best single oxylipin group model; and **(C)** smallest oxylipin panel model achieving AUC ≥ 0.85.

(16). For diagnostic and prognostic research, a good biomarker must have a large dynamic range within the population. In the current study, 22 oxylipins had concentrations in the linear quantification range in at least 98% of sampled adults, which allowed us to evaluate the most abundant enzymatic oxylipin pathways; however, excluded pathways generated by COX or aspirin and ROS.

Diagnostic and Prognostic Efficacy of Oxylipins in CAD

Currently used risk assessment scores of CAD, such as the 10-year Framingham general CVD risk score, have been developed for the general population and have shown limited efficacy in high risk CAD adult management (4). In adults with significant diseased coronary arteries, a five-oxylipin panel diagnosed three diseased arteries with 100% sensitivity and 70% specificity. During a median 5-year survival, a panel of two oxylipins predicted survival with 86% sensitivity and 91% specificity. The oxylipin panels improved three diseased artery diagnosis and survival prognosis compared with the 10-year Framingham general CVD risk score.

Clinical Relevance of Oxylipins in CAD

Coronary artery disease (CAD) limits nutrient and oxygen supply to generate sufficient energy in cardiomyocytes, which becomes an even bigger challenge as the number and severity of diseased coronary arteries increase or plaques rupture with subsequent thrombus formation (5). In the present study, adults with more diseased coronary arteries (≥70% stenosis) had lower plasma concentrations of hydroxylated omega-3 PUFA-derived epoxides, specifically we observed lower levels of 19,20-DiHDPA (**Figure 6**). To our knowledge, the link between oxylipin concentrations and number of diseased

coronary arteries has not been previously reported. The enzyme responsible for hydroxylation of epoxides is sEH, which is induced by hypoxia and has been proposed as potential pharmacological target for CAD (26–28). However, we cannot exclude the possibility that participants with CAD were already on medication that inhibited soluble CYP450 epoxide hydrolase. However, the gradual decrease in concentrations of LA-derived 12,13-DiHOME and DHA-derived DiHDPA with increasing diseased artery number support the hypothesis that the lower concentrations are a response to the hypoxia caused by arterial occlusions (29).

Five-year survival and no CABG surgery was linked to lower concentrations of oxygenated omega-6 PUFA LA and ARA, specifically lower concentrations of LA-derived mid-chain HODE and ARA-derived mid-chain HETE, which are either generated by oxygenation of lipoxygenases or hydroxylation of CYP1B1 (**Figure 6**). In support, elevated 15-HETE concentrations and LOX-15 enzymatic activity have been reported in ischemic heart disease and hypoxic human cardiomyocytes and cardiac endothelial cells (15), supporting our hypothesis that the elevated mid-chain HETE and HODE concentrations are a response to the hypoxia caused by the arterial occlusions. High concentrations of HETE, including 5-HETE, 12-HETE, and 15-HETE, were reported in atherosclerotic plaques, especially in those that were more likely to rupture (14). Elevated circulating concentrations of 5-HETE and 12-HETE were observed in individuals after cardiac surgery (16). Elevated concentrations of 5-HETE, 12-HETE, and 15-HETE were reported in individuals with acute cardiac syndrome (17). Elevated circulating concentrations of 5-HETE, 12-HETE, and 15-HETE were reported in individuals with CAD by Xu et al. (20), whereas only numerical increases were reported by Shishebor et al. (19) and Auguet

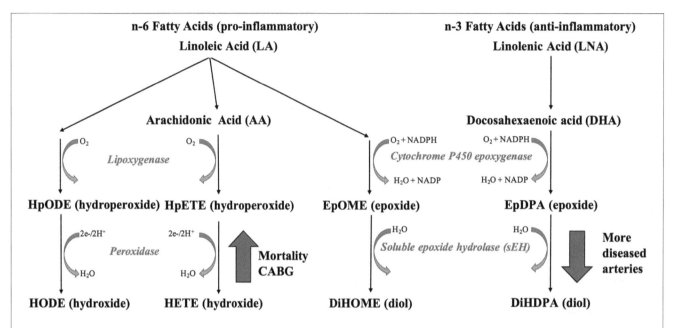

FIGURE 6 | The link between plasma oxylipins and coronary artery disease. Adults with more diseased coronary arteries ($\geq$70% stenosis) had lower plasma concentrations of hydroxylated omega-3 fatty acid-derived epoxygenated oxylipins, which was linked to decreased soluble epoxide hydrolase (sEH) activity. Nonsurviving adults with diseased coronary arteries had higher plasma concentration of oxygenated omega-6 fatty acids, which was linked to increased lipoxygenase or CYP1B1 activity.

et al. (21); the latter did not quantify 5-HETE. The role of elevated mid-chain HETE in cardiovascular dysfunction has been well documented, whereas less is known of the role of mid-chain HODE (3, 30, 31). Inhibition of the oxygenation step of the LOX pathway has been proposed as treatment option for CAD management (30), suggesting clinical relevance of the identified oxylipins as indicator of chronic hypoxia.

Limitations of the Study

First, the number of adults with CAD were relatively small and came from a high-risk group, which underwent coronary angiography, but in whom the presence and extent of CAD was clearly defined. Second, all but five adults with CAD were on medical therapy for treatment for hypertension, hyperlipidemia, and/or diabetes, which could have influenced the levels of oxylipins. Third, differences in collateral blood flow may have impacted oxylipin concentration, which was not assessed in this cohort. Fourth, most adults with CAD had to undergo revascularization shortly after angiography, which may impact later outcomes. Fifth, follow-up time was limited to <6 years, which impacted the number of outcomes. Sixth, diagnostic and prognostic oxylipin panels could not be validated due to the limited clearly defined population size.

SUMMARY AND CONCLUSION

In summary, we observed a link between plasma oxylipin concentrations and CAD severity. Concentrations of six oxylipins decreased with the number of diseased arteries; a panel of five oxylipins diagnosed three diseased arteries with 100% sensitivity and 70% specificity. Concentrations of five oxylipins were lower and one oxylipin was higher with survival; a panel of two oxylipins predicted survival during follow-up with 86% sensitivity and 91% specificity. Plasma oxylipins may assist in diagnosis and prognosis of CAD in high-risk adults in combination with standard risk assessment tools. Our promising results require confirmation in larger unselected populations.

AUTHOR CONTRIBUTIONS

DL, MG-J, GB, AA, DR, NA, CM, and SK: conceptualization. DL, MG-J, GB, AA, AV, JM, DJ, and CM: data curation. DL, MG-J, and GB: formal analysis and writing (original draft). MG-J, DJ, CM, and SK: funding acquisition. DL, MG-J, GB, AA, AV, JM, DJ, DR, NA, CM, and SK: investigation and writing (review and editing). DL, MG-J, GB, AA, DJ, CM, and SK: methodology. DL, MG-J, NA, CM, and SK: project administration. MG-J and GB: software and visualization. GB, DJ, CM, and SK: supervision. DL, MG-J, GB, DJ, CM, and SK: validation. All authors contributed to the article and approved the submitted version.

ACKNOWLEDGMENTS

We thank Jeffrey Morrè (Operational Manager, Oregon State University Mass Spectrometry Center) for technical assistance and advice.

REFERENCES

1. Roth GA, Johnson C, Abajobir A, Abd-Allah F, Abera SF, Abyu G, et al. Global, regional, and national burden of cardiovascular diseases for 10 causes, 1990 to 2015. *J Am Coll Cardiol.* (2017) 70:1–25. doi: 10.1016/j.jacc.2017.04.052

2. Pagidipati NJ, Gaziano TA. Estimating deaths from cardiovascular disease: a review of global methodologies of mortality measurement. *Circulation.* (2013) 127:749–56. doi: 10.1161/CIRCULATIONAHA.112.128413

3. Nayeem MA. Role of oxylipins in cardiovascular diseases. *Acta Pharmacol Sin.* (2018) 39:1142–54. doi: 10.1038/aps.2018.24

4. Hajar R. Risk factors for coronary artery disease: historical perspectives. *Heart Views.* (2017) 18:109–14. doi: 10.4103/HEARTVIEWS.HEARTVIEWS_106_17

5. Ambrose JA, Singh M. Pathophysiology of coronary artery disease leading to acute coronary syndromes. *F1000Prime Rep.* (2015) 7:8. doi: 10.12703/P7-08

6. Bentzon JF, Otsuka F, Virmani R, Falk E. Mechanisms of plaque formation and rupture. *Circ Res.* (2014) 114:1852–66. doi: 10.1161/CIRCRESAHA.114.302721

7. Rafieian-Kopaei M, Setorki M, Doudi M, Baradaran A, Nasri H. Atherosclerosis: process, indicators, risk factors and new hopes. *Int J Prev Med.* (2014) 5:927–46. https://www.ncbi.nlm.nih.gov/pubmed/25489440.

8. Zhong H, Yin H. Role of lipid peroxidation derived 4-hydroxynonenal (4-HNE) in cancer: focusing on mitochondria. *Redox Biol.* (2014) 4:193–9. doi: 10.1016/j.redox.2014.12.011

9. Gaweł S, Wardas M, Niedworok E, Wardas P. Dialdehyd malonowy (MDA) jako wskaźnik procesów peroksydacji w organizmie. *Wiad Lek.* (2004) 57:453–5.

10. Parthasarathy S, Raghavamenon A, Garelnabi MO, Santanam N. Oxidized low-density lipoprotein. *Methods Mol Biol.* (2010) 610:403–17. doi: 10.1007/978-1-60327-029-8_24

11. Catala A. Lipid peroxidation of membrane phospholipids generates hydroxy-alkenals and oxidized phospholipids active in physiological and/or pathological conditions. *Chem Phys Lipids.* (2009) 157:1–11. doi: 10.1016/j.chemphyslip.2008.09.004

12. Tourdot BE, Ahmed I, Holinstat M. The emerging role of oxylipins in thrombosis and diabetes. *Front Pharmacol.* (2014) 4:176. doi: 10.3389/fphar.2013.00176

13. Gabbs M, Leng S, Devassy JG, Monirujjaman M, Aukema HM. Advances in our understanding of oxylipins derived from dietary PUFAs. *Adv Nutr.* (2015) 6:513–540. doi: 10.3945/an.114.007732

14. Mallat Z, Nakamura T, Ohan J, Lesèche G, Tedgui A, Maclouf J, et al. The relationship of hydroxyeicosatetraenoic acids and F2-isoprostanes to plaque instability in human carotid atherosclerosis. *J Clin Invest.* (1999) 103:421–7. doi: 10.1172/JCI3985

15. Lundqvist A, Sandstedt M, Sandstedt J, Wickelgren R, Hansson GI, Jeppsson A, et al. The arachidonate 15-lipoxygenase enzyme product 15-HETE is present in heart tissue from patients with ischemic heart disease and enhances clot formation. *PLoS One.* (2016) 11:1–13. doi: 10.1371/journal.pone.0161629

16. Strassburg K, Huijbrechts AML, Kortekaas KA, Lindeman JH, Pedersen TL, Dane A, et al. Quantitative profiling of oxylipins through comprehensive LC-MS/MS analysis: application in cardiac surgery. *Anal Bioanal Chem.* (2012) 404:1413–26. doi: 10.1007/s00216-012-6226-x

17. Zu L, Guo G, Zhou B, Gao W. Relationship between metabolites of arachidonic acid and prognosis in patients with acute coronary syndrome. *Thromb Res.* (2016) 144:192–201. doi: 10.1016/j.thromres.2016.06.031

18. Caligiuri SPB, Aukema HM, Ravandi A, Lavallée R, Guzman R, Pierce GN. Specific plasma oxylipins increase the odds of cardiovascular and cerebrovascular events in patients with peripheral artery disease. *Can J Physiol Pharmacol.* (2017) 95:961–8. doi: 10.1139/cjpp-2016-0615

19. Shishehbor MH, Zhang R, Medina H, Brennan ML, Brennan DM, Ellis SG, et al. Systemic elevations of free radical oxidation products of arachidonic acid are associated with angiographic evidence of coronary artery disease. *Free Radic Biol Med.* (2006) 41:1678–83. doi: 10.1016/j.freeradbiomed.2006.09.001

20. Xu YJ, Ho WE, Xu F, Wen T, Ong CN. Exploratory investigation reveals parallel alteration of plasma fatty acids and eicosanoids in coronary artery disease patients. *Prostaglandins Other Lipid Mediat.* (2013) 106:29–36. doi: 10.1016/j.prostaglandins.2013.08.003

21. Auguet T, Aragonès G, Colom M, Aguilar C, Martín-Paredero V, Canela N, et al. Targeted metabolomic approach in men with carotid plaque. *PLoS One.* (2018) 13:1–11. doi: 10.1371/journal.pone.0200547

22. Pedersen TL, Newman JW. Establishing and performing targeted multi-residue analysis for lipid mediators and fatty acids in small clinical plasma samples. *Methods Mol Biol.* (2018) 1730:175–212. doi: 10.1007/978-1-4939-7592-1_13

23. La Frano MR, Hernandez-Carretero A, Weber N, Borkowski K, Pedersen TL, Osborn O, et al. Diet-induced obesity and weight loss alter bile acid concentrations and bile acid-sensitive gene expression in insulin target tissues of C57BL/6J mice. *Nutr Res.* (2017) 46:11–21. doi: 10.1016/j.nutres.2017.07.006

24. García-Jaramillo M, Lytle AK, Spooner HM, Jump BD. A lipidomic analysis of docosahexaenoic acid (22:6, ω3) mediated attenuation of western diet induced nonalcoholic steatohepatitis in male Ldlr$^{-/-}$ mice. *Metabolites.* (2019) 9:252. doi: 10.3390/metabo9110252

25. Housley L, Magana AA, Hsu A, Beaver LM, Wong CP, Stevens JF, et al. Untargeted metabolomic screen reveals changes in human plasma metabolite profiles following consumption of fresh broccoli sprouts. *Mol Nutr Food Res.* (2018) 62:e1700665. doi: 10.1002/mnfr.201700665

26. Morisseau C, Hammock BD. Impact of soluble epoxide hydrolase and epoxyeicosanoids on human health. *Annu Rev Pharmacol Toxicol.* (2012) 53:37–58. doi: 10.1146/annurev-pharmtox-011112-140244

27. Wagner KM, McReynolds CB, Schmidt WK, Hammock BD. Soluble epoxide hydrolase as a therapeutic target for pain, inflammatory and neurodegenerative diseases. *Pharmacol Ther.* (2017) 180:62–76. doi: 10.1016/j.pharmthera.2017.06.006

28. Imig JD. Prospective for cytochrome P450 epoxygenase cardiovascular and renal therapeutics. *Pharmacol Ther.* (2018) 192:1–19. doi: 10.1016/j.pharmthera.2018.06.015

29. Fleming I. The pharmacology of the cytochrome P450 epoxygenase/soluble epoxide hydrolase axis in the vasculature and cardiovascular disease. *Pharmacol Rev.* (2014) 66:1106–40. doi: 10.1124/pr.113.007781

30. Dobrian AD, Lieb DC, Cole BK, Taylor-Fishwick DA, Chakrabarti SK, Nadler JL. Functional and pathological roles of the 12- and 15-lipoxygenases. *Prog Lipid Res.* (2011) 50:115–31. doi: 10.1016/j.plipres.2010.10.005

31. Maayah ZH, El-Kadi AOS. The role of mid-chain hydroxyeicosatetraenoic acids in the pathogenesis of hypertension and cardiac hypertrophy. *Arch Toxicol.* (2016) 90:119–36. doi: 10.1007/s00204-015-1620-8

Novel Urinary Glycan Biomarkers Predict Cardiovascular Events in Patients with Type 2 Diabetes: A Multicenter Prospective Study With 5-Year Follow Up (U-CARE Study 2)

Koki Mise[1†], Mariko Imamura[1†], Satoshi Yamaguchi[1], Mayu Watanabe[1],*
Chigusa Higuchi[1], Akihiro Katayama[2], Satoshi Miyamoto[3], Haruhito A. Uchida[4],
Atsuko Nakatsuka[1], Jun Eguchi[1], Kazuyuki Hida[5], Tatsuaki Nakato[6], Atsuhito Tone[6],
Sanae Teshigawara[6], Takashi Matsuoka[7], Shinji Kamei[7], Kazutoshi Murakami[7],
Ikki Shimizu[8], Katsuhiro Miyashita[9], Shinichiro Ando[10], Tomokazu Nunoue[11],
*Michihiro Yoshida[3], Masao Yamada[12], Kenichi Shikata[3] and Jun Wada[1**]*

[1] Department of Nephrology, Rheumatology, Endocrinology and Metabolism, Okayama University Graduate School of Medicine, Dentistry and Pharmaceutical Sciences, Okayama, Japan, [2] Diabetes Center, Okayama University Hospital, Okayama, Japan, [3] Center for Innovative Clinical Medicine, Okayama University Hospital, Okayama, Japan, [4] Department of Chronic Kidney Disease and Cardiovascular Disease, Okayama University Graduate School of Medicine, Dentistry and Pharmaceutical Sciences, Okayama, Japan, [5] Department of Diabetology and Metabolism, National Hospital Organization Okayama Medical Center, Okayama, Japan, [6] Okayama Saiseikai General Hospital, Okayama, Japan, [7] Kurashiki Central Hospital, Kurashiki, Japan, [8] The Sakakibara Heart Institute of Okayama, Okayama, Japan, [9] Japanese Red Cross Okayama Hospital, Okayama, Japan, [10] Okayama City General Medical Center, Okayama, Japan, [11] Nunoue Clinic, Tsuyama, Japan, [12] GlycoTechnica Ltd., Yokohama, Japan

Correspondence:
Koki Mise
kokims-frz@okayama-u.ac.jp
orcid.org/0000-0003-0296-7429
Jun Wada
junwada@okayama-u.ac.jp
orcid.org/0000-0003-1468-5170

[†] These authors have contributed equally to this work

Background: Although various biomarkers predict cardiovascular event (CVE) in patients with diabetes, the relationship of urinary glycan profile with CVE in patients with diabetes remains unclear.

Methods: Among 680 patients with type 2 diabetes, we examined the baseline urinary glycan signals binding to 45 lectins with different specificities. Primary outcome was defined as CVE including cardiovascular disease, stroke, and peripheral arterial disease.

Results: During approximately a 5-year follow-up period, 62 patients reached the endpoint. Cox proportional hazards analysis revealed that urinary glycan signals binding to two lectins were significantly associated with the outcome after adjustment for known indicators of CVE and for false discovery rate, as well as increased model fitness. Hazard ratios for these lectins (+1 SD for the glycan index) were UDA (recognizing glycan: mixture of Man5 to Man9): 1.78 (95% CI: 1.24–2.55, $P = 0.002$) and Calsepa [High-Man (Man2–6)]: 1.56 (1.19–2.04, $P = 0.001$). Common glycan binding to these lectins was high-mannose type of N-glycans. Moreover, adding glycan index for UDA to a model including known confounders improved the outcome prediction [Difference of Harrel's C-index: 0.028 (95% CI: 0.001–0.055, $P = 0.044$), net reclassification improvement at 5-year risk increased by 0.368 (0.045–0.692, $P = 0.026$), and the Akaike information criterion and Bayesian information criterion decreased from 725.7 to 716.5, and 761.8 to 757.2, respectively].

Conclusion: The urinary excretion of high-mannose glycan may be a valuable biomarker for improving prediction of CVE in patients with type 2 diabetes, and provides the rationale to explore the mechanism underlying abnormal *N*-glycosylation occurring in patients with diabetes at higher risk of CVE.

Trial Registration: This study was registered with the University Hospital Medical Information Network on June 26, 2012 (Clinical trial number: UMIN000011525, URL: https://upload.umin.ac.jp/cgi-open-bin/ctr_e/ctr_view.cgi?recptno=R000013482).

Keywords: cardiovascular event, diabetes, lectins, N-glycans, urinary biomarkers

INTRODUCTION

Cardiovascular disease (CVD) is a global burden especially in low- and middle-income countries and the leading cause of disability and mortality (1). The understanding of CVD risk factors is quite important to establish the cardiovascular risk prediction models. The age, gender, body mass index (BMI), systolic blood pressure (SBP), diabetes mellitus, smoking, total cholesterol levels, and past cardiovascular events are established and also traditional risk factors in middle-aged and older individuals (2). Chronic kidney disease (CKD) is an emerging global health burden with prevalence of ~15% of adult populations and is independently associated with increased cardiovascular event (CVE) including stroke and peripheral arterial disease (PAD) besides the traditional risk factors (3, 4). The addition of albuminuria and estimated glomerular filtration rate (eGFR) to traditional risk factors is significantly associated with cardiovascular outcomes in meta-analysis of general population cohort (5, 6). In type 2 diabetes, the CVE risk prediction is potentially improved by novel biomarkers involved in the biological process, not explained by the traditional risk factors (7). The improvement of risk prediction is statistically evaluated by discrimination ability and reclassification. The area under the receiver operating characteristic (AUROC) or c-index is a measurement for discrimination capacity of classification model, while the net reclassification improvement (NRI) is a commonly used measure for the prediction increment by the addition of new biomarkers. In the Second Manifestations of ARTertial disease (SMART) and the European Prospective Investigation into Cancer and Nutrition-NL (EPIC-NL) (8), Action in Diabetes and Vascular Disease: Preterax and Diamicron Modified Release Controlled Evaluation (ADVANCE) study (9), and the Outcome Reduction With Initial Glargine Intervention (ORIGIN) trial (10), the 23, 16, and 284 serum or plasma biomarkers were evaluated as to whether these biomarkers independently improve the AUROC and NRI, respectively. The three biomarkers in SMART/EPIC-NL, six in ADVANCE, and 10 in ORIGIN were identified in the prediction of CVD composite outcomes. N-terminal pro-B-type natriuretic peptide (NT-proBNP) was only the common biomarker in two studies for the prediction of composite CVE. In addition to the candidate approach for the identification of biomarkers, non-biased screening using

metabolomic approach was also attempted such as amino acid (11) and lipid profiles (12).

The vigorous attempts were made for the identification of circulating biomarkers, and some of the urinary biomarkers were independently associated with CVE in patients with type 2 diabetes; however, they have failed to achieve significant incremental ability based on c-statistic and NRI (13–15). Urine albumin creatinine ratio (UACR) and eGFR are now regarded as the classical risk factors for CVE in type 2 diabetes; the concept of "cardiorenal syndrome" suggests that the identification of urinary biomarkers is promising approach. In the Urinary biomarker for Continuous And Rapid progression of diabetic nEphropathy (U-CARE) study, we performed urinary lectin microarray, measured urinary glycan signals binding to 45 lectins, and evaluated the potential for the prediction of 30% decline of eGFR or end-stage renal disease (ESRD) in the patients with type 2 diabetes (16). We found that the urinary glycan binding signals to *Sambucus nigra* (SNA), *Ricinus communis* (RCA120), *Dolichos biflorus* (DBA), *Agaricus bisporus* (ABA), *Artocarpus integrifolia* (Jacalin), and *Amaranthus caudatus* (ACA) improved the prediction of renal outcome in the models employing the known risk factors (16). The U-CARE study suggested that the global alterations of glycosylation of urinary protein are valuable disease progression markers and may be linked to disease mechanisms in diabetic kidney disease (DKD). The aim of this study (U-CARE Study 2) is to investigate in patients with type 2 diabetes the impact of urinary lectin microarray on the prediction of CVE by adding the glycan binding signals in the multivariate model containing the established risk factors of CVE.

MATERIALS AND METHODS

Study Design and Participants

This is a second report of the U-CARE Study, a prospective cohort study, which started in 2012. Precise study design was described previously (16). In the current study, among 688 patients with type 2 diabetes admitted to multi-institutions in Japan, 680 patients were enrolled. Eight patients were excluded in this study since they were diagnosed with slowly progressive type 1 diabetes during follow-up. The diagnosis of diabetes was based on the Japanese Diabetes Society criteria (17). This study was registered with the University Hospital Medical Information

Network in June 2012 (UMIN000011525). Written informed consent was obtained from all participants.

Laboratory Parameters and Definitions

Urinary glycans were measured by the evanescent-field fluorescence-assisted lectin microarray (18). In brief, we measured urinary levels of Cy3-labeled glycoprotein binding to 45 lectins coated on microplates. In a previous study, we demonstrated that net glycan intensity [Net-I; raw glycan intensity (Raw-I)—background intensity] more accurately predicted the 24-h urinary glycan in comparison with Net-I or Raw-I/urinary creatinine ratios (16, 19). Based on the evidence, we analyzed glycan indexes defined by Net-I and logarithmically transformed Net-I when they did not follow normal distribution.

In this study, CVD was defined as events requiring admission for treatment, excluding the events with arrhythmia, dilated cardiomyopathy, and valvular heart disease to focus attention on the atherosclerotic cardiovascular diseases. Stroke was defined as cerebral bleeding and infarction requiring admission for treatment, while PAD as an event requiring admission for open surgery and/or endovascular intervention. CVE was defined as any CVD, stroke, or PAD events. Mortality due to cardiovascular death or other causes was also assessed. BMI was calculated as weight divided by the square of height (kg/m^2). Hypertension was defined as a baseline blood pressure $\geq 140/90$ mmHg or use of antihypertensive drugs. GFR was estimated by the Japanese coefficient-modified Chronic Kidney Disease Epidemiology Collaboration equation. The baseline UACR (mg/gCr) was measured in a spot urine specimen, and normoalbuminuria, microalbuminuria, and macroalbuminuria were defined as UACR <30 mg/gCr, $30 \leq$ UACR < 300 mg/gCr, and 300 mg/gCr $\leq$ UACR, respectively. Hemoglobin A1c (HbA1c) data are presented as National Glycohemoglobin Standardization Program values according to the recommendations of the Japanese Diabetes Society and the International Federation of Clinical Chemistry (20). The grade of diabetic retinopathy was determined by an ophthalmologist at baseline. The average annual values of clinical parameters including HbA1c, SBP, and diastolic blood pressure (DBP) were obtained. The administration of statin, angiotensin-converting enzyme (ACE) inhibitor or angiotensin II type I receptor blocker (ARB), glucagon-like peptide-1 receptor agonists (GLP1), and sodium glucose transporter 2 (SGLT2) inhibitor during follow-up were also recorded. These data and previous CVE were compared between patients with and without outcome.

Study Endpoint

The primary endpoint was defined as incidence of CVE, and follow-up period was defined as the period from the initiation of observation to the earliest CVE, death, or last observation of clinical variables.

Statistical Analysis

Data were presented as percentages or the mean ± standard deviation (SD), as appropriate. All skewed variables were subjected to natural logarithmic transformation to improve normality before analysis. Correlations among glycan indexes

were evaluated by Pearson correlation analysis. The cumulative incidence rate of the primary outcome was estimated by Kaplan–Meier curves for urinary glycan quartiles in all patients, and incidence rates were compared with the log-rank test, including trend test among quartile groups. The Cox proportional hazards model was used to calculate the hazard ratio (HR) and 95% confidence interval (CI) for the event-censored endpoint. HR and 95% CI for the 1 SD increase of glycan index were individually calculated in each model. In the multivariate model, HRs were adjusted for age, gender, BMI, SBP, low-density lipoprotein (LDL) cholesterol, HbA1c, eGFR, and previous CVE at baseline. These covariates were selected as potential confounders on the basis of biological plausibility and previous reports (15, 21). False discovery rates (FDRs) for 45 glycan indexes were calculated by the Benjamini–Hochberg procedure in these Cox regression analyses to control the expected proportion of false rejections (22). The level of FDR was defined as 0.05. Time-dependent area under curve (AUC) in multivariate Cox regression analysis was obtained by integration of AUC in every 0.2 year from 0.5 year-observation calculated by 500 bootstrap sampling (23). We also compared Harrell's concordance index (c-index) between multivariate Cox proportional hazards models with or without glycan biomarkers. In addition, the Akaike information criterion (AIC) and Bayesian information criterion (BIC) in the multivariate Cox regression models were calculated to compare the model fitness. Furthermore, improvement in discriminating the 5-year risk of the study outcome was assessed by analyses of AUROC, category-free NRI, and absolute integrated discrimination improvement (IDI), as reported elsewhere (24, 25). The 95% CIs for the differences of the Harrell's c-index and AUROC, category-free NRI, and IDI were computed from 5,000 bootstrap samples to adjust for optimism bias. Two-tailed P-values < 0.05 were considered as statistically significant. Analyses and creation of graphs were performed with Stata SE software (version 14.0, StataCorp LP) and Origin (version 2018, OriginLab).

RESULTS

Observation Period and Outcome Incidence

The median follow-up period was 4.8 years [interquartile range (IQR): 3.6–5.1 years]. During follow-up, the primary endpoint (CVE) occurred in 62 patients (9%), and 21 patients (3%) died. CVE was the cause of two patient deaths. Detailed information of CVE and other causes of death are shown in **Supplementary Tables 1, 2.**

Clinical Characteristics

The clinical characteristics of all participants at baseline are displayed in **Table 1.** Their age was 63 ± 11 years (mean ± SD), 61% of the patients were men, and 24% of them had previous CVE. The median duration of diabetes was 11.1 years (IQR: 6.2–17.7), and baseline HbA1c was 7.1 ± 1.1% (54.3 ± 12.0 mmol/mol). Under 56% of statin use, the baseline LDL and non-high-density lipoprotein (non-HDL) cholesterol levels were 100.1 ± 25.3 and 126.5 ± 30.6 mg/dl, respectively.

TABLE 1 | Baseline clinical parameters.

Clinical parameters		All patients (n = 680)
Age (years)		63 ± 11
Male (%)		61
BMI (kg/m^2)		25.6 ± 4.6
Prior CVD/stroke/PAD (%)		17/9/1
Prior cardiovascular event (%)		24
Duration of DM (years)*		11.1 (6.2 > 17.7)
HbA1c	(%)	7.1 ± 1.1
	(mmol/mol)	54.3 ±12.0
Triglyceride (mg/dl)*		116 (81–163)
Total cholesterol (mg/dl)		180.5 ± 31.9
LDL cholesterol (mg/dl)		100.1 ± 25.3
Non-HDL cholesterol (mg/dl)		126.5 ± 30.6
Uric acid (mg/dl)		5.4 ± 1.4
SBP (mmHg)		131.0 ± 17.0
DBP (mmHg)		74.7 ± 10.9
Hypertension (%)[†]		70
Retinopathy (NDR/SDR/prePDR/PDR, %)[‡]		67/17/6/10
eGFR (ml/min/1.73 m^2)		71.0 ± 17.7
CKD GFR Categories (G1/G2/G3a/G3b/G4/G5, %)		10/69/11/6/3/1
UACR (mg/gCr)*		17.7 (7.8–74.1)
Normo/Micro/Macro (%)		63/25/12
Any type of antihypertensive agents (%)		62
ACE inihibitor or ARB (%)		53
Calcium channel blocker (%)		38
Number of antihypertensive agents*		1 (0–2)
Treatment for diabetes		
(Diet only/OHA/Insulin, %)		4/64/32
Drug treatment for hyperglycemia		32/10/35/28/15/49/7
(SU/GLIN/BG/αGI/TZD/DPP4-I/GLP1, %)		
Drug treatment for dyslipidemia/statin use (%)		64/56

*BMI, body mass index; CVD, cardiovascular disease requiring admission for treatment; Stroke, cerebral bleeding or infarction requiring admission for treatment; PAD, peripheral arterial disease requiring admission for intervention or surgery; Cardiovasular event, any event of CVD, Stroke, and PAD; HbA1c, hemoglobin A1c; Duration of DM, estimated duration of diabetes mellitus; LDL cholesterol, low-density lipoprotein cholesterol; non-HDL cholesterol, non high-density lipoprotein cholesterol; SBP, systolic blood pressure; DBP, diastolic blood pressure; Retinopathy, diabetic retinopathy; NDR/SDR/prePDR/PDR, non diabetic retinopathy, simple diabetic retinopathy, pre proliferative diabetic retinopathy, and proliferative diabetic retinopathy, respectively; eGFR, estimated glomerular filtration rate, CKD GFR Categories; G1: ≥90 ml/min/1.73 m^2, G2: 60–90 ml/min/1.73 m^2, G3a: 45–59 ml/min/1.73 m^2, G3b: 30–44 ml/min/1.73 m^2, G4: 15–29 ml/min/1.73 m^2; UACR, urinary albumin creatinine ratio; Normo/Micro/Macro, normoalbuminuria, microalbuminuria, and macroalbuminuria, respectively; ACE inhibitor or ARB, treatment with an angiotensin-converting enzyme inhibitor or angiotensin II type I receptor blocker, respectively; Diet only, diet regimen only; OHA, oral hypoglycemic agent; Insulin therapy, treatment with insulin (including basal-supported oral therapy); SU, sulfonylurea; GLIN, meglitinide anologs; BG, biguanide (Metformin); αGI, alpha-glucosidase inhibitors; TZD, thiazolidinediones; DPP4-I, DPP-4 inhibitors; GLP1, glucagon-like peptide 1 receptor agonists; SGLT2, sodium glucose transporter 2. *Median (interquartile range). [†]Hypertension was defined as blood pressure ≥140/90 mmHg or any antihypertensive drug treatment. [‡]Data from 664 patients (98%) were available.*

Similarly, 62% of the patients received antihypertensive agents, average blood pressures were SBP (131.0 ± 17.0 mmHg) and DBP (74.7 ± 10.9 mmHg). The mean baseline eGFR

was 71.0 ± 17.7 ml/min/1.73 m^2 and median UACR was 17.7 mg/gCr (IQR: 7.8–74.1). The average annual HbA1c, SBP, and DBP levels, and percentage of the use of ACE inhibitor or ARB, and GLP-1 receptor agonist during follow-up were not significantly different between the patients with and without outcome. Statin use during observation was significantly higher, and the use of SGLT2 inhibitor was significantly lower in patients with outcome compared with those without outcome (**Supplementary Table 3**).

Relation Between Primary Endpoint and Glycan Binding to the Lectin Panel

Unadjusted and adjusted HRs for glycan binding to the panel of 45 lectins with different specificities and the reported structure of the glycan binding to each lectin are shown in **Figure 1** and **Supplementary Table 4**. The urinary glycan binding signals to 13 lectins [*Pisum sativum* (PSA), *Lens culinaris* (LCA), *Aleuria aurantia* (AAL), SNA, *Tanthes japonica* (TJAI), RCA120, *Narcissus pseudonarcissus* (NPA), *Canavalia ensiformis* (ConA), *Galanthus nivalis* (GNA), *Hippeastrum hybrid* (HHL), *Tulipa gesneriana* (TxLCI), *Urtica dioica* (UDA), and *Calystegia sepium* (Calsepa)] were significantly associated with the outcome in either of the univariate and multivariate models. Among them, both glycan binding signals to UDA and Calsepa were selected based on the FDR <0.05 in the multivariate models. We fitted a series of multivariate Cox regression models, which include (i) only covariates, (ii) covariates + UACR, (iii) covariates + glycan signals (binding to UDA or Capsela), and (iv) covariates + UACR + glycan signal (**Table 2**). Then, the improvement of model fitness was evaluated based on the reduction of both AIC and BIC criteria. These criteria were minimized at model (iii) for both of UDA and Capsela, which were considered the best fitting model, that is, the two glycans were more substantially improved model fitness, and the addition of UACR did not exhibit improvement of model fitting. Glycan signals for UDA and Calsepa were not incorporated into the model at the same time to avoid multicolinearity because of the high correlation with each other (r = 0.87).

The relationships between the glycan indexes and outcome remained largely unchanged when treated of statin, ACE inhibitor or ARB, and SGLT2 inhibitor during the follow-up period, and the average annual HbA1c, average annual SBP, and baseline non-HDL cholesterol were incorporated into the multivariate model (**Supplementary Table 5**). As shown in **Supplementary Table 4**, UDA and Calsepa are known to bind to a mixture of Man5 to Man9 and to High-Man (Man2-6), respectively. The common recognized glycans are classified into intermediate and immature products of N-glycan synthesis (26).

Time-Dependent Area Under Curve and Harrell's C-Index in Cox Regression Model With or Without Urinary Glycans

Time-dependent AUCs and Harrell's C indexes in multivariate Cox regression model with or without glycan binding signals to UDA and Calsepa are displayed in **Figures 2A,B**. Overall, AUCs during observation were higher in models with those

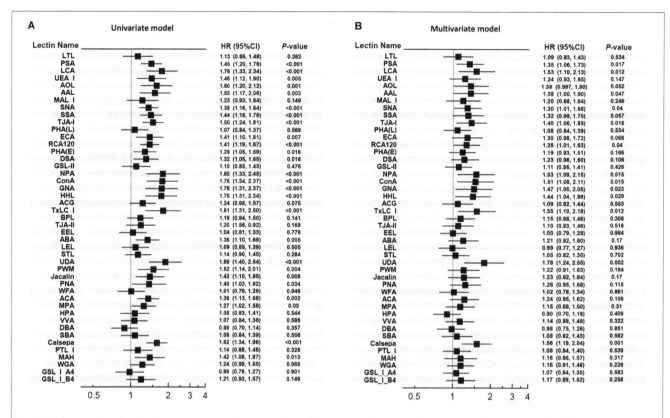

FIGURE 1 | Univariate and multivariate Cox proportional hazard models for the outcome. **(A)** Univariate Cox proportional hazard models. **(B)** Multivariate Cox proportional hazard models. HR per 1 SD increase in each glycan index is shown. In the multivariate model, HR was adjusted for age, gender, body mass index, systolic blood pressure, hemoglobin A1c, low-density lipoprotein cholesterol, estimated glomerular filtration rate, past cardiovascular event at baseline. HR, hazard ratio; 95% CI, 95% confidence interval.

TABLE 2 | Comparison of hazard ratio and model fitting between multivariate models with or without UACR and urinary glycans for UDA and Calsepa.

Markers	Multivariate model					Markers	Multivariate model with UACR				
	HR	95% CI	P-value	AIC	BIC		HR	95% CI	P-value	AIC	BIC
None	–	–	–	725.7	761.8	UACR	1.32	0.99–1.75	0.058	724.1	764.8
UDA	1.78	1.24–2.55	0.002	716.5	757.2	UDA	1.70	1.16–2.49	0.006	718.0	763.2
Calsepa	1.56	1.19–2.04	0.001	718.0	758.7	Calsepa	1.50	1.11–2.02	0.009	719.6	764.8

Covariates in multivariate model: age, gender, body mass index, systolic blood pressure, hemoglobin A1c, low density cholesterol levels, estimated glomerular filtration rate, and past cardiovascular event at baseline. Each glycan index was employed into the multivariate model with or without log transformed UACR. UACR, urinary albumin creatinine ratio; HR, hazard ratio; 95% CI, 95% confidence interval; AIC, Akaike's information criterion; BIC, Bayesian information criterion; UDA, Urtica dioica; Calsepa, Calystegia sepium.

glycan indexes than in model without them, while the Harrell's C-index was significantly higher only in the model containing glycan binding signal to UDA than in model without the glycans [Harrell's C-index for model without UDA: 0.766 (95% CI: 0.705–0.828), Harrell's C-index for model with UDA: 0.794 (0.739–0.850), and the difference in Harrell's C-index: 0.028 (0.001–0.055, $P = 0.044$)].

Cumulative Incidence Rate of the Primary Outcome in Urinary Glycan Quartiles

Kaplan–Meier curves stratified according to quartiles for baseline urinary glycan binding to UDA and Calsepa are shown in

Figure 3. The cumulative incidence rate of the outcome was significantly higher in the higher quartile for urinary glycan binding to UDA and Calsepa than in the lower quartiles [P for trend: <0.001 for UDA (**Figure 3A**) and <0.0001 for Calsepa (**Figure 3B**)].

5-Year Risk Classification Ability of Urinary Glycan Binding to Urtica Dioica and Calystegia Sepium

The difference of AUROC between logistic regression models with or without urinary markers, category-free NRI, absolute IDI for predicting the primary outcome at 5-year follow-up time

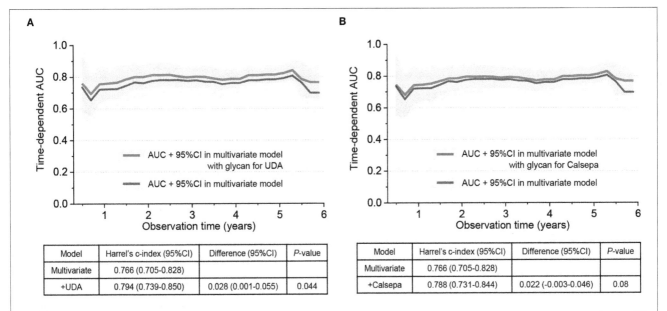

FIGURE 2 | Time-dependent area under curve (AUC) and Harrell's C-index in Cox regression model with or without urinary glycans binding to UDA and Calsepa. **(A)** AUC and Harrell's C-index with or without urinary glycans binding to UDA. **(B)** AUC and Harrell's C-index with or without urinary glycans binding to Calsepa. In the multivariate Cox regression model without glycan, age, gender, body mass index, systolic blood pressure, hemoglobin A1c, low-density lipoprotein cholesterol, estimated glomerular filtration rate, past cardiovascular event at baseline were incorporated as adjusted variables. On the other hand, multivariate model with glycan includes the same covariates and any of two glycans binding to UDA and Calsepa. UDA, *Urtica dioica*; Calsepa, *Calystegia sepium*.

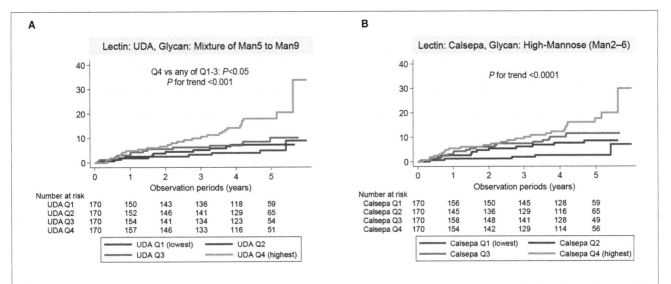

FIGURE 3 | Cumulative incidence rate of the outcome. **(A)** Cumulative incidence rate in patients stratified according to the quartiles of urinary glycan indexes for UDA. **(B)** Cumulative incidence rate in patients stratified according to the quartiles of urinary glycan indexes for Calsepa. The cumulative incidence rate was significantly higher in patients with higher glycan indexes than in those with lower glycan indexes (UDA: *P* for trend <0.001, Calsepa: *P* for trend <0.0001). Among quartile groups for UDA, cumulative incidence rate was significantly higher in highest quartile group (Q4) compared with lower quartile groups (Q1–3) (*P* < 0.05). The log-rank test was used for failure analysis. UDA, *Urtica dioica*; Calsepa, *Calystegia sepium*; Man, Mannose.

obtained by adding UACR and the glycan indexes for UDA and Calsepa are summarized in **Table 3**. Adding of either glycan indexes to the multivariate model significantly improved the ability of discrimination and reclassification such as AUROC and NRI [difference in AUROC: 0.031 (95% CI: 0.001–0.062,

$P = 0.045$) for UDA, 0.027 (0.001–0.053, $P = 0.040$) for Calsepa, category-free NRI: 0.368 (0.045–0.692, $P = 0.026$) for UDA, and 0.388 (0.099–0.677, $P = 0.008$) for Calsepa], whereas either of the two glycan indexes did not significantly improve integrated discrimination [IDI: 0.024 (-0.009–0.056, $P = 0.16$) for UDA

TABLE 3 | AUROC, category-free NRI, and IDI for predicting the 5-year outcome with UACR and urinary glycan binding to UDA and Calsepa.

	AUROC (95% CI)	Difference of AUROC (95% CI)	P-value	Category-free NRI (95% CI)	P-value	IDI (95% CI)	P-value
Only covariates	0.774 (0.711–0.837)						
With UACR	0.790 (0.732–0.849)	0.017 (−0.002–0.035)	0.083	0.269 (−0.027–0.564)	0.075	0.005 (−0.014–0.024)	0.59
With glycan to UDA (Mixture of Man5 to Man9)	0.805 (0.748–0.862)	0.031 (0.001–0.062)	0.045	0.368 (0.045–0.692)	0.026	0.024 (−0.009–0.056)	0.16
With glycan to Calsepa [High-Man (Man2-6)]	0.801 (0.744–0.857)	0.027 (0.001–0.053)	0.040	0.388 (0.099–0.677)	0.008	0.021 (−0.010–0.053)	0.18

Covariates: age, gender, body mass index, systolic blood pressure, hemoglobin A1c, low density cholesterol levels, estimated glomerular filtration rate, and past cardiovascular event at baseline.
AUROC, The area under a receiver operating characteristic; NRI, net reclassification improvement; IDI, integrated discrimination improvement; UACR, urine albumin creatinine ratio; 95% CI, 95% confidence interval; UDA, Urtica dioica; Calsepa, Calystegia sepium; Man, Mannose.

and 0.021 (−0.010–0.053, $P = 0.18$) for Calsepa]. On the other hand, adding UACR did not show any significance on the incremental prediction [difference in AUROC: 0.017 (−0.002–0.035, $P = 0.083$), category-free NRI: 0.269 (−0.027–0.564, $P = 0.075$), and IDI: 0.005 (−0.014–0.024, $P = 0.59$)].

DISCUSSION

The urine glycan binding signals to UDA (mixture of Man5 to Man9) and Calsepa [High-Man (Man2-6)] improved model fitness scores for discrimination ability (Harrell's C index and AUROC), reclassification (NRI), and log-likelihood/complexity (AIC and BIC) when they were incorporated into the multivariate Cox and logistic regression model employing traditional risk factors. The strength of the current study was that the two urinary glycan signals were the novel urinary markers, which could provide the new mechanism of CVE in diabetes. They demonstrated the incremental predictive power with statistical significance, and they might be better markers than UACR. In previous studies of patients with type 2 diabetes, several urinary markers such as urinary kidney injury molecule 1, urinary neutrophil gelatinase-associated lipocalin, urinary liver-type fatty acid-binding protein, and urinary COOH-terminal propeptide of collagen VI, have been investigated for predicting CVE (13, 15, 27). However, none of them showed the statistical significance of model discrimination or reclassification in the multivariate model including known risk factors. Although it has been shown that UACR is associated with CVE independent of established confounders, its incremental predictive ability is limited (21). In our study, UACR had a marginal impact on the outcome in the multivariate Cox regression analysis [HR for logUACR: 1.32 (95% CI: 0.99–1.75), $P = 0.058$, **Table 2**], while it failed to demonstrate the significant values of AUROC, NRI, and IDI (**Table 3**) in the multivariate models, which was compatible with the previous results (21). In contrast to UACR, glycan indexes for UDA and Calsepa showed statistical significance of the incremental prediction as mentioned above. In addition, model fitness scores, i.e., AIC and BIC, were clearly better than

that of UACR. Therefore, these novel glycan indexes might be superior to UACR for predicting CVE in patients with type 2 diabetes.

Interestingly, UDA and Calsepa recognize the high mannose glycan structures (**Supplementary Figure 1**). In endoplasmic reticulum (ER), Glc3Man9GlcNAc2 is transferred to the NXT/NXS sites of protein, Glc residues removed by glucosidases, and Man9GlcNAc2 converted to Man8GlcNAc2 by ER α-mannosidase I (MAN1B1). The glycoproteins are then transferred to cis-Golgi; the additional Man residues are removed until Man5GlcNAc2 is generated. Man5GlcNAc2 is a key intermediate for the pathway to hybrid and complex N-glycans in trans-Golgi and trans-Golgi network by the removal of mannose residues by Golgi mannosidases, while some of Man5GlcNAc2 also escapes further modification, and mature membrane or secreted glycoprotein carries Man5-9GlcNAc2, i.e., high mannose structures (**Supplementary Figure 1A**) (26). In the glycan analysis by urine lectin microarray, the elevation of high mannose and complex type of N-glycans in urine glycoproteins are tightly linked to the development of composite CVE.

The high-throughput plasma or serum N-glycan profiling studies using hydrophilic interaction liquid chromatography (HILIC) of peptide-N-glycosidase F digested and fluorescently labeled N-glycans were reported, and 46 N-glycan peaks (GP1-GP46) were demonstrated (28–32). In the patients with normo- and hyperglycemia during acute inflammation, the comparison of N-glycan profile demonstrated that increased branched, galactosylated, and sialylated tri- and tetraantennary N-glycans are associated with the development of type 2 diabetes (28). In Ghanaian population, branched, trigalactosylated, antennary fucosylated, and triantennary N-glycans (**Supplementary Figure 1B**) were increased in the patients with type 2 diabetes (29). A lower relative abundance of simple biantennary N-glycans and a higher abundance of branched, galactosylated, and sialylated complex N-glycans were increased both in type 1 (31) and type 2 (30) diabetes, and similar trends with increased levels of complex N-glycans (GP12, GP16, and GP22) were seen for higher UACR and greater annual loss of eGFR (29, 31). Recently, in the prospective European Prospective Investigation of Cancer (EPIC)—Potsdam cohort ($n = 27,548$), the increased levels of complex N-glycans, GP5 in women, and GP16, GP23, and GP29 in men, improved the accuracy of risk prediction score for CVD (32).

Independent of serum or plasma N-glycan profiling, our efforts to identify the biomarkers to improve the prediction of DKD and CVD outcomes have been directed to the clinical studies using urinary glycan profiling by lectin microarray in the patients with type 2 diabetes (16, 33). Previously, we found that urinary glycan profiling by lectin microarray demonstrated the considerable changes in glycan binding signals during the progression of DKD in urine samples rather than serum samples (16, 33). The changes in glycan profile in urine samples may reflect the glycosylation changes in glycoproteins produced in kidney tissues or the changes in selective permeabilities of blood-derived glycoproteins through glomerular capillaries. In addition, the lectins are long-standing experimental tools to identify the glycan structures, which enable lectin microarray to detect the broad range of glycans compared with HILIC or other methods using mass analysis. For instance, the capture of O-glycans and neutral N-glycans such as high-mannose type and hybrid type N-glycans (**Supplementary Figure 1C**) are extremely difficult in HILIC (34). Furthermore, only 20 µl of urine samples is required, and the single step of Cy3 labeling without enzymatic treatments achieve the less-time consuming and high-throughput analyses. By taking these advantages of urine lectin microarray, we successfully identified that the glycan binding signals to high mannose or mannose-recognizing lectins, UDA and Calsepa, contributed the improvement of the prediction models using established risk factors for CVE. In the previous study, we identified that the glycan-binding signals to SNA, RCA120, DBA, ABA, Jacalin, and ACA significantly improved the prediction models for 30% decline in eGFR or ESRD, and these lectins mainly recognized the O-glycan structures, suggesting the specificity of the analyses with lectin microarray (16). Furthermore, the application of those eight lectins for the urine samples of the patients with type 2 diabetes provides a useful diagnostic tool for the future risk of the CVD and DKD progression.

Novel Mechanism of the Atherosclerotic Cardiovascular Event in Diabetes

The current clinical study provides the insight into the mechanism for the progression of atherosclerosis in type 2 diabetes. The detection of high mannose N-glycans, i.e., immature forms of N-glycans, in the urine samples in the patients with type 2 diabetes suggests the abnormalities in the processing and maturation of N-glycans in the ER and Golgi. In the ER, Glc1Man9GlcNAc2 N-glycans are properly folded by the assistance of calnexin and calreticulin, while the misfolded Man9GlcNAc2 is recognized by ER-degradation-enhancing α mannosidase I-like (EDEM) leading to ER degradation (26). The inhibition of ER α-mannosidase I (MAN1B1), which mediates the conversion of Man9GlcNAc2 to Man8GlcNAc2, was reported to enhance high mannose intercellular adhesion molecule-1

expression on endothelial cell surface (35). The impairment of quality control of glycoproteins and mannosidase activity in ER may cause the accumulation of high mannose N-glycans in ER. In addition, the knockout of the triple gene encoding Golgi α1,2-mannosidases (MAN1A1, MAN1A2, and MAN1B1) resulted in the production of high mannose N-glycans (36). The defects in the Golgi α1,2-mannosidases are also candidate mechanisms to produce high mannose N-glycans. The link between high mannose N-glycans and CVE further suggested the new mechanism for the progression of atherosclerosis in type 2 diabetes. High mannose N-glycans induced on endothelial cells by oscillatory shear stress, or tumor necrosis factor-α mediates the monocytic recruitment (37), and hypercholesterolemic patients exhibited higher plasma levels of a cluster of high-mannose and complex/hybrid N-glycans (38).

Study Limitations

One of the key limitations in this study is that this was a multi-center observational study, and the therapeutic strategy of diabetes and its complications in each participant was not exactly standardized, which might have affected the incidence of the outcome. However, the sensitivity analyses revealed that the impact of glycan indexes for UDA and Calsepa on the outcome did not largely change even when the various treatment factors during follow-up periods were incorporated into the multivariate Cox regression models (**Supplementary Table 5**). In addition, we might not be able to adjust for other possible confounders in the multivariate models. Several blood biomarkers, such as NT-proBNP and high-sensitivity troponin T, have been established as useful markers for predicting CVE (9, 39). It remains unknown whether glycan indexes for UDA and Calsepa are significantly associated with the outcome independent of those biomarkers. Nevertheless, we hope that these novel urinary markers predict CVE independent of other confounders since these glycan markers could reflect the novel mechanism of CVE as mentioned above.

CONCLUSIONS

The glycan profiling by urine lectin microarray demonstrated that the elevation of high mannose and complex type of N-glycans in urine glycoproteins is tightly linked to the development of CVE. UDA and Calsepa in lectin microarray may be a useful diagnostic tool for the prediction of CVD risk in patients with type 2 diabetes. The evidence linking the increased high mannose and complex type of N-glycans to the incidence of CVE in patients with diabetes suggests that the disease mechanisms and therapeutic targets are related to organellar dysfunction in the ER and Golgi, as well as to the progression of atherosclerosis.

AUTHOR CONTRIBUTIONS

KMis conceived the study, formulated the analysis plan, performed the statistical analyses, collected the clinical data, performed the urinary lectin microarray, and wrote the manuscript. MI collected and assessed all the clinical data. SY measured the urinary glycan binding signals to lectins and collected the clinical data. MW, CH, AK, SM, HU, AN, JE, KH, TN, AT, ST, TM, SK, KMu, IS, KMiy, SA, TN, and KS recruited the patients and assessed the data. MYo supported the statistical analyses. MYa measured the urinary glycan binding signals to lectins, analyzed the urinary lectin microarray data, and wrote the manuscript. JW conceived the study, supervised the data collection, analyzed the data, and edited the manuscript. All authors contributed to the interpretation of the data, critical revision of the manuscript, and approval of the final version of the manuscript.

ACKNOWLEDGMENTS

We are grateful to Drs. Ichiro Nojima, Yuzuki Kano, Yuriko Yamamura, and Yasuhiro Onishi for collecting data. We are also grateful to Daniele Spinelli for helpful comments on the analyses.

REFERENCES

1. Muthee TB, Kimathi D, Richards GC, Etyang A, Nunan D, Williams V, et al. Factors influencing the implementation of cardiovascular risk scoring in primary care: a mixed-method systematic review. *Implement Sci.* (2020) 15:57. doi: 10.1186/s13012-020-01022-x

2. van Bussel EF, Hoevenaar-Blom MP, Poortvliet RKE, Gussekloo J, van Dalen JW, van Gool WA, et al. Predictive value of traditional risk factors for cardiovascular disease in older people: a systematic review. *Prev Med.* (2020) 132:105986. doi: 10.1016/j.ypmed.2020.105986

3. Go AS, Chertow GM, Fan D, McCulloch CE, Hsu CY. Chronic kidney disease and the risks of death, cardiovascular events, and hospitalization. *N Engl J Med.* (2004) 351:1296–305. doi: 10.1056/NEJMoa041031

4. Tonelli M, Muntner P, Lloyd A, Manns BJ, Klarenbach S, Pannu N, et al. Risk of coronary events in people with chronic kidney disease compared with those with diabetes: a population-level cohort study. *Lancet.* (2012) 380:807–14. doi: 10.1016/S0140-6736(12)60572-8

5. Chronic Kidney Disease Prognosis, Matsushita K, van der Velde M, Astor BC, Woodward M, Levey AS, et al. Association of estimated glomerular filtration rate and albuminuria with all-cause and cardiovascular mortality in general population cohorts: a collaborative meta-analysis. *Lancet.* (2010) 375:2073–81. doi: 10.1016/S0140-6736(10)60674-5

6. Matsushita K, Coresh J, Sang Y, Chalmers J, Fox C, Guallar E, et al. Estimated glomerular filtration rate and albuminuria for prediction of cardiovascular outcomes: a collaborative meta-analysis of individual participant data. *Lancet Diabetes Endocrinol.* (2015) 3:514–25. doi: 10.1016/S2213-8587(15)00040-6

7. Bachmann KN, Wang TJ. Biomarkers of cardiovascular disease: contributions to risk prediction in individuals with diabetes. *Diabetologia.* (2018) 61:987–95. doi: 10.1007/s00125-017-4442-9

8. van der Leeuw J, Beulens JW, van Dieren S, Schalkwijk CG, Glatz JF, Hofker MH, et al. Novel biomarkers to improve the prediction of cardiovascular event risk in type 2 diabetes mellitus. *J Am Heart Assoc.* (2016) 5:e003048. doi: 10.1161/JAHA.115.003048

9. Looker HC, Colombo M, Agakov F, Zeller T, Groop L, Thorand B, et al. Protein biomarkers for the prediction of cardiovascular disease in type 2 diabetes. *Diabetologia.* (2015) 58:1363–71. doi: 10.1007/s00125-015-3535-6

10. Gerstein HC, Pare G, McQueen MJ, Haenel H, Lee SF, Pogue J, et al. Identifying novel biomarkers for cardiovascular events or death in people with dysglycemia. *Circulation.* (2015) 132:2297–304. doi: 10.1161/CIRCULATIONAHA.115.015744

11. Welsh P, Rankin N, Li Q, Mark PB, Wurtz P, Ala-Korpela M, et al. Circulating amino acids and the risk of macrovascular, microvascular and mortality outcomes in individuals with type 2 diabetes: results from the ADVANCE trial. *Diabetologia.* (2018) 61:1581–91. doi: 10.1007/s00125-018-4619-x

12. Alshehry ZH, Mundra PA, Barlow CK, Mellett NA, Wong G, McConville MJ, et al. Plasma lipidomic profiles improve on traditional risk factors for the prediction of cardiovascular events in type 2 diabetes mellitus. *Circulation.* (2016) 134:1637–50. doi: 10.1161/CIRCULATIONAHA.116.023233

13. Vaduganathan M, White WB, Charytan DM, Morrow DA, Liu Y, Zannad F, et al. Relation of serum and urine renal biomarkers to cardiovascula risk in patients with type 2 diabetes mellitus and recent acute coronary syndromes (from the EXAMINE trial). *Am J Cardiol.* (2019) 123:382–91. doi: 10.1016/j.amjcard.2018.10.035

14. Rotbain Curovic V, Hansen TW, Eickhoff MK, von Scholten BJ, Reinhard H, Jacobsen PK, et al. Urinary tubular biomarkers as predictors of kidney function decline, cardiovascular events and mortality in microalbuminuric type 2 diabetic patients. *Acta Diabetol.* (2018) 55:1143–50. doi: 10.1007/s00592-018-1205-0

15. Rasmussen DGK, Hansen TW, von Scholten BJ, Nielsen SH, Reinhard H, Parving HH, et al. Higher collagen VI formation is associated with all-cause mortality in patients with type 2 diabetes and microalbuminuria. *Diabetes Care.* (2018) 41:1493–500. doi: 10.2337/dc17-2392

16. Mise K, Imamura M, Yamaguchi S, Teshigawara S, Tone A, Uchida HA, et al. Identification of novel urinary biomarkers for predicting renal prognosis in patients with type 2 diabetes by glycan profiling in a multicenter prospective cohort study: U-CARE study 1. *Diabetes Care.* (2018) 41:1765–75. doi: 10.2337/dc18-0030

17. Seino Y, Nanjo K, Tajima N, Kadowaki T, Kashiwagi A, Araki E, et al. Report of the committee on the classification and diagnostic criteria of diabetes mellitus. *J Diabetes Invest.* (2010) 1:212–28. doi: 10.1111/j.2040-1124.2010.00074.x

18. Kuno A, Uchiyama N, Koseki-Kuno S, Ebe Y, Takashima S, Yamada M, et al. Evanescent-field fluorescence-assisted lectin microarray: a new strategy for glycan profiling. *Nat Methods.* (2005) 2:851–6. doi: 10.1038/nmeth803

19. Kawakita C, Mise K, Onishi Y, Sugiyama H, Yoshida M, Yamada M, et al. Novel urinary glycan profiling by lectin array serves as the biomarkers for predicting renal prognosis in patients with IgA nephropathy. *Sci Rep.* (2021) 11:3394. doi: 10.1038/s41598-020-77736-1

20. Kashiwagi A, Kasuga M, Araki E, Oka Y, Hanafusa T, Ito H, et al. International clinical harmonization of glycated hemoglobin in Japan: from Japan diabetes society to national glycohemoglobin standardization program values. *J Diabetes Invest.* (2012) 3:39–40. doi: 10.1111/j.2040-1124.2012.00207.x

21. Scirica BM, Mosenzon O, Bhatt DL, Udell JA, Steg PG, McGuire DK, et al. Cardiovascular outcomes according to urinary albumin and kidney disease in patients with type 2 diabetes at high cardiovascular risk: observations from the SAVOR-TIMI 53 trial. *JAMA Cardiol.* (2018) 3:155–63. doi: 10.1001/jamacardio.2017.4228

22. Benjamini Y, Hochberg Y. Controlling the false discovery rate: a practical and powerful approach to multiple testing. *J Roy Stat Soc B.* (1995) 57:289–300. doi: 10.1111/j.2517-6161.1995.tb02031.x

23. Cattaneo M, Malighetti P, Spinelli D. Estimating receiver operative characteristic curves for time-dependent outcomes: the stroccurve package. *Stata J.* (2018) 17:1015–23. doi: 10.1177/1536867X1701700415

24. Pencina MJ, D'Agostino RB Sr, D'Agostino RB Jr, Vasan RS. Evaluating the added predictive ability of a new marker: from area under the ROC curve to reclassification and beyond. *Stat Med.* (2008) 27:157–72; discussion 207–12. doi: 10.1002/sim.2929

25. Pencina MJ, D'Agostino RB, Pencina KM, Janssens AC, Greenland P. Interpreting incremental value of markers added to risk prediction models. *Am J Epidemiol.* (2012) 176:473–81. doi: 10.1093/aje/kws207

26. Stanley P, Taniguchi N, Aebi M. N-Glycans. In: Varki A, Cummings RD, Esko JD, Stanley P, Hart GW, Aebi M, et al., editors. *Essentials of Glycobiology*. Cold Spring Harbor Laboratory Press: Cold Spring Harbor, NY (2015). p. 99–111.

27. Panduru NM, Forsblom C, Saraheimo M, Thorn LM, Gordin D, Elonen N, et al. Urinary liver-type fatty acid binding protein is an independent predictor of stroke and mortality in individuals with type 1 diabetes. *Diabetologia.* (2017) 60:1782–90. doi: 10.1007/s00125-017-4328-x

28. Keser T, Gornik I, Vuckovic F, Selak N, Pavic T, Lukic E, et al. Increased plasma N-glycome complexity is associated with higher risk of type 2 diabetes. *Diabetologia.* (2017) 60:2352–60. doi: 10.1007/s00125-017-4426-9

29. Adua E, Memarian E, Russell A, Trbojevic-Akmacic I, Gudelj I, Juric J, et al. High throughput profiling of whole plasma N-glycans in type II diabetes mellitus patients and healthy individuals: a perspective from a Ghanaian population. *Arch Biochem Biophys.* (2019) 661:10–21. doi: 10.1016/j.abb.2018.10.015

30. Adua E, Anto EO, Roberts P, Kantanka OS, Aboagye E, Wang W. The potential of N-glycosylation profiles as biomarkers for monitoring the progression of type II diabetes mellitus towards diabetic kidney disease. *J Diabetes Metab Disord.* (2018) 17:233–46. doi: 10.1007/s40200-018-0365-3

31. Bermingham ML, Colombo M, McGurnaghan SJ, Blackbourn LAK, Vuckovic F, Pucic Bakovic M, et al. N-Glycan profile and kidney disease in type 1 diabetes. *Diabetes Care.* (2018) 41:79–87. doi: 10.2337/dc17-1042

32. Wittenbecher C, Stambuk T, Kuxhaus O, Rudman N, Vuckovic F, Stambuk J, et al. Plasma N-Glycans as emerging biomarkers of cardiometabolic risk: a prospective investigation in the EPIC-potsdam cohort study. *Diabetes Care.* (2020) 43:661–8. doi: 10.2337/dc19-1507

33. Inoue K, Wada J, Eguchi J, Nakatsuka A, Teshigawara S, Murakami K, et al. Urinary fetuin-A is a novel marker for diabetic nephropathy in type 2 diabetes identified by lectin microarray. *PLoS ONE.* (2013) 8:e77118. doi: 10.1371/journal.pone.0077118

34. Gargano AFG, Schouten O, van Schaick G, Roca LS, van den Berg-Verleg JH, Haselberg R, et al. Profiling of a high mannose-type N-glycosylated lipase using hydrophilic interaction chromatography-mass spectrometry. *Anal Chim Acta.* (2020) 1109:69–77. doi: 10.1016/j.aca.2020.02.042

35. Regal-McDonald K, Xu B, Barnes JW, Patel RP. High-mannose intercellular adhesion molecule-1 enhances CD16(+) monocyte adhesion to the endothelium. *Am J Physiol Heart Circ Physiol.* (2019) 317:H1028–H38. doi: 10.1152/ajpheart.00306.2019

36. Jin ZC, Kitajima T, Dong W, Huang YF, Ren WW, Guan F, et al. Genetic disruption of multiple alpha1,2-mannosidases generates mammalian cells producing recombinant proteins with high-mannose-type N-glycans. *J Biol Chem.* (2018) 293:5572–84. doi: 10.1074/jbc.M117.813030

37. Scott DW, Chen J, Chacko BK, Traylor JG, Jr., Orr AW, et al. Role of endothelial N-glycan mannose residues in monocyte recruitment during atherogenesis. *Arterioscler Thromb Vasc Biol.* (2012) 32:e51–9. doi: 10.1161/ATVBAHA.112.253203

38. Bai L, Li Q, Li L, Lin Y, Zhao S, Wang W, et al. Plasma high-mannose and complex/hybrid N-Glycans are associated with hypercholesterolemia in humans and rabbits. *PLoS ONE.* (2016) 11:e0146982. doi: 10.1371/journal.pone.0146982

39. Scirica BM, Bhatt DL, Braunwald E, Raz I, Cavender MA, Im K, et al. Prognostic implications of biomarker assessments in patients with type 2 diabetes at high cardiovascular risk: a secondary analysis of a randomized clinical trial. *JAMA Cardiol.* (2016) 1:989–98. doi: 10.1001/jamacardio.2016.3030

7

Prognostic Value of Natriuretic Peptides for All-Cause Mortality, Right Ventricular Failure, Major Adverse Events and Myocardial Recovery in Advanced Heart Failure Patients Receiving a Left Ventricular Assist Device

Eva Janssen, J. Wouter Jukema, Saskia L. M. A. Beeres, Martin J. Schalij and Laurens F. Tops*

Department of Cardiology, Leiden University Medical Center, Leiden, Netherlands

*Correspondence:
Laurens F. Tops
l.f.tops@lumc.nl

Aims: Major adverse event (MAE) rates during left ventricular assist device (LVAD) therapy in advanced heart failure (HF) patients are high, and impair quality of life and survival. Prediction and risk stratification of MAEs in order to improve patient selection and thereby outcome during LVAD therapy is therefore warranted. Circulating natriuretic peptides (NPs) are strong predictors of MAEs and mortality in chronic HF patients. However, whether NPs can identify patients who are at risk of MAEs and mortality or tend toward myocardial recovery after LVAD implantation is unclear. The aim of this systematic review is to analyze the prognostic value of circulating NP levels before LVAD implantation for all-cause mortality, MAEs and myocardial recovery after LVAD implantation.

Methods and Results: Electronic databases were searched for studies analyzing circulating NP in adults with advanced HF before LVAD implantation in relation to mortality, MAEs, or myocardial recovery after LVAD implantation. Twenty-four studies published between 2008 and 2021 were included. Follow-up duration ranged from 48 hours to 5 years. Study sample size ranged from 14 to 15,138 patients. Natriuretic peptide levels were not predictive of all-cause mortality. However, NPs were predictive of right ventricular failure (RVF) and MAEs such as ventricular arrhythmias, moderate or severe aortic regurgitation, and all-cause rehospitalization. No relation between NPs and myocardial recovery was found.

Conclusion: This systematic review found that NP levels before LVAD implantation are not predictive of all-cause mortality after LVAD implantation. Thus, NP levels may be of limited value in patient selection for LVAD therapy. However, NPs help in risk stratification of MAEs and may be used to identify patients who are at risk for RVF, ventricular arrhythmias, moderate or severe aortic regurgitation, and all-cause rehospitalization after LVAD implantation.

Keywords: left ventricular assist device, circulating biomarkers, natriuretic peptides, adverse events, prognosis

INTRODUCTION

The prognosis of advanced heart failure (HF) is poor, with annual mortality rates over 50%, and limited treatment options (1). Cardiac transplantation is the most effective treatment, although its availability is limited due to insufficient number of donor organs and strict eligibility criteria. Left ventricular assist devices (LVADs) are an alternative treatment option through mechanical unloading of the failing left ventricle (LV). To date, LVAD therapy is increasingly used as destination therapy in patients not eligible for transplantation. Patient selection and timing of LVAD implantation is guided by the profiles of the Interagency Registry for Mechanically Assisted Circulatory Support (INTERMACS) classifying patients with advanced heart failure (2).

The most recent INTERMACS report has shown a 1-year survival rate of 79–80% in patients receiving continuous flow (CF)-LVAD therapy (3, 4). Major adverse event (MAE) and rehospitalization rates are high, and impair quality of life and survival (4, 5). These MAEs include neurologic event (defined as stroke or transient ischemic attack), gastrointestinal bleeding, major infection, and right heart failure (RVF) occurring 13–20, 20–25, 40–43, and 29–38% at 1 year after CF-LVAD implantation, respectively (4). All-cause rehospitalization rates were 21–23% (4). Device explantation for LV myocardial recovery is rare with 3.1% at 3 years, and <5% at 5 years follow-up (3, 6). It would be beneficial to identify patients prone to myocardial recovery, and consider adjustments of their pharmacological treatment (7). To identify patients at risk of MAEs and early mortality would be of great importance. Treatment options for MAEs are limited and often ineffective, having corresponding high mortality rates. Thus, prediction and risk stratification of MAEs before LVAD implantation is warranted in order to improve patient selection, and thereby outcome of LVAD therapy. Measurement of circulating biomarkers such as natriuretic peptides (NPs) may help in risk stratification.

Three subtypes of NP are known; atrial natriuretic peptide (ANP), B-type natriuretic peptide (BNP), and C-type natriuretic peptide (CNP) (8, 9). Natriuretic peptides mainly reflect the hemodynamic burden of the failing heart, and are regulated by volume overload and neuro-hormonal stimulation. Prehormone pro-BNP is released by cardiomyocytes in reaction to mechanical stretch and myocardial ischemia. Upon secretion into the circulation it is cleaved in biologically active BNP and its inactive remnant N-terminal proBNP (NT-proBNP) (**Figure 1**) (8–12). Levels of NP are influenced by various factors including age, gender, comorbidities, renal function, pulmonary disease, and obesity (13–15). Heart failure medication, including beta-blockers, diuretics, and inotropes affect NP levels, reflecting the improvement in hemodynamic state induced by these therapies. The novel HF drug sacubitril/valsartan influences BNP and NT-proBNP levels differently, in particular during the first 8–10 weeks after initiation. Whereas, the use of sacubitril/valsartan, a neprilysin inhibitor, may increase the circulating levels of BNP, it does not affect the circulating levels of NT-proBNP since the latter is not a substrate of neprilysin inhibition. Nonetheless, both BNP and NT-proBNP have prognostic value during treatment

with sacubitril/valsartan (8, 16). Finally, it has been demonstrated that a large percentage of measured circulating BNP or NT-proBNP is in fact their prehormone proBNP. Therefore, BNP, NT-proBNP, and proBNP measurements from different assays are not reliably comparable due to their differences in cross-reactivity (17, 18).

In the American College of Cardiology/American Heart Association guideline, BNP and NT-proBNP have a class IA recommendation to establish disease severity and prognosis of patients with chronic HF (2). Hutfless et al. showed that preoperative BNP levels are strong predictors of postoperative need for intra-aortic balloon pump, longer postoperative hospital stay, and higher 1-year mortality in patients undergoing open heart surgery (19). Furthermore, the prognostic value of NP levels related to all-cause mortality, adverse events, and rehospitalization in chronic HF patients has been well-established (20–24).

Whether preoperative NP levels can improve patient selection for LVAD therapy by identifying patients who are at risk for early all-cause mortality, right ventricular failure (RVF), or MAEs, and can identify patients who tend toward myocardial recovery after LVAD implantation, is not yet systematically evaluated. In this review, we sought to systematically evaluate the prognostic value of circulating NP levels in advanced HF patients before LVAD implantation for all-cause mortality, RVF, MAEs including rehospitalization, and myocardial recovery after successful LVAD implantation.

METHODS

This systematic review is written in accordance with the Preferred Reporting Items for Systematic Reviews and Meta-analyses (PRISMA) guideline (**Supplementary Material 1**). Since individual patient data are not included, institutional review board approval was not required.

Literature Search and Selection

Seven electronic databases were searched: MEDLINE, Web of Science Core Collection, Cochrane Reviews, Cochrane Trials, PubMed, Factiva, and Embase. The following (MeSH) terms were used: "left ventricular assist device," "ventricular assist device," "mechanical circulatory support," "biomarkers," "natriuretic peptide," "B-type natriuretic peptide," "brain natriuretic peptide," "pro B-type natriuretic peptide," "pro brain natriuretic peptide," "NT-pro B-type natriuretic peptide," "N-terminal pro B-type natriuretic peptide," and "N-terminal pro brain natriuretic peptide." The search was restricted to human studies published in English up to January 1st, 2021. Study selection criteria were predefined as described in **Table 1**.

The authors of this manuscript screened the titles and abstracts of all studies retrieved from the literature search. Potentially relevant studies, or studies whose relevance could not be ascertained based on the abstract, were screened full text. A single assessor screened each article full text for inclusion. Corresponding authors were contacted to obtain full data not covered in the publication.

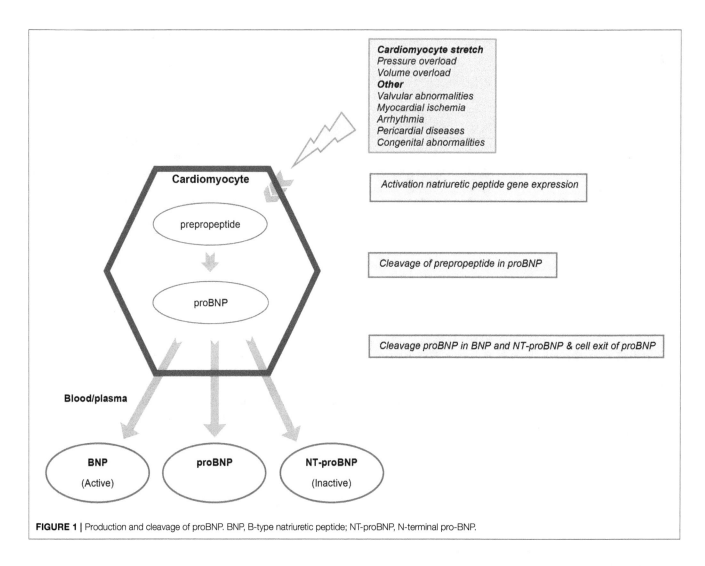

FIGURE 1 | Production and cleavage of proBNP. BNP, B-type natriuretic peptide; NT-proBNP, N-terminal pro-BNP.

TABLE 1 | Inclusion–and exclusion criteria.

Inclusion

Patient population: humans > 18 years with advanced HF who will receive left ventricular assist device therapy

Outcome(s): all-cause mortality, right ventricular failure, major adverse events, myocardial recovery

Prognostic factor: circulating natriuretic peptide levels measured before LVAD implantation

Language: English

Exclusion

Reviews, editorials, case reports, abstracts

Data Collection
Extracted data included details of the patient population, etiology of HF, type of VAD, device strategy, timing of blood sampling for NPs measurement, type of NPs, cut-off points of NPs (when available), type of statistical analysis, adjusted variables for multivariate analysis, and duration of follow-up.

The outcomes all-cause mortality, RVF, MAEs (including all-cause planned and unplanned rehospitalization) and myocardial recovery, and their describing definitions were extracted. Major adverse events were defined according to the "2020 Updated definitions of adverse events for trials and registries of mechanical circulatory support" (25). In the current review, the following MAEs were included: ventricular arrhythmia (VA), aortic regurgitation (AR), "combined adverse events" (including episode of VA, HF, chest pain, bleeding, infection, thrombosis, pump-related problems, biliary disfunction, elective procedures), complicated postoperative stay, and all-cause rehospitalization.

Study Quality
The Newcastle–Ottawa Scale (NOS) for observational cohorts was used to assess the quality of all included studies (26). The NOS score was then converted into Agency for Healthcare Research and Quality standards (AHRQ); good, fair, and poor (27).

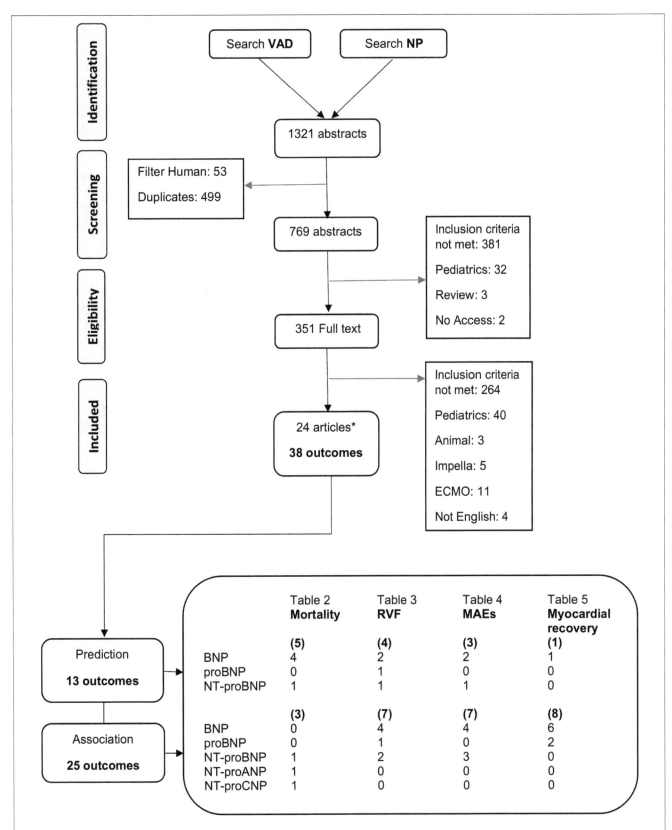

FIGURE 2 | PRISMA flow diagram for literature search and study selection process. *Several articles contain multiple circulating NP or outcomes. ANP, atrial natriuretic peptide; BNP, B-type natriuretic peptide; CNP, C-type natriuretic peptide; ECMO, extracorporeal membrane oxygenation; MAEs, major adverse events; NP, natriuretic peptide; NT-proBNP, N-terminal pro-BNP; RVF, right ventricular failure; VAD, ventricular assist device.

RESULTS

Literature Search

The literature search and selection process is presented in the PRISMA flow diagram in **Figure 2**. The literature search retrieved 1,321 citations from the seven electronic databases. After duplicates were removed, 769 citations went through title and abstract screening, of which 351 articles were screened full text. A total of 745 citations were excluded; the majority did not meet the inclusion criteria regarding advanced HF, reporting any kind of endpoint, receiving LVAD therapy, or measurement of circulating NPs prior to device implantation. Eventually, 24 articles passed full text screening and were included in this review.

Study Characteristics

The included studies were published between 2008 and 2020, and were from countries in Europe, the United States of America, and Japan. Twenty-three of the included studies were retrospective cohort studies. The 24 studies were fairly heterogenous reporting on multiple subtypes of NP, and various and multiple outcomes. This resulted in a total of 38 outcomes in all studies, where predictive relations were studied in 13 and associative relations in 25 (**Figure 2**). Follow-up duration ranged from 48 hours up to 5 years after LVAD implantation. Study sample sizes ranged from 14 to 15,138 patients. Natriuretic peptides were extracted from various materials (blood or plasma), measured with different assays, and presented in diverse measuring units. The upper

TABLE 2 | Baseline characteristics and outcomes of included studies for all-cause mortality.

References	NP	Timing NP days	Design N	LVAD/CF N (%)	DT/BTT N (%)	Male gender N (%)	Age years	ICM N (%)	FU days	Definition outcome mortality	Statistics	Relation NPs—mortality
						Predictive relation						
Papathanasiou et al. (28)	BNP- Log pg/ml	2	RS 103	103 (100) 103 (100)	69 (67) 34 (33)	82 (80)	59 (11)[†]	56 (54)	180	All-cause mortality	HR, 95%CI	1.27 (0.94–1.71) $p = 0.12$
											HR, 95%CI	1.35 (0.92–1.96)[‡] $p = 0.12$
										All-cause mortality or rehospitalization	HR, 95%CI	*1.10 (0.87–1.37) $p = 0.45$*
											HR, 95%CI	*1.00 (0.76–1.33)[‡] $p = 0.98$*
Sato et al. (29)	BNP- Log pg/ml	1	RS 83	83 (100) 18 (22)	83 (100) 0 (0)	63 (76)	39 ± 12	3 (4)	90	All-cause mortality	HR, 95%CI	1.00 (0.99–1.00) $p = 0.673$
Yoshioka et al. (30)	BNP pg/ml	-	RS 41	41 (100) 6 (15)	0 (0) 41 (100)	29 (71)	39 ± 2	3 (7)	90	All-cause mortality	OR, 95%CI	1.00 (0.99–1.00) $p = 0.246$
Shiga et al. (31)	BNP pg/ml	-	RS 47	47 (100) 0 (0)	0 (0) 47 (100)	35 (75)	39 ± 15	12 (26)	730	All-cause mortality	OR, 95%CI	1.000 (1.000–1.001) $p = 0.576$
	BNP ≥1,000 pg/ml										OR, 95%CI	1.143 (0.382–3.421) $p = 0.812$
Topilsky et al. (32)	NT-proBNP per 100 increase pg/ml	1	R- 83	83 (100) 83 (100)	56 (67) 27 (23)	81 (98)	63 ± 12	45 (54)	30	Mortality	OR, 95%CI	1.03 (1.01–1.06) **$p = 0.003$**
						Associative relation						**Survivors vs. non-survivors Median (range)**
Cabiati et al. (33)	NT-proBNP pg/ml	Hospital admission	RS 17	17 (100) 17 (100)	- -	16 (94)	51 (47–63)[†]	5 (28)	28	All-cause mortality	χ2 test	986.10 vs. 5721.00 **$p = 0.028$**
	NT-proANP nmol/l	Hospital admission	RS 17	17 (100) 17 (100)	- -	16 (94)	51 (47–63)[†]	5 (28)	28	All-cause mortality	χ2 test	8.04 vs. 11.20 $p = 0.832$
	NT-proCNP pg/ml	Hospital admission	RS 17	17 (100) 17 (100)	- -	16 (94)	51 (47–63)[†]	5 (28)	28	All-cause mortality	χ2 test	85.92 vs. 52.07 $p = 0.322$

Age in years is described in Mean ± SD, except for [†] Median (range).
[‡] Adjusted for age, male gender, DT, EF, creatinine, CKD, ECLS, IABP, invasive ventilation, inotropes.
BNP, B-type natriuretic peptide; BTT, bridge to transplant; CKD, chronic kidney disease; CF, continuous flow; CI confidence interval; DT, destination therapy; ECLS, Extra Corporeal Life Support; EF, ejection fraction; FU, follow up; HR, hazards ratio; IABP, intra-aortic balloon pump; ICM, ischemic cardiomyopathy; Log, log transformed, LVAD, left ventricular assist device; NP, natriuretic peptide; NT-proBNP; N-terminal pro-B-type NP; N, number; OR, odds ratio; R, retrospective cohort; S, single center; SD, standard deviation; vs., versus.
The bold p-values indicate statistical significance.

TABLE 3 | Baseline characteristics and outcomes of included studies for right ventricular failure.

References	NP	Timing NP days	Design N	LVAD/CF N (%)	DT/BTT N (%)	Male gender N (%)	Age years	ICM N (%)	FU Days	Definition outcome RVF	Statistics	Relation NPs—RVF
Predictive relation												
Shiga et al. (34)	BNP- Log pg/ml / BNP ≥1,200 pg/ml	-	RS 79	79 (100) / 20 (25)	0 (0) / 79 (100)	58 (73)	39 ± 14	14 (18)	PO	ECMO, or need for RVAD	OR, 95%CI / OR, 95%CI	1.001 (1.000–1.001) **p = 0.043** / 8.409 (0.922–76.73) p = 0.059
Kato et al. (35)	BNP >1,232 ng/ml	≤5	RS 61	61 (100) / 30 (49)	- / -	52 (85)	54 ± 13	25 (41)	2–14	NO inhalation >48 h, and/or restarting/ inotropic support >14 days, or need for RVAD	OR, 95%CI / OR, 95%CI	1.021 (1.000–1.042) **p = 0.035** / 1.021(1.000–1.027)‡ **p = 0.0357**
Loghmanpour et al. (36)	proBNP -	-	RM 10909	10909 (100) / 10909 (100)	3811 (35) / 6901 (63)	8,606 (78)	(50–69)†	4,466 (41)	2–14	Pharmacological management of RVF/PVR, cr need for RVAD	Bayesian model; 176 variables	**6th most powerful predictor out of 176**
Potapov et al. (37)	NT-proBNP >10,000 pg/ml	1	R- 54	54 (100) / 37 (69)	- / -	49 (91)	52 (32–69)†	6 (11)	2	In absence of cardiac tamponade 2 criteria, MAP ≤55 mmHg, CVP ≥16 mmHg, mixed VS ≤55%, CI <2 L/min/m², IS >20 h, or need for RVAD	OR, 95%CI	1 (1–1.002) p = 0.1
												RVF vs. no RVF Mean ± SD
Associative relation												
Kapelios et al. (38)	BNP pg/ml	-	RS 20	20 (100) / 20 (100)	20 (100) / 0 (100)	19 (95)	54 ± 10	12 (60)	1,241 ± 694*	>1 year: inotrope: iv or inhaled vasodilator (>7days), tqo of the four criteria; CVP >18 mmHg or mean RAP >18 mmHg, CI <2.3 L/min/m², ascites/ peripheral edema, CVP>, or need for RVAD	Paired t-test	1,819 ± 1,492 vs. 1,359 ± 1,611 p = 0.52
Kato et al. (35)	BNP pg/ml	≤5	RS 61	61 (100) / 30 (49)	- / -	52 (85)	54 ± 13	25 (41)	2–14	NO inhalation >48 h, and/or restarting/ inotropic support >14 days, or need for RVAD	Paired t-test	1895.1 ± 1551.1 vs. 1250.5 ± 1045.2 p = 0.0572
Shiga et al. (34)	BNP- Log pg/ml	-	RS 79	79 (100) / 20 (25)	0 (0) / 79 (100)	58 (73)	39 ± 14	14 (18)	PO	ECMO, or need for RVAD	χ2 test	7.55 ± 0.60 vs. 6.76 ± 0.90 **p = 0.041**
Deswarte et al. (39)	BNP pg/ml	-	RM 14	14 (100) / 14 (100)	14 (100) / 0 (0)	-	63 (37–69)†	7 (50)	30	Inotropic support ≤14days, death caused by RVF, or need for RVAD	Mann-Whitney U-test	1,792 (992–8,500) vs. 1,710 (701–3,643)§ p > 0.05#
Pettinari et al. (40)	proBNP -	-	R- 59	59 (100) / 59 (100)	4 (7) / 55 (93)	53 (90)	48 ± 15	31 (52)	PO	Need for RVAD	Mann-Whitney U-test	11,034 ± 9,620 vs. 4,667 ± 3,082 p = 0.06

(Continued)

Handbook of Cardiovascular Biomarkers: Pathophysiology and Disease Management

TABLE 3 | Continued

References	NP	Timing NP days	Design N	LVAD/CF N (%)	DT/BTT N (%)	Male gender N (%)	Age years	ICM N (%)	FU Days	Definition outcome RVF	Statistics	Relation NPs–RVF
Hennig et al. (41)	NT-proBNP pg/ml	1	RS 40	40 (100) 22 (55)	0 (0) 40 (100)	38 (95)	54 ± 13	–	2	In absence of cardiac tamponade two criteria: MAP ≤55 mmHg, CVP ≥16 mmHg, mixed VS ≤55%, CI <2 L/min/m², IS >20 h; or need for RVAD	Mann-Whitney U-test or χ2 test	17,174 vs. 6,322[†] **p = 0.032**
Potapov et al. (37)	NT-proBNP pg/ml	1	R- 54	54 (100) 37 (69)	– –	49 (91)	52 (32–69)[†]	6 (11)	2	In absence of cardiac tamponade two criteria: MAP ≤55 mmHg, CVP ≥16 mmHg, mixed VS ≤55%, CI <2 L/min/m², IS >20 h; or need for RVAD	Mann-Whitney U-test or t-test	13,026 (8,800–17,566) vs. 4,699 (925–10,433)[†] **p = 0.003**

Age in years is described in Mean ± SD, except for [†] Median (range).
[†] Adjusted for PAP, RAP, RVSWI, tBili, RV FAC, serum OPN.
[*] Mean ± SD.
[§] Mean (interquartile range).
[#] Exact p-value unknown.
BNP, B-type natriuretic peptide; BTT, bridge to transplant; CF, continuous flow; CI, cardiac index; CI confidence interval; CVP, central venous pressure; DT, destination therapy; ECMO, Extracorporeal membrane oxygenation; FU, follow up; h, hours; HR, hazards ratio; ICM, ischemic cardiomyopathy; IS, inotropic support; Log, log transformed; LVAD, left ventricular assist device; M, multicenter; MAP, mean arterial pressure; N, number; NO, nitric oxide; NP, natriuretic peptide; NT-proBNP; N-terminal pro-B-type NP; OPN, osteopontin; OR, odds ratio; PAP, pulmonary artery pressure; PO, postoperative; PVR, pulmonary vascular resistance; R, retrospective cohort; RVAD, right ventricular assist device; RVF, right ventricular failure; RV FAC, right ventricular fractional area change; RVSWI, right ventricular stroke work index; S, single center; SD, standard deviation; tBili, total bilirubin concentration; vs., versus; VS, venous saturation.
The bold p-values indicate statistical significance.

cut off levels for normal NP levels varied from one study to the other. It should be pointed out that NP levels, unless log transformed, are non-normal distributed. Nevertheless, several studies included in this review chose to report NP levels non-log transformed. Descriptive statistic, mean ± standard deviation (SD), was used for log transformed NP measurements. Median and (interquartile) range was used for non-log transformed NP measurements. Groups were compared using various analyses depending on how continuous variables were expressed and how many groups were compared. Univariate and multivariate Cox regression was used for survival analyses expressed in hazard ratio. Univariate and multivariate logistic regression was used to estimate the strength of the effect of NPs expressed in odds ratio. The quality assessed by the NOS was "good" in all studies (**Supplementary Material 2**).

Study Results

The 24 studies assessing the relation between NP levels before LVAD implantation and all-cause mortality, RVF, MAEs, and myocardial recovery after implantation are summarized in **Tables 2–5**.

All-Cause Mortality

Five studies analyzed the predictive value of NPs for all-cause mortality, of which 4 studies included BNP and 1 study included NT-proBNP (**Table 2**). None of the studies found BNP levels before LVAD implantation predictive of all-cause mortality (28–31). In contrast, NT-proBNP levels before LVAD implantation were predictive of 30-days all-cause mortality (32). The study by Cabiati et al. looked at an associative relation and found that NT-proBNP was associated with 4-weeks all-cause mortality, while NT-proANP and NT-proCNP were not (33).

Right Ventricular Failure

Four studies assessed the predictive value of NPs for RVF (two studies BNP, one study proBNP, and one study NT-proBNP) (**Table 3**) (34–37). All studies had at least the outcome "need for right ventricular assist device (RVAD)." Study sample size was 54–79, with the exception of the study by Loghmanpour et al. with a large study population of $N = 10,909$ (34–37). The two studies analyzing BNP demonstrated that BNP levels before LVAD implantation were predictive of the need of RVAD postoperatively up to 14 days (34, 35). In the study of Shiga et al. it was demonstrated that BNP levels ≥1,200 pg/ml were not predictive of RVF, while in the study by Kato et al. BNP levels ≥1,232 ng/ml were an independent predictor of RVF after 2–14 days (34, 35). In a Bayesian prediction model, proBNP levels had high predictive value for RVF in 2–14 days after LVAD implantation (36). NT-proBNP levels before LVAD implantation were not predictive of RVF within 48 hours post-operatively (37). Importantly, this study by Potapov et al. used a cut-off value of NT-proBNP >10,000 pg/ml (37). Of the seven studies analyzing an associative relation, four analyzed BNP, one analyzed proBNP, and two analyzed NT-proBNP (34, 35, 37–41). Shiga et al. found that BNP levels were associated with "need for RVAD" within the postoperative period (34). Both Hennig et al. and Potapov et al. found that NT-proBNP was associated with RVF within 48 hours

TABLE 4 | Baseline characteristics and outcomes of included studies for major adverse events.

References	NP	Timing NP days	Design N	LVAD/CF N (%)	DT/BTT N (%)	Male gender N (%)	Age years	ICM N (%)	FU Days	Definition outcome MAEs	Statistics	Relation NPs—MAEs
Predictive Relation												
Truby et al. (42)	BNP >500 ng/l	-	RM 10603	10,279 (97) 10,603 (100)	4,474 (42) 6,047 (57)	8,246 (78)	>60 (45)*	4,738 (45)	730	Moderate or severe AR	HR, 95%CI	1.48 (1.23–1.77) **p < 0.001**
Hellman et al. (43)	BNP max. pg/ml	122	RS 74	74 (100) 74 (100)	- -	49 (66)	56	30 (41)	15	VA: VF, VT, or asymptomatic NSVT	OR, 95%CI	1.5–5.1‡ **p = 0.0008**
Hasin et al. (44)	NT-proBNP per 1,000 increase pg/ml	Hospital admission	RS 88	115 (100) 115 (100)	73 (63) 42 (37)	96 (83)	62 (53–69)†	56 (49)	511 ± 329#	Less rehospitalization: Cardiac (VA, HF, chest pain), bleeding, infection, thrombosis, pump related, biliary, elective, other	HR, 95%CI	0.98 (0.96–0.99) **p = 0.022** 0.98 (0.96–1.00)§ **p = 0.022**
												Outcome vs. no outcome Median (range)
Associative Relation												
Truby et al. (42)	BNP ng/l	-	RM 10603	10,279 (97) 10,603 (100)	4,474 (42) 6047 (57)	8,246 (78)	>60 (45)*	4,738 (45)	730	Moderate or severe AR	Kruskal-Wallis test	915 (489–1783) vs. 756 (382–1421) **p = 0.001**
Hegarova et al. (45)	BNP ng/l	1	PS 136	136 (100) 136 (100)	0 (0) 136 (100)	121 (89)	51 (23–72)†	54 (40)	298 (159–456)†	Less adverse events; HF, infection, pump thrombosis	Mann-Whitney U-test	1440.4 vs. 2405.5# **p = 0.001**
	BNP ng/l	1	PS 59	59 (100) 59 (100)	0 (0) 59 (100)	51 (86)	51 (23–72)†	23 (39)	298 (159–456)†	Rehospitalization	Mann-Whitney U-test	1118.7 vs. 1762.1# p = 0.056
Hellman et al. (43)	BNP pg/ml	122	RS 74	74 (100) 74 (100)	- -	49 (66)	56	30 (41)	15	VA: VF, VT, or asymptomatic NSVT	Mann-Whitney U-test	2,373 vs. 1,309 **p = 0.0016**
Hasin et al. (46)	NT-proBNP pg/ml	Hospital admission	RS 72	72 (100) 72 (100)	21 (29)	63 (87)	63 (53–69)†	36 (50)	14	Complicated postoperative stay: IC > 5days, ventilator support > 2days, total hospital stay >14 days	Mann-Whitney U-test	4,786 (2,232–13,790) vs. 3,199 (869–11,803) p = 0.224
	NT-proBNP Log pg/ml											1.14 (0.46–2.16) vs. 1.09 (0.32–3.30)‡‡ p = 0.725
	NT-proBNP pg/ml	1	RS 72	72 (100) 72 (100)	21 (29)	63 (87)	63 (53–69)†	36 (50)	14	Complicated postoperative stay: IC >5 days, ventilator support >2 days, total hospital stay >14 days	Mann-Whitney U-test	3,446 (1,801–8,101) vs. 3,431 (932–5,113) p = 0.187
	NT-proBNP Log pg/ml											1.11 (0.52–2.72) vs. 0.98 (0.49–2.16)‡‡ p = 0.410
Hasin et al. (44)	NT-proBNP Per 1,000 expressed pg/ml	Hospital admission	RS 115‡	115 (100) 115 (100)	73 (63) 42 (37)	96 (83)	62 (53–69)†	56 (49)	511 ± 329#	Less rehospitalization: Cardiac (VA, HF, chest pain), bleeding, infection, thrombosis, pump related, biliary, elective, other	Wilcoxon signed rank test	4.3 (2.4–8.3) vs. 4.7 (3.0–8.1) **p = 0.022**

Age in years is described in Mean ± SD, except for *Percentage with age > 60 years and †Median (range).

‡Adjusted for VT in the past, ICD, CAD, and age.

§Adjusted for age, gender, and age.

#Mean ± SD.

‡‡Adjusted for age, gender, and glomerular filtration rate.

AR, aortic regurgitation; BNP, B-type natriuretic peptide; BTT, bridge to transplant; CAD, coronary artery disease; CF, continuous flow; FU, follow up; HF, heart failure; HR, hazards ratio; IC, intensive care; ICD, internal cardiac defibrillator; ICM, ischemic cardiomyopathy; Log, log transformed; LVAD, left ventricular assist device; M, multicenter; MAEs, major adverse events; Max, maximal level measured; NP, natriuretic peptide; NT-proBNP; N-terminal pro-B-type NP; N, number; OR, odds ratio; P, prospective cohort; R, retrospective cohort; S, single center; SD, standard deviation; VA, ventricular arrhythmia; VF, ventricular fibrillation; (NS)VT, non-sustained ventricular tachycardia; vs., versus.

The bold p-values indicate statistical significance.

TABLE 5 | Baseline characteristics and outcomes of included studies for left ventricular (LV) myocardial recovery.

References	NP	Timing NP Days	Design N	LVAD/CF N (%)	DT/BTT N (%)	Male gender N (%)	Age Years	ICM N (%)	FU Days	Definition outcome Myocardial recovery	Statistics	Relation NPs—Myocardial recovery
												Predictive relation
Imamura et al. (47)	BNP- Log pg/ml	1	RS 27	27 (100) 22 (81)	0 (0) 27 (100)	21 (78)	35 ± 14	0 (0)	183	LVRR (EF ≥35%)	OR, 95%CI	0.753 (0.021-27.17) p = 0.877
											Associative relation	**Myocardial recovery vs. no myocardial recovery Mean ± SD**
Topkara et al. (6)	BNP pg/ml	–	RM 13454	13,454 (100) 13,454 (100)	5,257 (39) 3,714 (28)	10,567 (79)	51.5 ± 13	6,241 (46)	1,096	Device explant vs. no device explant	Unpaired t-test	926.7 ± 860.9 vs. 1169.9 ± 1097.6 **p = 0.024**
			RM 8805	8,805 (100) 8,805 (100)	351 (46)	6,918 (79)	57.1 ± 14	3942 (29)	1,096	LVRR (EF ≥40%) vs. no LVRR (EF <30%)	Unpaired t-test	1240.9 ± 149.5 vs. 1157.4 ± 1086.1 p = 0.199
	proBNP pg/ml	–	RM 13454	13,454 (100) 13,454 (100)	241 (32) 5,257 (39)	10,567 (79)	51.5 ± 13	6241 (46)	1,096	Device explant vs. no device explant	Unpaired t-test	4642.4 ± 7323.3 vs. 6787.2 ± 7887.3 p = 0.153
			RM 8805	8,805 (100) 8,805 (100)	3,714 (28) 351 (46) 241 (32)	6,918 (79)	57.1 ± 14	3942 (29)	1,096	LVRR (EF ≥40%) vs. no LVRR (EF <30%)	Unpaired t-test	9880.8 ± 11664.4 vs. 6617.3 ± 7737.5 **p = 0.003**
Wever-Pinzon et al. (48)	BNP pg/ml	–	RM 15138	14,287 (94) 13,987 (92)	5601 (37) 4,284 (28)	11,877 (78)	50	27 (14)	1,826	Device explant or deactivation	X² test	742 (377-1090) vs. 825 (412-1565)* p = 0.10
Imamura et al. (47)	BNP- Log pg/ml	1	RS 27	27 (100) 22 (81)	0 (0) 27 (100)	21 (78)	35 ± 14	0 (0)	183	LVRR (EF ≥35%)	Unpaired t-test	2.8 ± 0.2 vs. 2.8 ± 0.3 p = 0.882
Imamura et al. (49)	BNP- Log pg/ml	1	R- 60	60 (100) 34 (57)	0 (0) 60 (100)	48 (80.0)	40.1 ± 12	0 (0)	183	LVRR (EF ≥35%) or device explant	Unpaired t-test	2.92 ± 0.30 vs. 2.89 ± 0.36 p = 0.793
Mano et al. (50)	BNP pg/ml	–	RS 41	41 (100) 0 (0)	0 (0) 41 (100)	28 (68)	30.1 ± 10	0 (0)	365	Device explant	Unpaired t-test	1140 ± 660 vs. 1282 ± 1074 p = 0.76

Age in years is described in Mean ± SD.

*Median (IRQ).

BNP, B-type natriuretic peptide; BTT, bridge to transplant; CF, continuous flow; CI, confidence interval; DT, destination therapy; FU, follow up; HR, hazards ratio; ICM, ischemic cardiomyopathy; Log, log transformed; LVAD, left ventricular assist device; LVRR, left ventricular reverse remodeling; M, multicenter; NP, natriuretic peptide; NT-proBNP, N-terminal pro-B-type NP; N, number; OR, odds ratio; R, retrospective cohort; S, single center; SD, standard deviation; vs., versus.

The bold p-values indicate statistical significance.

postoperatively (37, 41). The remaining studies did not find an association between NP levels and RVF, although in some studies results were close to statistical significance (35, 38–40).

Major Adverse Events

A total of five studies assessed the predictive or associative relation between NPs and MAEs. The following MAEs were identified in these studies: VA, AR, "combined adverse events" (including episode of VA, HF, chest pain, bleeding, infection, thrombosis, pump-related problems, biliary disfunction, elective procedures), complicated postoperative stay, and all-cause rehospitalization. Three studies analyzed whether NPs were predictive of MAEs, of which two studies assessed BNP and one study assessed NT-proBNP (**Table 4**). All studies found that BNP and NT-proBNP levels before LVAD implantation were predictive of MAEs (42–44). Hellman et al. demonstrated that BNP was an independent predictor for VA within 15 days post-operative (43). In a large study by Truby et al. BNP >500 ng/l was predictive of the development of moderate or severe AR (42). NT-proBNP measured at "hospital admission" before LVAD implantation was an independent predictor for rehospitalization due to cardiac, bleeding, infection, thrombosis, pump related, biliary, or "elective" events (44). Of the studies reporting on associative relations, three studies analyzed BNP levels and two studies analyzed NT-proBNP levels (42, 44–46). In these studies, BNP levels before LVAD implantation were associated with MAEs between 2 weeks up to 2 years (42, 43, 45). In a sub-analysis, Hegarova et al. demonstrated that although BNP was associated with adverse events up to 1.5 years after initial discharge, it was not associated with subsequent rehospitalizations (45). The two studies analyzing NT-proBNP levels found that it was not associated with complicated post-operative stay. However, it was associated with less rehospitalization for combined adverse events (44, 46).

Myocardial Recovery

Only one study assessed the predictive value of NP for myocardial recovery (**Table 5**). This study found that BNP levels before LVAD implantation were not predictive of LV recovery after 6 months (47). Five studies reported on associative relations between NP and myocardial recovery. All studies analyzed BNP levels, whereas Topkara et al. additionally investigated proBNP levels. Besides the large study by Topkara et al. none of the included studies found an association between BNP and LV recovery (6, 47–50).

DISCUSSION

To the best of our knowledge, this is the first systematic review assessing the prognostic value of circulating NP levels in advanced HF patients receiving LVAD therapy. The main findings are as follows:

1. B-type natriuretic peptide is not predictive of all-cause mortality at a follow-up of 3 months or longer. Evidence regarding NT-proBNP is insufficient to draw a reliable conclusion.

2. B-type natriuretic peptide is predictive of RVF in the postoperative period after the first 48 hours. In contrast, NT-proBNP seems associated with RVF within 48 hours after LVAD implantation.

3. B-type natriuretic peptide and NT-proBNP levels appear to be predictive of various MAEs, and related to rehospitalization up to 1.5 years after LVAD implantation.

4. B-type natriuretic peptide is not predictive of, and most likely not associated with, myocardial recovery.

All-Cause Mortality

None of the studies found that BNP levels before LVAD implantation are predictive of all-cause mortality up to 2 years after implantation. In contrast, Topilsky et al. demonstrated that preoperative NT-proBNP levels are predictive of 1-month mortality after LVAD implantation (32). The study by Papathanasiou et al. analyzing BNP, had a similar study sample size and baseline characteristics compared to the study by Topilsky et al., but did not report a significant predictive relation (28). The differences in type of NPs and length of follow-up may have contributed to this contradictory finding. The follow-up duration may be an important factor, as both studies analyzing 1-month mortality found a significant relation (32, 33). This may suggest that NPs are related to early postoperative mortality, but lose their prognostic value for all-cause mortality at longer follow-up. Of note, both studies analyzed NT-proBNP, and to date no studies are available analyzing BNP levels in relation to 1-month mortality after LVAD implantation. Whether BNP and NT-proBNP have different prognostic power regarding all-cause mortality after LVAD implantation needs to be investigated in future prospective studies.

In the studies included in this review, BNP levels are not predictive of all-cause mortality after LVAD implantation. This is an interesting finding, since NPs (including BNP and NT-proBNP) are strong predictors of all-cause mortality in HF patients (2, 20–22). In addition, BNP levels are independent predictors of mortality in advanced HF patients receiving cardiac resynchronization defibrillator (CRT-D) therapy (51, 52). It may well be that NPs are not so much a predictor of mortality risk after LVAD implantation, but rather a reflection of disease severity. Furthermore, the change in prognostic value of NPs may be caused by several mechanisms related to the LVAD itself. The device unloads the LV, thereby reducing pressure and stretch of cardiomyocytes. Reduced myocardial stretch may lead to lower NP levels. Decreased NP levels are related to a lower mortality risk (53). In parallel with the improvements in hemodynamics and prognosis provided by the LVAD, NT-proBNP levels decrease after LVAD implantation (27, 49). However, they remain abnormal and elevated compared to the levels in chronic HF patients, suggesting that key pathological changes on cellular myocardial level remain, despite LVAD support (49). This may partly be explained by the fact that the flow mechanisms of the devices, including lack of pulsatility and high rotation speed of the LVAD disc or propeller, influence several physiological processes connected to NPs, like neurohormonal changes and sympathetic and renin-angiotensin-aldosterone activity (27, 49, 51). These processes may result in altered NP release. Therefore, the prognostic value of NP levels before LVAD implantation may be changed by the therapy itself. Nonetheless, several studies have shown that NP measurements and their fluctuations during LVAD therapy are strongly related to adverse outcome including mortality (28, 29, 45). These findings may suggest, that NP levels before implantation and during LVAD support may not have similar predictive value for all-cause mortality, as the hemodynamic support provided by the LVAD may change NP levels and the accompanied mortality risk.

Finally, another explanation for the lack of predictive value of NPs regarding all-cause mortality could be the erratic course of LVAD therapy. Major adverse event rates are high and correspond to high mortality rates. The studies included in this review that found no relation between NPs and all-cause mortality had a follow-up duration of 90, 180, and 730 days after LVAD implantation. Competing risk analyses should have been performed to account for the effect of MAEs on mortality. However, none of the studies included in this review provided these analyses. This statistic error could explain why in the included studies NPs are not predictive for mortality, but appear to have predictive value for various MAEs.

Right Ventricular Failure

Four studies investigated whether NP levels were predictive of RVF after LVAD implantation. Due to the large study by Loghmanpour et al. the sample size of the studies (BNP, proBNP) reporting a positive predictive value for RVF was 11.049 patients, whereas the total sample size of the studies (NT-proBNP) which reported no predictive value was 54 patients (34–37). All studies analyzing BNP and proBNP were predictive, whereas the study by Potapov et al. analyzing NT-proBNP was not. It should be noted that this is only one study with a small study population (37). Nevertheless, this finding may be linked to the type of NPs that was investigated. In addition, this could be explained by the follow-up duration. Potapov et al. investigated RVF within 48 hours postoperatively, whereas all other studies analyzed RVF after the first 48 hours post LVAD implantation (34–37). Furthermore, it should be noted that in all studies, the definition of RVF included "need for RVAD." Since the decision to use an RVAD after LVAD implantation may vary based on clinical practice, this may change the definition of outcome and thereby the prognostic value of NPs for prediction of RVF.

It is well-known that RVF after LVAD implantation severely impairs prognosis. In the INTERMACS registry, RVF represented the specific cause of death in 4% of all patients (4). The interaction between the LVAD, the right ventricle (RV), and NP system is complex. Preoperative elevated NP levels, inflammatory markers and cytokines may represent a worse hemodynamic status and therefore a higher susceptibility to RVF after LVAD implantation (41). At the same time, it has been suggested that elevations in neurohumoral markers and cytokines may directly influence RV function, contributing to the development of RVF (41).

One study included in our review analyzed late RVF after LVAD implantation, and found no relation of BNP levels before LVAD implantation to late RVF (mean follow-up of 3.4 years) (38). This may be explained by the fact that development of RVF during long-term support is most likely multi-factorial. Different from the LV, the RV does not exhibit significant reverse structural remodeling despite reduced RV afterload during LVAD support (54–56). Kato et al. demonstrated that the CF-LVAD impairs the physiological contractility of cardiomyocytes by the non-pulsatile mode of LV unloading, which over time could lead to decreased RV compliance and contractility (40, 57). Furthermore, interventricular septum displacement caused by suction of the CF-LVAD may result in RV dysynchrony and also reduced cooptation of the tricuspid valve. In long-term LVAD therapy, this may gradually increase tricuspid regurgitation and subsequent increase RV preload. Over time these factors could contribute to the development of late RVF (38). Future studies should address preoperative circulating NP levels in relation to these different factors, in order to better predict RVF during long-term LVAD support.

Major Adverse Events

In the INTERMACS registry, the most frequently reported MAEs after LVAD implantation are infection, neurologic events, RVF, device malfunction including pump thrombosis, and multiple system organ failure (4). However, apart from RVF, there were no studies available that assessed the relation between NPs and these specific MAEs. The studies included in this review assessed the relation between NP levels before LVAD implantation and MAEs including VA, AR, "combined adverse events," complicated postoperative stay, and all-cause rehospitalization. All studies that were included found that NP (BNP and NT-proBNP) levels before LVAD implantation are predictive of diverse MAEs occurring in the postoperative period within 15 days up to 2 years follow-up, and rehospitalizations within 1.5 year after LVAD implantation (42–44).

Ventricular Arrhythmia

Hellman et al. demonstrated that high BNP levels before LVAD implantation are a powerful predictor for VA up to 15 days (43). Several mechanisms may explain this finding. BNP levels reflect ventricular stretch and hypertrophy, which over time results in tissue fibrosis and other changes of the myocardium that may be a substrate for VA (58). The LVAD unloads the failing heart, but cannot initiate reverse remodeling within 15 days. Thus, the substrate for VA remains, as does the prognostic value of BNP before LVAD implantation. Another possible explanation may be that high BNP levels are associated with elevated levels of cytokines and catecholamines, resulting in prolongation of the action potential and enhanced calcium entry, causing QTc prolongation and promoting arrhythmogenesis, eventually triggering VA (43, 59).

Aortic Regurgitation

During CF-LVAD therapy, up to 15% of the patients may develop moderate to severe AR, with significant impact on morbidity and mortality (42). The study by Truby et al. identified BNP levels >500 ng/L as a predictor in a univariate analysis of a cox proportional hazard model for the development of moderate or severe AR after 2 years of LVAD therapy. However, BNP levels were not taken into account in the multivariate analysis of AR development (42). Factors like body mass index, sex, and destination therapy strategy appear to be stronger predictors of development of moderate or severe AR than BNP levels (42). Nevertheless, this study points out that BNP identifies patients who are vulnerable for adverse events. In patients with AR, NPs are predictive of the development of HF and mortality (60). However, no studies are available that assess the prognostic value of NPs in relation to AR in (advanced) HF patients. Therefore, more studies are needed to get mechanistic insights into the relation between NPs and AR in HF patients receiving LVAD therapy.

Rehospitalization and Combined Adverse Events

Two studies analyzed rehospitalization after initial discharge, of which Hasin et al. found higher NT-proBNP before LVAD implantation predictive for, and associated with, less rehospitalization for any MAE (44). Hegarova et al. demonstrated that higher BNP levels were associated with less or no combined adverse events that required outpatient care or rehospitalization. In a sub-analysis, the authors found that BNP levels were not able to differentiate between combined adverse events that required rehospitalization and those that did not (45). Interestingly, both studies demonstrated that higher NP levels before LVAD implantation were related to less combined adverse events (44, 45). This finding may be related to the kind of MAE. Hasin et al. found that cardiac events (30.4%) including VA, HF, and chest pain, and bleeding events (29.6%) were the main reasons for rehospitalization, whereas Hegarova et al. found that pump thrombosis (29%) and decompensated HF (26%) were the most frequent adverse events (44, 45). These findings suggest that NP levels before LVAD implantation within a certain range may be predictive for rehospitalization of specific MAEs.

Myocardial Recovery

Among the articles considered in this systematic review, five studies investigated the relation of NPs with myocardial recovery. Imamura et al. demonstrated that BNP before LVAD implantation was not predictive for LV ejection fraction recovery (47). The study by Topkara et al. demonstrated that NP levels (BNP, proBNP) were associated with myocardial recovery, while the other studies did not (6, 47–50). The total sample size in the four studies that found no association was just slightly larger than the sample size of the one study that did, mainly due to the large studies by Topkara et al. (6) and Wever-Pinzon et al. (48). Both authors extracted their data from the INTERMACS registry, had comparable inclusion criteria, baseline characteristics, outcome and median follow-up. Nevertheless, they found conflicting results. This may be related to the fact that Wever-Pinzon et al. additionally included patients implanted with pulsatile-flow LVADs, and a relatively high number of INTERMACS level 1 patients, who were in critical cardiogenic shock at time of device implantation (48). The higher number of INTERMACS level 1 patients may explain the higher levels of BNP found within the recovery group, and may diminish the associative relation between lower levels of BNP and myocardial recovery. Taken together, these reports are indicative for the fact that NPs may not be a specific marker for cardiac recovery, but rather reflect

the general physical condition and the severity of HF in advanced HF patients receiving LVAD therapy.

Limitations

Although we systematically assessed the evidence for NP and its role as prognostic biomarker in advanced HF patients who receive LVAD therapy, our study is not devoid of its own limitations. According to the NOS score, most studies included in our review were of good quality. However, a number of these studies had a small patient population and therefore low statistical power. The heterogenous nature of the data in terms of timing of NP measurements, subtypes of NP, follow-up time, statistical analyses, and end-points pre-empted us from performing a meta-analysis and derive definitive conclusions. In addition, in a number of studies included in this review, the predictive value of NPs in LVAD patients was not the main hypothesis. We were not able to asses all end-points because of limited literature, and several end-points had heterogenous and subjective definitions, such as "need for RVAD" for the definition of RVF. Although it is generally accepted that NP levels are influenced by gender, age, BMI, comorbidities, kidney disease, and HF medication, most studies did not take all variables into account. In addition, some bias was created as the manuscripts from the same authors, and several studies analyzing multiple subtypes of NP or end-points, were included.

Future Perspective

Given the high incidence of MAEs after LVAD implantation, optimization of patient selection is crucial in order to improve outcome after LVAD implantation. Circulating NP levels may have some power predicting MAEs, RVF and rehospitalization during LVAD therapy. However, new, more promising, circulating biomarkers have been identified for prognostication of MAEs and mortality in HF patients (15, 61–64). Multi-biomarker panels seem to improve the prognostic power of these biomarkers. Emdin et al. compared a multi-biomarker panel [NT-proBNP, soluble suppression of tumorigenicity-2 (sST2), high-sensitive troponin T (hs-TnT)] with a single biomarker (NT-proBNP). Relative risk for all-cause mortality was higher among patients with elevated levels of all multi-panel biomarkers compared to patients with elevated levels of a single biomarker (NT-proBNP, sST2, hs-TnT; RR 9.5 vs. NT-proBNP; RR 2.3, respectively) (65). Ahmad et al. showed that novel biomarkers, such as galectin-3 (GAL-3), ST2, growth differentiation factor-15 (GDF-15), high sensitive C-reactive protein (hs-CRP), and copeptin, when stratified by baseline NT-proBNP levels in their cohort of advanced HF patients, were more sensitive of maladaptive processes than traditional laboratory markers with established prognostic significance, such as red blood cell distribution width, creatinine, blood urea nitrogen, and sodium, which remained within normal limits (66). These studies show that novel biomarkers and their multi-biomarker panels may reflect disease severity more accurately than currently used metrics (65–67). In addition, these novel biomarkers provide a unique insight into the pathophysiologic changes of HF as they reflect the different maladaptive processes involved e.g., oxidative stress, fibrosis, and inflammation (68).

Therefore, novel biomarkers may be considered for screening of patients with advanced HF requiring CF-LVAD therapy, and monitoring of LVAD patients. The present systematic review demonstrates that in order to improve generalizability and interpretation, large prospective studies with predefined outcome, and follow-up duration analyzing preimplantation NPs, multi-biomarker panels and their changes over time are warranted. Validated assays in consecutive patients should be used, and detailed cardiovascular profiles should be created to systematically define pathologies contributing to the levels of NP and other circulating biomarkers.

CONCLUSIONS

This systematic review demonstrates that BNP levels before LVAD implantation are not predictive of all-cause mortality after LVAD implantation. The implantation of an LVAD appears to alter prognosis and NP levels to such an extent that prognosis for mortality stratified by NP levels before LVAD implantation is not applicable after LVAD implantation. However, NP levels appear to identify advanced HF patients who are at risk for postoperative RVF and MAEs, such VA, AR, and rehospitalization. More studies regarding the timing of NP measurements, using different subtypes of NPs within prospective cohorts with predetermined endpoints and follow-up are needed to confirm the prognostic value of NPs in advanced HF patients who will receive LVAD therapy.

AUTHOR CONTRIBUTIONS

EJ: conceptualization: lead, formal analysis: lead, investigation: equal, methodology: equal, project administration: lead, software: equal, writing–original draft: lead, writing–review & editing: equal. JJ: conceptualization: lead, investigation: equal, methodology: equal, supervision: lead, writing-original draft: equal, writing–review & editing: equal. SB: conceptualization: lead, methodology: equal, supervision: equal, writing–original draft: equal, writing–review & editing: equal. MS: conceptualization: equal, supervision: equal, writing-original draft: equal, writing–review & editing: equal. LT: conceptualization: lead, formal analysis: equal, methodology: equal, supervision: lead, writing- original draft: lead, writing–review & editing: lead. All authors contributed to the article and approved the submitted version.

REFERENCES

1. Ahmad T, Patel CB, Milano CA, Rogers JG. when the heart runs out of heartbeats: treatment options for refractory end-stage heart failure. *Circulation.* (2012) 125:2948–55. doi: 10.1161/CIRCULATIONAHA.112.097337
2. Yancy CW, Jessup M, Bozkurt B, Butler J, Casey DE Jr, Colvin MM, et al. 2017 ACC/AHA/HFSA focused update of the 2013 ACCF/AHA guideline for the management of heart failure: a report of the American college of cardiology/American heart association task force on clinical practice guidelines and the heart failure society of America. *J Am Coll Cardiol.* (2017) 70:776–803. doi: 10.1016/j.jacc.2017.04.025
3. Teuteberg JJ, Cleveland JC Jr, Cowger J, Higgins RS, Goldstein DJ, Keebler M, et al. The society of thoracic surgeons intermacs 2019 annual report: the changing landscape of devices and indications. *Ann Thorac Surg.* (2020) 109:649–60. doi: 10.1016/j.athoracsur.2019.12.005
4. Kormos RL, Cowger J, Pagani FD, Teuteberg JJ, Goldstein DJ, Jacobs JP, et al. The society of thoracic surgeons intermacs database annual report: evolving indications, outcomes, and scientific partnerships. *Ann Thorac Surg.* (2019) 107:341–53. doi: 10.1016/j.athoracsur.2018.11.011
5. Kirklin JK, Pagani FD, Kormos RL, Stevenson LW, Blume ED, Myers SL, et al. Eighth annual INTERMACS report: special focus on framing the impact of adverse events. *J Heart Lung Transplant.* (2017) 36:1080–6. doi: 10.1016/j.healun.2017.07.005
6. Topkara VK, Garan AR, Fine B, Godier-Furnemont AF, Breskin A, Cagliostro B, et al. Myocardial recovery in patients receiving contemporary left ventricular assist devices: results from the interagency registry for mechanically assisted circulatory support (INTERMACS). *Circ Heart Fail.* (2016) 9 e003157.doi: 10.1161/CIRCHEARTFAILURE.116.003157
7. Hon JK, Yacoub MH. Bridge to recovery with the use of left ventricular assist device and clenbuterol. *Ann Thorac Surg.* (2003) 75:S36–41. doi: 10.1016/S0003-4975(03)00460-0
8. Motiwala SR, Januzzi JL. The role of natriuretic peptides as biomarkers for guiding the management of chronic heart failure. *Clin Pharmacol Ther.* (2013) 93:57–67. doi: 10.1038/clpt.2012.187
9. Levin ER, Gardner DG, Samson WK. Natriuretic peptides. *NEJM.* (1998) 339:321–8. doi: 10.1056/NEJM199807303390507
10. Kinnunen P, Vuolteenaho O, Ruskoaho H. Mechanisms of atrial and brain natriuretic peptide release from rat ventricular myocardium: effect of stretching. *Endocrinology.* (1993) 132:1961–70. doi: 10.1210/endo.132.5.8477647
11. Weber M, Hamm C. Role of B-type natriuretic peptide (BNP) and NT-proBNP in clinical routine. *Heart.* (2006) 92:843–9. doi: 10.1136/hrt.2005.071233
12. Piek A, Du W, de Boer RA, Sillje HHW. Novel heart failure biomarkers: why do we fail to exploit their potential? *Crit Rev Clin Lab Sci.* (2018) 55:246–63. doi: 10.1080/10408363.2018.1460576
13. Savic-Radojevic A, Pljesa-Ercegovac M, Matic M, Simic D, Radovanovic S, Simic T. Novel biomarkers of heart failure. *Adv Clin Chem.* (2017) 79:93–152. doi: 10.1016/bs.acc.2016.09.002
14. Madamanchi C, Alhosaini H, Sumida A, Runge MS. Obesity and natriuretic peptides, BNP and NT-proBNP: mechanisms and diagnostic implications for heart failure. *Int J Cardiol.* (2014) 176:611–7. doi: 10.1016/j.ijcard.2014.08.007
15. Chow SL, Maisel AS, Anand I, Bozkurt B, de Boer RA, Felker GM, et al. Role of biomarkers for the prevention, assessment, and management of heart failure: a scientific statement from the American heart association. *Circulation.* (2017) 135:e1054–91. doi: 10.1161/CIR.0000000000000490
16. Myhre PL, Vaduganathan M, Claggett B, Packer M, Desai AS, Rouleau JL, et al. B-Type natriuretic peptide during treatment with sacubitril/valsartan: the PARADIGM-HF trial. *J Am Coll Cardiol.* (2019) 73:1264–72. doi: 10.1016/j.jacc.2019.01.018
17. Saenger AK, Rodriguez-Fraga O, Ler R, Ordonez-Llanos J, Jaffe AS, Goetze JP, et al. Specificity of B-type natriuretic peptide assays: cross-reactivity with different BNP, NT-proBNP, and proBNP peptides. *Clin Chem.* (2017) 63:351–8. doi: 10.1373/clinchem.2016.263749
18. Lam CS, Burnett JC Jr, Costello-Boerrigter L, Rodeheffer RJ, Redfield MM. Alternate circulating pro-B-type natriuretic peptide and b-type natriuretic peptide forms in the general population. *J Am Coll Cardiol.* (2007) 49:1193–202. doi: 10.1016/j.jacc.2006.12.024
19. Hutfless R, Kazanegra R, Madani M, Bhalla MA, Tulua-Tata A, Chen A, et al. Utility of B-type natriuretic peptide in predicting postoperative complications and outcomes in patients undergoing heart surgery. *J Am Coll Cardiol.* (2004) 43:1873–9. doi: 10.1016/j.jacc.2003.12.048

20. Oremus M, Don-Wauchope A, McKelvie R, Santaguida PL, Hill S, Balion C, et al. BNP and NT-proBNP as prognostic markers in persons with chronic stable heart failure. *Heart Failure Rev.* (2014) 19:471–505. doi: 10.1007/s10741-014-9439-6

21. Doust JA, Pietrzak E, Dobson A, Glasziou PP. How well does B-type natriuretic peptide predict death and cardiac events in patients with heart failure: systematic review. *Brit Med J.* (2005) 330:625–7. doi: 10.1136/bmj.330.7492.625

22. Huang YT, Tseng YT, Chu TW, Chen J, Lai MY, Tang WR, et al. N-terminal pro b-type natriuretic peptide (NT-pro-BNP)–based score can predict in-hospital mortality in patients with heart failure. *Sci Rep.* (2016) 6:29590. doi: 10.1038/srep29590

23. Januzzi JL Jr, Maisel AS, Silver M, Xue Y, DeFilippi C. Natriuretic peptide testing for predicting adverse events following heart failure hospitalization. *Congest Heart Fail.* (2012) 18:S9–13. doi: 10.1111/j.1751-7133.2012.00306.x

24. Savarese G, Musella F, D'Amore C, Vassallo E, Losco T, Gambardella F, et al. Changes of natriuretic peptides predict hospital admissions in patients with chronic heart failure: a meta-analysis. *JACC: Heart Failure.* (2014) 2:148–58. doi: 10.1016/S0735-1097(14)60737-3

25. Kormos RL, Antonides CFJ, Goldstein DJ, Cowger JA, Starling RC, Kirklin JK, et al. Updated definitions of adverse events for trials and registries of mechanical circulatory support: a consensus statement of the mechanical circulatory support academic research consortium. *J Heart Lung Transplant.* (2020) 39:735–50. doi: 10.1016/j.healun.2020.03.010

26. Moskalewicz A, Oremus M. No clear choice between newcastle-ottawa scale and appraisal tool for cross-sectional studies to assess methodological quality in cross-sectional studies of health-related quality of life and breast cancer. *J Clin Epid.* (2020) 120:94–103. doi: 10.1016/j.jclinepi.2019.12.013

27. Berkman ND, Lohr KN, Morgan LC, Richmond E, Kuo TM, Morton S, et al. *Reliability Testing of The Ahrq Epc Approach to Grading The Strength of Evidence in Comparative Effectiveness Reviews.* Rockville: AHRQ Methods for Effective Health Care (2012).

28. Papathanasiou M, Pizanis N, Tsourelis L, Koch A, Kamler M, Rassaf T, et al. Dynamics and prognostic value of B-type natriuretic peptide in left ventricular assist device recipients. *J Thorac Dis.* (2019) 11:138–44. doi: 10.21037/jtd.2018.12.43

29. Sato T, Seguchi O, Iwashima Y, Yanase M, Nakajima S, Hieda M, et al. Serum brain natriuretic peptide concentration 60 days after surgery as a predictor of long-term prognosis in patients implanted with a left ventricular assist device. *ASAIO J.* (2015) 61:373–8. doi: 10.1097/MAT.0000000000000234

30. Yoshioka D, Sakaguchi T, Saito S, Miyagawa S, Nishi H, Yoshikawa Y, et al. Predictor of early mortality for severe heart failure patients with left ventricular assist device implantation: significance of INTERMACS level and renal function. *Circ J.* (2012) 76:1631–8. doi: 10.1253/circj.CJ-11-1452

31. Shiga T, Kinugawa K, Hatano M, Yao A, Nishimura T, Endo M, et al. Age and preoperative total bilirubin level can stratify prognosis after extracorporeal pulsatile left ventricular assist device implantation. *Circ J.* (2011) 75:121–8. doi: 10.1253/circj.CJ-10-0770

32. Topilsky Y, Oh JK, Shah DK, Boilson BA, Schirger JA, Kushwaha SS, et al. Echocardiographic predictors of adverse outcomes after continuous left ventricular assist device implantation. *JACC: Cardiovasc Imaging.* (2011) 4:211–22. doi: 10.1016/j.jcmg.2010.10.012

33. Cabiati M, Caruso R, Caselli C, Frigerio M, Prescimone T, Parodi O, et al. The natriuretic peptide time-course in end-stage heart failure patients supported by left ventricular assist device implant: focus on NT-proCNP. *Peptides.* (2012) 36:192–8. doi: 10.1016/j.peptides.2012.05.018

34. Shiga T, Kinugawa K, Imamura T, Kato N, Endo M, Inaba T, et al. Combination evaluation of preoperative risk indices predicts requirement of biventricular assist device. *Circ J.* (2012) 76:2785–91. doi: 10.1253/circj.CJ-12-0231

35. Kato TS, Chokshi A, Singh P, Khawaja T, Iwata S, Homma S, et al. Markers of extracellular matrix turnover and the development of right ventricular failure after ventricular assist device implantation in patients with advanced heart failure. *J Heart Lung Transplant.* (2012) 31:37–45. doi: 10.1016/j.healun.2011.10.007

36. Loghmanpour NA, Kormos RL, Kanwar MK, Teuteberg JJ, Murali S, Antaki JF. A bayesian model to predict right ventricular failure following

37. Potapov EV, Stepanenko A, Dandel M, Kukucka M, Lehmkuhl HB, Weng Y, et al. Tricuspid incompetence and geometry of the right ventricle as predictors of right ventricular function after implantation of a left ventricular assist device. *J Heart Lung Transplant.* (2008) 27:1275–81. doi: 10.1016/j.healun.2008.08.012

38. Kapelios CJ, Charitos C, Kaldara E, Malliaras K, Nana E, Pantsios C, et al. Late-onset right ventricular dysfunction after mechanical support by a continuous-flow left ventricular assist device. *J Heart Lung Transplant.* (2015) 34:1604–10. doi: 10.1016/j.healun.2015.05.024

39. Deswarte G, Kirsch M, Lesault PF, Trochu JN, Damy T. Right ventricular reserve and outcome after continuous-flow left ventricular assist device implantation. *J Heart Lung Transplant.* (2010) 29:1196–8. doi: 10.1016/j.healun.2010.05.026

40. Pettinari M, Jacobs S, Rega F, Verbelen T, Droogne W, Meyns B. Are right ventricular risk scores useful? *Eur J Cardiothorac Surg.* (2012) 42:621–6. doi: 10.1093/ejcts/ezs104

41. Hennig F, Stepanenko AV, Lehmkuhl HB, Kukucka M, Dandel M, Krabatsch T, et al. Neurohumoral and inflammatory markers for prediction of right ventricular failure after implantation of a left ventricular assist device. *Gen Thorac Cardiovasc Surg.* (2011) 59:19–24. doi: 10.1007/s11748-010-0669-9

42. Truby LK, Garan AR, Givens RC, Wayda B, Takeda K, Yuzefpolskaya M, et al. Aortic insufficiency during contemporary left ventricular assist device support: analysis of the INTERMACS registry. *JACC Heart Fail.* (2018) 6:951–60. doi: 10.1016/j.jchf.2018.07.012

43. Hellman Y, Malik AS, Lin H, Shen C, Wang IW, Wozniak TC, et al. B-type natriuretic peptide levels predict ventricular arrhythmia post left ventricular assist device implantation. *Artificial Organs.* (2015) 39:1051–5. doi: 10.1111/aor.12486

44. Hasin T, Marmor Y, Kremers W, Topilsky Y, Severson CJ, Schirger JA, et al. Readmissions after implantation of axial flow left ventricular assist device. *J Am Coll Cardiol.* (2013) 61:153–63. doi: 10.1016/j.jacc.2012.09.041

45. Hegarova M, Kubanek M, Netuka I, Maly J, Dorazilova Z, Gazdic T, et al. Clinical correlates of b-type natriuretic peptide monitoring in outpatients with left ventricular assist device. *Biomed Pap Med Fac Univ Palacky Olomouc Czech Repub.* (2017) 161:68–74. doi: 10.5507/bp.2017.003

46. Hasin T, Kushwaha SS, Lesnick TG, Kremers W, Boilson BA, Schirger JA, et al. Early trends in N-terminal pro-brain natriuretic peptide values after left ventricular assist device implantation for chronic heart failure. *Am J Cardiol.* (2014) 114:1257–63. doi: 10.1016/j.amjcard.2014.07.056

47. Imamura T, Kinugawa K, Nitta D, Kinoshita O, Nawata K, Ono M. Preoperative iodine-123 meta-iodobenzylguanidine imaging is a novel predictor of left ventricular reverse remodeling during treatment with a left ventricular assist device. *J Artif Organs.* (2016) 19:29–36. doi: 10.1007/s10047-015-0857-6

48. Wever-Pinzon O, Drakos SG, McKellar SH, Horne BD, Caine WT, Kfoury AG, et al. Cardiac recovery during long-term left ventricular assist device support. *J Am Coll Cardiol.* (2016) 68:1540–53. doi: 10.1016/j.jacc.2016.07.743

49. Imamura T, Kinugawa K, Hatano M, Fujino T, Muraoka H, Inaba T, et al. Preoperative beta-blocker treatment is a key for deciding left ventricular assist device implantation strategy as a bridge to recovery. *J Artificial Organs.* (2014) 17:23–32. doi: 10.1007/s10047-013-0748-7

50. Mano A, Nakatani T, Oda N, Kato T, Niwaya K, Tagusari O, et al. Which factors predict the recovery of natural heart function after insertion of a left ventricular assist system? *J Heart Lung Transplant.* (2008) 27:869–74. doi: 10.1016/j.healun.2008.05.007

51. El-Saed A, Voigt A, Shalaby A. Usefulness of brain natriuretic peptide level at implant in predicting mortality in patients with advanced but stable heart failure receiving cardiac resynchronization therapy. *Clin Cardiol.* (2009) 32:E33–8. doi: 10.1002/clc.20490

52. Shalaby AA, Abraham WT, Fonarow GC, Bersohn MM, Gorcsan J III, Lee LY, et al. Association of BNP and troponin levels with outcome among cardiac resynchronization therapy recipients. *Pacing Clin Electrophysiol.* (2015) 38:581–90. doi: 10.1111/pace.12610

53. Zile MR, Claggett BL, Prescott MF, McMurray JJ, Packer M, Rouleau JL, et al. Prognostic implications of changes in n-terminal pro-B-type natriuretic peptide in patients with heart failure. *J Am Coll Cardiol.* (2016) 68:2425–36. doi: 10.1016/j.jacc.2016.09.931

54. Maybaum S, Mancini D, Xydas S, Starling RC, Aaronson K, Pagani FD, et al. Cardiac improvement during mechanical circulatory support–a prospective multicenter study of the LVAD working group. *Circulation.* (2007) 115:2497–505. doi: 10.1161/CIRCULATIONAHA.106.633180

55. Klotz S, Naka Y, Oz MC, Burkhoff D. Biventricular assist device-induced right ventricular reverse structural and functional remodeling. *J Heart Lung Transplant.* (2005) 24:1195–201. doi: 10.1016/j.healun.2004.08.005

56. Drakos SG, Wever-Pinzon O, Selzman CH, Gilbert EM, Alharethi R, Reid BB, et al. Magnitude and time course of changes induced by continuous-flow left ventricular assist device unloading in chronic heart failure: insights into cardiac recovery. *J Am Coll Cardiol.* (2013) 61:1985–94. doi: 10.1016/j.jacc.2013.01.072

57. Kato TS, Chokshi A, Singh P, Khawaja T, Cheema F, Akashi H, et al. Effects of continuous-flow versus pulsatile-flow left ventricular assist devices on myocardial unloading and remodeling. *Circulation Heart Fail.* (2011) 4:546–53. doi: 10.1161/CIRCHEARTFAILURE.111.962142

58. Tapanainen JM, Lindgren KS, Makikallio TH, Vuolteenaho O, Leppaluoto J, Huikuri HV. natriuretic peptides as predictors of non-sudden and sudden cardiac death after acute myocardial infarction in the beta-blocking era. *J Am Coll Cardiol.* (2004) 43:757–63. doi: 10.1016/j.jacc.2003.09.048

59. Vrtovec B, Knezevic I, Poglajen G, Sebestjen M, Okrajsek R, Haddad F. Relation of B-type natriuretic peptide level in heart failure to sudden cardiac death in patients with and without QT interval prolongation. *Am J Cardiol.* (2013) 111:886–90. doi: 10.1016/j.amjcard.2012.11.041

60. Pizarro R, Bazzino OO, Oberti PF, Falconi ML, Arias AM, Krauss JG, et al. Prospective validation of the prognostic usefulness of b-type natriuretic peptide in asymptomatic patients with chronic severe aortic regurgitation. *J Am Coll Cardiol.* (2011) 58:1705–14. doi: 10.1016/j.jacc.2011.07.016

61. Aimo A, Januzzi JL Jr, Bayes-Genis A, Vergaro G, Sciarrone P, Passino C, et al. Clinical and prognostic significance of sST2 in heart failure: JACC review topic of the week. *J Am Coll Cardiol.* (2019) 74:2193–203. doi: 10.1016/j.jacc.2019.08.1039

62. Barutaut M, Fournier P, Peacock WF, Evaristi MF, Dambrin C, Caubère C, et al. sST2 adds to the prognostic value of Gal-3 and BNP in chronic heart failure. *Acta Cardiol.* (2019) 75:739–47. doi: 10.1080/00015385.2019.1669847

63. Bettencourt P, Ferreira-Coimbra J, Rodrigues P, Marques P, Moreira H, Pinto MJ, et al. Towards a multi-marker prognostic strategy in acute heart failure: a role for GDF-15. *ESC Heart Fail.* (2018) 5:1017–22. doi: 10.1002/ehf2.12301

64. Salah K, Stienen S, Pinto YM, Eurlings LW, Metra M, Bayes-Genis A, et al. Prognosis and NT-proBNP in heart failure patients with preserved versus reduced ejection fraction. *Heart.* (2019) 105:1182–9. doi: 10.1136/heartjnl-2018-314173

65. Emdin M, Aimo A, Vergaro G, Bayes-Genis A, Lupón J, Latini R, et al. sST2 predicts outcome in chronic heart failure beyond NT-proBNP and high-sensitivity troponin T. *J Am Coll Cardiol.* (2018) 72:2309–20. doi: 10.1016/j.jacc.2018.08.2165

66. Ahmad T, Fiuzat M, Felker GM, O'Connor C. Novel biomarkers in chronic heart failure. *Nat Rev Cardiol.* (2012) 9:347–59. doi: 10.1038/nrcardio.2012.37

67. Mathieu K, Ibrahim E-B, Michael B, Martin B, Ibrahim A. Biomarkers in cardiomyopathies and prediction of sudden cardiac death. *Curr Pharm Biotechnol.* (2017) 18:472–81. doi: 10.2174/1389201018666170623125842

68. Frangogiannis NG. Cardiac fibrosis: cell biological mechanisms, molecular pathways and therapeutic opportunities. *Mol Aspects Med.* (2019) 65:70–99. doi: 10.1016/j.mam.2018.07.001

8

Echocardiographic, Biochemical and Electrocardiographic Correlates Associated with Progressive Pulmonary Arterial Hypertension

Ahmed Zaky[1], Iram Zafar[1], Juan Xavier Masjoan-Juncos[1], Maroof Husain[1], Nithya Mariappan[1], Charity J. Morgan[2], Tariq Hamid[3], Michael A. Frölich[1], Shama Ahmad[1] and Aftab Ahmad[1]*

[1] Department of Anesthesiology and Perioperative Medicine, University of Alabama at Birmingham, Birmingham, AL, United States, [2] Department of Biostatistics, University of Alabama at Birmingham, Birmingham, AL, United States, [3] Division of Cardiovascular Disease, Department of Medicine, University of Alabama at Birmingham, Birmingham, AL, United States

*Correspondence:
Aftab Ahmad
aftabahmad@uabmc.edu

Background: Pulmonary arterial hypertension (PAH) is a progressive proliferative vasculopathy associated with mechanical and electrical changes, culminating in increased vascular resistance, right ventricular (RV) failure, and death. With a main focus on invasive tools, there has been an underutilization of echocardiography, electrocardiography, and biomarkers to non-invasively assess the changes in myocardial and pulmonary vascular structure and function during the course of PAH.

Methods: A SU5416-hypoxia rat model was used for inducing PAH. Biventricular functions were measured using transthoracic two-dimensional (2D) echocardiography/Doppler (echo/Doppler) at disease onset (0 week), during progression (3 weeks), and establishment (5 weeks). Similarly, electrocardiography was performed at 0, 3, and 5 weeks. Invasive hemodynamic measurements and markers of cardiac injury in plasma were assessed at 0, 3, and 5 weeks.

Results: Increased RV systolic pressure (RVSP) and rate of isovolumic pressure rise and decline were observed at 0, 3, and 5 weeks in PAH animals. EKG showed a steady increase in QT-interval with progression of PAH, whereas P-wave height and RS width were increased only during the initial stages of PAH progression. Echocardiographic markers of PAH progression and severity were also identified. Three echocardiographic patterns were observed: a steady pattern (0–5 weeks) in which echo parameter changed progressively with severity [inferior vena cava (IVC) expiratory diameter and pulmonary artery acceleration time (PAAT)], an early pattern (0–3 weeks) where there is an early change in parameters [RV fractional area change (RV-FAC), transmitral flow, left ventricle (LV) output, estimated mean PA pressure, RV performance index, and LV systolic eccentricity index], and a late pattern (3–5 weeks) in which there is only a late rise at advanced stages of PAH (LV diastolic eccentricity index). RVSP correlated with PAAT, PAAT/PA ejection times, IVC diameters, RV-FAC, tricuspid systolic excursion, LV systolic eccentricity and output, and transmitral flow. Plasma myosin light chain (Myl-3) and cardiac troponin I (cTnI) increased progressively across the three time points. Cardiac troponin T (cTnT) and fatty acid-binding protein-3 (FABP-3) were significantly elevated only at the 5-week time point.

Conclusion: Distinct electrocardiographic and echocardiographic patterns along with plasma biomarkers were identified as useful non-invasive tools for monitoring PAH progression.

Keywords: pulmonary arterial hypertension, echocardiography, disease progression, electrocardiography, SU5416, cardiac troponin T, cardiac troponin I, FABP-3

INTRODUCTION

Pulmonary arterial hypertension (PAH) is a progressive proliferative vasculopathy affecting small pulmonary arterioles culminating in increased vascular resistance and right ventricular afterload (1). According to a recent task force report, assessing RV function is an ongoing challenge (2).

Failure of the RV to adapt to increased afterload is the principal cause of death in patients with pulmonary hypertension (PH) (3, 4). Factors reflecting RV dysfunction by cardiac catheterization such as cardiac index and mean right atrial pressure are significant predictors of survival in patients with PAH (3). Additionally, a failing RV causes poor prognosis even if pulmonary vascular resistance is reduced (5), demonstrating the importance of evaluating and maintaining RV function in PAH patients.

Despite the prognostic significance of the RV status in PH, gaps still remain in the assessment of RV function and structure both during the course of the disease and during treatment (6). This stems in part from the lack of well-established clinical determinants of RV function, and the complex structure and orientation of the RV in the anterior chest that hampers a straightforward assessment using conventional imaging modalities (2, 7). Previous attempts to evaluate progression of PAH in animal models were limited in that invasive measurements were carried out at one time point with an underutilization of echocardiography to assess the pulmonary vasculature and the left ventricle during the course of PAH (6). While advanced imaging techniques can provide a better assessment of RV function, a vast number of clinicians still rely on conventional imaging modalities. Furthermore, less attention has been given to the assessment of the electrical

function and trend of biomarker progression during the course of PAH. Understanding the biochemical, electrocardiographic, and echocardiographic patterns during the course of PAH may guide clinical management of patients with PAH and help identify patients at an early stage of the disease when therapies could potentially be more effective (8). Furthermore, recent change in the clinical diagnosis of PAH using a threshold of mean pulmonary artery pressure (mPAP) from >25 to >20 mmHg underscores the efforts in diagnosing PAH at an early stage (9, 10).

To address these gaps, we sought to perform a comprehensive analysis to assess electrical, biochemical, and mechanical changes that occur in the heart and in the pulmonary circulation during the progression of PAH in a SU5416-hypoxia rat model. Our objective is to identify sensitive indices that can be obtained and monitored non-invasively in the early diagnosis of PAH and during the course of PAH.

METHODS

Animal Model of Pulmonary Arterial Hypertension

All animal experiments were performed under the University of Alabama Institutional Animal Care and Use Committee approval and in accordance with the National Institutes of Health Guide for the care and use of laboratory animals. This manuscript adheres to the ARRIVE guidelines. PAH was induced in rats using an established model (11). Briefly, adult male Sprague–Dawley rats weighing 160–200 g were injected subcutaneously with SU-5416 (20 mg/kg), a vascular endothelial growth factor receptor 2 (VEGFR-2) inhibitor, and exposed to normobaric hypoxia (10% O_2) for 3 weeks (SuHyx rats). They were then returned to normoxia (21% O_2, room air) for two additional weeks. For invasive measurements, separate sets of animals were used for the control, 3- and 5-week time points groups. For echocardiographic measurements, the same animals were used for the control (0 week), 3- and 5-week measurements. The number of animals used in each measurement is indicated in the figure legends. Experiments in each group were carried out independently for a minimum of two times.

Hemodynamic Measurements

Hemodynamic measurements were performed in rats under 2% isoflurane anesthesia using a 1.4 F high-fidelity Millar catheter as described by us before (12). Using a Biopac data acquisition system and AcqKnowledge III software (ACQ 3.2), the rate of

---

Abbreviations: HV D, hepatic vein diastolic; HV S/D, hepatic vein systolic/diastolic; IVC_EXP, inferior vena cava expiratory diameter; IVC_INSP, inferior vena cava inspiratory diameter; LV CO, left ventricle cardiac output; LVSV, left ventricle stroke volume; LV-EIs, left ventricle eccentricity index systolic; LV-Eid, left ventricle eccentricity index diastolic; LV-VCFr, left ventricle circumferential shortening; MPAP, mean pulmonary artery pressure; MV(E/A), early diastolic mitral velocity/late diastolic mitral velocity; PAAT, pulmonary artery acceleration time; PAET, pulmonary artery ejection time; RVEDV, right ventricle end diastolic volume; RVESV, right ventricle end systolic volume; RVEDP, right ventricle end diastolic pressure; RVESP, right ventricle end systolic pressure; RV-EF, right ventricle ejection fraction; RV-FAC, right ventricle fractional area change; RV-FWT, right ventricle free wall thickness; RV-MPI, right ventricle myocardial performance index; RV-CO, right ventricle cardiac output; RVSV, right ventricle stroke volume; TAPSE, tricuspid annular plane systolic excursion; TV-Sa, tricuspid valve systolic wave.

rise of ventricular pressure during systole ($dP/dT_{maximum}$) and subsequent fall during diastole ($dP/dT_{minimum}$) were measured. Systemic blood pressure was also monitored using the same catheter inserted in the carotid artery. In animals where echocardiography was carried out, invasive measurements were performed at the end of the 5-week protocol before the animals ($n = 10$) were euthanized. Separate sets of animals were used for invasive measurements of naïve ($n = 17$) and 3-week exposed animals ($n = 11$).

Immunofluorescence Staining

Animals were euthanatized, and the left lung was inflation fixed with low-melting agarose and immersed in a solution of 10% formalin in ethanol for up to 48 h. The tissues were then processed for paraffin embedding. Five-micrometer-thick sections were cut on positively charged slides, and deparaffinization and antigen retrieval was performed. Sections were then blocked in 5% normal goat serum and incubated overnight with anti-von Willebrand factor (vWF) antibody (Dako cat# A0082) and anti-alpha smooth muscle actin (α-SMA) (Abcam cat# 18147). After washing with TBST (Tris-buffered saline with 0.025% Triton-X100), fluorescence tagged secondary antibodies, anti-rabbit Alexa fluor 488 (vWF), and anti-mouse Alexa fluor 594 (α-SMA) were applied, and sections were incubated for 1 h. Sections were then washed, rinsed with PBS, and mounted with VECTASHIELD containing DAPI (Vector laboratories). Images were captured at ×20 using the BZ-X800 Keyence microscope.

Cardiac Biomarker Measurements

Levels of cardiac and skeletal muscle markers of injury were measured in the plasma of rats from 0-, 3-, and 5-week time points using the meso scale discovery (Rockville, MD, USA) muscle injury panel 1 kit. A multiplex assay to quantitate plasma levels of cTnI (cardiac troponin I), cTnT (cardiac troponin T), FABP3 (fatty acid-binding protein 3), Myl3 (myosin light chain 3), and sTnI (skeletal troponin I) were carried out using standards and as per protocol of the manufacturer.

Echocardiography and Electrocardiography

Transthoracic echocardiography and electrocardiography were performed in anesthetized animals (2% isoflurane) as described by us before (12). Echocardiography was performed prior to, at 3 and 5 weeks post exposure using a Vevo2100 high-resolution ultrasound system (Visual Sonics Inc., Toronto, ON, Canada) using a 13- to 24-MHz linear transducer (MS-250). Rats were placed supine on the warmed stage (37°C) of the echocardiography system. Two-dimensional cardiac images were acquired from the parasternal long- and short-axis, apical, subcostal, and suprasternal views using M-mode and B-modes at mid papillary level and averaged to determine the RV and LV dimensions at end systole and end diastole as described (13).

The RV and LV volumes, cardiac output, fractional shortening, fractional area of change, and ejection fraction were obtained according to guidelines (14). The LV systolic and diastolic eccentricity index was calculated as the ratio of the LV anteroposterior dimension and the septolateral dimension. The parasternal pulmonary artery view was obtained, and pulsed wave Doppler was used to measure flow across the RV outflow tract. End systolic diameter of the pulmonary artery was measured, and the end systolic diameter of the pulmonary artery to the end systolic diameter of ascending aorta ratio (stiffness index) was calculated. Apical four-chamber views with B- and M-modes were obtained to determine tricuspid annular plane systolic excursion (TAPSE). Pulsed wave Doppler was used to determine transmitral and transtricuspid early (E) and atrial (A) wave peak velocities, isovolumic relaxation time (IVRT), E-wave deceleration time, and isovolumic contraction time, with the ratio of E to A calculated across both the mitral and tricuspid valves. A tricuspid regurgitant jet was sought to estimate the RVSP when discernable (15). Tissue Doppler imaging was used to determine lateral mitral and tricuspid annular diastolic peak early (E'), late atrial (A'), systolic (S') annular velocities, and (E) to (E') ratios were calculated. Myocardial performance index (MPI) for both ventricles was calculated from the spectral Doppler tracing of transmitral and transtricuspid flows as described (16). A subcostal inferior vena caval view was obtained, and the inferior vena caval diameter was measured at end inspiration and end exhalation. Pulsed wave Doppler was used to assess hepatic venous blood flow.

For electrocardiography, a two-channel electrocardiography was performed on anesthetized rats prior to, at 3 and 5 weeks post exposure. To obtain ECG tracings, bipolar platinum electrodes were positioned in the thorax (subcutaneous tissue) directly in derivation DII. To determine the intervals RR, PR, QT, corrected QT (QTc), and QRS complex, a period of 10 s was analyzed in the ECG tracing of each animal. The QT interval was measured starting from the onset of the QRS complex until the end of the T wave, which is the return of the T wave to the baseline. QTc was obtained using Bazett's formula (QTc $= QT/HRR$) (17). Parameters were analyzed using previously described procedures (18).

Statistical Analyses

Values were expressed as mean ±SEM. Statistical analyses were performed using Prism software. Repeated measures one-way ANOVA was used to test for differences in each parameter at 0, 3, and 5 weeks. For statistically significant parameters, post-hoc pairwise t-tests were conducted using Tukey's method for correcting for multiple comparisons. To assess the relationship between invasively measured RVSP and echocardiographic parameters, control and study animals were pooled, and Pearson correlations were calculated. Fisher's z transformation was used to calculate 95% confidence intervals. Due to the large number of tested parameters, a Bonferroni correction was applied to adjust for multiple comparisons.

RESULTS

Invasive Hemodynamics

A rat SuHyx model of PAH was used as described before (11). Right ventricular systolic pressure (RVSP) and hypertrophy were measured at 0, 3, and 5 weeks to confirm progression and

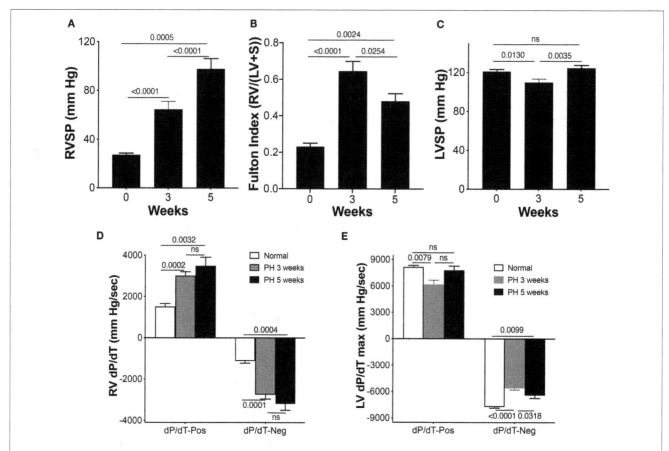

FIGURE 1 | Right ventricle (RV) pressures and electrocardiographic parameters in pulmonary arterial hypertension (PAH) rats. Pulmonary arterial hypertension was induced in rats as described in the Methods section. **(A)** The RV systolic pressure (RVSP) was measured in separate sets of control animals and animals at 3 and 5 weeks during the development of PAH, $n = 10$–17 animals/group. **(B)** Fulton Index ($n = 6$–9 animals/group). **(C)** Left ventricle systolic pressure (LVSP), $n = 10$–17 animals/group. **(D)** Rates of rise and decline of the RV pressure in systole (above baseline) and in diastole (below baseline) (dP/dT) were recorded, $n = 10$–17 animals/group. **(E)** Rates of rise and decline of the LV pressure in systole (above baseline) and in diastole (below baseline) (dP/dT) were recorded, $n = 9$–17 animals/group.

establishment of PH. **Figure 1A** demonstrates a steady increase in RVSP in the PAH rats at 3 and 5 weeks, when compared with the controls. As expected in this model, the chronic increase in RV afterload led to RV hypertrophy shown by an increase in the Fulton index both at 3 and 5 weeks compared with controls (**Figure 1B**). Hypertrophy was more at the 3-week time point compared with the 5-week time point. LV systolic pressure (LVSP) remained unaltered in the PAH group at 5 weeks but was decreased at the 3-week time point (**Figure 1C**). The rate of rise of RV pressure during ejection and post ejection phases of the cardiac cycle was used to assess the contractile and relaxation properties of the RV. RV dP/dT$_{maximum}$ was substantially elevated in the PAH animals at 3 and 5 weeks when compared with the controls (**Figure 1D**). Similarly, the RV dP/dT$_{minimum}$ at 3 and 5 weeks were increased in the PAH animals when compared with the controls (**Figure 1D**). Since RV dysfunction can alter LV contractility, we measured the LV dP/dT. Interestingly, LV dP/dT positive did not differ from the control at 5 weeks, but there was a decrease at the 3-week time point (**Figure 1E**).

However, the LV dP/dT negative in the PAH group at 3 and 5 weeks were both diminished when compared with the controls (**Figure 1E**).

Electrocardiography
Polarization characteristics of the heart chambers resulting from adaptation and maladaptation were assessed using electrocardiography (EKG). Representative tracing at all three time points shows changes with progression of PAH (**Figure 2A**). A significant prolongation in the corrected QT interval (QTc), an increase in the amplitude of P and T waves, and a widening of the QRS complex were observed in the PAH animals across the three time points, 0, 3, and 5 weeks (**Figures 2B–G**).

Lung Histology and Cardiac Markers of Injury
To validate PAH pathology, the lung sections were stained for vWF and α-SMA to highlight changes in the intima and media of the arteries, respectively, during disease progression. As

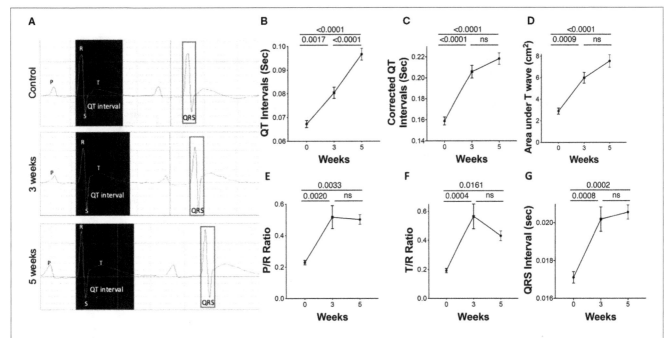

FIGURE 2 | Electrocardiographic parameters during PAH progression in rats. Pulmonary arterial hypertension was induced in rats as described in the Methods. A 2-channel electrocardiography (EKG) was utilized to record parameters. **(A)** Representative EKG tracings, showing **(B)** uncorrected QT intervals, **(C)** corrected QT intervals, **(D)** area under the T wave, **(E)** P/R ratio, **(F)** T/R ratio, and **(G)** QRS interval was also performed. $N = 7–10$ animals/group.

expected, the lung histology showed increased muscularization of the arteries with time demonstrating the progressive nature of the disease in this model (**Figures 3A–C**). Markers of cardiac injury are known to increase in pulmonary hypertension. cTnI increased linearly with disease progression (**Figure 3D**). Similarly, myosin light chain 3 (Myl3), a ventricular and slow skeletal muscle isoform, also increased linearly with disease progression (**Figure 3H**). Cardiac troponin T, however, increased only at the 5-week time point (**Figure 3E**). As expected, sTnI did not change with disease severity (**Figure 3F**). FABP3 (aka: H-FABP; heart type fatty acid-binding protein) increased only at the 5-week time point (**Figure 3G**).

Echocadiographic Estimation of Pulmonary Pressures and Pulmonary Vascular Resistance

In addition to the invasive RVSP, we also measured non-invasive surrogates of PH using echo Doppler across three time points. PAAT and PAAT/PAET were reduced with disease progression (**Figures 4A,C**). A non-significant reduction in PAET from baseline to 3 weeks occurred (**Figure 4B**). Calculated values of mPAP using PAAT increased significantly at 3 weeks of PH. Although, mPAP was expected to increase with progression of PH, calculated values did not increase further between 3 and 5 weeks (**Figure 4D**). The PA diameter as assessed by echocardiography progressively increased across the three time points. The PA distensibility index was significantly increased at 3 weeks with no further increase at 5 weeks (**Figure 4E**). Increased PA resistance and a reduction in compliance of

large PAs cause premature systolic PA wave reflection resulting in flow deceleration and a mid-systolic notch. A mid-systolic notch was discernable with progressive PAH at 5 weeks (**Figure 4F**).

Right Ventricle Function and Structure

RV fractional area of change (RV-FAC) and ejection fraction (EF) reflect global RV systolic function. Tricuspid annular plane systolic excursion (TAPSE) and tricuspid valve systolic wave (TV-Sa) can serve as surrogates of the systolic function of the RV. Although, variable, RV systolic function was significantly reduced with progression of PAH. RV-FAC was significantly reduced at 3 weeks and continued to decline over 5 weeks (**Figure 4G**). Both EF and TAPSE, as measured by M-mode echocardiography tended to decrease with PH but were not statistically significant (**Figures 4H,I**). TV-Sa was significantly reduced starting at 3 weeks (**Figure 4J**). Similarly, RV myocardial performance index (RV-MPI), a measure of global systolic and diastolic RV function (19), was also increased at 3 weeks with no further change from 3 to 5 weeks (**Figure 4K**). Interestingly, RVSV did not change across the three time points (**Figure 4L**). However, a non-statistical reduction in RV cardiac output (RV-CO) at an early time point was observed (**Figure 4M**).

Increased RV pressure overload results in RV hypertrophy. The RV free wall thickness (RV-FWT), an indicator of RV hypertrophy, was significantly increased at 3 weeks. Furthermore, modest non-significant FWT changes occurred at 3- to 5-week time point (**Figure 4N**). An increase in FWT is consistent

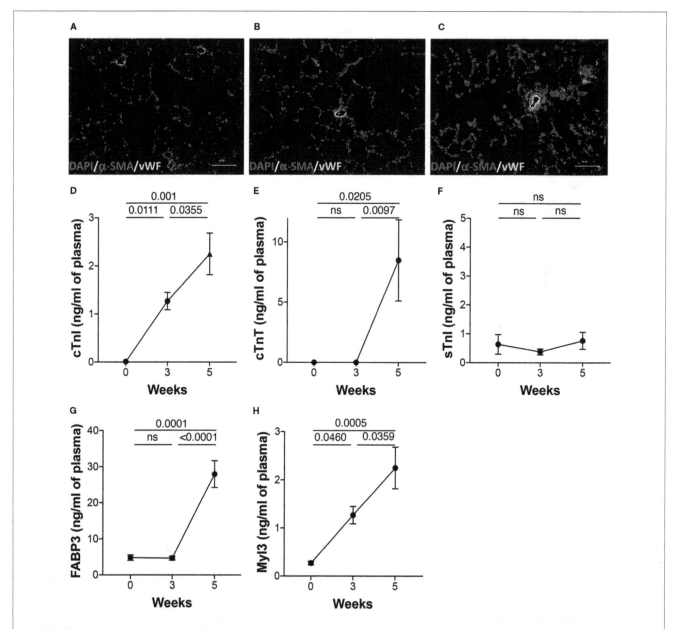

FIGURE 3 | Lung histology and plasma biomarkers of cardiac injury. PAH was induced in rats over a 5-week period as described in the Methods. **(A–C)** Representative images of the lung sections from the three time points stained for anti-vWF and anti-αSMA as described in details in the Methods. DAPI was used as a counterstain to visualize nuclei in tissue. Plasma was collected from separate sets of animals from naïve (0 day), 3 and 5 weeks post-induction of PAH. Markers of injury were estimated in the plasma using a multiplexed, meso scale discovery platform for **(D)** cardiac troponin I (cTnI), **(E)** cardiac troponin T (cTnT), **(F)** skeletal troponin I (sTnI), **(G)** fatty acid binding protein 3 (FABP3), and **(H)** myosin light chain 3 (Myl3). $N = 5–9$ animals/group.

with increased Fulton index at 3 and 5 weeks. No significant change in the RV diastolic function (RV E/A ratio, E′, or E/E′) was noticed across the three time points (data not shown).

Inferior Vena Cava and Hepatic Venous Flows

The hepatic venous (HV) flows and IVC diameter indicate the flow upstream from the PA and can be altered in PAH.

The IVC diameters progressively increased from 0 to 5 weeks (**Figures 5A,B**). An increase in RV-EDP can lead to an increase in the amplitude of the HV atrial reversal waveform. A non-significant reduction in the S/D over time was observed (**Figure 5C**). Peak velocity of the HV atrial reversal wave was also increased (**Figure 5D**).

Left Ventricle Function and Structure

The progressive increase in RV afterload can compromise LV function, structure, and filling. The inter-ventricular septum

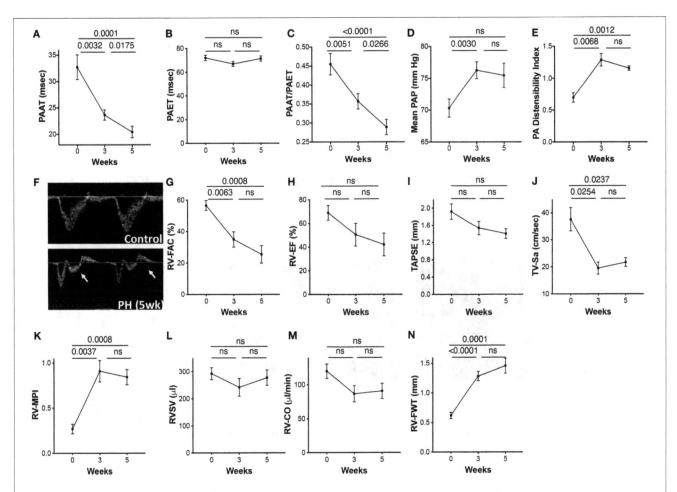

FIGURE 4 | Echocardiographic parameters of the pulmonary artery and the RV during progression of PAH. PAH was induced in rats over a 5-week period as described in the Methods. Echocardiographic images were acquired prior to induction of PH (0 day) and at 3 and 5 weeks post-induction. **(A)** Pulmonary artery acceleration time (PAAT), **(B)** pulmonary artery ejection time (PAET), **(C)** PAAT/PAET ratio, **(D)** calculated mean pulmonary artery pressure (mPAP), and **(E)** PA distensibility index, calculated as the ratio of the PA diameter (obtained from parasternal RV outflow tract view) to ascending aortic diameter from parasternal long axis flow at end diastole. **(F)** Pulse wave Doppler tracings showing the PA flow obtained from parasternal RV outflow view. Arrow shows the PA mid systolic notch. Each animal served as its own control at previous time points. A 2-dimensional echocardiographic examination of the RV was also performed from multiple acoustic views. **(G)** RV fractional area of change (RV-FAC) was measured from the transgastric midpapillary view, **(H)** RV-EF, **(I)** Tricuspid annular plane systolic excursion (TAPSE), **(J)** Tricuspid peak annular systolic velocity (TV-Sa), and **(K)** RV myocardial performance index (RV-MPI). **(L)** RVSV and **(M)** RV-CO were calculated from the parasternal long axis view. **(N)** RV free wall thickness (FWT) was measured from the apical four-chamber views. $N = 10$ animals/group.

was flattened with a leftward shift (**Figure 6A**). The LV eccentricity index systolic (LV-EIs) and the LV eccentricity index diastolic (LV-EId) increased progressively from baseline to 5 weeks (**Figures 6B,C**). A significant reduction in the LV filling was demonstrated by a reduced E and E/A from baseline to week 3, with a trend toward further reduction afterward (**Figures 6D,H**). LV cardiac output (LV-CO) was significantly reduced at week 3 with modest changes thereafter (**Figure 6E**). LV-SV was reduced at 3 weeks with no additional change with increased severity of PAH (**Figure 6F**). There was a significant reduction in the LV velocity of circumferential shortening (LV-VCFr) at 5 weeks (**Figure 6G**). In summary, reduced LV filling and output early in the disease was followed by reduction in the LV contractility at more advanced stage of PAH.

Correlation Between Echocardiographic Variables and Invasively Measured Right Ventricular Systolic Pressure

Pooled analyses of the study and control animals revealed significant correlation between invasively measured RVSP and each of the following parameters: pulmonary artery acceleration time (PAAT), PAAT/PAET (pulmonary artery ejection time), IVC diameter, RV-FAC, TAPSE, LV-EIs, LV-CO, LV-SV, and trans-mitral E/A (**Table 1**).

DISCUSSION

Using serial measurements, we identified distinct patterns of EKG, and biochemical and echocardiographic parameters that

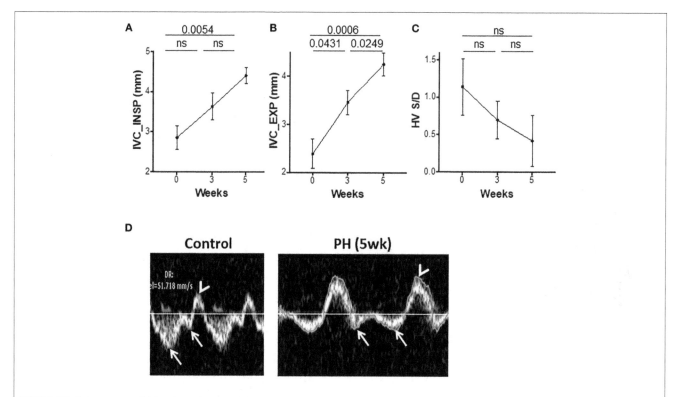

FIGURE 5 | Inferior vena cava (IVC) and hepatic venous flows during progression of PAH. IVC diameters at end inspiration **(A)** and end expiration **(B)** and the ratio of hepatic venous systolic to diastolic peak velocities **(C)** were measured from the subcostal view. **(D)** Representative echocardiographic images showing hepatic venous flow pattern with a reversal of systolic to diastolic peak velocity ratio (arrows) and prominent atrial reversal peak velocity wave (arrowhead) in control and animals with PH. $N = 10$ animals/group.

together can potentially be used to detect PAH early, monitor PAH progression, and assess RV dysfunction and its response to treatment. Knowledge of these patterns addresses the current gap in practice that focuses primarily on PAP reduction rather than on holistically reversing myocardial and vascular remodeling (2). Echocardiographic markers showed three different patterns representative of the pulmonary vascular and cardiac remodeling that takes place during the course of PAH; a steady pattern in which there is a progressive change of the echo parameters across the three time points of PAH (IVC end inspiratory, IVC end expiratory diameter, and PAAT), an early change in which there is an early reduction [RV-FAC, TV-Sa, MV(E/A), LV-CO, LVSV] or increase (mPAP by PAAT, RV-MPI, LV-EIs) followed by a plateau at severe PH, and a late pattern in which there is only a late rise at severe stages of PAH (LV-EId). In the same animal model, plasma biomarkers of cardiac injury showed two different patterns. Plasma levels of Myl-3 and cTnI steadily increased across the three time points compared with FABP-3 and cTnT that showed only a late rise at the 5-week time point. Grouping these variables into "patterns" overcomes some of their individual limitations in terms of their temporal relationship to the severity and progression of PAH.

PAH is characterized by a decrease in pulmonary vascular compliance and an increase in PVR causing initial adaptive compensation followed by a maladaptive decompensatory phase of the RV failure (20). The patterns identified in our study

capture some of these mechanisms. The presence of mid-systolic notching on the RV outflow tract spectral Doppler observed at the 5-week time point can be used as a qualitative marker of the reduction in the PA compliance responsible for the increase in pulsatile load of the RV, which precedes the increase in PVR. It can also be used as a qualitative surrogate of the RV/PA uncoupling, an important measure in determining the RV maladaptation in PAH (21).

With progressive increase in mPAP, less time is spent during ejection, and a faster rise in peak systolic pressure occurs due to a rapid closure of the pulmonary valve, causing reduction in PAAT and PAAT/PAET ratio (22). The reduction in PAAT is indicative of increased PVR and is a consistent finding in preclinical and clinical PH, further supporting its reliability in monitoring the disease progression (22). Although, there has been some success in echocardiographically estimated mPAP, consistent determination of estimates remain a challenge (23, 24).

RV hypertrophy is the hallmark of PAH, and an increase in the RV free wall thickness (FWT) signifies an important compensatory mechanism by which the RV reduces its wall stress induced by the increase in pressure overload. Here we used the RV-FWT as a surrogate of RV hypertrophy rather than measuring the RV mass, given the limitations of measuring the RV mass by M-mode echocardiography (14). These findings were confirmed by Fulton index measurements and are consistent with other reports (25) and may represent a compensatory mechanism. The

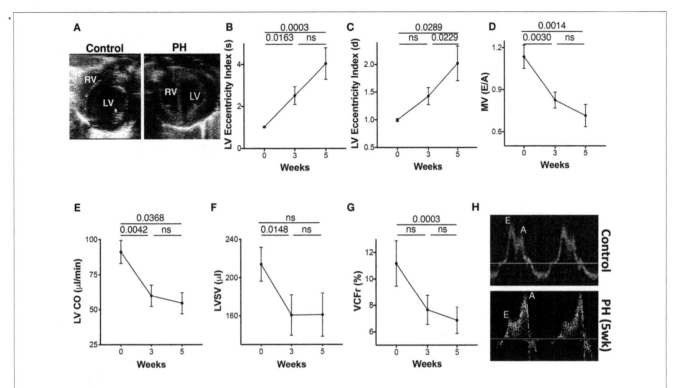

FIGURE 6 | Echocardiographic parameters of the left ventricle (LV) during progression of PAH. **(A)** Apical view of the chambers showing the RV and LV. LV eccentricity index image showing a reduction in the septolateral diameter in relation to the antero-inferior diameter of the LV. Eccentricity index was calculated from the transgastric midpapillary short axis view as the ratio of the antero-inferior diameter to the septolateral diameter of the LV. **(B)** LV eccentricity index in systole, **(C)** LV eccentricity index in diastole, **(D)** Transmitral ratio of peak early to late diastolic wave velocity, **(E)** CO, **(F)** SV, and **(G)** LV velocity of circumferential shortening as measured from the parasternal long axis view at 0, 3, and 5 weeks of PH induction. **(H)** Echocardiographic tracings showing mitral valve flow in control (top) and PH (bottom) animals. $N = 10$ animals/group.

RV contractility as measured by dP/dT_{max} increased significantly during the early phase of PAH development and consistent with other reports (26, 27). However, changes from 3 to 5 weeks were not significant despite a significant increase in RVSP and may represent the maladaptive phase of PAH. High RV dP/dT_{max} positive values were observed in PH patients even with evidence of RV failure (28). In advanced stages of PAH, dP/dT may be more dependent on the RV mass, HR, and intracavitary pressure rather than myocardial contractility (29).

Increased PA pressures can alter hepatic venous (HV) flows and IVC diameter leading to a reduction in the forward flow from the HV to the RV. An increase in IVC diameter reflects an increase in back pressure from the right atrium as a result of increase in RV afterload and can serve as a prognostic indicator of PH (30). Hepatic venous flow was shown to plateau after 3 weeks reflecting sensitivity only during the initial phases of development of PAH. This reflects the variable presentation of PAH in terms of the development of RV failure, elevation of the RV-EDP, occurrence of significant TR, and occurrence of atrial fibrillation (AF). Although, TR is a consistent finding in humans with PH, we were unable to discern a consistent tricuspid regurgitant jet due to technical limitations in image acquisition in rats.

We analyzed the correlation between the echocardiographic markers of progression of PAH and RVSP in order to assess their association with the severity of PAH. Markers associated with severity of PAH may be used for prognostication, whereas those associated with progression of PAH may be sought for monitoring of the disease progression and response to therapy. The correlation of TAPSE with RVSP confirms its prognostic significance and is consistent with previous reports. However, its failure to reduce beyond 3 weeks of PAH progression can be explained by the RV assuming a more spherical configuration during advanced stages of PAH and that TAPSE, being representative of the longitudinal motion of the RV and only of the free wall of the TV annulus, may be less contributing to RV ejection at this advanced stage of PAH. We are aware of the limitations of M-mode echocardiography in measuring RVEF compared with 3D echocardiography, which we did not possess at the time of the study. Similarly, RV-FAC, while being a prognostic marker of PAH, may not be an ideal marker of progression since it lacks representation of the RV outflow tract and may not represent the intrinsic contractility of the RV. Overall, echocardiography is a valuable tool in monitoring the severity and progression of PAH and may be helpful in its early diagnosis.

In the model, serial changes in the LV with progressive PAH were also characterized. The rise in LVSP pattern is consistent with previous reports (31). Flattening of the inter-ventricular septum with a leftward shift is also consistent with other studies

TABLE 1 | Correlation of echocardiographic variable with right ventricular systolic pressure (RVSP).

Variable	Correlation coefficient	p-Value
HV D	−0.44	0.053
HV S/D	−0.45	0.044
HV S2	−0.06	0.792
IVC_INSP	0.31	0.185
IVC-EXP	0.56	0.010
LV CO	−0.65	0.002
LV eccentricity index d	0.52	0.027
LV eccentricity index s	0.58	0.013
MPAP (common)	−0.62	0.055
MPAP (PAAT <120 ms)	−0.39	0.271
MV (E/A)	−0.77	<0.001
PA distensibility index	0.56	0.045
PAAT	−0.63	0.004
PAET	0.26	0.266
PAAT/PAET	−0.64	0.003
RV-EF	−0.34	0.208
RV-FAC	−0.60	0.005
RV mass	0.12	0.671
RV-MPI	0.48	0.053
RV-CO	−0.51	0.075
RVSV	−0.52	0.066
LVSV	−0.58	0.007
TAPSE	−0.50	0.025
TV-Sa	−0.09	0.714

(32). This reduces LV septo-lateral dimension compared with antero-inferior dimension at end systole and diastole reflecting ventricular interdependence (33). The initial pattern of reduced filling is evidenced by a decrease in transmitral E/A and an increase in LV-EIs and LV-EId, followed by a reduction in LV-CO and LV-SV, and ending with a reduction in contractility as shown by reduced VCFr. The latter is considered a less load-dependent index of systolic function compared with LV-EF (34).

In our EKG studies, progressive prolongation in QT-interval reflects an abnormality in ventricular depolarization or repolarization, which may predispose to ventricular arrhythmias reportedly common in PH (35). Prolongation of QT-interval has been shown to correlate with cardiac remodeling, in addition to being an independent predictor of mortality in PH (36). Increased QT-interval and wide RS-interval observed in our studies were also consistent with other reports where QRS prolongation was associated with clinical severity and mortality in patients with PH (37, 38). An increase in the QRS interval is a sign of intraventricular electrical conduction delay, likely due to ventricular dys-synchrony resulting from RV hypertrophy and dilation. Increased amplitude of the P wave is a sign of atrial enlargement likely related to right atrial enlargement secondary to elevated RVSP and secondary to PH (18). These EKG findings of raised right atrial pressure, intraventricular conduction delay, and propensity for ventricular arrhythmias are consistent with adverse outcomes in PH (39).

Makers of cardiac injury are frequently used in stratification of disease. Our findings of increased levels of cTnT and FABP3 only during the late stages of PAH suggests their potential use as markers of disease severity. It is therefore not surprising that both of these markers were shown to correlate with major adverse events and were also predictors of mortality (40, 41). On the other hand, cTnI levels increased linearly with PAH progression suggesting its potential use as a sensitive marker of disease progression and in response to therapies. We also found that Myl3, another marker of cardiotoxicity (42, 43), also increased with disease severity and can also be potentially used as a sensitive marker of PH progression.

In summary, recognizing biochemical, electrocardiographic, and echocardiographic patterns of PAH progression and severity may help in the monitoring and prognostication of RV function in PAH. Despite limitations, echocardiography is invaluable not only in diagnosing PAH but also in follow-up. There is a need for a "collective" assessment of the entire cardiovascular system in PAH. More studies are needed to mechanistically correlate electrical, vascular, and mechanical remodeling to non-invasive echo- and electrocardiographic findings.

AUTHOR CONTRIBUTIONS

AZ and AA helped conceive the idea, design the study, analyze the data, and write the manuscript. IZ, MH, and NM helped acquire and analyze the data and review and write the manuscript. JM-J and TH helped analyze the data and review and write the manuscript. CM and MF helped with the statistical analysis of the data and reviewed and edited the manuscript. All authors contributed to the article and approved the submitted version.

ACKNOWLEDGMENTS

The authors are grateful to Wayne Bradley for performing the echocardiography measurements. We thank Dr. Dan Berkowitz for providing valuable feedback.

REFERENCES

1. van de Veerdonk MC, Bogaard HJ, Voelkel NF. The right ventricle and pulmonary hypertension. *Heart Fail Rev.* (2016) 21:259–71. doi: 10.1007/s10741-016-9526-y
2. Lahm T, Douglas IS, Archer SL, Bogaard HJ, Chesler NC, Haddad F, et al. Assessment of right ventricular function in the research setting: knowledge gaps and pathways forward. An Official American Thoracic Society research statement. *Am J Respir Crit Care Med.* (2018) 198:e15–43. doi: 10.1164/rccm.201806-1160ST
3. Boucly A, Weatherald J, Savale L, Jais X, Cottin V, Prevot G, et al. Risk assessment, prognosis and guideline implementation in pulmonary arterial hypertension. *Eur Respir J.* (2017) 50:e1700889. doi: 10.1183/13993003.00889-2017
4. Hemnes AR, Champion HC. Right heart function and haemodynamics in pulmonary hypertension. *Int J Clin Pract Suppl.* (2008) 160:11–9. doi: 10.1111/j.1742-1241.2008.01812.x

5. van de Veerdonk MC, Kind T, Marcus JT, Mauritz GJ, Heymans MW, Bogaard HJ, et al. Progressive right ventricular dysfunction in patients with pulmonary arterial hypertension responding to therapy. *J Am Coll Cardiol.* (2011) 58:2511–9. doi: 10.1016/j.jacc.2011.06.068

6. Voelkel NF, Quaife RA, Leinwand LA, Barst RJ, McGoon MD, Meldrum DR, et al. Right ventricular function and failure: report of a National Heart, Lung, and Blood Institute working group on cellular and molecular mechanisms of right heart failure. *Circulation.* (2006) 114:1883–91. doi: 10.1161/CIRCULATIONAHA.106.632208

7. Badano LP, Ginghina C, Easaw J, Muraru D, Grillo MT, Lancellotti P, et al. Right ventricle in pulmonary arterial hypertension: haemodynamics, structural changes, imaging, and proposal of a study protocol aimed to assess remodelling and treatment effects. *Eur J Echocardiogr.* (2010) 11:27–37. doi: 10.1093/ejechocard/jep152

8. Galie N, Humbert M, Vachiery JL, Gibbs S, Lang I, Torbicki A, et al. 2015 ESC/ERS Guidelines for the diagnosis and treatment of pulmonary hypertension: the joint task force for the diagnosis and treatment of pulmonary hypertension of the European Society of Cardiology (ESC) and the European Respiratory Society (ERS): Endorsed by: Association for European Paediatric and Congenital Cardiology (AEPC), International Society for Heart and Lung Transplantation (ISHLT). *Eur Respir J.* (2015) 46:903–75. doi: 10.1183/13993003.01032-2015

9. Maron BA, Kovacs G, Vaidya A, Bhatt DL, Nishimura RA, Mak S, et al. Cardiopulmonary hemodynamics in pulmonary hypertension and heart failure: JACC review topic of the week. *J Am Coll Cardiol.* (2020) 76:2671–81. doi: 10.1016/j.jacc.2020.10.007

10. Simonneau G, Montani D, Celermajer DS, Denton CP, Gatzoulis MA, Krowka M, et al. Haemodynamic definitions and updated clinical classification of pulmonary hypertension. *Eur Respir J.* (2019) 53:e1801913. doi: 10.1183/13993003.01913-2018

11. Taraseviciene-Stewart L, Kasahara Y, Alger L, Hirth P, Mc Mahon G, Waltenberger J, et al. Inhibition of the VEGF receptor 2 combined with chronic hypoxia causes cell death-dependent pulmonary endothelial cell proliferation and severe pulmonary hypertension. *FASEB J.* (2001) 15:427–38. doi: 10.1096/fj.00-0343com

12. Ahmad S, Masjoan Juncos JX, Ahmad A, Zaky A, Wei CC, Bradley WE, et al. Bromine inhalation mimics ischemia-reperfusion cardiomyocyte injury and calpain activation in rats. *Am J Physiol Heart Circ Physiol.* (2019) 316:H212–23. doi: 10.1152/ajpheart.00652.2017

13. Liu J, Rigel DF. Echocardiographic examination in rats and mice. *Methods Mol Biol.* (2009) 573:139–55. doi: 10.1007/978-1-60761-247-6_8

14. Rudski LG, Lai WW, Afilalo J, Hua L, Handschumacher MD, Chandrasekaran K, et al. Guidelines for the echocardiographic assessment of the right heart in adults: a report from the American Society of Echocardiography endorsed by the European Association of Echocardiography, a registered branch of the European Society of Cardiology, and the Canadian Society of Echocardiography. *J Am Soc Echocardiogr.* (2010) 23:685–713; quiz 86–8. doi: 10.1016/j.echo.2010.05.010

15. Steckelberg RC, Tseng AS, Nishimura R, Ommen S, Sorajja P. Derivation of mean pulmonary artery pressure from non-invasive parameters. *J Am Soc Echocardiogr.* (2013) 26:464–8. doi: 10.1016/j.echo.2013.01.006

16. Tei C, Ling LH, Hodge DO, Bailey KR, Oh JK, Rodeheffer RJ, et al. New index of combined systolic and diastolic myocardial performance: a simple and reproducible measure of cardiac function–a study in normals and dilated cardiomyopathy. *J Cardiol.* (1995) 26:357–66. doi: 10.1016/S0894-7317(05)80111-7

17. Tattersall ML, Dymond M, Hammond T, Valentin JP. Correction of QT values to allow for increases in heart rate in conscious Beagle dogs in toxicology assessment. *J Pharmacol Toxicol Methods.* (2006) 53:11–9. doi: 10.1016/j.vascn.2005.02.005

18. Konopelski P, Ufnal M. Electrocardiography in rats: a comparison to human. *Physiol Res.* (2016) 65:717–25. doi: 10.33549/physiolres.933270

19. Levy PT, Sanchez Mejia AA, Machefsky A, Fowler S, Holland MR, Singh GK. Normal ranges of right ventricular systolic and diastolic strain measures in children: a systematic review and meta-analysis. *J Am Soc Echocardiogr.* (2014) 27:549–60.e3. doi: 10.1016/j.echo.2014.01.015

20. Vonk-Noordegraaf A, Haddad F, Chin KM, Forfia PR, Kawut SM, Lumens J, et al. Right heart adaptation to pulmonary arterial hypertension: physiology and pathobiology. *J Am Coll Cardiol.* (2013) 62(Suppl. 25):D22–33. doi: 10.1016/j.jacc.2013.10.027

21. Ghuysen A, Lambermont B, Kolh P, Tchana-Sato V, Magis D, Gerard P, et al. Alteration of right ventricular-pulmonary vascular coupling in a porcine model of progressive pressure overloading. *Shock.* (2008) 29:197–204. doi: 10.1097/shk.0b013e318070c790

22. Tossavainen E, Soderberg S, Gronlund C, Gonzalez M, Henein MY, Lindqvist P. Pulmonary artery acceleration time in identifying pulmonary hypertension patients with raised pulmonary vascular resistance. *Eur Heart J Cardiovasc Imaging.* (2013) 14:890–7. doi: 10.1093/ehjci/jes309

23. Parasuraman S, Walker S, Loudon BL, Gollop ND, Wilson AM, Lowery C, et al. Assessment of pulmonary artery pressure by echocardiography-A comprehensive review. *Int J Cardiol Heart Vasc.* (2016) 12:45–51. doi: 10.1016/j.ijcha.2016.05.011

24. Naing P, Kuppusamy H, Scalia G, Hillis GS, Playford D. Non-invasive assessment of pulmonary vascular resistance in pulmonary hypertension: current knowledge and future direction. *Heart Lung Circ.* (2017) 26:323–30. doi: 10.1016/j.hlc.2016.10.008

25. Vitali SH, Hansmann G, Rose C, Fernandez-Gonzalez A, Scheid A, Mitsialis SA, et al. The Sugen 5416/hypoxia mouse model of pulmonary hypertension revisited: long-term follow-up. *Pulm Circ.* (2014) 4:619–29. doi: 10.1086/678508

26. Hsu S, Houston BA, Tampakakis E, Bacher AC, Rhodes PS, Mathai SC, et al. Right ventricular functional reserve in pulmonary arterial hypertension. *Circulation.* (2016) 133:2413–22. doi: 10.1161/CIRCULATIONAHA.116.022082

27. Wang Z, Schreier DA, Hacker TA, Chesler NC. Progressive right ventricular functional and structural changes in a mouse model of pulmonary arterial hypertension. *Physiol Rep.* (2013) 1:e00184. doi: 10.1002/phy2.184

28. Stein PD, Sabbah HN, Anbe DT, Marzilli M. Performance of the failing and non-failing right ventricle of patients with pulmonary hypertension. *Am J Cardiol.* (1979) 44:1050–5. doi: 10.1016/0002-9149(79)90168-1

29. Levine HJ, Gaasch WH. *The Ventricle : Basic and Clinical Aspects.* Boston: Nijhoff; Hingham, MA: Distributors for North America, Kluwer Academic (1985). p. ix, 345. doi: 10.1007/978-1-4613-2599-4

30. Watanabe R, Amano H, Saito F, Toyoda S, Sakuma M, Abe S, et al. Echocardiographic surrogates of right atrial pressure in pulmonary hypertension. *Heart Vessels.* (2019) 34:477–83. doi: 10.1007/s00380-018-1264-8

31. Sztuka K, Jasinska-Stroschein M. Animal models of pulmonary arterial hypertension: a systematic review and meta-analysis of data from 6126 animals. *Pharmacol Res.* (2017) 125(Pt. B):201–14. doi: 10.1016/j.phrs.2017.08.003

32. Kim BS, Heo R, Shin J, Lim YH, Park JK. E/E' and D-shaped left ventricle severity in patients with increased pulmonary artery pressure. *J Cardiovasc Imaging.* (2018) 26:85–92. doi: 10.4250/jcvi.2018.26.e6

33. Egemnazarov B, Schmidt A, Crnkovic S, Sydykov A, Nagy BM, Kovacs G, et al. Pressure overload creates right ventricular diastolic dysfunction in a mouse model: assessment by echocardiography. *J Am Soc Echocardiogr.* (2015) 28:828–43. doi: 10.1016/j.echo.2015.02.014

34. Mizuno R, Fujimoto S, Saito Y, Okamoto Y. Detection of latent anthracycline-induced cardiotoxicity using left ventricular end-systolic wall stress-velocity of circumferential fiber-shortening relationship. *Heart Vessels.* (2014) 29:384–9. doi: 10.1007/s00380-013-0375-5

35. Smith B, Genuardi MV, Koczo A, Zou RH, Thoma FW, Handen A, et al. Atrial arrhythmias are associated with increased mortality in pulmonary arterial hypertension. *Pulm Circ.* (2018) 8:1–9. doi: 10.1177/2045894018790316

36. Rich JD, Thenappan T, Freed B, Patel AR, Thisted RA, Childers R, et al. QTc prolongation is associated with impaired right ventricular function and predicts mortality in pulmonary hypertension. *Int J Cardiol.* (2013) 167:669–76. doi: 10.1016/j.ijcard.2012.03.071

37. Sun PY, Jiang X, Gomberg-Maitland M, Zhao QH, He J, Yuan P, et al. Prolonged QRS duration: a new predictor of adverse outcome in idiopathic pulmonary arterial hypertension. *Chest.* (2012) 141:374–80. doi: 10.1378/chest.10-3331

38. Temple IP, Logantha SJ, Absi M, Zhang Y, Pervolaraki E, Yanni J, et al. Atrioventricular node dysfunction and ion channel transcriptome in

pulmonary hypertension. *Circ Arrhythm Electrophysiol.* (2016) 9:e003432. doi: 10.1161/CIRCEP.115.003432

39. Raymond RJ, Hinderliter AL, Willis PW, Ralph D, Caldwell EJ, Williams W, et al. Echocardiographic predictors of adverse outcomes in primary pulmonary hypertension. *J Am Coll Cardiol.* (2002) 39:1214–9. doi: 10.1016/S0735-1097(02)01744-8

40. Qian HY, Huang J, Yang YJ, Yang YM, Li ZZ, Zhang JM. Heart-type fatty acid binding protein in the assessment of acute pulmonary embolism. *Am J Med Sci.* (2016) 352:557–62. doi: 10.1016/j.amjms.2016.08.018

41. Filusch A, Giannitsis E, Katus HA, Meyer FJ. High-sensitive troponin T: a novel biomarker for prognosis and disease severity in patients with pulmonary arterial hypertension. *Clin Sci.* (2010) 119:207–13. doi: 10.1042/CS2010 0014

42. Schultze AE, Main BW, Hall DG, Hoffman WP, Lee HY, Ackermann BL, et al. A comparison of mortality and cardiac biomarker response between three outbred stocks of Sprague Dawley rats treated with isoproterenol. *Toxicol Pathol.* (2011) 39:576–88. doi: 10.1177/019262331140 2219

43. Berna M, Ackermann B. Increased throughput for low-abundance protein biomarker verification by liquid chromatography/tandem mass spectrometry. *Anal Chem.* (2009) 81:3950–6. doi: 10.1021/ac900 2744

9

Circulating Neprilysin Level Predicts the Risk of Cardiovascular Events in Hemodialysis Patients

Hyeon Seok Hwang[1], Jin Sug Kim[1], Yang Gyun Kim[1], Yu Ho Lee[2], Dong-Young Lee[3], Shin Young Ahn[4], Ju-Young Moon[1], Sang-Ho Lee[1], Gang-Jee Ko[4*] and Kyung Hwan Jeong[1*]

[1] Division of Nephrology, Department of Internal Medicine, KyungHee University, Seoul, South Korea, [2] Division of Nephrology, Department of Internal Medicine, CHA Bundang Medical Center, CHA University, Seongnam, South Korea, [3] Division of Nephrology, Department of Internal Medicine, Veterans Health Service Medical Center, Seoul, South Korea, [4] Division of Nephrology, Department of Internal Medicine, Korea University College of Medicine, Seoul, South Korea

*Correspondence:
Gang-Jee Ko
lovesba@korea.ac.kr
Kyung Hwan Jeong
aprilhwan@naver.com

Background: Neprilysin inhibition has demonstrated impressive benefits in heart failure treatment, and is the current focus of interest in cardiovascular (CV) and kidney diseases. However, the role of circulating neprilysin as a biomarker for CV events is unclear in hemodialysis (HD) patients.

Methods: A total of 439 HD patients from the K-cohort were enrolled from June 2016 to April 2019. The plasma neprilysin level and echocardiographic findings at baseline were examined. The patients were prospectively followed up to assess the primary endpoint (composite of CV events and cardiac events).

Results: Plasma neprilysin level was positively correlated with left ventricular (LV) mass index, LV end-systolic volume, and LV end-diastolic volume. Multivariate linear regression analysis revealed that neprilysin level was negatively correlated with LV ejection fraction ($\beta = -2.14$; $p = 0.013$). The cumulative event rate of the composite of CV events was significantly greater in neprilysin tertile 3 ($p = 0.049$). Neprilysin tertile 3 was also associated with an increased cumulative event rate of cardiac events ($p = 0.016$). In Cox regression analysis, neprilysin tertile 3 was associated with a 2.61-fold risk for the composite of CV events [95% confidence interval (CI), 1.37–4.97] and a 2.72-fold risk for cardiac events (95% CI, 1.33–5.56) after adjustment for multiple variables.

Conclusions: Higher circulating neprilysin levels independently predicted the composite of CV events and cardiac events in HD patients. The results of this study suggest the importance of future studies on the effect of neprilysin inhibition in reducing CV events.

Keywords: cardiovascular disease, hemodialysis, neprilysin, atherosclerosis, left ventricular systolic dysfunction

INTRODUCTION

Cardiovascular (CV) disease is a major cause of death in patients undergoing hemodialysis (HD) treatment, and an extremely high rate of CV complications has been reported in these patients (1, 2). HD patients are consistently exposed to risk factors for uremia, hemodynamic overload, and sympathetic and neurohumoral activation (3, 4). Furthermore, HD treatment itself induces metabolic derangement and electrolyte shift in cardiomyocytes, episodic cardiac ischemia, and fibrosis (5, 6). Therefore, HD patients experience repetitive cardiac injuries, and these adverse processes induce cardiac dysfunction, structural changes, and remodeling, which are key factors for high CV morbidity and mortality rates.

Natriuretic peptides have been introduced into the dialysis setting, based on their pathophysiologic role in heart failure, to assess for myocardial ischemia, systolic dysfunction, and risk of future cardiac events (7, 8). Natriuretic peptides have a wide range of CV effects contributing to natriuresis, vasodilation, and blood pressure regulation. Neprilysin is the key enzyme responsible for their degradation, and its inhibition enhances the effect of natriuretic peptides on the CV system (9, 10). Previous reports have identified that neprilysin exists in soluble form in the bloodstream, and demonstrated that circulating neprilysin plays a central role in neurohormonal regulation, CV remodeling, and CV dysfunction (11–13). The neprilysin is also anticipated to be a promising biotarget for the reduction of CV risk in patients with chronic kidney disease (CKD) and cross-sectional study showed the usefulness of neprilysin for heart failure diagnosis in dialysis patients (14–18). However, almost studies exploring the neprilysin in patients with CKD enrolled the patients who were not receiving dialysis, and no evidence exists on circulating neprilysin as a pathologic surrogate to predict the incident CV events in patients undergoing HD treatment.

Therefore, we performed this study to test the hypothesis that plasma neprilysin levels are independently associated with an increased risk for future CV events in HD patients. We also investigated circulating neurohormonal markers and echocardiographic parameters to determine their relationships with neprilysin level.

MATERIALS AND METHODS

Study Population

All data in this study were obtained from the registry of the K-cohort, which is a multicenter, prospective cohort of HD patients in Korea. The inclusion and exclusion criteria have been previously described (19). A total of 637 patients were recruited between June 2016 and April 2019, and 439 patients with whole plasma samples at the time of study enrollment were included in this study.

The study protocol was approved by the local ethics committee (KHNMC 2016-04-039), and the study was conducted in accordance with the principles of the Second Declaration of Helsinki. All participants involved in the study signed written informed consent forms before enrollment.

Data Collection and Definitions

Demographic factors, comorbid conditions, laboratory data, dialysis information, and concomitant medication were collected at the time of inclusion. Information on patient comorbidities was derived to calculate the Charlson comorbidity index score (20). Blood samples for laboratory test and biomarkers were drawn before the start of HD in a mid-week dialysis session. Laboratory data were collected, and delivered $spKt/V$ (K, dialyzer clearance; t, time; V, urea distribution volume) was assessed using the conventional method (21). Body mass

index was calculated as body weight divided by the square of body height.

The patients were classified into three groups based on the circulating level of neprilysin: tertile 1, < 107.0 pg/ml; tertile 2, 107.0–237.5 pg/ml; and tertile 3, ≥ 237.5 pg/ml. All patients were prospectively followed up after baseline assessments. The patient follow-up was censored at the time of transfer to peritoneal dialysis, kidney transplantation, follow-up loss, or patient consent withdrawal.

Laboratory Measures

Plasma samples for neurohormonal assessment were collected using ethylenediaminetetraacetic acid-treated tubes at the time of study entry. After centrifugation for 15 min at 1000 g at room temperature, the samples were stored at $-80°C$ until use. Enzyme-linked immunosorbent assay was performed using Magnetic Luminex® Screening Assay multiplex kits (R&D Systems Inc., Minneapolis, MN, USA) to measure B-type natriuretic peptide (BNP), N-terminal-pro-B-type natriuretic peptide (NT-proBNP), interleukin-6 (IL-6), and galectin-3. Neprilysin levels were measured using a modified sandwich immunoassay (product no. SK00724-01; Aviscera Biosciences, Santa Clara, CA, USA). All patient samples were quantified for relevant markers; however, IL-6 was only measured in a subset of patients due to sample availability. IL-6 level was measured in 331 (75.4%) patients [128 (87.1%) patients in neprilysin tertile 1, 115 (78.8%) patients in neprilysin tertile 2, and 88 (60.3%) patients in neprilysin tertile 3]. The proportion of IL-6-measured patients was significantly lower in patients with neprilysin tertile 3 ($p < 0.001$). hsCRP was measured using immunoturbidimetric method on Beckman Coulter AU5800 Analyzers (Brea, CA, USA).

Echocardiographic Measures

Of all patients, 355 (80.1%) patients received echocardiographic examination [123 (83.7%) in tertile 1, 113 (77.4%) in tertile 2, and 119 (81.5%) in tertile 3]. The echocardiographic data was collected from clinical report. M-mode and 2D measurements were conducted by trained sonographers or cardiologist in accord with methods recommended by the American Society of Echocardiography (22). Echocardiographic examiners were blinded to the clinical data and biomarker measurements and cardiologists adjudicate and confirm all echocardiographic findings. LV end-diastolic diameter (LVDd), LV end-systolic diameter (LVDs), LV posterior wall thickness (PWT), and interventricular septal thickness (IVST) was measured in M-mode plane. LV mass was estimated using the Devereux formula and body surface area was used to index the LV mass. LV end-diastolic volume (LVEVd), LV end-systolic volume (LVEVs), LV ejection fraction (LVEF), and left atrial dimensions were determined in apical two- and four-chamber views. Peak early diastolic flow velocity (E) and peak late diastolic flow velocity (A) were determined from the mitral valve inflow velocity curve in pulsed wave Doppler. Peak early diastolic tissue velocity (E′) was measured from the septal aspect of the mitral annulus in tissue Doppler. The ratio of E to A wave (E/A) and E to E$'$ (E/E$'$) was calculated.

Outcome Measures

The primary study endpoint was a composite of incident CV events, including cardiac and non-cardiac vascular events. Cardiac events were defined as acute coronary syndrome, heart failure, ventricular arrhythmia, cardiac arrest, and sudden death. Non-cardiac events included cerebral infarction, cerebral hemorrhage, and peripheral vascular occlusive diseases requiring revascularization or surgical intervention. All mortality events from any cause were recorded and carefully reviewed. The secondary endpoints were levels of circulating neurohormonal markers and echocardiographic parameters, and their correlations with neprilysin level were analyzed.

Statistical Analysis

Data are expressed as mean $\pm$ standard deviation (SD) or median [interquartile range (IQR)]. Kolmogorov-Smirnov test was used to assess the normality of the distribution of the variables. Differences among the three groups were identified using analysis of variance or Kruskal-Wallis test. Tukey *post hoc* test and Mann-Whitney *U*-test with Bonferroni correction were used to identify differences between more than two groups. Categorical variables were compared using the chi-square test or Fisher's exact test. Log-transformed values of high-sensitivity C-reactive protein (hsCRP) levels were used in regression analysis because of a skewed distribution. The values of neprilysin levels were log-transformed for linear regression analysis, and 1 SD was used for hazard ratio (HR) calculations. Spearman's analyses were used to evaluate the correlation between neprilysin level and continuous variables. The association between neprilysin level and LVEF was identified using linear regression analysis. A Cox proportional hazard model was constructed to identify independent variables related to CV events or patient death. Multivariate models included significantly associated parameters according to their weight in univariate testing and clinically fundamental parameters. Baseline characteristics and laboratory data was compared between patients with and without incident cardiac event to adjust the multivariate model (**Supplementary Table 1**). Charlson comorbidity score, prevalence of CV event history, hemoglobin level, and plasma NT-proBNP level was significantly different between two groups. All of these parameters were included in multivariate Cox model. We tried to adjust baseline cardiac remodeling status using NT-proBNP or BNP, because echocardiographic data is not fully investigated in this study. Statistical analyses were performed using SPSS software (version 22.0; SPSS, IBM Corp., Armonk, NY, USA). *p*-values < 0.05 were considered significant.

RESULTS

Baseline Demographic Characteristics and Laboratory Data

The median neprilysin level was 155.2 (IQR 88.6, 304.2) pg/ml in all studied patients. According to tertile, the median

TABLE 1 | Baseline demographic and laboratory data of the study population.

	Tertiles of neprilysin level			P-value
	Tertile 1 < 107.0 pg/ml (*n* = 147)	**Tertile 2** 107.0–237.5 pg/ml (*n* = 146)	**Tertile 3** ≥ 237.5 pg/ml (*n* = 146)	
Age (years)	64.9 ± 12.1	61.5 ± 11.4*	58.7 ± 14.2*	<0.001
Male (%)	109 (74.1)	92 (63.0)	91 (62.3)	0.055
Body mass index (kg/m^2)	23.43 ± 3.82	22.99 ± 3.90	23.43 ± 4.55	0.567
HD duration (years)	4.66 ± 6.01	3.63 ± 5.07	2.91 ± 4.54*	0.017
Diabetes (%)	77 (52.4)	88 (60.3)	84 (57.5)	0.383
History of CV event (%)	64 (43.5)	62(42.5)	59 (40.4)	0.859
Charlson comorbidity score	4.10 ± 1.71	4.13 ± 1.21	3.97 ± 1.55	0.616
Hemoglobin (g/dl)	10.55 ± 1.28	10.46 ± 1.14	10.39 ± 1.26	0.529
Albumin (g/dl)	3.77 ± 0.33	3.82 ± 0.30	3.84 ± 0.34	0.156
LDL-cholesterol (mg/dl)	76.08 ± 25.62	77.72 ± 28.50	75.46 ± 24.84	0.752
hsCRP (mg/dl)	1.42 (0.20, 3.49)	0.92 (0.19, 3.54)	0.70 (0.19, 2.80)	0.149
Predialysis SBP (mmHg)	144.3 ± 18.9	141.3 ± 19.9	142.3 ± 21.8	0.421
Ultrafiltration (L)	2.25 ± 1.11	2.14 ± 1.07	2.29 ± 1.07	0.462
spKt/V	1.59 ± 0.46	1.55 ± 0.31	1.58 ± 0.25	0.634
ESA use (%)	131 (89.1)	132 (91.0)	136 (93.2)	0.479
BNP (pg/ml)	50.6 (16.3, 91.0)	37.3 (7.6, 86.6)	35.4 (7.6, 88.5)	0.384
NT-proBNP (pg/ml)	286 (200, 442)	330 (189, 475)	317 (198, 477)	0.542
IL-6 (pg/ml)	3.3 (2.2, 5.8)	3.0 (1.9, 4.8)	2.7 (2.1, 4.2)*	0.032
Galectin-3 (ng/ml)	17.2 (15.0, 19.8)	17.5 (15.0, 20.5)	19.0 (15.4, 22.0)*	0.029

IL-6 was measured in 331 (75.4%) patients.
*p < 0.05 vs. tertile 1.
HD, hemodialysis; CV, cardiovascular; LDL, low-density lipoprotein; hsCRP, high-sensitivity C-reactive protein; SBP, systolic blood pressure; spKt/V, single-pool Kt/V; ESA, erythropoietin-stimulating agent; BNP, brain natriuretic peptide; NT-proBNP, N-terminal-pro-B-type natriuretic peptide; MMP-2, matrix metalloproteinase-2.

neprilysin level was 68.4 (IQR 45.2, 89.2) pg/ml in tertile 1 (*n* = 147), 155.9 (IQR 127.2, 184.4) pg/ml in tertile 2 (*n* = 146), and 424.0 (IQR 303.4, 741.6) pg/ml in tertile 3 (*n* = 146). The baseline patient demographics, clinical characteristics, and laboratory results are described in **Table 1**. Patients in tertile 3 of neprilysin level were younger and had a shorter duration of dialysis therapy than those in neprilysin tertile 1. Twenty (4.6%) patients with heart failure were enrolled in this study. Heart failure with preserved LVEF was observed in 6 (1.4%) patients and heart failure with reduced LVEF in 14 (3.2%) patients. Laboratory data and dialysis characteristics did not show significant differences. Among the circulating neurohormonal markers, galectin-3 showed a significantly higher level in patients in neprilysin tertile 3 than in patients in the other tertiles.

TABLE 2 | Correlation of neprilysin level with circulating cardiac markers and echocardiographic parameters.

	Correlation coefficient	P-value
Circulating neurohormonal marker		
BNP (pg/ml)	−0.092	0.055
NT-proBNP (pg/ml)	0.003	0.949
hsCRP (mg/dl)	−0.105	0.029
IL-6 (pg/ml)	−0.134	0.014
Galectin-3 (ng/ml)	0.124	0.009
Echocardiographic parameters		
LV mass index (g/m^2)	0.129	0.043
LVDs (mm)	0.068	0.235
LVDd (mm)	0.063	0.235
LVESV (ml)	0.137	0.035
LVEDV (ml)	0.137	0.035
LVEF (%)	−0.185	< 0.001
IVST (mm)	0.046	0.470
PWT (mm)	−0.023	0.690
E/E'	0.019	0.778
E/A	0.024	0.731
LA dimension (mm)	−0.048	0.445

Echocardiography was examined in 355 (80.9%) patients.
BNP, B-type natriuretic peptide; NT-proBNP, N-terminal-pro-B-type natriuretic peptide; MMP-2, matrix metalloproteinase-2; LV, left ventricle; LVDs, left ventricular end-systolic diameter; LVDd, left ventricular end-diastolic diameter; LVESV, left ventricular end-systolic volume; LVEDV, left ventricular end-diastolic volume; IVST, interventricular septal thickness in diastolic; PWT LV, posterior wall thickness in diastolic; LVEF, left ventricle ejection fraction; LA, left atrium.

Correlation of Neprilysin Level With Circulating Cardiac Markers and Echocardiographic Parameters

The correlations between the levels of neprilysin and circulating neurohormonal markers are shown in **Table 2** and **Supplementary Figure 1**. The plasma levels of BNP and NT-proBNP did not show a significant correlation with neprilysin level. A significant positive correlation was found between galectin-3 and neprilysin levels, and the circulating levels of hsCRP and IL-6 were negatively correlated with neprilysin level. However, all coefficient values and distribution patterns suggested that the correlation power was not strong.

The baseline echocardiographic measurements are described in **Supplementary Table 2**. LVEF was significantly different across tertiles, and the lowest LVEF was observed in patients in neprilysin tertile 3. Posterior wall thickness and the E/A ratio showed different mean values among the neprilysin tertiles. To investigate the relationship between neprilysin level and cardiac structures, the correlation between neprilysin level and echocardiographic parameters was evaluated (**Table 2**). LV systolic and diastolic diameters, LV wall thickness, and diastolic parameters were not correlated with circulating neprilysin level. A significant negative correlation was observed between LVEF and neprilysin level. LV mass index, LVESV, and LVEDV were positively correlated with neprilysin level. However, the coefficient values and distribution patterns of variables indicated weak correlation power (**Supplementary Figure 2**).

TABLE 3 | Relationship between the baseline parameters and LVEF.

	Unstandardized β	95% CI	P-value
Age (years)	0.03	−0.40, 0.10	0.417
Male	−0.57	−2.36, 1.22	0.531
History of CV event	−2.93	−4.68, −1.18	0.002
Hemoglobin (g/dl)	0.56	−0.12, 1.24	0.107
NT-proBNP (pg/ml)	−0.003	−0.007, 0.001	0.112
Ultrafiltration (L)	−0.54	−1.35, 0.27	0.193
Neprilysin (pg/ml)	−2.14	−3.83, −0.45	0.013

Of the all studied patients, 355 (80.9%) patients were examined with echocardiography. CV, cardiovascular; NT-proBNP, N-terminal-pro-B-type natriuretic peptide.

Relationship Between Plasma Neprilysin Level and Left Ventricular Ejection Fraction in Hemodialysis Patients

Univariate and multivariate linear regression models were constructed to determine the association between neprilysin level and LV systolic function. In univariate analysis, LVEF was significantly associated with history of CV events ($\beta = -2.89$; $p = 0.001$), NT-proBNP level ($\beta = -0.01$; $p = 0.023$), and neprilysin level ($\beta = -2.19$; $p = 0.011$). Hemoglobin level ($\beta = 0.50$; $p = 0.155$) and ultrafiltration volume ($\beta = -0.65$; $p = 0.115$) showed borderline significance in association with neprilysin level. The multivariate linear regression model is shown in **Table 3**. History of CV events ($\beta = -2.93$; $p = 0.002$) and neprilysin level ($\beta = -2.14$; $p = 0.013$) were independent determinants of LVEF in HD patients.

Prognostic Utility of Neprilysin Level in Hemodialysis Patients

During a mean follow-up of 30.1 months, 61 deaths (13.9%) and 66 CV events (15.0%) occurred. Of the CV events, acute coronary syndrome occurred in 27 patients, heart failure occurred in 6 patients, ventricular arrhythmia occurred in 4 patients, cardiac arrest occurred in 9 patients, sudden death occurred in 6 patients, cerebral vascular accidents occurred in 8 patients, and peripheral vascular occlusive diseases occurred in 6 patients. The cumulative event rate of the composite of CV events was significantly greater in neprilysin tertile 3 ($p = 0.049$; **Figure 1A**). Neprilysin tertile 3 was associated with a greater cumulative event rate of cardiac events ($p = 0.016$; **Figure 1B**). The cumulative event rate of patient death did not differ among patients in the different neprilysin tertiles ($p = 0.127$).

Univariable Cox regression analysis revealed that plasma neprilysin tertile 3 was significantly associated with an increased risk for the composite of CV events [HR, 2.10; 95% confidence interval (CI), 1.14–3.88; $p = 0.017$; **Table 4**]. This association remained significant after adjustment for multiple variables (HR, 2.61; 95% CI, 1.37–4.97; $p = 0.004$). Neprilysin increment per 1 SD also had an independent risk for composite events (HR, 1.40; 95% CI, 1.17–1.66; $p < 0.001$). To further investigate the risk for the composite of CV events, the HRs for cardiac events and non-cardiac vascular events were evaluated. Patients in neprilysin tertile 3 had a significant risk for cardiac events

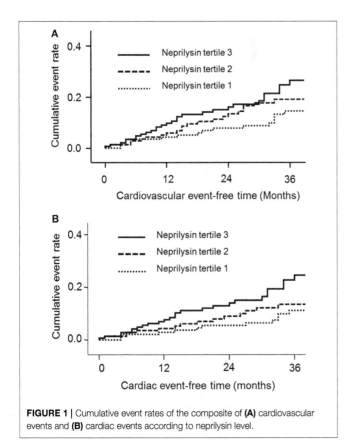

FIGURE 1 | Cumulative event rates of the composite of **(A)** cardiovascular events and **(B)** cardiac events according to neprilysin level.

TABLE 4 | Hazard ratios of neprilysin tertiles for cardiovascular events.

	No. event (%)	HR (95% CI), crude	HR (95% CI), adjusted
Composite of CVE			
Neprilysin tertile 1	16 (10.9)	Reference	Reference
Neprilysin tertile 2	21 (14.4)	1.46 (0.76, 2.81)	1.77 (0.90, 3.49)
Neprilysin tertile 3	29 (19.9)	2.10* (1.14, 3.88)	2.61* (1.37, 4.97)
Neprilysin per SD		1.32* (1.11, 1.57)	1.40* (1.17, 1.66)
Cardiac event			
Neprilysin tertile 1	12 (8.2)	Reference	Reference
Neprilysin tertile 2	16 (11.0)	1.45 (0.70, 2.98)	1.56 (0.72, 3.36)
Neprilysin tertile 3	26 (17.8)	2.54* (1.28, 5.05)	2.72* (1.33, 5.56)
Neprilysin per SD		1.37* (1.14, 1.64)	1.44* (1.20, 1.74)
Non-cardiac vascular event			
Neprilysin tertile 1	4 (2.7)	Reference	Reference
Neprilysin tertile 2	7 (4.8)	1.84 (0.54, 6.27)	2.56 (0.68, 9.72)
Neprilysin tertile 3	4 (2.7)	1.00 (0.25, 4.02)	1.47 (0.34, 6.30)
Neprilysin per SD		1.26 (0.89, 1.78)	1.27 (0.90, 1.78)
Patient death			
Neprilysin tertile 1	29 (19.7)	Reference	Reference
Neprilysin tertile 2	16 (11.0)	0.59 (0.32, 1.09)	0.75 (0.40, 1.42)
Neprilysin tertile 3	16 (11.0)	0.60 (0.33, 1.11)	0.81 (0.43, 1.55)
Neprilysin per SD		0.81 (0.52, 1.26)	0.88 (0.60, 1.29)

All analyses are adjusted for the following: age, sex, body mass index, Charlson comorbidity index, hemoglobin, hsCRP, NT-proBNP, ESA use, HD duration, spKt/V. hsCRP, high-sensitivity C-reactive protein; NT-proBNP, N-terminal-pro-B-type natriuretic peptide; ESA, erythropoietin-stimulating agent; HD, hemodialysis; spKt/V, single-pool Kt/V.
*p < 0.05.

after adjustment for multiple covariates (HR, 2.72; 95% CI, 1.33–5.56; $p = 0.006$) and neprilysin increment per 1 SD was also associated with the risk of cardiac events (HR, 1.44; 95% CI, 1.20–1.74; $p < 0.001$). However, neprilysin level per tertile or per 1 SD increment did not show a significant risk for non-cardiac events and patient death. We re-construct multivariate Cox hazard model including BNP as covariates, instead of NT-proBNP. Neprilysin tertile 3 and neprilysin increment per 1 SD was significantly associated with higher risk of CV composite and cardiac events (**Supplementary Table 3**).

DISCUSSION

Our prospective observational cohort study demonstrated that an increased level of neprilysin was associated with a greater cumulative event rate of CV composites and cardiac events. In addition, higher levels of neprilysin increased the risk for incident CV composites and cardiac events after adjustment for multiple covariates. Plasma neprilysin level was positively correlated with galectin-3 circulating level, LV dimension, and LV mass index. In addition, an independent negative relationship was observed between neprilysin level and LVEF. These findings suggest that neprilysin is a novel biomarker for assessing the risk of CV events, and that it is associated with cardiac structural and functional changes in HD patients.

Interestingly, we found a weakly negative correlation between neprilysin and the inflammatory markers hsCRP and IL-6. Inflammatory substrates are known to be degradable by neprilysin, and we presumed that higher levels of neprilysin are associated with a reduced inflammatory state. However, the correlation power between neprilysin and inflammatory marker was weak, suggesting that the inhibitory interaction was not substantial in HD patients (9, 23). The additional incidental finding was negative correlation between neprilysin levels and age ($\rho = -0.167$; $p < 0.001$). The reason of this finding is not clear, but we presumed that the correlation between circulating neprilysin level and age is dependent on population characteristics, because the correlations coefficients were changeable in different patient categories (11, 24, 25).

Galectin-3 is a contributing factor to cardiac fibrosis, and a biomarker for LV remodeling and heart failure progression (26–28). Our results showed that neprilysin level was positively correlated with galectin-3 level. In addition, LV internal volume and LV mass index increased as the plasma level of neprilysin increased. These findings suggest that circulating neprilysin level reflects the pathologic deformation of cardiac structures. However, correlation power indicated the weak relationship between neprilysin and echocardiographic parameters. Therefore, we construct linear regression model to find out independent relationship between neprilysin and LVEF. We observed that neprilysin level was associated with lower LVEF after multiple adjustment. These findings suggest that neprilysin is a noticeable indicator of LV systolic dysfunction and cardiac remodeling in HD patients.

The use of cardiac biomarkers in clinical practice allows clinicians to identify high-risk patients for incident CV events. Although BNP and NT-proBNP have been widely used in patients with heart failure, their use in HD patients is challenging because of high individual variations, increased plasma levels without any evidence of cardiac disease, more than normal values in 90% of HD patients, and wide differences in cutoff value for risk stratification in diverse studies (29–31). Therefore, alternative cardiac biomarkers are required in dialysis care, and neprilysin is of particular interest because it is a new biotarget for innovative therapeutic strategies in heart failure (10, 32). Our study revealed that plasma neprilysin levels were significantly associated with increased rates of CV composites and cardiac events. The association remained significant after adjustment for multiple established CV risk factors, including NT-proBNP. These findings suggest that higher neprilysin levels contribute to incident CV risk independently of traditional CV risk factors and that neprilysin is a valuable biomarker for CV risk prediction in patients undergoing HD treatment.

Although we found a significant predictive ability of neprilysin for adverse CV outcomes in HD patients, recent studies on non-dialysis-dependent CKD revealed that high neprilysin levels did not predict poor CV outcomes (33). We presumed that these divergent results might originate from the greater activation of natriuretic peptide systems in HD patients. Because HD patients usually have higher degrees of cardiac remodeling than non-dialysis-dependent CKD patients, the activation of natriuretic peptides is more pronounced in HD patients (34–36). Therefore, the clinical importance of neprilysin in HD patients may become larger with activated natriuretic peptides. This explanatory assumption is also supported by the discrepant results in different heart failure settings. Previous studies have reported that circulating neprilysin level is predictive of CV death in patients with heart failure with acute decompensation or reduced LVEF, but is not associated with CV outcomes in patients with heart failure with preserved LVEF (11, 12, 37, 38).

This study had some limitations. Echocardiographic parameters and IL-6 levels were not measured in some patients. The lower proportion of IL-6-measured patients in neprilysin tertile 3 may be possible to cause the bias in correlation analysis.

Furthermore, given the limited number of events, we could not perform individual analyses for heart failure, although HD patients are at a higher risk for congestion (39). In addition, we measured neprilysin concentration only, and neprilysin activity was not measured. It was reported in a previous study that neprilysin activity, but not concentration, provided diagnostic information about heart failure in dialysis patients (18). Lower neprilysin activity combining with multi-markers helped to determine the presence of heart failure. Therefore, measurement of neprilysin activity might provide additional data on the risk of incident CV event. Further studies with neurohormonal peptides, neprilysin concentration and activity may improve predictability of CV complication in HD patients.

CONCLUSION

Circulating neprilysin level was correlated with pathologic remodeling of echocardiographic structures and independently associated with lower LVEF. Higher circulating neprilysin levels were associated with a greater risk of the composite of CV events and cardiac events in HD patients. Our results suggest the importance of future studies on the implication of neprilysin inhibition for HD patients.

AUTHOR CONTRIBUTIONS

HSH conceived the research question conceived and designed the analysis. JSK, YGK, YHL, D-YL, J-YM, JYM, and S-HL undertook data collection conducted the study. HSH, G-JK, and KHJ drafted the manuscript. All authors reviewed the results and commented on the manuscript. All authors read and approved the final manuscript.

ACKNOWLEDGMENTS

This work was supported by Patient-Centered Clinical Research Coordinating Center funded by the Ministry of Health and Welfare, Republic of Korea (H19C0481, HC19C0041).

REFERENCES

1. Cheung AK, Sarnak MJ, Yan G, Dwyer JT, Heyka RJ, Rocco MV, et al. Atherosclerotic cardiovascular disease risks in chronic hemodialysis patients. *Kidney Int.* (2000) 58:353-62. doi: 10.1046/j.1523-1755.2000.00173.x

2. Thompson S, James M, Wiebe N, Hemmelgarn B, Manns B, Klarenbach S, et al. Cause of death in patients with reduced kidney function. *J Am Soc Nephrol.* (2015) 26:2504-11. doi: 10.1681/ASN.2014070714

3. Meeus F, Kourilsky O, Guerin AP, Gaudry C, Marchais SJ, London GM. Pathophysiology of cardiovascular disease in hemodialysis patients. *Kidney Int Suppl.* (2000) 76:S140-7. doi: 10.1046/j.1523-1755.2000.07618.x

4. Rangaswami J, McCullough PA. Heart failure in end-stage kidney disease: pathophysiology, diagnosis, and therapeutic strategies. *Semin Nephrol.* (2018) 38:600-17. doi: 10.1016/j.semnephrol.2018.08.005

5. Odudu A, McIntyre CW. An update on intradialytic cardiac dysfunction. *Semin Dial.* (2016) 29:435-41. doi: 10.1111/sdi.12532

6. McIntyre CW. Effects of hemodialysis on cardiac function. *Kidney Int.* (2009) 76:371-5. doi: 10.1038/ki.2009.207

7. Wang AY, Lam CW, Yu CM, Wang M, Chan IH, Zhang Y, et al. N-terminal pro-brain natriuretic peptide: an independent risk predictor of cardiovascular congestion, mortality, and adverse cardiovascular outcomes in chronic peritoneal dialysis patients. *J Am Soc Nephrol.* (2007) 18:321-30. doi: 10.1681/ASN.2005121299

8. Wang AY. Clinical utility of natriuretic peptides in dialysis patients. *Semin Dial.* (2012) 25:326-33. doi: 10.1111/j.1525-139X.2012.01079.x

9. Bayes-Genis A, Barallat J, Richards AM. A test in context: neprilysin: function, inhibition, and biomarker. *J Am Coll Cardiol.* (2016) 68:639-53. doi: 10.1016/j.jacc.2016.04.060

10. McMurray JJ, Packer M, Desai AS, Gong J, Lefkowitz MP, Rizkala AR, et al. Angiotensin-neprilysin inhibition versus enalapril in heart failure. *N Engl J Med.* (2014) 371:993-1004. doi: 10.1056/NEJMoa1409077

11. Bayes-Genis A, Barallat J, Galan A, de Antonio M, Domingo M, Zamora E, et al. Soluble neprilysin is predictive of cardiovascular death and heart failure hospitalization in heart failure patients. *J Am Coll Cardiol.* (2015) 65:657-65. doi: 10.1016/j.jacc.2014.11.048

12. Bayes-Genis A, Barallat J, Pascual-Figal D, Nunez J, Minana G, Sanchez-Mas J, et al. Prognostic value and kinetics of soluble neprilysin in acute heart failure: a pilot study. *JACC Heart Fail.* (2015) 3:641-4. doi: 10.1016/j.jchf.2015.03.006

13. Wang Y, Zhou R, Lu C, Chen Q, Xu T, Li D. Effects of the angiotensin-receptor neprilysin inhibitor on cardiac reverse remodeling: meta-analysis. *J Am Heart Assoc.* (2019) 8:e012272. doi: 10.1161/JAHA.119.012272

14. Haynes R, Zhu D, Judge PK, Herrington WG, Kalra PA, Baigent C. Chronic kidney disease, heart failure and neprilysin inhibition. *Nephrol Dial Transplant.* (2020) 35:558-64. doi: 10.1093/ndt/gfz058

15. Judge P, Haynes R, Landray MJ, Baigent C. Neprilysin inhibition in chronic kidney disease. *Nephrol Dial Transplant.* (2015) 30:738-43. doi: 10.1093/ndt/gfu269

16. James M, Manns B. Neprilysin inhibition and effects on kidney function and surrogates of cardiovascular risk in chronic kidney disease. *Circulation.* (2018) 138:1515-8. doi: 10.1161/CIRCULATIONAHA.118.036523

17. Lyle MA, Iyer SR, Redfield MM, Reddy YNV, Felker GM, Cappola TP, et al. Circulating neprilysin in patients with heart failure and preserved ejection fraction. *JACC Heart Fail.* (2020) 8:70-80. doi: 10.1016/j.jchf.2019.07.005

18. Claus R, Berliner D, Bavendiek U, Vodovar N, Lichtinghagen R, David S, et al. Soluble neprilysin, NT-proBNP, and growth differentiation factor-15 as biomarkers for heart failure in dialysis patients (SONGBIRD). *Clin Res Cardiol.* (2020) 109:1035-47. doi: 10.1007/s00392-020-01597-x

19. Hwang HS, Kim JS, Kim YG, Lee SY, Ahn SY, Lee HJ, et al. Circulating PCSK9 level and risk of cardiovascular events and death in hemodialysis patients. *J Clin Med.* (2020) 9:244. doi: 10.3390/jcm9010244

20. Charlson ME, Pompei P, Ales KL, MacKenzie CR. A new method of classifying prognostic comorbidity in longitudinal studies: development and validation. *J Chronic Dis.* (1987) 40:373-83. doi: 10.1016/0021-9681(87)90171-8

21. Gotch FA. Kinetic modeling in hemodialysis. In: Nissenson AR, Fine RN, Gentile DE, editors. *Clinical Dialysis.* 3rd ed. Norwalk, CT: Appleton and Lange (1995). pp. 156-88.

22. Lang RM, Badano LP, Mor-Avi V, Afilalo J, Armstrong A, Ernande L, et al. Recommendations for cardiac chamber quantification by echocardiography in adults: an update from the American Society of Echocardiography and the European Association of Cardiovascular Imaging. *J Am Soc Echocardiogr.* (2015) 28:1-39.e14. doi: 10.1016/j.echo.2014.10.003

23. Chen Y, Burnett JC, Jr. Biochemistry, therapeutics, and biomarker implications of neprilysin in cardiorenal disease. *Clin Chem.* (2017) 63:108-15. doi: 10.1373/clinchem.2016.262907

24. Pavo N, Arfsten H, Cho A, Goliasch G, Bartko PE, Wurm R, et al. The circulating form of neprilysin is not a general biomarker for overall survival in treatment-naive cancer patients. *Sci Rep.* (2019) 9:2554. doi: 10.1038/s41598-019-38867-2

25. Reddy YNV, Iyer SR, Scott CG, Rodeheffer RJ, Bailey K, Jenkins G, et al. Soluble neprilysin in the general population: clinical determinants and its relationship to cardiovascular disease. *J Am Heart Assoc.* (2019) 8:e012943. doi: 10.1161/JAHA.119.012943

26. Ho JE, Liu C, Lyass A, Courchesne P, Pencina MJ, Vasan RS, et al. Galectin-3, a marker of cardiac fibrosis, predicts incident heart failure in the community. *J Am Coll Cardiol.* (2012) 60:1249-56. doi: 10.1016/j.jacc.2012.04.053

27. de Boer RA, Voors AA, Muntendam P, van Gilst WH, van Veldhuisen DJ. Galectin-3: a novel mediator of heart failure development and progression. *Eur J Heart Fail.* (2009) 11:811-7. doi: 10.1093/eurjhf/hfp097

28. Lok DJ, Lok SI, Bruggink-Andre de la Porte PW, Badings E, Lipsic E, van Wijngaarden J, et al. Galectin-3 is an independent marker for ventricular remodeling and mortality in patients with chronic heart failure. *Clin Res Cardiol.* (2013) 102:103-10. doi: 10.1007/s00392-012-0500-y

29. Vickery S, Price CP, John RI, Abbas NA, Webb MC, Kempson ME, et al. B-type natriuretic peptide (BNP) and amino-terminal proBNP in patients with CKD: relationship to renal function and left ventricular hypertrophy. *Am J Kidney Dis.* (2005) 46:610-20. doi: 10.1053/j.ajkd.2005.06.017

30. Booth J, Pinney J, Davenport A. N-terminal proBNP–marker of cardiac dysfunction, fluid overload, or malnutrition in hemodialysis patients? *Clin J Am Soc Nephrol.* (2010) 5:1036-40. doi: 10.2215/CJN.09001209

31. Fahim MA, Hayen A, Horvath AR, Dimeski G, Coburn A, Johnson DW, et al. N-terminal pro-B-type natriuretic peptide variability in stable dialysis patients. *Clin J Am Soc Nephrol.* (2015) 10:620-9. doi: 10.2215/CJN.09060914

32. Velazquez EJ, Morrow DA, DeVore AD, Duffy CI, Ambrosy AP, McCague K, et al. Angiotensin-neprilysin inhibition in acute decompensated heart failure. *N Engl J Med.* (2019) 380:539-48. doi: 10.1056/NEJMoa1812851

33. Emrich IE, Vodovar N, Feuer L, Untersteller K, Nougue H, Seiler-Mussler S, et al. Do plasma neprilysin activity and plasma neprilysin concentration predict cardiac events in chronic kidney disease patients? *Nephrol Dial Transplant.* (2019) 34:100-8. doi: 10.1093/ndt/gfy066

34. Roberts MA, Hare DL, Sikaris K, Ierino FL. Temporal trajectory of B-type natriuretic peptide in patients with CKD stages 3 and 4, dialysis, and kidney transplant. *Clin J Am Soc Nephrol.* (2014) 9:1024-32. doi: 10.2215/CJN.08640813

35. Horii M, Matsumoto T, Uemura S, Sugawara Y, Takitsume A, Ueda T, et al. Prognostic value of B-type natriuretic peptide and its amino-terminal proBNP fragment for cardiovascular events with stratification by renal function. *J Cardiol.* (2013) 61:410-6. doi: 10.1016/j.jjcc.2013.01.015

36. Paoletti E, De Nicola L, Gabbai FB, Chiodini P, Ravera M, Pieracci L, et al. Associations of left ventricular hypertrophy and geometry with adverse outcomes in patients with CKD and hypertension. *Clin J Am Soc Nephrol.* (2016) 11:271-9. doi: 10.2215/CJN.06980615

37. Goliasch G, Pavo N, Zotter-Tufaro C, Kammerlander A, Duca F, Mascherbauer J, et al. Soluble neprilysin does not correlate with outcome in heart failure with preserved ejection fraction. *Eur J Heart Fail.* (2016) 18:89-93. doi: 10.1002/ejhf.435

38. O'Connor CM, deFilippi C. PARAGON-HF - why we do randomized, controlled clinical trials. *N Engl J Med.* (2019) 381:1675-6. doi: 10.1056/NEJMe1912402

39. Campbell DJ. Long-term neprilysin inhibition - implications for ARNIs. *Nat Rev Cardiol.* (2017) 14:171-86. doi: 10.1038/nrcardio.2016.200

10

Echocardiographic Prognosis Relevance of Attenuated Right Heart Remodeling in Idiopathic Pulmonary Arterial Hypertension

Qin-Hua Zhao [1†], Su-Gang Gong [1†], Rong Jiang [1†], Chao Li [2], Ge-Fei Chen [3], Ci-Jun Luo [1], Hong-Ling Qiu [1], Jin-Ming Liu [1], Lan Wang [1,2*] and Rui Zhang [1,2*]

[1] Department of Pulmonary Circulation, Shanghai Pulmonary Hospital, Tongji University School of Medicine, Shanghai, China, [2] Tongji University School of Medicine, Shanghai, China, [3] Department of Biosciences and Nutrition, Karolinska Institutet, Stockholm, Sweden

*Correspondence:
Rui Zhang
zgr1219@163.com
Lan Wang
wanglan198212@163.com

† These authors have contributed equally to this work

Background: Right ventricular (RV) function is a great determination of the fate in patients with pulmonary arterial hypertension (PAH). Monitoring RV structure back to normal or improvement should be useful for evaluation of RV function. The aims of this study were to assess the prognostic relevance of changed right heart (RH) dimensions by echocardiography and attenuated RH remodeling (ARHR) in idiopathic PAH (IPAH).

Methods: We retrospectively analyzed 232 consecutive adult IPAH patients at baseline assessment and included RH catheterization and echocardiography. ARHR at the mean 20 ± 12 months' follow-up was defined by a decreased right atrium area, RV mid-diameter, and left ventricular end-diastolic eccentricity index. The follow-up end point was all-cause mortality.

Results: At mean 20 ± 12 months' follow-up, 33 of 232 patients (14.2%) presented with ARHR. The remaining 199 surviving patients were monitored for another 25 ± 20 months. At the end of follow-up, the survival rates at 1, 3, and 5 years were 89, 89, and 68% in patients with ARHR, respectively, and 84, 65 and 41% in patients without ARHR (log-rank $p = 0.01$). ARHR was an independent prognostic factor for mortality. Besides, ARHR was available to further stratify patients' risk assessment through the French PAH non-invasive-risk criteria.

Conclusions: Echocardiographic ARHR is an independent determinant of prognosis in IPAH at long-term follow-up. ARHR might be a useful tool to indicate the RV morphologic and functional improvement associated with better prognostic likelihood.

Keywords: pulmonary arterial hypertension, right heart remodeling, echocardiography, biomarkers, prognosis

INTRODUCTION

Pulmonary arterial hypertension (PAH) was a progressive disease that affected both pulmonary vasculature and heart. Although the initial damage in PAH may involve the pulmonary vasculature, the prognosis of patients with PAH is closely related to the right ventricular (RV) function (1–3). RV function is a great clinical determinant of the fate in patients with severe pulmonary hypertension

(PH) (4, 5). The right heart (RH) failure may be a consequence of increased afterload in PH. An adapted right ventricle showed slightly dilated with preserved stroke volume and systolic function, whereas a maladapted right ventricle is dilated with reduced systolic function and increased dimensions (5, 6). Therefore, the changes of RV dimensions were inevitable and associated with pulmonary hemodynamics. Monitoring RV dimension could predict clinical worsening even at apparent clinical stability in PAH (7).

Echocardiography is an essential and non-invasive component estimated the role of RV function in PAH. Imaging modalities would be ideal to validate potential RV function and allow the creation of prediction scores to identify risk of mortality (8–10). Badagliacca et al. have reported the reversal of RH remodeling (RHRR) was associated with an improved outcome in idiopathic PAH (IPAH) patients by assessing right atrium (RA) area, left ventricular systolic eccentricity index (LV-EI), and RV end-diastolic area (11). Moreover, several clinical common echocardiographic variables were associated with mortality risk such as RV mid-diameter (RVMD) and tricuspid annular plane systolic excursion (12–14).

In the present study, we try to reassess and recalculate the efficacy of RH dimension's changes through general clinical echocardiographic parameters. Here, we defined a new model of attenuated RH remodeling (ARHR) using a decrease in RA area, RVMD, and left ventricular end-diastolic eccentricity index (LV-EId). Each of these echocardiographic parameters has been reported to be a determinant of prognosis in PAH (10, 11, 13). We proposed a hypothesis that ARHR created by a decrease in RA area, RVMD, and LV-EId would be associated with mortality and clinic outcomes.

MATERIALS AND METHODS
Study Subjects and Design
Two hundred thirty-two consecutive treatment-naive adult IPAH patients (≥18 years of age at diagnosis) were enrolled and monitored at the time of their first right heart catheterization (RHC) in Shanghai Pulmonary Hospital from November 2010 to January 2018. IPAH was diagnosed according to guideline standard: a mean pulmonary artery pressure (mPAP) ≥25 mmHg and pulmonary vascular resistance (PVR) >3 Woods units at rest in the presence of a normal pulmonary artery wedge pressure (≤15 mmHg) on RHC (15, 16). In accordance with criteria, the respiratory function tests, perfusion lung scan, computed

Abbreviations: BMI, body mass index; CI, cardiac index; IPAH, idiopathic pulmonary arterial hypertension; LAESD, left atrium end-systolic diameter; LV A wave PW, pulsed wave left ventricular A wave; LVEDD, left ventricular end-diastolic diameter; LVEF, left ventricular ejection fraction; LV-EId, left ventricular end-diastolic eccentricity index; LVESD, left ventricular end-systolic diameter; LV E wave PW, pulsed wave left ventricular E wave; mPAP, mean pulmonary arterial pressure; 6MWD, 6-min walking distance; NT-proBNP, N-terminal fragmental of pro–brain natriuretic peptide; PAWP, pulmonary artery wedge pressure; PASP, pulmonary arterial systolic pressure; PVR, pulmonary vascular resistance; RA area, right atrium area; RAP, right atrial pressure; RVLD, right ventricular longitudinal diameter; RVMD, right ventricular mid diameter; TAPSE, tricuspid annular plane systolic excursion; SvO2, mixed venous oxygen saturation; WHO FC, World Health Organization functional class.

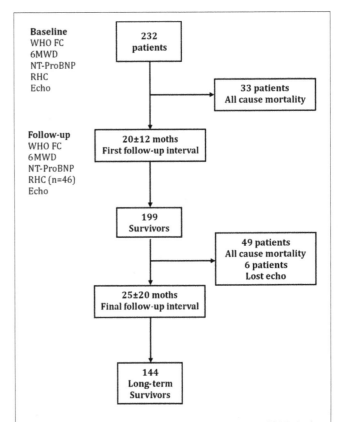

FIGURE 1 | Study design flowchart. Echo, echocardiography; 6MWD, 6-min walking distance; NT-proBNP, N-terminal fragmental of pro–brain natriuretic peptide; RHC, right heart catheterization; WHO FC, World Health Organization functional class.

tomography scan, and echocardiography were used. If patients had definite causes of PAH, such as connective tissue disease and congenital heart disease, portopulmonary hypertension, chronic pulmonary thromboembolism, PH due to left heart diseases and lung diseases, and/or hypoxemia, they could be excluded.

The baseline assessment at the time of diagnosis included medical history, physical examination, 6-min walking distance (6MWD), N-terminal fragmental of pro–brain natriuretic peptide (NT-proBNP), RHC, and echocardiography. During the first follow-up interval (mean follow-up time 20 ± 12 months), 33 patients died for all cause. The follow-up parameters included physical examination, 6MWD, NT-proBNP, echocardiography, and RHC (only 46 patients received RHC test). The 199 remaining survivors were reevaluated at a mean 25 ± 20 months until December 2018 (**Figure 1**). The major end point was all-cause mortality. The study was conformed according to the principles of the Declaration of Helsinki and was approved by the ethics committee of Shanghai Pulmonary Hospital (no. K16-293). Written informed consent signatures were obtained from all patients.

RHC and Echocardiographic Assessment
Pulmonary hemodynamics were examined in triplicate at end-expiration using triple-lumen balloon-tipped thermodilution

Swan–Ganz catheters. Cardiac output was detected by thermodilution (15, 16). Baseline echocardiographic measurements were performed within 24–48 h of the RHC. All echocardiographic data were acquired using commercially available equipment (Vivid 7, GE Healthcare) in standard views. The results were reviewed by at least three echocardiographic experts. Measurements were obtained from the mean of three consecutive beats based on the American Society of Echocardiography guidelines (17). The echo parameters and derived assessments that we focused on common and widely available for daily clinical practice, including RA area, RVMD, RV longitudinal diameter (RVLD), right atrial pressure (RAP), left atrium end-systolic diameter (LAESD), left ventricular end-diastolic diameter (LVEDD), left ventricular ejection fraction (LVEF), LV-EId, left ventricular end-systolic diameter (LVESD), pulmonary arterial systolic pressure (PASP), tricuspid annular plane systolic excursion (TAPSE), and presence of pericardial effusion. Spectral continuous-wave Doppler signal of tricuspid regurgitation corresponding to the RV-RA pressure gradient. SPAP was calculated as the sum of the estimated RAP and the peak pressure gradient between the peak RV and RA, as estimated by application of the modified Bernoulli equation to peak velocity represented by the tricuspid regurgitation Doppler signal. Early diastolic transmitral flow velocity (E) and late diastolic transmitral flow velocity (A) were measured by Doppler echocardiography. ARHR was defined by echocardiographic parameters of RA area, RVDM, and LV-EId, according to Cox proportional hazards regression for mortality risk at follow-up.

RVMD was defined as transversal RV diameter in the middle third of RV inflow, approximately hallway between the maximal basal diameter and the apex, at the level of papillary muscles at end-diastole (18). RA area is traced at the end of ventricular systole from the lateral aspect of the tricuspid annulus to the septal aspect, excluding the area between the leaflets and annulus, as well as the inferior vena cava, superior vena cava, and RA appendage (17). LV-EId was measured in the parasternal short-axis view at end-diastole. This index was calculated as D2/D1, where D2 is the minor-axis dimension of the left ventricle parallel to the septum, and D1 is the minor-axis dimension perpendicular to and bisecting the septum (3). TAPSE is measured by M-mode echocardiography with the cursor optimally aligned along the direction the tricuspid lateral annulus in the apical four-chamber view (18).

Statistical Analysis

Continuous variables were expressed as means with corresponding standard deviations, and categorical variables were expressed as numbers and percentages. The proportions were compared with the χ^2 test. If the data were normally distributed, two-group comparisons were performed with unpaired or paired, two-tailed t-test for means. If the data were not normally distributed, non-parametric two-sided Mann–Whitney U test was used. Bivariate linear analysis was to evaluate the correction between the change of NT-proBNP, 6MWD, and RA area, RVMD, and LV-EId during the follow-up, fitting curve was used a quadratic model with mean value 95% confidence interval.

Cox proportional hazards regression was used to determine risk factors for mortality at follow-up and to identify the association among patient characters and outcomes. For optimal cutoff value for mortality, RA area, RVMD, and LV-EId were generated by receiver operating characteristic (ROC) curves. The Cox proportional hazards regression used to derive a risk calculator assigning weighted for three echo parameters. An integer score of RA area was assigned a value of 1 for the β-coefficient associated with a hazard ratio (HR) of 1.009. Integer scores of 1.621 for RVMD and 2.033 for LV-EId were created assigning values of 1.5 and 2.0, respectively. The total sum of three echo parameters was used for each patient based on the number of the echo cutoff value. Univariate and multivariate logistic regression analyses were chosen to identify clinical and hemodynamic determinants of ARHR. Multivariate analysis to WHO FC I–II, 6MWD, and NT-proBNP for model 1 was created, and WHO FC I–II plus ARHR for model 2. The C-statistic was calculated for each model and model discrimination by R version 2.11.1 (19).

The French non-invasive low-risk criterion was calculated based on the number of non-invasive criteria to derive the original model 1, including WHO FC I–II, 6MWD >440 m, NT-proBNP <300 ng/L (20). The French non-invasive low-risk criteria score was used for Cox regression analysis to predict mortality (model 1), and model 2 was added the echo score. Survival analyses were performed using the Kaplan–Meier method and were compared by means of the log-rank test. For all analyses, $p < 0.05$ was considered statistically significant. All calculations were performed using the SPSS 14.0 statistical software package (Statistical Package for the Social Sciences, Chicago, IL, USA).

RESULTS

Baseline Clinical and Hemodynamic Characteristics of Patients

The baseline clinical, hemodynamic, and echocardiographic features of the IPAH patients are summarized in **Table 1**. Among 232 patients with IPAH, 147 (71%) were women, and 153 (66%) in WHO FC III and IV, with impaired exercise capacity and severe PH hemodynamic status. The echocardiography examination at baseline presented severe RV dilatation and systolic function reduction. Most patients had mild to moderate tricuspid regurgitation.

During mean 20 ± 12 follow-up interval, 33 patients (14%) died, including 26 deaths directly related to RH failure, 5 sudden deaths, and 2 cases not able to be ascertained. Compared with the remaining 199 patients, these patient deaths at baseline were more severe and had advanced disease, such as PVR (16 ± 10 vs. 13 ± 6 Woods unit, $p = 0.01$), RAP (9 ± 6 vs. 6 ± 5 mmHg, $p = 0.03$), S_VO_2 (60 ± 9 vs. 64 ± 9 %, $p = 0.02$), mPAP (62 ± 17 vs. 58 ± 15 mmHg, $p = 0.24$), CI (2.4 ± 0.8 vs. 2.7 ± 0.8 L/min per m^2, $p = 0.16$), NT-proBNP (1,341 ± 974 vs. 964 ± 1,092 ng/L, $p = 0.03$), WHO FC (3.0 ± 0.6 vs. 2.6 ± 0.6, $p = 0.04$), and 6MWD (356 ± 106 vs. 394 ± 110 m, $p = 0.09$).

TABLE 1 | Baseline clinical, hemodynamic, and echocardiographic characteristics of patients with IPAH.

Variable	Mean ± SD or no. (%) (n = 232)
Age, years	40 ± 15
Female, n (%)	147 (71)
BMI, kg/m^2	22 ± 4.7
WHO FC, n (%)	
Class I–II	79 (34)
Class III	142 (61)
Class IV	11 (5)
6MWD, m	390 ± 107
NT-proBNP, ng/L	997± 1,088
Hemodynamics	
RAP, mmHg	7 ± 4.9
mPAP, mmHg	59 ± 15
PAWP, mmHg	8 ± 3.1
CI, L/min per m^2	2.6 ± 0.8
PVR, Woods units	14 ± 6.5
S$_V$O$_2$, %	62 ± 9.1
Echocardiography	
RA area, cm^2	25 ± 11
RVMD, cm	4.5 ± 0.8
LV-EId	1.6 ± 0.4
RVLD, cm	6.5 ± 0.9
RA major axis dimension, cm	5.3 ± 1.0
RA minor axis dimension, cm	4.9 ± 1.2
LVESD, cm	2.2 ± 0.5
LVEDD, cm	3.8 ± 0.6
LAESD, cm	3.1 ± 0.5
TAPSE, mm	17 ± 3.4
LV-E wave PW, cm/s	54.9 ± 18.7
LV-A wave PW, cm/s	58.9 ± 17.1
LVEF, %	74 ± 8.4
PASP, mmHg	86 ± 23
RAP, mmHg	7 ± 3
Pericardial effusion, n (%)	63 (27)
Initial specific therapies, n (%)	
No specific/CCB therapy	16 (7)
Monotherapy	145 (63)
ERA	35 (15)
PDE5i	98 (42)
Prostanoid	12 (5)
Dual combination	71 (31)

Values are expressed as medians (interquartile range) or n (%), unless otherwise stated. BMI, body mass index; CCB, calcium channel blocker; CI, cardiac index; ERA, endothelin receptor antagonist; IPAH, idiopathic pulmonary arterial hypertension; LAESD, left atrium end-systolic diameter; LV A wave PW, pulsed wave left ventricular A wave; LVEDD, left ventricular end-diastolic diameter; LVEF, left ventricular ejection fraction; LV-EId, left ventricular end-diastolic eccentricity index; LVESD, left ventricular end-systolic diameter; LV E wave PW, pulsed wave left ventricular E wave; mPAP, mean pulmonary arterial pressure; 6MWD, 6-min walking distance; NT-proBNP, N-terminal fragmental of pro–brain natriuretic peptide; PAWP, pulmonary artery wedge pressure; PASP, pulmonary arterial systolic pressure; PDE5i, phosphodiesterase type 5 inhibitor; PVR, pulmonary vascular resistance; RA area, right atrium area; RAP, right atrial pressure; RVLD, right ventricular longitudinal diameter; RVMD, right ventricular mid diameter; TAPSE, tricuspid anular plane systolic excursion; SvO2, mixed venous oxygen saturation; WHO FC, World Health Organization functional class.

Clinical and echocardiographic information was available for 199 survivors at the mean first follow-up interval.

Clinical and Echocardiographic Findings at First Follow-Up

At the first follow-up reevaluation, the 199 surviving patients had a relative improvement in clinical condition (6MWD, +37 ± 71 m, $p = 0.02$; NT-proBNP, −361 ± 652 ng/L, $p = 0.025$; WHO FC, −0.2 ± 0.1, $p = 0.53$) and hemodynamics (PVR, −3.3 ± 1.9 Woods unit, $p = 0.004$; mPAP, −10.6 ± 9.3 mmHg, $p = 0.03$; CI, +0.5 ± 0.2 L/min per m^2, $p = 0.005$; RAP, −2.0 ± 1.5 mmHg, $p = 0.39$; S$_V$O$_2$, +5.9 ± 4.0 %, $p = 0.13$; follow-up RHC samples were from 46 patients). Importantly, these patients had a significant improvement of most echocardiographic parameters (RA area, −4.2 ± 3.8 cm^2, $p = 0.010$; RVMD, −0.3 ± 0.1 cm, $p = 0.015$; LV-EId, 0.09 ± 0.04, $p = 0.03$; TAPSE, +0.24 ± 0.49, $p = 0.027$; RA major axis dimension, 0.17 ± 0.37 cm, $p = 0.001$; RA minor axis dimension, 0.19 ± 0.33 cm, $p = 0.011$; LVEF, 6.0 ± 3.0 %, $p < 0.001$; LV-E wave, 8.0 ± 3.4 cm/s, $p = 0.001$; LV-E wave, 2.2 ± 4.5 cm/s, $p = 0.51$; pericardial effusion 8% regression, $p = 0.002$) compared with their baseline data.

ARHR and Determinants

At univariate analysis, absolute changes from baseline to the first follow-up assessment in RA area (HR, 1.009; 95% confidence interval, 0.991–1.027; $p = 0.01$), RVMD (HR, 1.621; 95% confidence interval, 1.083–2.427; $p = 0.01$), and LV-EId (HR, 2.033; 95% confidence interval, 0.386–3.524; $p = 0.02$) were predictive of all-cause death in the subsequent period. The optimal cutoff points by ROC analysis protective against all-cause death were −5.8 cm^2 (sensitivity, 75%; specificity, 66%) for RA area change, −0.7 cm (sensitivity, 77%; specificity, 68%) for RVMD change, and −0.4 (sensitivity, 86%; specificity, 67%) for LV-EIs change.

A score was created deriving integers according to the HRs of the latter echo variables. Based on the achievement of change cutoff points of echo parameters, patients are categorized by the echo score. One hundred thirty-four patients (67.3%) had a score between 0 and 2.0 (0 or 1 protective changes cutoff point of echo parameters), 30 (15.1%) had a score between 2.5 and 3.5 (achievement of 2-echo-parameters cutoff point), and 35 (17.6%) had a score between 4.0 and 4.5 (achievement of all 3-echo-parameters cutoff point). The score between 4.0 and 4.5 was selected as a comprehensive criterion for ARHR. Conversely, a score <4.0 was defined as without ARHR. There were no significant differences in clinical and echocardiographic parameters between patients with or without subsequent ARHR at the first follow-up interval (**Table 2**). At the first follow-up, a significant correlation was present between the change of NT-proBNP and improvement of RA area ($r^2 = 0.51$, $p = 0.009$) and RVMD ($r^2 = 0.45$, $p = 0.001$) (**Figure 2**). Two examples of patients with and without ARHR at the first follow-up are demonstrated at **Figure 3**.

ARHR and Prognosis

After the first follow-up evaluation, the remaining 199 surviving patients were monitored for a mean of 25 ± 20 months. During

TABLE 2 | Clinical, hemodynamic, and echocardiographic characteristics of two patient groups based on ameliorative right heart remodeling at first follow-up interval.

Variable	No ARHR (n = 164)	ARHR (n = 35)	p-value
Age, years	42 ± 17	37 ± 11	0.16
Female, n (%)	131 (75)	18 (75)	0.89
WHO FC, n (%)			0.22
Class I–II	56 (32)	9 (38)	
Class III	108 (62)	14 (58)	
Class IV	11 (6)	1 (4)	
6MWD, m	415 ± 115	389 ± 131	0.92
NT-proBNP, ng/L	805 ± 1,141	1,023 ± 1,297	0.74
Echocardiography			
RA area, cm²	28 ± 12	23 ± 13	0.06
RVMD, cm	5.1 ± 0.9	4.5 ± 0.8	0.28
LV-EId	1.6 ± 0.5	1.5 ± 0.3	0.24
RVLD, cm	6.6 ± 0.8	6.5 ±0.7	0.59
RA major axis dimension, cm	5.5 ± 1.4	6.2 ± 1.3	0.72
RA minor axis dimension, cm	5.0 ± 1.4	5.3 ± 1.4	0.79
LVESD, cm	2.0 ± 0.6	1.5 ± 0.4	0.14
LVEDD, cm	3.7 ± 0.7	3.2 ±0.2	0.13
LAESD, cm	3.1 ± 0.5	3.0 ± 0.3	0.34
TAPSE, mm	17 ±4.2	13 ± 6.6	0.46
LV-E wave PW, cm/s	61.6 ± 18.1	58.2 ± 21.1	0.44
LV-A wave PW, cm/s	61.7 ± 19.4	71.7 ± 10.7	0.86
LVEF, %	78 ± 9.6	81 ± 6.7	0.40
PASP, mmHg	83 ± 24	90 ± 12	0.49
RAP, mmHg	7 ±3	8 ± 5	0.21
Pericardial effusion, n (%)	53 (30)	13 (54)	0.22
Initial specific therapies, n (%)			
No specific/CCB therapy	6 (3)	1 (4)	
Monotherapy			
ERA	25 (14)	4 (17)	
PDE5i	47 (27)	5 (21)	
Prostanoid	7 (4)	1 (4)	
Dual combination	88 (50)	13 (54)	

Values are expressed as medians (interquartile range) or n (%), unless otherwise stated. ARHR, attenuated right heart remodeling; CCB, calcium channel blocker; ERA, endothelin receptor antagonist; LAESD, left atrium end-systolic diameter; LV A wave PW, pulsed wave left ventricular A wave; LVEDD, left ventricular end-diastolic diameter; LVEF, left ventricular ejection fraction; LV-EId, left ventricular end-diastolic eccentricity index; LVESD, left ventricular end-systolic diameter; LV E wave PW, pulsed wave left ventricular E wave; 6MWD, 6-min walking distance; NT-proBNP, N-terminal fragmental of pro–brain natriuretic peptide; PASP, pulmonary arterial systolic pressure; PDE5i, phosphodiesterase type 5 inhibitor; RA area, right atrium area; RVLD, right ventricular longitudinal diameter; RVMD, right ventricular mid diameter; TAPSE, tricuspid anular plane systolic excursion; WHO FC, World Health Organization functional class.

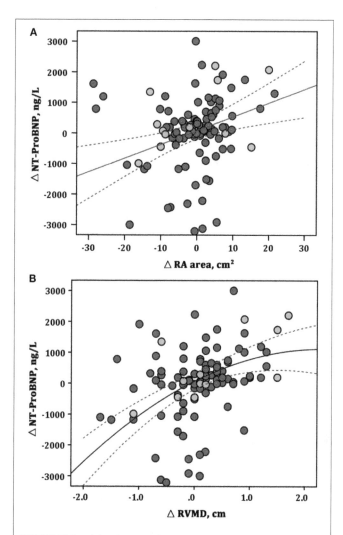

FIGURE 2 | Correlations between the changes in RA area, RVMD, and NT-proBNP at the first follow-up assessment. **(A)** ΔRA area vs. Δ NT-proBNP (linear model: $r^2 = 0.51$, $p = 0.009$); **(B)** ΔRVMD vs. Δ NT-proBNP (linear model: $r^2 = 0.45$, $p = 0.001$). Green circles represent the patients with ARHR; blue circles, without ARHR. NT-proBNP, N-terminal fragmental of pro–brain natriuretic peptide; RA, right area; RVMD, right ventricular mid diameter.

this period, there were 55 patient deaths. The total survival rate at the final follow-up assessment was 85, 70, and 53% at 1, 3, and 5 years of follow-up, respectively.

As shown in **Table 3**, we generated two Cox regression models at the follow-up assessment. Model 1 demonstrated that WHO FC I and II and NT-proBNP were independent predictors of

death. Model 2 was created by adding the echo score according to the 3 echo parameters, showing the ARHR and WHO I and II were significantly protective factors independently from other variables. Accordingly, there were a greater proportion of patients attaining ARHR in WHO FC I–II group and lesser proportion of ARHR patients in WHO FC III ($p = 0.01$) (**Figure 4**). No ARHR patients were in the WHO FC IV group.

The survival curves at final follow-up of 199 surviving patients classified according to ARHR are shown in **Figure 5**. Patients with ARHR had a better long-term survival than others (log-rank $p = 0.01$). The cumulative survival rates at 1, 3, and 5 years of follow-up were 89, 89, and 68% in patients with ARHR, respectively, and 84, 65, and 41% in patients without ARHR.

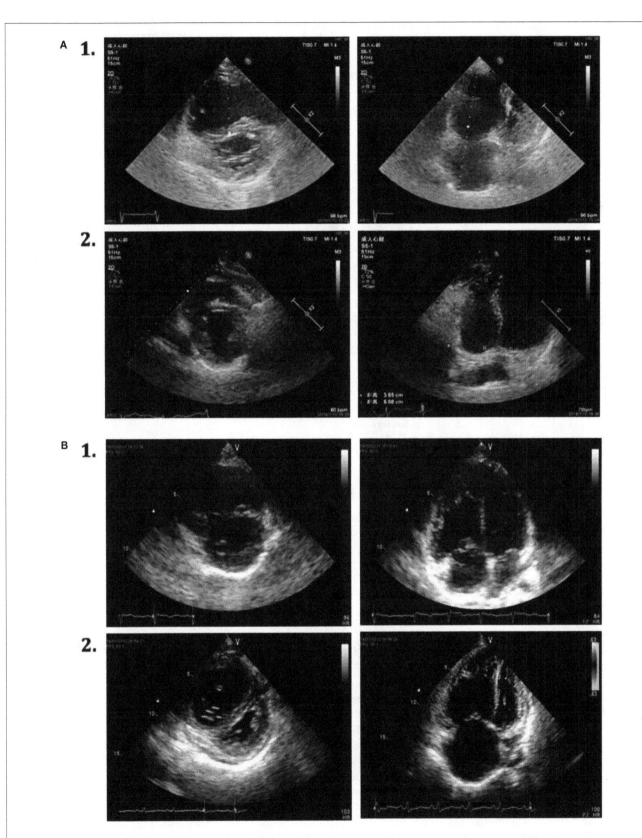

FIGURE 3 | Echocardiographic parasternal short-axis view and apical four-chamber view in 2 patients with IPAH. **(A)** 1. The characteristics at baseline. 2. Attenuated right heart remodeling of the same patient at the first follow-up assessment. **(B)** 1. The characters at baseline. 2. Without attenuated right heart remodeling of the same patient at the first follow-up assessment.

TABLE 3 | Cox regression models for dead prediction at the first follow-up evaluation: model 1 and model 2.

Variable	Unit	HR (95% confidence interval)	p-value	C-statistic (95% confidence interval)
Model 1				0.60 (0.52–0.73)
WHO I–II		0.46 (0.21–0.97)	0.0001	
6MWD	1	0.99 (0.98–1.02)	0.07	
NT-proBNP	1	1.46 (1.27–3.14)	0.002	
Model 2				0.75 (0.69–0.82)
WHO I–II		0.55 (0.21–0.98)	0.0001	
Echo score[a]				
0-2	REF			
2.5–3.5		0.80 (0.39–1.96)	0.45	
4–4.5 (ARHR)		0.42 (0.21–0.88)	0.004	

ARHR, attenuated right heart remodeling; CI, confidence interval; HR, hazard ratio; 6MWD, 6-min walking distance; NT-proBNP, N-terminal fragmental of pro–brain natriuretic peptide; WHO FC, World Health Organization functional class.
[a]Echo score, score based on protective changes in echo parameters by ROC curve analysis cutoff value.

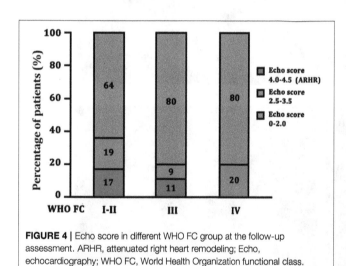

FIGURE 4 | Echo score in different WHO FC group at the follow-up assessment. ARHR, attenuated right heart remodeling; Echo, echocardiography; WHO FC, World Health Organization functional class.

ARHR Combined With French Non-invasive Low-Risk Criteria

To explore the adding value of ARHR on a well-generated risk evaluation tool, we repeated the analysis building a first model 1 according to the number of French non-invasive low-risk criteria (WHO FC I–II; 6MWD >440 m; NT-proBNP <300 ng/L). The ARHR echo score was then added to model 2 was and showed prognostic strength power (**Table 4**). The survival of the four groups are shown in **Figure 6**, based on the combination of French non-invasive low-risk criteria (3 criteria vs. 0–2 criteria) and ARHR (echo score 4.0–4.5 vs. <4.0). Patients with ARHR and French non-invasive criterion 0 had the best prognosis; 1-, 3-, and 5-year survival rates were all 100%. Patients without ARHR (score <4) and French non-invasive criteria 0–2 presented worst survival, and 1-, 3-, and 5-year survival rates were 78, 63, and 46%, respectively. However, we did not

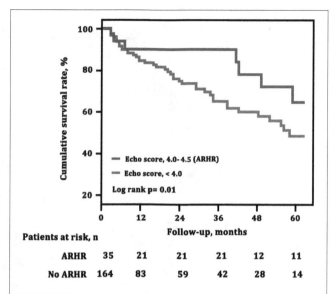

FIGURE 5 | Survival estimates of patients with and without attenuated right heart remodeling (ARHR). Green line (echo score, 4.0–4,5) represents the survival of patients with ARHR; blue line (echo score, <4.0) represents the survival of patients without ARHR.

TABLE 4 | Cox regression models for dead prediction according to the French non-invasive risk assessment and echo.

Variable	Unit	HR (95% confidence interval)	p-value	C-statistic (95% confidence interval)
Model 1				0.61 (0.53–0.73)
French non-invasive low-risk criteria[a]				
3 criteria	REF			
1–2 criteria		3.03 (1.10–4.28)	0.031	
0 criteria		2.77 (0.84–3.15)	0.041	
Model 2				0.72 (0.67–0.80)
French non-invasive low-risk criteria				
3 criteria	REF			
1–2 criteria		2.77 (1.06–3.04)	0.092	
0 criteria		2.97 (0.89–3.85)	0.042	
Echo score[b]				
0–2	REF			
2.5–3.5		0.83 (0.22–1.79)	0.655	
4–4.5 (ARHR)		0.39 (0.12–0.77)	0.012	

[a]French non-invasive low-risk criteria: based on the number of non-invasive criteria (WHO FC I–II; 6MWD >440 m; NT-proBNP <300 ng/L).
[b]Echo score: score based on protective changes in echo parameters by ROC curve analysis cutoff value.

find significant difference between the combination of ARHR (score 4.0–4.5) and French non-invasive criterion 0–2 and those of non-ARHR (score <4.0) and French non-invasive criteria 3 (**Figure 6**).

DISCUSSION

Echocardiographic RV imaging combined with pulmonary hemodynamics was a good framework to interpret the prognosis

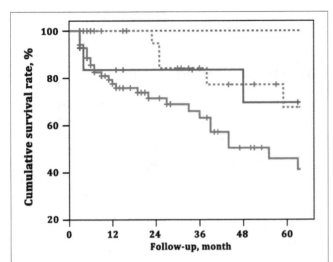

FIGURE 6 | Survival estimates of the four groups of patients based on the combination of French non-invasive low-risk criteria and attenuated right heart remodeling (ARHR). Blue dashed line represents French non-invasive criterion 3 and echo score 4.0–4.5. Red solid line represents French non-invasive criteria 0–2 and echo score 4.0–4.5. Blue solid line represents French non-invasive criterion 3 and echo score <4.0. Red dashed line represents French non-invasive criteria 0–2 and echo score <4.0.

of patients with IPAH (1, 4). Monitoring the change of RV dimensions back to normal or improvement should be useful for evaluation of the RV function. Therefore, it is noteworthy to find a practical echocardiographic predictor tool to remind prognosis. In our study, we defined an ARHR model and found that at the first reevaluation (a) ARHR was an independent predictor of mortality; and (b) ARHR combined with French non-invasive criterion could better predict the outcome of death. The RHRR might serve as a tool for pending prognosis in patients with IPAH.

RA area, RVMD, and LV-EId selected in this study were conventional and important echocardiography indices (12, 17, 21–24). For example, RA area >18 cm^2 was considered as one of the preferred parameters for end-diastole RA enlargement (17). RA enlargement reflected the severity of RH failure and predicted adverse outcomes in patients with severe primary PH (3). A study from Badagliacca's team used RA area as one of the determinants of RV reverse remodeling (10). Therefore, our findings supposed the change of RA area was also a marker of RA dilatation. If there is RV dilatation, RVMD should be measured to respond the chronic volume and/or pressure overload (22). In our study, RV size was measured from a four-chamber view, where RVMD was easily obtained and markers of RV dilatation. The third important parameter in this study is LV-EId, reflecting the degree of septal shift in diastole (3, 10). Echocardiography showed improved LV-EId in proportion to treatment-induced decrease in PVR (24). Taken together, the shift in RV remodeling during the development of PAH is not well elucidated. It is challenging to determine the best parameters for reflecting RV failure progression (25). ARHR in this study might be an indication with reversal of RH dimensions.

It is recognized that the change of RV structure is the main predictor of poor clinical outcomes in PAH (22). There was no

more than 18% of IPAH patients presented with ARHR after a mean of 20 ± 12 months in our study, despite that more than 93% of patients had received PAH-specific therapies. This result is similar with the study on RHRR in IPAH patients after 1-year targeted treatment, which implies that the reversal of RV remodeling is hard and complex (10). At first follow-up time, both the disease severity and echocardiographic indicators seemed to have no significant difference between ARHR and no-ARHR group. However, the patients with ARHR had better long-term survival, as longstanding increase of RV afterload will overwhelm the compensatory mechanisms of the RV (26). Not surprisingly, the patients' hemodynamic status of pulmonary circulation is not always consistent with the changes of RV structure and function. Despite hemodynamics deterioration in patients with PAH, RV contractility is usually increased and not decreased (4, 27, 28). Consequently, the amount of work for the RV remained unaltered, leading to a clinical improvement but unchanged prognosis (29). Therefore, non-invasive imaging of RV dimensions and function is important to the longitudinal monitoring of patients with PAH and continued understanding of the response of RV to pulmonary vascular remodeling (30).

French PH registry permitted to use three non-invasive variables to assess the low-risk criteria score, such as WHO FC, 6MWD, and BNP/NT-proBNP (20). However, it remained unclear whether the addition of other non-invasive modes, such as echocardiography, to the three non-invasive criteria could further improve the prognostic utility (20, 31, 32). Notably, in our study, echocardiography-determined ARHR was able to further stratify patients assessed with French non-invasive low-risk criteria score, suggesting a better prognosis for those patients achieving ARHR. The 1-, 3-, and 5-year survival rates were all 100% in patients with ARHR and French non-invasive criterion 0, compared with 78%, 63%, and 46% in patients with no ARHR (score <4) and French non-invasive criteria 1–4, respectively. Therefore, our results indicated that non-invasive French low-risk criteria combined with echocardiography ARHR would be a preferable predictor model for mortality in patients with IPAH.

Certainly, several echocardiographic parameters were related to long-term prognosis, such as TAPSE, PASP, etc. (12, 33, 34). However, changes in TAPSE or PASP were not predictive of mortality at univariate analysis in our first follow-up time. This is attributable to the limitation of TAPSE assuming that the displacement of a single segment represents the function of a complex 3D, considering the RV shape is more "regular" (35, 36). Indeed, patients in our study underwent more pronounced increases in RV afterload (severe RV dilation), especially for non-ARHR patients who did not have significant improvement for systolic function. Thus, echocardiography is still a comprehensive and multiple tool for non-invasive assessment of the RH.

STUDY LIMITATIONS

There are several limitations to this study. First, this is a retrospectively study in a single center, and the sample size is not large enough with a potential selection bias. The follow-up intervals of PAH patients were not fixed and varied. Second, the follow-up intervals of patients are not standardized and lack of RHC hemodynamic testing. It is different to further analyze the relationship between the change of hemodynamic parameters and ARHR. Then, we did not select the best ROC curve cutoff values for subsequent analysis to avoid the potential risk of a type I error. Finally, there are limitations to the quantification of RH morphology and function using two-dimensional echocardiography. In the future, we need more and accurate parameters to evaluate RV function.

CONCLUSIONS

In summary, our study demonstrated that echocardiographic ARHR created by RA area, RVMD, and LV-EId was an independent predictor of long-term prognosis in patients with IPAH. Similarly, ARHR integrated with French non-invasive criterion could better predict the risk for mortality. ARHR might be a useful tool to indicate RV morphologic and functional improvement associated with better prognostic likelihood. Whether this increases the proportion of patients with ARHR remained to be further confirmed in prospective and multicenter assessments.

AUTHOR CONTRIBUTIONS

RZ and LW were directly involved in the patients' recruitment and care, contributed to the study design, study conduct and supervision, scientific overview, data analysis, and editing of the manuscript. Q-HZ, S-GG, and RJ contributed to patient enrolment, data analysis, scientific interpretation, drafting, and editing the original manuscript. CL, G-FC, C-JL, H-LQ, and J-ML contributed to recruitment of participants, data collection and curation, and formal analysis. All authors have reviewed the manuscript and approved the final version for submission.

ACKNOWLEDGMENTS

The authors acknowledge the contribution of all investigators who participated in this study. We also thank the patients who participated in the study.

REFERENCES

1. van Wolferen SA, Marcus JT, Boonstra A, Marques KM, Bronzwaer JG, Spreeuwenbera MD, et al. Prognostic value of right ventricular mass, volume, and function in idiopathic pulmonary arterial hypertension. *Eur Heart J.* (2007) 28:1250–7. doi: 10.1093/eurheartj/ehl477

2. Sachdev A, Villarraga HR, Frantz RP, McGoon MD, Hsiao JF, Maalouf JF, et al. Right ventricular strain for prediction of survival in patients with pulmonary arterial hypertension. *Chest.* (2011) 139:1299–309. doi: 10.1378/chest. 10-2015

3. Raymond RJ, Hinderliter AL, Willis PW, Palph D, Caldwell EJ, Williams W, et al. Echocardiographic predictors of adverse outcomes in primary pulmonary hypertension. *J Am Coll Cardiol.* (2002) 39:1214–9. doi: 10.1016/s0735-1097(02) 01744-8

4. Vonk-Noordegraaf A, Chin KM, Haddad F, Hassoun PM, Hemnes AR, Hopkins SR, et al. Pathophysiology of the right ventricle and of the pulmonary circulation in pulmonary hypertension: an update. *Eur Respir J.* (2019) 53:1801900. doi: 10.1183/13993003.019 00-2018

5. Vonk-Noordegraaf A, Haddad F, Chin KM, Forfia PR, Kwaut SM, Lumens J, et al. Right heart adaptation to pulmonary arterial hypertension: physiology and pathobiology. *J Am Coll Cardiol.* (2013) 62:D22–33. doi: 10.1016/j.jacc.2013.10.027

6. Badagliacca R, Poscia R, Pezzuto B, Nocioni M, Mezzapesa M, Francone M, et al. Right ventricular remodeling in idiopathic pulmonary arterial hypertension: adaptive versus maladaptive morphology. *J Heart Lung Transplant.* (2015) 34:395–403. doi: 10.1016/j.healun.2014. 11.002

7. van de Veerdonk MC, Marcus JT, Westerhof N, Westerhof N, deMan FS, Boonstra A, et al. Signs of right ventricular deterioration in clinically stable patients with pulmonary arterial hypertension. *Chest.* (2015) 147:1063–71. doi: 10.1378/chest.14-0701

8. Amsallem M, Sweatt AJ, Aymami MC, Kuznetsova T, Selej M, Lu HQ, et al. Right heart end-systolic remodeling index strongly predicts outcomes in pulmonary arterial hypertension: comparison with validated models. *Circ Cardiovasc Imaging.* (2017) 10:e005771. doi: 10.1161/CIRCIMAGING.116. 005771

9. Fine NM, Chen LB, Bastiansen PM, Frantz RP, Pellikka PA, Oh JK, et al. Outcome prediction by quantitative right ventricular function assessment in 575 subjects evaluated for pulmonary hypertension. *Circ Cardiovasc Imaging.* (2013) 6:711–21. doi: 10.1161/CIRCIMAGING.113.000640

10. Naeije R, Manes A. The right ventricle in pulmonary arterial hypertension. *Eur Respir Rev.* (2014) 23:476–87. doi: 10.1183/09059180.00007414

11. Badagliacca R, Poscia R, Pezzuto B, Papa S, Reali M, Pesce F, et al. Prognostic relevance of right heart reverse remodeling in idiopathic pulmonary arterial hypertension. *J Heart Lung Transplant.* (2017) 2498:32041–7. doi: 10.1016/j.healun.2017.09.026

12. Shelburne NJ, Parikh KS, Chiswell K, Shaw LK, Sivak J, Arges K, et al. Echocardiographic assessment of right ventricular function and response to therapy in pulmonary arterial hypertension. *Am J Cardiol.* (2019) 124:1298–304. doi: 10.1016/j.amjcard.2019.07.026

13. El-Yafawi R, Rancourt D, Hacobian M, Atherton D, Cohen MC, Wirth JA. Pulmonary hypertension subjects exhibit right ventricular transient exertional dilation during supine exercise stress echocardiography. *Pulm Circ.* (2019) 9:2045894019851904. doi: 10.1177/2045894019851904

14. Saeed S, Smith J, Grigoryan K, Lysne V, Rajani R, Chambers JB. The tricuspid annular plane systolic excursion to systolic pulmonary artery pressure index: association with all-cause mortality in patients with moderate or severe tricuspid regurgitation. *Int J Cardiol.* (2020) 317:176–80. doi: 10.1016/j.ijcard.2020.05.093

15. Galie N, Hoeper MM, Humbert M, Torbicki A, Vachiery JL, Barbera JA, et al. Guidelines for the diagnosis and treatment of pulmonary hypertension: the Task Force for the Diagnosis and Treatment of Pulmonary Hypertension of the European Society of Cardiology (ESC) and the European Respiratory Society (ERS), endorsed by the International Society of Heart and Lung Transplantation (ISHLT). *Eur Heart J.* (2009) 30:2493–537. doi: 10.1093/eurheartj/ehp297

16. Galie N, Humbert M, Vachiery JL, Gibbs S, Lang I, Torbicki A, et al. 2015 ESC/ERS Guidelines for the diagnosis and treatment of pulmonary hypertension: the Joint Task Force for the Diagnosis and Treatment of Pulmonary Hypertension of the European Society of Cardiology (ESC) and the European Respiratory Society (ERS): Endorsed by: Association for European Paediatric and Congenital Cardiology (AEPC), International Society for Heart and Lung Transplantation (ISHLT). *Eur Respir J.* (2015) 46:903–75. doi: 10.1183/13993003.01032-2015

17. Rudski LG, Lai WW, Afilalo J, Hua L, Handschumacher MD, Chandrasekaran K, et al. Guidelines for the echocardiographic assessment of the right heart in adults: a report from the American Society of Echocardiography endorsed by the European Association of Echocardiography, a registered branch of the European Society of Cardiology, and the Canadian Society of Echocardiography. *J Am Soc Echocardiogr.* (2010) 23:685–713. doi: 10.1016/j.echo.2010.05.010

18. Lang RM, Badano LP, Mor-Avi V, Afilalo J, Armstrong A, Ernande L, et al. Recommendations for cardiac chamber quantification by echocardiography in adults: an update from the American Society of Echocardiography and the European Association of Cardiovascular Imaging. *J Am Soc Echocardiogr.* (2015) 28:1–39. e14. doi: 10.1016/j.echo.2014.10.003

19. Jayaram N, Beekman RH, Benson L, Holzer R, Jenkins K, Kennedy KF, et al. Adjusting for risk associated with pediatric and congenital cardiac catheterization: a report from the NCDR IMPACT Registry. *Circulation.* (2015) 132:1863–70. doi: 10.1161/CIRCULATIONAHA.114.014694

20. Boucly A, Weatherald J, Savale L, Jais X, Cottin V, Prevot G, et al. Risk assessment, prognosis and guideline implementation in pulmonary arterial hypertension. *Eur Respir J.* (2017) 50:1700889. doi: 10.1183/13993003.00889-2017

21. D'Alto M, Scognamiglio G, Dimopoulos K, Bossone E, Vizza D, Romeo E, et al. Right heart and pulmonary vessels structure and function. *Echocardiography.* (2015) 32 Suppl1:S3–10. doi: 10.1111/echo.12227

22. Cassady SJ, Ramani GV. Right heart failure in pulmonary hypertension. *Cardiol Clin.* (2020) 38:243–55. doi: 10.1016/j.ccl.2020.02.001

23. Haddad F, Hunt S, Rosenthal DN, Murphy DJ. Right ventricular function in cardiovascular disease, part I: anatomy, physiology, aging, and functional assessment of the right ventricle. *Circulation.* (2008) 117:1436–48. doi: 10.1161/CIRCULATIONAHA.107.653576

24. D'Alto M, Badaliacca RB, Argiento P, Romeo E, Farro A, Papa S, et al. Risk redution and right heart reverse remodeling by upfront triple combination therapy in pulmonary arterial hypertension. *Chest.* (2020) 157:376–83. doi: 10.1016/j.chest.2019.09.009

25. Schuba B, Michel S, Guenther S, Weig T, Emaser J, Schneider C, et al. Lung transplatation in patients with severe pulmonary hypertension-focus on right ventricular remodelling. *Clin Transplant.* (2019) 33:e13586. doi: 10.1111/ctr.13586

26. van der Bruggen CEE, Tedford RJ, Handoko ML, van der Velden J, de Man FS. RV pressure overload: from hypertrophy to failure. *Cardiovasc Res.* (2017) 113:1423–32. doi: 10.1093/cvr/cvx145

27. Spruijt OA, de Man F, Groepenhoff H, Oosterveer F, Westerhof N, Vonk-Noordegraaf A, et al. The effects of exercise on right ventricular contractility and right ventricular-arterial coupling in pulmonary hypertension. *Am J Respir Crit Care Med.* (2015) 191:1050–7. doi: 10.1164/rccm.201412-2271OC

28. Moceri P, Bouvier P, Baudouy D, Dimopoulos K, Cerboni P, Wort SJ, et al. Cardiac remodelling amongst adults with various aetiologies of pulmonary arterial hypertension including Eisenmenger syndrome-implications on survival and the roe of right ventricular transverse strain. *Eur Heart J Cardiovasc Imaging.* (2017) 18:1262–70. doi: 10.1093/ehjci/jew277

29. Noordegraaf AV, Bogaard HJ. Restoring the right ventricle. *Chest.* (2020) 157:251–2. doi: 10.1016/j.chest.2019.10.022

30. Harrison A, Hatton N, Ryan JJ. The right ventricule under pressure: evaluating the adaptive and maladaptive changes in the right ventricle in pulmonary arterial hypertension using echocardiography (2013 Grover Conference series). *Pulm Circ.* (2015) 5:29–47. doi: 10.1086/679699

31. Hoeper MM, Pittrow D, Opitz C, Gibbs JS, Rosenkranz S, Grunig E, et al. Risk assessement in pulmonary arterial hypertension. *Eur Respir J.* (2018) 51:1702606. doi: 10.1183/13993003.02606-2017

32. Benza RL, Farber HW, Selej M, Gomberg-Maitland M. Assessing risk in pulmonary arterial hypertension: what we know, what we don't. *Eur Respir J.* (2017) 50:1701353. doi: 10.1183/13993003.01353-2017

33. Wright LM, Dwyer N, Celermajer D, Kritharides L, Marwick TH. Follow-up of pulmonary hypertension with echocardiography. *JACC Cardiovasc Imaging.* (2016) 9:733–46. doi: 10.1016/j.jcmg.2016.02.022

34. Wright LM, Dwyer N, Wahi S, Marwick TH. Relative importance of baselien and longitudinal evaluation in the follow-up of vasodilator therapy in pulmonary arterial hypertension. *JACC Cardiovasc Imaging.* (2019) 12:2103–11. doi: 10.1016/j.jcmg.2018.08.017

35. Mauritz GJ, Kind T, Marcus JT, Bogaard HJ, van deVeerdonk M, Postmus PE, et al. Progressive changes in right ventricular geometric shortening and long-term survival in pulmonary arterial hypertension. *Chest.* (2012) 141:935–43. doi: 10.1378/chest.10-3277

36. Hoette S, Creuze N, Gunther S, Montani D, Savale L, Jais X, et al. RV fractional area change and TAPSE as predictors of severe right ventricular dysfunction in pulmonary hypertension: a CMR study. *Lung.* (2018) 196:157–64. doi: 10.1007/s00408-018-0089-7

An Robust Rank Aggregation and Least Absolute Shrinkage and Selection Operator Analysis of Novel Gene Signatures in Dilated Cardiomyopathy

Xiao Ma, Changhua Mo, Liangzhao Huang, Peidong Cao, Louyi Shen and Chun Gui*

Department of Cardiology, First Affiliated Hospital of Guangxi Medical University, Nanning, China

*Correspondence:
Chun Gui
guichun@yahoo.com

Objective: Dilated cardiomyopathy (DCM) is a heart disease with high mortality characterized by progressive cardiac dilation and myocardial contractility reduction. The molecular signature of dilated cardiomyopathy remains to be defined. Hence, seeking potential biomarkers and therapeutic of DCM is urgent and necessary.

Methods: In this study, we utilized the Robust Rank Aggregation (RRA) method to integrate four eligible DCM microarray datasets from the GEO and identified a set of significant differentially expressed genes (DEGs) between dilated cardiomyopathy and non-heart failure. Moreover, LASSO analysis was carried out to clarify the diagnostic and DCM clinical features of these genes and identify dilated cardiomyopathy derived diagnostic signatures (DCMDDS).

Results: A total of 117 DEGs were identified across the four microarrays. Furthermore, GO analysis demonstrated that these DEGs were mainly enriched in the regulation of inflammatory response, the humoral immune response, the regulation of blood pressure and collagen–containing extracellular matrix. In addition, KEGG analysis revealed that DEGs were mainly enriched in diverse infected signaling pathways. Moreover, Gene set enrichment analysis revealed that immune and inflammatory biological processes such as adaptive immune response, cellular response to interferon and cardiac muscle contraction, dilated cardiomyopathy are significantly enriched in DCM. Moreover, Least absolute shrinkage and selection operator (LASSO) analyses of the 18 DCM-related genes developed a 7-gene signature predictive of DCM. This signature included ANKRD1, COL1A1, MYH6, PERELP, PRKACA, CDKN1A, and OMD. Interestingly, five of these seven genes have a correlation with left ventricular ejection fraction (LVEF) in DCM patients.

Conclusion: Our present study demonstrated that the signatures could be robust tools for predicting DCM in clinical practice. And may also be potential treatment targets for clinical implication in the future.

Keywords: dilated cardiomyopathy, Robust Rank Aggregation, novel gene signatures, Least absolute shrinkage and selection operator analysis, PERELP

INTRODUCTION

Dilated cardiomyopathy (DCM), characterized by left ventricular or bicentricular enlargement and myocardial systolic dysfunction, is the main cause of systolic heart failure and heart transplantation in about 40 million people worldwide (1, 2). The etiology of dilated cardiomyopathy is still not clear, and it is generally believed that people with genetic background of dilated cardiomyopathy are usually infected with Coxsackie virus, adenovirus and influenza virus, and then resulting cardiac inflammation and immune damage jointly lead to the occurrence and development of dilated cardiomyopathy (3, 4). In recent decades, many strategies including early diagnosis, more accurate typing, evidence-based treatment, rigorous follow-up, and the use of advanced anti-heart failure drugs, have improved the quality of life and long-term survival of patients with dilated cardiomyopathy (5, 6). However, patients with dilated cardiomyopathy presenting

with symptoms of heart failure have a poor clinical prognosis, with a 5-year mortality rate of ~20% in these patients (7, 8). At present, the pathogenesis of dilated cardiomyopathy is still poorly understood.

Advances in gene chips and high-throughput sequencing help to identify the key role of potential core genes and small molecule in the biological process of a variety of diseases (9, 10). Many studies have used microarray chip technology to measure the gene and non-coding RNA expression profile of dilated cardiomyopathy, providing the gene expression pattern of the myocardial tissue of dilated cardiomyopathy. For example, Zhang et al. used bioinformatics method to reanalyze gene expression profile and potential functional network in cardiac tissue of patients with dilated cardiomyopathy (11). Tao et al. also reported four hub lncRNAs in the DCM-related module, which helped to enhance the understanding of DCM pathophysiological process and reveal its potential treatment targets (12). However, most of the gene signatures were analyzed from a single data set,

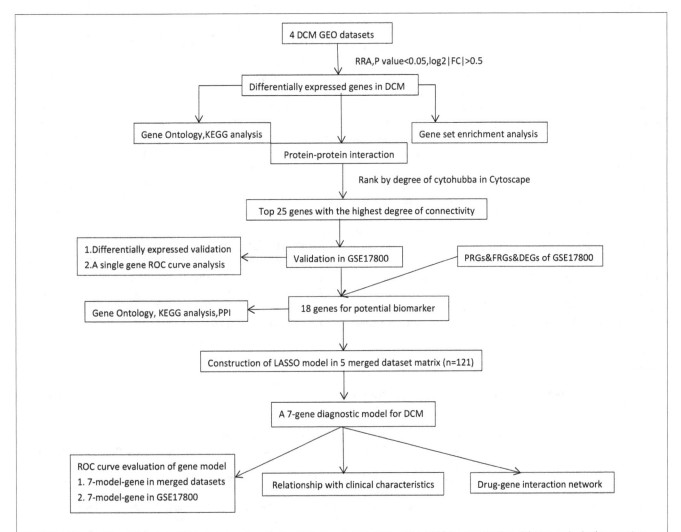

FIGURE 1 | The workflow of the study. DCM, dilated cardiomyopathy; RRA, Robust Rank Aggregation; LASSO, Least absolute shrinkage and selection operator; DEGs, differentially expressed genes; KEGG, Kyoto Encyclopedia of Genes and Genomes; PPI, protein-protein interaction; Con, control normal cardiac tissues; ROC, receiver operating characteristic; FRGs, ferroptosis-related genes; PRGs, pyroptosis-related genes.

and a limited number of patients have been included in most previous studies, which may compromise the prediction power or reliability. In-depth exploration of the public datasets can reveal disease related genes and develop a efficient risk gene signature in combination with clinicopathological characteristics (13), which can help to form a promising tool for predicting status of DCM and individualized therapy.

To explore potential pathogenesis and therapeutic targets of DCM, a series of analysis based on microarray chip data were performed. we developed a 7-gene DCM derived diagnosis signature (DCMDDS) distinguished DCM from NC with high specificity and sensitivity in both the training and validation cohorts. Besides, we performed gene-clinical feature correlation analysis on the 7-gene DCMDS, and predicted potential therapeutic targets via the DGIdb database. The present study provided new diagnostic markers and potential gene-based targeted treatment drug for DCM.

METHODS
Data Download
The workflow of the present study was shown in **Figure 1**. Four gene expression profiles of DCM, including GSE3585, GSE9800, GSE21610, and GSE42955, were downloaded from the Gene Expression Omnibus (GEO) (http://www.ncbi.nlm.nih.gov/geo accessed on 17 June 2021) and used to identify DEGs between DCM and normal cardiac (NC) tissue samples (**Table 1**). The criteria for selecting these datasets included: (1) Gene expression data must be available for both DCM and NCT samples, (2) at least 5,000 genes must be included when the microarray platform is used for expression profiling. In general, DCM is defined by patients with clinical features of a left ventricular end-diastolic diameter over than 56 mm and a left ventricular ejection fraction (LVEF) <50% (14). Exclusion criteria were genetic DCM or any cardiovascular, life-limiting systemic condition or an infectious or tumoral condition that may influence the definition of DCM. Of the five datasets (including the GSE17800 dataset below) with DCM, only four provided DCM definition (GSE3585 GSE17800, GSE21610 and GSE42955), and both datasets used the above criteria. In the GSE9800, a patient's DCM status was provided

without specifying how it was defined. GEO belongs to public databases. The patients involved in the database have obtained ethical approval. Users can download these relevant data for free for research and publish relevant articles. A majority of data are based on open source data, so there are no ethical issues and other conflicts of interest.

Data Preprocessing and Identification of Robust Differentially Expressed Genes (DEGs)
R software (version 3.6.1) was performed to process and statistically analyze the expression files. We downloaded the series matrix files of datasets from GEO. The R package "limma" (15) was utilized to normalize the data and find DEGs, and a volcano map of DEGs was drawn using the "ggplot2" package (16) to show the DEGs. We then used RRA to integrate the results of those 4 datasets to find the most significant DEGs (17). The P value of each gene indicated its ranking in the final gene list, and genes with adjusted $P < 0.05$ and log2|FC| > 0.5 were considered as significant DEGs in the RRA analysis.

Enrichment Analyses of GO and KEGG Pathway
Gene Ontology (GO) analysis and Kyoto Encyclopedia of Genes and Genomes (KEGG) analysis of DEGs were calculated using clusterProfiler package. clusterProfiler was a package of R software that was designed to compare and visualize functional profiles among gene clusters (18). A P value < 0.05 was considered to be significant, and the identified significant analyses were sorted by gene counts. Subsequently, the R package "RCircos" (version 1.2.1) (19) was used to visualize the expression patterns of different microarrays and chromosomal locations for the top 40 DEGs sorted by their P value.

Gene Set Enrichment Analysis
We performed gene set enrichment analysis (GSEA) using the gene expression matrix through the "clusterProfiler" package. "c2.cp.kegg.v7.0.symbols.gmt" was selected as the reference gene set (20). A false discovery rate (FDR) < 0.25 and $P < 0.05$ were considered significant enrichment.

TABLE 1 | The characteristic baseline of microarray.

Series accession	Normal(n)	DCM(n)	Samples	Platform	Author ref	Application
GSE3585	5	7	left ventricular tissue samples	GPL96 Affymetrix Human Genome U133A Array	Barth AS et al.	Integrated Analysis
GSE42955	5	12	left ventricle tissue samples	GPL6244 Affymetrix Human Gene 1.0 ST Array	Molina-Navarro MM et al.	Integrated Analysis
GSE9800	2	12	Left ventricular tissue samples	GPL887 Agilent-012097 Human 1A Microarray G4110B	Ohtsuki M et al.	Integrated Analysis
GSE21610	8	22	Left ventricular tissue samples	GPL570 [HG-U133_Plus_2] Affymetrix Human Genome U133 Plus 2.0 Array	Patrick Schwientek. et al.	Integrated Analysis
GSE17800	8	40	Myocardial biopsies tissue samples	GPL570 [HG-U133_Plus_2] Affymetrix Human Genome U133 Plus 2.0 Array	Sabine Ameling et al.	Validation and clinical relevance analysis

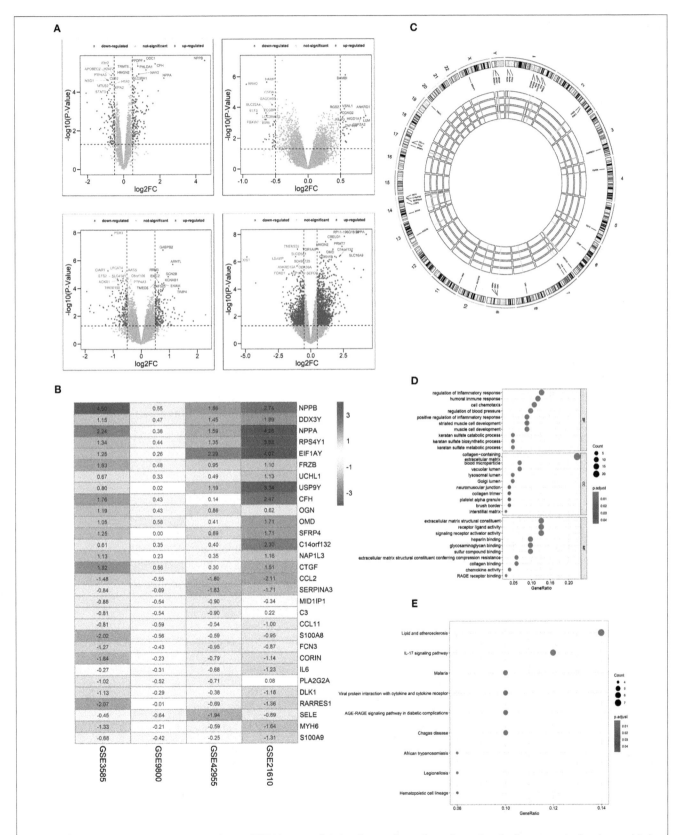

FIGURE 2 | Identification of differentially expressed genes (DEGs) between dilated cardiomyopathy cardiac and normal cardiac tissues samples from four unrelated cohorts. **(A)** Volcano plots of datasets GSE3585 and GSE9800 (upper panel), and GSE21610 and GSE42955 (lower panel) from the GEO database. DEGs with

(Continued)

FIGURE 2 | |log2 (Fold change)| > 0.5 would be listed, additionally. **(B)** Heatmap of the top 15 downregulated and the top 15 upregulated genes from Robust Rank Aggregation analysis of four datasets. Each column represents a dataset and each row a gene. The number in each rectangle represents the value of log2 (fold change). The gradual color ranging from blue to red represents the changing process from down- to up-regulation (DCM vs. Control). **(C)** Circular visualization of expression patterns and chromosomal positions of the top 40 DEGs. The outer circle represents chromosomes, and lines coming from each gene point to their specific chromosomal locations. **(D)** GO enrichment analyses of differentially expressed genes (DEGs) between localized DCM and normal cardiac samples. **(E)** KEGG pathway analyses of differentially expressed genes (DEGs) between localized DCM and normal cardiac samples. DCM, dilated cardiomyopathy; GO, Gene Ontology; KEGG, Kyoto Encyclopedia of Genes and Genomes. The size of each dot represents the count of genes, and the color represents the p-value.

Protein-Protein Interaction (PPI) Network

The PPI network was constructed with a threshold of medium confidence ≥ 0.4 through the Search Tool for the Retrieval of Interacting Genes (STRING) database (21). Cytoscape software (v3.6.1; http://www.cytoscape.org/) was used to visualize the network. Then, the top 25 genes with highest connectivity in the network were identified by DEGREE in cytoHubba (22).

The Identification and Validation of Hub Genes

The mRNA levels of high connectivity genes were verified in datasets GSE17800 and Student's t test was used to compare the expression levels of DCM and control groups. A list of 259 ferroptosis-related genes (FRGs) was identified through the ferroptosis database (FerrDb; http://www.zhounan.org/ferrdb) (23), a publicly available database of ferroptosis regulators, markers, and disease associations. A list of 34 pyroptosis-related genes (PRGs) from prior reviews and studies were also extracted (24, 25). The DEGs of GSE17800 was performed by limma package. And then, the DEGs in GSE17800 were intersected with FRGs/PRGs to obtain potential hub genes related to ferroptosis or pyroptosis. The high connectivity genes after validation and hub FRGs/PRGs were imported into the NCBI website for evaluating the expression abundance in normal human cardiac via high-throughput sequencing. Then, the gene expression with a threshold of RPKM in cardiac tissue ≥ 5 in NCBI Gene expression column was regarded as hub gene. To evaluate the identified ability of hub genes in DCM, ROC curve analysis were conducted in the GSE17800 data set through pROC package (26).

Construction of a Diagnostic Model and Correlation Analysis for DCM

To investigate whether the hub genes could be applied for predicting DCM occurrence, five datasets from the GEO database, GSE3585, GSE42955, GSE9800, GSE21610 and GSE17800, were pooled together, and the combined dataset was then adjusted for batch effect through the "ComBat" function of sva (version 3.34.0) R package (27) and assigned as the training set. The transcriptional profile of GSE17800 which included 40 DCM and 8 no-heart failure (NHF) samples, was used for the validation of the model. The predictability of the model was then evaluated by area under the curve (AUC) of ROC. The "ggstatsplot" package (https://indrajeetpatil.github.io/ggstatsplot/) was used to perform Spearman correlation analysis on diagnostic markers and the "ggplot2" package was used to visualize the results. A two-sided $p < 0.05$ was considered to be statistically significant.

RESULTS

Integrated Screening for Robust DCM-Associated Genes

Four GEO datasets were used for the identification of robust DCM-associated genes (**Table 1**). Using the "limma" R package, we normalized expression data from datasets GSE3585, GSE9800, GSE21610, and GSE42955, and identified 253, 60, 2078, and 370 DEGs between DCM and normal cardiac tissues respectively, with a cut-off of $p < 0.05$ and log2|FC| > 0.5 (**Figure 2A**). Integration of all genes by the RRA method resulted in 117 DEGs ($|log2FC| \geq 0.5$, $p < 0.05$), 100 of which were upregulated and 17 downregulated in DCM.

The top 15 upregulated and the top 15 downregulated genes in CRPC are shown as hierarchical cluster heatmaps (**Figure 2B**). For the top 40 DEGs between DCM and normal cardiac tissues, their expression patterns across the four datasets used for analysis, along with their chromosomal locations are shown in a circos plot (**Figure 2C**). The location of these 40 DEGs involves almost all chromosomes except for the 12, 15, 16, 18, 20, 21, 22 chromosome. The top three upregulated genes included NPPB, NPPA, and EIF1AY, and they are located on chromosomes 2, 6, 1, 17, and 2, respectively. The top three downregulated genes (CCL2, SERPINA3,RARRES1) are located on chromosomes 17, 14,and 3, respectively.

GO enrichment and KEGG pathway analyses were performed to further elucidate the potential biological function and the promising signaling pathways involving the entire 117 DEGs. With GO function analysis, we discovered that the DEGs are mostly enriched in biological process (BP), including the regulation of inflammatory response, the humoral immune response, the regulation of blood pressure, keratan sulfate metabolic process, and the striated muscle cell development. With regard to CC, the DEGs are enriched in the collagen–containing extracellular matrix, vacuolar lumen, blood microparticle, lysosomal lumen. As for molecular function, extracellular matrix structural constituent, signaling receptor activator activity, collagen binding and RAGE receptor binding (**Figure 2D**). In the KEGG pathway analysis, the DEGs participated in diverse infected signaling pathways, including Malaria, African trypanosomiasis, and Viral protein interaction with cytokine and cytokine receptor, Chagas disease and Legionellosis, and some immune-associated pathways such as the IL-17 signaling pathway (**Figure 2E**).

Gene Set Enrichment Analysis

Gene set enrichment analysis was also used to revealed the potential molecular mechanisms of DCM based on all gene

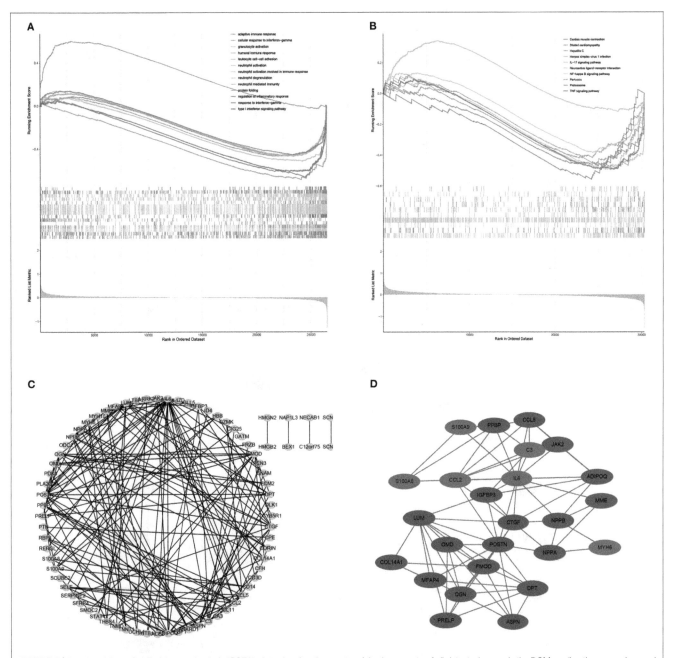

FIGURE 3 | Results of Gene Set Enrichment Analysis (GSEA) plots showing the most enriched gene sets of all detected genes in the DCM cardiac tissues and normal cardiac tissues in an integrated analysis of four datasets. **(A)** The top three most significant up-regulated enriched gene sets in the biological processes: protein folding, humoral immune response, regulation of inflammatory response. **(B)** The top three most significant up-regulated enriched gene sets in the Kyoto Encyclopedia of Genes and Genomes analysis: Herpes simplex virus 1 infection, Neuroactive ligand–receptor interaction, IL−17 signaling pathway. **(C)** PPI network of differentially expressed genes (DEGs). **(D)** Hub gene of differentially expressed genes.

information in the gene expression matrix. The enrichment analysis of gene sets revealed that compared to control samples, immune and inflammatory biological processes such as adaptive immune response, cellular response to interferon–gamma, neutrophil activation, protein folding, regulation of inflammatory response are significantly enriched in DCM (**Figure 3A**). The enriched KEGG pathways of GSEA showed that cardiac muscle contraction, dilated cardiomyopathy, hepatitis C, herpes simplex virus 1 infection

and TNF signaling pathway are significantly enriched in DCM (**Figure 3B**).

PPI Network Analysis and Screening the Top 25 Genes With Highest Connectivity

STRING is an online tool for investigating and integrating interaction between proteins (21). PPI network of these genes was obtained after imputing the DEGs into the online tool. STRING (**Figures 3C, 4A**). In order to identify the top highest connectivity

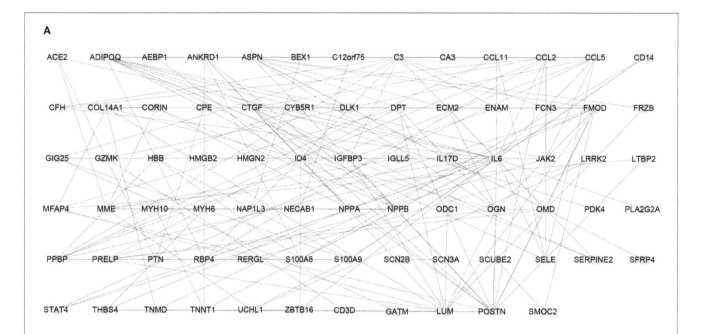

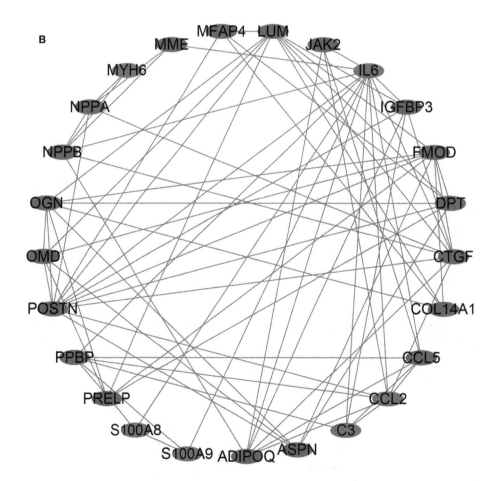

FIGURE 4 | Protein-protein interaction (PPI) network. **(A)** PPI network of 117 differentially expressed genes (DEGs). **(B)** subnetwork of top 25 genes with the highest degree of connectivity from the PPI network. Node color reflects the degree of connectivity (Red color represents a higher expression, and blue color represents a lower expression).

TABLE 2 | The clinical characteristics of GSE17800 in dilated cardiomyopathy.

Parameter	DCM group (N = 40)	Control group (N = 8)	p value
Age, years	50.21 ± 9.35	43.13 ± 14.76	0.084
Gender (Male/Female)	28/12	6/2	0.887
BMI, kg/m^2	27.88 ± 4.57	26.33 ± 5.26	0.303
LVEF, %	33.3 ± 6.4	59.8 ± 8.0	<0.001
LVIDD, mm	69.8 ± 8.0	51.4 ± 3.1	<0.001
Virus(Positive/Negative)	22/18	0/8	0.000
Inflammation	22 ± 23 or 18(12–22)	10 ± 3 or 10(8–13)	<0.001

BMI, body mass index; LVEF, left ventricular ejection fraction; LVIDD, left ventricular internal diameter at end-diastole.

25 genes in the network, the PPI network was imported into Cytoscape. And then, the top 25 genes with the highest degree of connectivity were calculated and extracted. Subsequently, the top 25 genes with the highest degree of connectivity were inputted into STRING to detect the interaction between proteins encoded by these genes (**Figures 3D, 4B**).

Validation of the Expression of the Top 25 Genes With Highest Connectivity in Independent Patient Cohorts

There are 48 cardiac tissue samples including 40 DCM tissues and eight control tissues in GSE17800 dataset. This microarray also reported the information of patient's clinical features (**Table 2**). Independent patient cohorts fron GSE17800 dataset was used to verify the top 25 genes mRNA levels in DCM, which indicated that expression of ANKRD1, ASPN, CTGF, DPT, FMOD, MFAP4, OMD, JAK2, NPPA, NPPB and IGFBP3 was also significantly up-regulated and MYH6 was significantly down-regulated in DCM cardiac tissues as compared to normal cardiac tissues (**Figure 5**).

The Identification of Hub Genes and Functional Annotation Analysis

GSE17800 was also processed as previous. DEGs between DCM and normal cardiac tissues in GSE17800 were 1410. To explore potential ferroptosis or pyroptosis related genes in dilated cardiomyopathy, we intersected FRGs and PRGs with GSE17800's DEGS, and obtained 6 ferroptosis related differential genes including YY1AP1, CDKN1A, SRC, SESN2, CBS, and HSPB1 and 2 pyroptosis related differential genes including PRKACA and COL1A1 (**Figure 6A**). Next, the 13 high connectivity genes after validation and 8 FRGs/PRGs above were further import into NCBI respectively to test their expressive abundance in normal cardiac tissues. These genes with over than 5 mean RPKM were regarded as the hub genes (**Figure 6B**). To reveal potential biological process of these hub genes, GO and KEGG analyses were conducted. The most significant GO terms for biological process, keratan sulfate catabolic process, and keratan sulfate biosynthetic process, as well as KEGG pathways, were shown in **Figures 6C–G**. These analysis showed that these

hub genes were mainly involved in keratan sulfate process, heart process and cGMP metabolic process. The PPI network of the 18 hub genes was also performed, which showed an interaction among them (except for YY1AP1) (**Figure 6H**).

Several Hub Genes Play a Diagnostic Role in DCM

A ROC curve analysis was performed to evaluated the diagnostic value of these hub genes in DCM. The results indicated that many genes, including ASPN ($AUC = 0.841$, $P < 0.0001$), COL1A2 ($AUC = 0.809$, $P < 0.0001$), DPT ($AUC = 0.844$, $P < 0.0001$), MYH6 ($AUC = 0.894$, $P < 0.0001$),NPPA ($AUC = 0.863$, $P < 0.0001$), NPPB ($AUC = 0.903$, $P < 0.0001$), PRELP ($AUC = 0.816$, $P < 0.0001$), PRKACA ($AUC = 0.822$, $P < 0.0001$) and YY1AP1 ($AUC = 0.891$, $P < 0.0001$), can efficiently distinguish DCM cardiac tissues from normal cardiac tissues (**Figures 7A–I**).

LAASO Model for Predicting DCM and Correlation of Clinicopathological Features and Model Genes

We extracted the expression profile of 18 hub genes from the merged datasets to construct LASSO model (**Figures 8A,B**). Through the LASSO, 7 genes were identified with non-zero regression coefficients, and the value of lambda.min = 0.03037093. ROC curve analysis indicated that the AUC of the 7-gene-based model was 0.938 in the merged gene set, which suggesting LASSO model may be used as a biomarker of DCM (**Figure 8C**). This model was further validated in a validation set (GSE17800) with AUC= 1 (**Figure 8D**).

Correlation heatmap of the 7 model genes and clinical factors revealed that LVEF had a significant positive correlation with MYH6 and had a significant negative correlation with LVIDD, ANKRD1, PRELP, COL1A1, CDKN1A. LVIDD had a significant negative correlation with MYH6 and had a significant positive correlation with inflammation, ANKRD1. Age and MYH6 had a significant negative correlation. The expression of MYH6 mRNA levels is associated with virus infection (**Figures 8E–J**).

Identification of the Potential Drugs

DGIdb was applied to determine the potential therapy drug that could reverse the expression of model gene in DCM. As shown in the drug–gene interaction network (**Figures 9A–D**), 18 drugs or molecular compounds included deoxycytidine, irinotecan hydrochloride, and cyclosporine, which differentially regulated the expression of ferroptosis-related gene CDKN1A. In addition, OMECAMTIV MECARBIL (INN), a cardiac specific myosin activator, was found to interact with MYH6. Further, collagenase clostridium histolyticum and antiplasmin regulated COL1A1 and 10 drugs or molecular compounds that included fasudil, SB-220025, SB-202190 and AST-487 regulated pyroptosis related gene PRKACA.

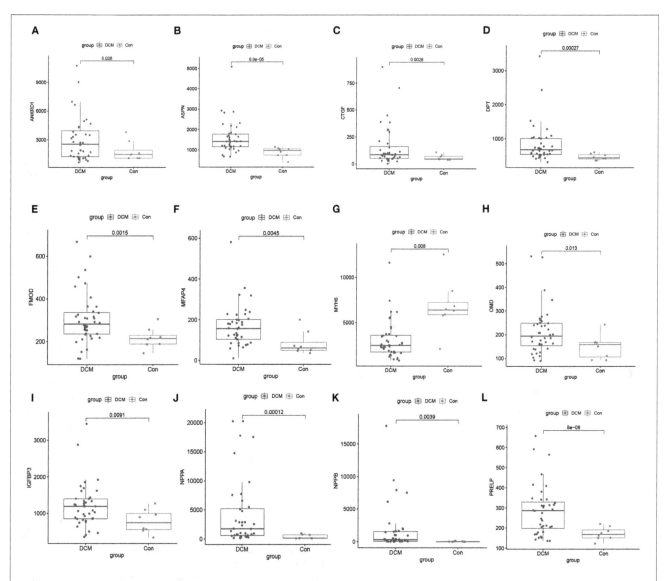

FIGURE 5 | Validation of top 25 genes with the highest degree of connectivity in GSE17800. The expression of genes **(A)** ANKRD1, **(B)** ASPN, **(C)** CTGF, **(D)** DPT, **(E)** FMOD1, **(F)** MFAP4, **(H)** OMD, **(I)** IGFBP3, **(J)** NPPA, **(K)** NPPB, **(L)** PRELP significantly upregulated, and **(G)** MYH6 significantly down regulated in the DCM in comparison to control group. DCM, dilated cardiomyopathy; Con, control group.

DISCUSSION

The pathogenesis of DCM, a complex and heterogeneous disease, remains unclear (28). Although many investigators have used microarray and RNA-seq to detect novel biomarkers and therapeutic targets for DCM, inconsistencies were seen between the DEGs found in different studies. To our knowledge, our work is the first to use RRA combined with LASSO regression model to explore novel hub genes associated with DCM. Previous studies compared gene expression profiles between DCM and non-heart failure samples for the dataset to explore hub gene and pathogenesis in DCM. However, these studies did not conduct link between gene expression and DCM clinical characteristics. This study integrated 4 qualified DCM datasets from GEO into the RRA method to identify DCM-associated genes and

develop expression-based molecular signatures to predict DCM, some of which, such as NPPB (29) and ASPN (30), have been reported to be biomarkers of DCM or play an important role in its pathogenesis. In addition, associations of developed signatures with the clinicopathological characteristics of DCM were also evaluated.

Different from previous studies, GO analysis of differential genes in this study mainly involves the regulation of inflammatory response, immune response, keratinin sulfate processing and muscle cell contraction. And KEGG pathway analysis is mainly involved diverse infected signaling pathways, including Malaria, African trypanosomiasis, and Viral protein interaction with cytokine and cytokine receptor, Chagas disease and Legionellosis, and some immune-associated pathways such as the IL-17 signaling pathway. In addition, GSEA clarified a

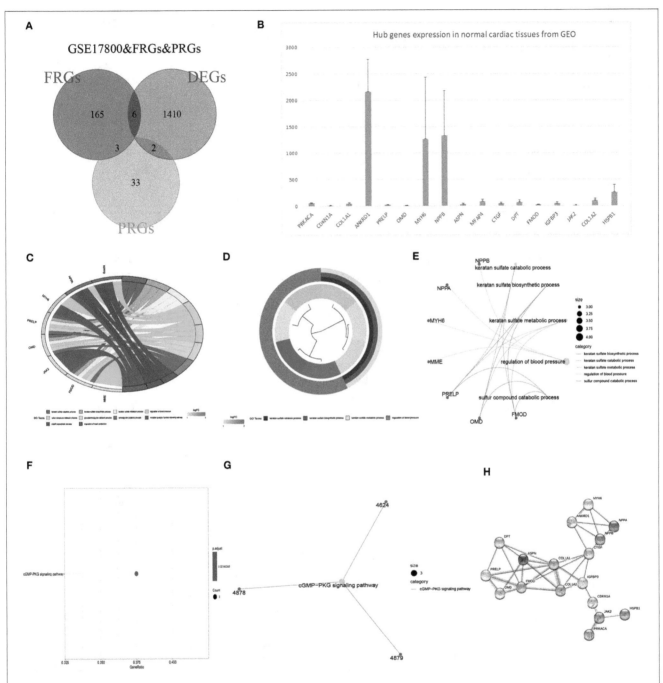

FIGURE 6 | The identification of DCM related genes and their functional analysis. **(A)** Venn diagram of ferroptosis-related genes, pyroptosis-related genes and DEGs in GSE17800. **(B)** The expression of potential biomarker genes including top 25 genes validated in GSE17800 and overlapping DEGs of ferroptosis-related genes, pyroptosis-related genes based on NCBI. **(C)** Chord plot shows the distribution of core genes in different GO-enriched functions. Symbols of core genes are presented on the left side of the graph with their fold change values mapped by color scale. **(D)** The top three significantly enriched Gene Ontology terms associated with potential biomarker genes. Gene involvement in the GO terms was determined by colored connecting lines. **(E)** Cluego network diagram shows the relationship between the potential biomarker genes and GO terms. **(F)** The bubble chart showed the KEGG pathway analyses of potential biomarker genes in DCM. **(G)** Cluego network diagram shows the relationship between the potential biomarker genes and KEGG terms. **(H)** PPI network of 18 potential biomarker genes.

new perspective for this study. It demonstrated that immune responses, such as adaptive immune response, cellular response to interferon–gamma, type I interferon signaling pathway, and inflammation responses including leukocyte cell-cell adhesion,

neutrophil activation, neutrophil degranulation are involved in the pathophysiological process of dilated cardiomyopathy. Also, DCM process, some kinds of infections and two immune-related disease pathways that include IL-17 signaling pathway and TNF

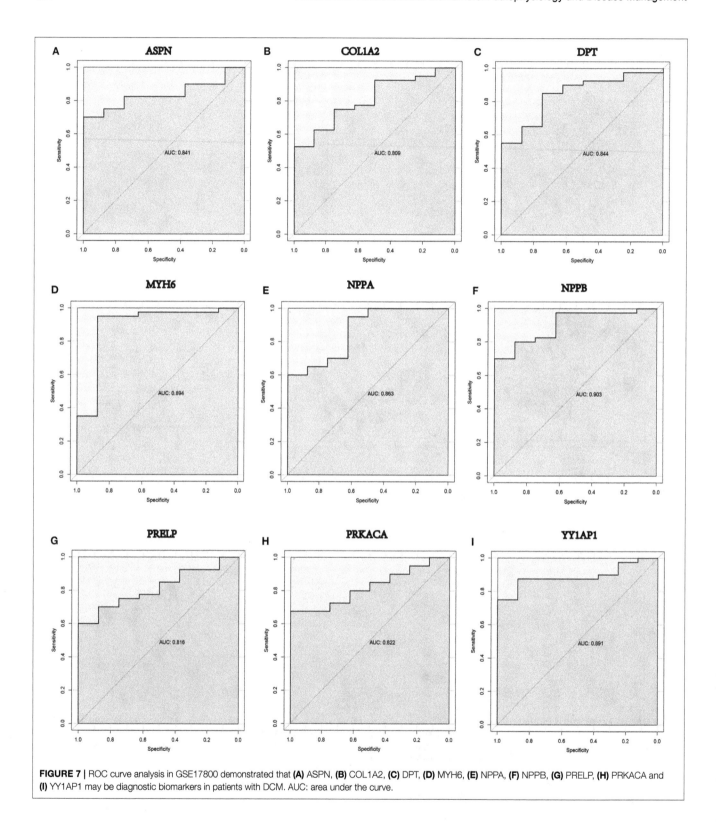

FIGURE 7 | ROC curve analysis in GSE17800 demonstrated that **(A)** ASPN, **(B)** COL1A2, **(C)** DPT, **(D)** MYH6, **(E)** NPPA, **(F)** NPPB, **(G)** PRELP, **(H)** PRKACA and **(I)** YY1AP1 may be diagnostic biomarkers in patients with DCM. AUC: area under the curve.

signaling pathway were involved. These confirmed that infection, inflammation and immune responses play important role in the development DCM.

Ferroptosis is reliant on a large number of cellular iron, interfering with the homeostasis of redox reactions, and eventually promoting cell death (31). Literature has indicated that iron-dependent ferroptosis is implicated in many cardiomyopathies (32). However, no studies have shown that ferroptosis is involved in the development of dilated cardiomyopathy; Moreover, pyroptosis is also another form

An Robust Rank Aggregation and Least Absolute Shrinkage and Selection Operator Analysis of Novel Gene...

125

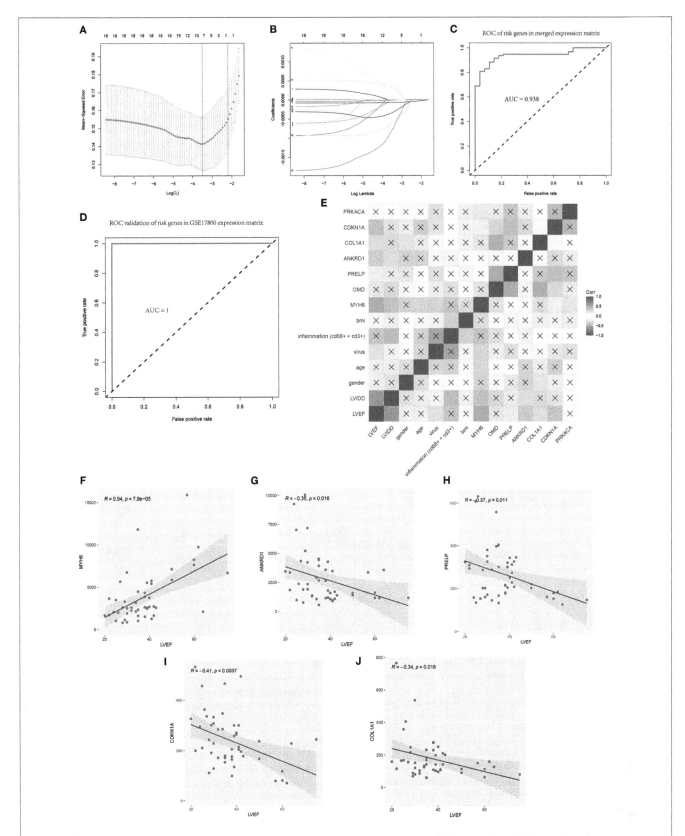

FIGURE 8 | A model for predicting DCM and correlation of clinicopathological features and model genes. **(A)** Least absolute shrinkage and selection operator (LASSO) logistic regression algorithm to screen diagnostic markers and risks genes in merged data matrix of five datasets. **(B)** Parameters of Lasso path and

(Continued)

FIGURE 8 | corresponding selected features of each fold. **(C)** ROC curve analysis of the 7-gene-based model in merged data matrix of five datasets (training set). **(D)** ROC curve analysis of the 7-gene-based model in GSE17800(validation set). **(E)** Correlation heat map of risks genes and clinicopathological features in datasets GSE17800. The depth of the color represents the strength of the correlation; red represents a positive correlation, blue represents a negative correlation. The "x" means irrelevance. Correlation analysis of left ventricular ejection fraction (LVEF) and **(F)** MYH6, **(G)** ANKRD1, **(H)** PRELP, **(I)** CDKN1A and **(J)** COL1A1.

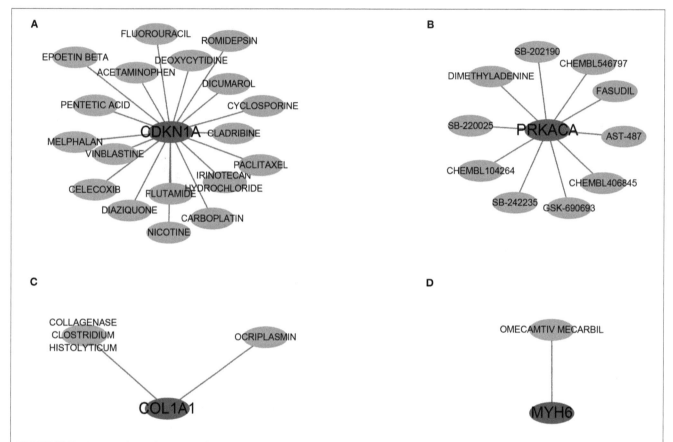

FIGURE 9 | The drug-gene interaction network. The dark red circle nodes in the center are the genes, and pale red nodes around are the drugs. **(A)** The interaction network of CDKN1A and its targeted compounds and drugs. **(B)** The interaction network of PRKACA and its targeted compounds and drugs. **(C)** The interaction network of COL1A1 and its targeted compounds and drugs. **(D)** The interaction network of MYH6 and its targeted compounds and drugs.

of cell death, which has only been shown in one study that NLRP3 inflammasome-mediated pyroptosis contributes to the pathogenesis of non-ischemic dilated cardiomyopathy (33). Therefore, the present study also for the first time reported ferroptosis related gene CDKN1A and pyroptosis related gene PRKACA may be involved in the development and progression of dilated cardiomyopathy.

We preliminarily obtained the possible core genes through protein interaction network and iron death or cell apoptosis related differential gene screening, and then carried out independent data set verification and expression abundance verification, and finally obtained the included 18 core genes. The 18 genes included up-regulated genes CDKN1A, COL1A1, ANKRD1, PRELP, OMD, NPPB, NPPA, ASPN, MFAP4, CTGF, DPT, FMOD, IGFBP3, JAK2, PRKACA and COL1A2, as well as down-regulated genes MYH6 and YY1AP1, which were mainly enriched in keratan sulfate process and cGMP–PKG signaling pathway through GO and KEGG analyses. some of them were demonstrated to exert essential roles in the pathogenesis of

DCM (34–37). Among these hub genes, we further explore their diagnostic value in DCM, and found that nine genes have certain diagnostic value for dilated cardiomyopathy (AUC > 80%). Among them, NPPA (natriuretic peptide A) and NPPB (natriuretic peptide B) belong to the natriuretic peptide family, which encoded atrial natriuretic peptide (ANP) and brain natriuretic peptide (BNP) respectively (36). The natriuretic peptide family is a general name of a group of peptides secreted mainly by the cardiovascular system to regulate hydroelectrolyte balance, reduce cardiac afterload, and dilate blood vessels through natriuretic diuresis (38). In heart failure, NPPB is expressed at a high level in DCM, and patients with higher BNP level have a worse cardiac function (39, 40).

Combined LASSO and the forward stepwise selection analyses of the 18 genes resulted in the most robust model with the fewest genes capable of predicting DCM, a panel of seven genes including ANKRD1, PRELP, PRKACA, COL1A1, OMD, MYH6 and CDKN1A significantly correlates with DCM. This seven-gene panel was named DCM derived diagnostic signature

(DCMDDS), and the DCMDDS score is based on the seven genes' expression levels and regression coefficients. The model was validated in 5 patient cohorts, comprising more than 120 patients. Interestingly, five of the seven DCMDDS genes were associated with left ventricular ejection fraction based on their expression levels and correlation coefficients, as demonstrated by the Spearman correlation analysis. Among DCMDDS genes, MYH6, ANKRD1 and COL1A1 have been showed to participated in the development of DCM, while PRELP, PRKACA, CDKN1A and OMD seldomly reported.

PERELP, proline and arginine rich end leucine rich repeat protein, is a member of the leucine-rich repeat (LRR) family of extracellular matrix proteins in connective tissue (41). It is unclear whether PERELP plays a role in DCM and other cardiomyopathy. Data from the Human Protein Atlas (HPA) revealed that PRELP is secreted to the extracellular matrix and may anchor basement membranes to the underlying connective tissue (42), suggesting its potential function in maintaining normal cellular structure. Besides, previous studies have suggested that PERELP has prognostic value in hepatocellular carcinoma and regulates the extracellular matrix and collagen mineralization in the bone system (43, 44).

PRKACA is a gene encoding the cAMP-dependent protein kinase A (PKA) catalytic subunits alpha. PKA can directly phosphorylate the cytoplasmic receptor NLRP3 and attenuate its ATPase function, which showed a relationship to pyroptosis (45). Therefore, PRKACA was regarded as a pyroptosis-related gene (24). Prolonged and elevated cyclic adenylyl monophosphate (cAMP) levels have been observed in both heart failure and several cardiomyopathy, while PKA is promptly activated by increasing intracellular concentrations of cAMP synthesized by adenylyl Cyclases (46, 47). These revealed that regulating PKA phosphorylation may be a therapeutic strategy for certain stages of progressive and congestive heart failure (48). However, its role in DCM still not be reported.

CDKN1A (cyclin-dependent kinase inhibitor 1A) encodes p21, plays an important role in the pathological process of P53-mediated ferroptosis (49). CDKN1A is a potent cell cycle inhibitor that mediates post-natal cardiomyocyte cell cycle arrest. Although no reported in DCM, CDKN1A is implicated in LMNA-mediated cellular stress responses, and the mutation of LMNA is one of the important mechanisms DCM (50, 51). Moreover, Shah et al. also found the mutations in the CDKN1A gene in the blood of patients with heart failure (52).

OMD (Osteomodulin) is a leucine- and aspartic acid-rich keratan sulfate proteoglycan, which belongs to the small leucine-rich proteoglycan family (SLRP) family (53). A recent study shown that OMD could directly bind to Type I collagen, further regulating the diameter and shape of collagen fbrils (54). Interestingly, the results of the present study also suggest a positive correlation between OMD and COL1A1, and its functional analysis mainly involved in extracellular matrix processes. Extracellular matrix fibrosis is regarded as an important process in the development of DCM (55). Therefore, targeted OMD gene therapy may be a potential therapeutic strategy for dilated cardiomyopathy. Guo et al. also found that Osteomodulin is a potential genetic target for hypertrophic cardiomyopathy (56).

To found the potential effective therapy for DCM, DGIdb database was used to exam therapeutic agents that might reverse the abnormally expression of DCMDDS genes. OMECAMTIV MECARBIL (INN), previously codenamed CK-1827452, is a cardiac specific myosin activator. It is clinically tested for its role in the treatment of left ventricular systolic heart failure (57). In the present study, MYH6 was down-regulated in DCM, while OMECAMTIV MECARBIL can target and activate it. This means that MYH6 may be one of the important targeted gene of OMECAMTIV MECARBIL in the treatment of heart failure. COL1A1, one of the component collagen type I, is the main component of extracellular matrix. Elevated expression levels of COL1A1 will lead to fibrosis of extracellular matrix of cardiac muscle (58). Collagenase clostridium histolyticum and antiplasmin might be a effective anti-fibrosis therapy approach in DCM via targeting COL1A1. The roles of the drugs or molecular compounds above in DCM still need to be further explored as potential therapeutic targets.

There were several limitations in our study. First, due to limited conditions, myocardial biopsy tissue specimens were not obtained to carry out basic experiments for verification. Nevertheless, we used a multi-chip combined analysis method and validated in external DCM samples to ensure the accuracy of the bioinformatics analysis in the study. In addition, in our analysis results, NPPA, NPPB, COL1A2, ASPN, ANKRD1 and CTGF were all confirmed to be closely related to heart failure in dilated cardiomyopathy in various studies. Second, the sample size of our multi-chip combined analysis was significantly expanded. However, due to the difficulty and high risk of myocardial tissue biopsy, the sample size of the data set in our study was still relatively small. Third, although we explored the relationship between genes and clinical factors, we failed to obtain prognostic information from datasets, and we could not further explore the relationship between DCMDDS genes and patient outcomes.

In summary, by combining RRA, LASSO, and other bioinformatics tools, this study identified 117 robust DEGs between DCM and NFH samples, many of which were not reported in previous studies. A 7-gene panel derived from the 117 DCM-associated genes comprised of a diagnostic model predictive of DCM. Five of the seven genes were closely related to left ventricular ejection fraction. Therefore, these gene signatures may help develop DCM biomarkers via large-scale randomized clinical trials.

AUTHOR CONTRIBUTIONS

XM, CM, and CG designed the present study, which was performed by XM, CM, and PC. XM and LH made substantial contributions to acquisition and analysis of data. XM and LS also made contributions to interpretation of data. XM wrote the initial draft of the manuscript. LH revised it critically for important intellectual content. All authors have participated sufficiently in the work to take public responsibility for appropriate portions of the content and approved the manuscript, as well as agreed to be accountable for all aspects of the work. All authors read and approved the final manuscript.

REFERENCES

1. Merlo M, Cannatà A, Gobbo M, Stolfo D, Elliott PM, Sinagra G. Evolving concepts in dilated cardiomyopathy. *Eur J Heart Fail.* (2018) 20:228–39. doi: 10.1002/ejhf.1103
2. Tayal U, Prasad S, Cook SA. Genetics and genomics of dilated cardiomyopathy and systolic heart failure. *Genome Med.* (2017) 9:20. doi: 10.1186/s13073-017-0410-8
3. Verdonschot J, Hazebroek M, Merken J, Debing Y, Dennert R, Rocca HPBL, et al. Relevance of cardiac parvovirus B19 in myocarditis and dilated cardiomyopathy: review of the literature. *Eur J Heart Fail.* (2016) 18:1430–41. doi: 10.1002/ejhf.665
4. Ameling S, Herda LR, Hammer E, Steil L, Teumer A, Trimpert C, et al. Myocardial gene expression profiles and cardiodepressant autoantibodies predict response of patients with dilated cardiomyopathy to immunoadsorption therapy. *Eur Heart J.* (2013) 34:666–75. doi: 10.1093/eurheartj/ehs330
5. Merlo M, Pivetta A, Pinamonti B, Stolfo D, Zecchin M, Barbati G, et al. Long-term prognostic impact of therapeutic strategies in patients with idiopathic dilated cardiomyopathy: changing mortality over the last 30 years. *Eur J Heart Fail.* (2014) 16:317–24. doi: 10.1002/ejhf.16
6. Merlo M, Pyxaras SA, Pinamonti B, Barbati G, Di Lenarda A, Sinagra G. Prevalence and prognostic significance of left ventricular reverse remodeling in dilated cardiomyopathy receiving tailored medical treatment. *J Am Coll Cardiol.* (2011) 57:1468–76. doi: 10.1016/j.jacc.2010.11.030
7. Gulati A, Jabbour A, Ismail TF, Guha K, Khwaja J, Raza S, et al. Association of fibrosis with mortality and sudden cardiac death in patients with nonischemic dilated cardiomyopathy. *JAMA.* (2013) 309:896–908. doi: 10.1001/jama.2013.1363
8. Køber L, Thune JJ, Nielsen JC, Haarbo J, Videbæk L, Korup E, et al. Defibrillator implantation in patients with non ischemic systolic heart failure. *N Engl J Med.* (2016) 375:1221–30. doi: 10.1056/NEJMoa1608029
9. Li N, Wu H, Geng R, Tang Q. Identification of core gene biomarkers in patients with diabetic cardiomyopathy. *DisMarkers.* (2018) 2018:6025061. doi: 10.1155/2018/6025061
10. Chen R, Ge T, Jiang W, Huo J, Chang Q, Geng J, et al. Identification of biomarkers correlated with hypertrophic cardiomyopathy with co-expression analysis. *J Cell Physiol.* (2019) 234:21999–2008. doi: 10.1002/jcp.28762
11. Zhang H, Yu Z, He J, Hua B, Zhang G. Identification of the molecular mechanisms underlying dilated cardiomyopathy via bioinformatic analysis of gene expression profiles. *Exp Ther Med.* (2017) 13:273–9. doi: 10.3892/etm.2016.3953
12. Tao L,Yang L, Huang X, Hua F, Yang X. Reconstruction and analysis of the lncRNA-miRNA-mRNA network based on competitive endogenous RNA reveal functional lncrnas in dilated cardiomyopathy. *Front Genet.* (2019) 10:1149. doi: 10.3389/fgene.2019.01149
13. Liu X, Yin M, Liu X, Da J, Zhang K, Zhang X, et al. Analysis of hub genes involved in distinction between aged and fetal bone marrow mesenchymal stem cells by robust rank aggregation and multiple functional annotation methods. *Front Genet.* (2020) 11:573877. doi: 10.3389/fgene.2020.573877
14. Calderon-Dominguez M, Belmonte T, Quezada-Feijoo M, Ramos M, Calderon-Dominguez J, Campuzano O, et al. Plasma microrna expression profile for reduced ejection fraction in dilated cardiomyopathy. *Sci Rep.* (2021) 11:7517. doi: 10.1038/s41598-021-87086-1
15. Ritchie ME, Phipson B, Wu D, Hu Y, Law CW, Shi W, et al. limma powers differential expression analyses for RNA-sequencing and microarray studies. *Nucleic Acids Res.* (2015) 43:e47. doi: 10.1093/nar/gkv007
16. Raaphorst RV, Kjos M, Veening J. Bactmap: an r package for integrating, analyzing and visualizing bacterial microscopy data. *Mol Microbiol.* (2020) 113:297–308. doi: 10.1111/mmi.14417

ACKNOWLEDGMENTS

We acknowledge GEO database for providing their platforms and contributors for uploading their meaningful datasets.

17. Kolde R, Laur S, Adler P, Vilo J. Robust rank aggregation for gene list integration and meta-analysis. *Bioinformatics.* (2012) 28:573–80. doi: 10.1093/bioinformatics/btr709
18. Yu G, Wang L, Han Y, He Q. clusterProfiler: an R package for comparing biological themes among gene clusters. *OMICS.* (2012) 16:284–7. doi: 10.1089/omi.2011.0118
19. Zhang H, Meltzer P, Davis S. RCircos: an R package for Circos 2D track plots. *BMC Bioinformatics.* (2013) 14:244. doi: 10.1186/1471-2105-14-244
20. Liberzon A, Birger C, Thorvaldsdóttir H, Ghandi M, Mesirov JP, Tamayo P. The Molecular Signatures Database (MSigDB) hallmark gene set collection. *Cell Syst.* (2015) 1:417–25. doi: 10.1016/j.cels.2015.12.004
21. Szklarczyk D, Morris JH, Cook H, Kuhn M, Wyder S, Simonovic M, et al. The STRING database in 2017: quality-controlled protein-protein association networks, made broadly accessible. *Nucleic Acids Res.* (2017) 45:D362–8. doi: 10.1093/nar/gkw937
22. Hu J, Zhou L, Song Z, Xiong M, Zhang Y, Yang Y, et al. The identification of new biomarkers for bladder cancer: a study based on TCGA and GEO datasets. *J Cell Physiol.* (2019) 1–12. doi: 10.1002/jcp.28208
23. Zhou N, Bao J. FerrDb: a manually curated resource for regulators and markers of ferroptosis and ferroptosis-disease associations. *Database (Oxford).* (2020) 2020:baaa021. doi: 10.1093/database/baaa021
24. Ye Y, Dai Q, Qi H. A novel defined pyroptosis-related gene signature for predicting the prognosis of ovarian cancer. *Cell Death Discov.* (2021) 7:71. doi: 10.1038/s41420-021-00451-x
25. Zhang L, Zhang L, Huang Z, Xing R, Li X, Yin S, et al. αIncreased HIF-1 in knee osteoarthritis aggravate synovial fibrosis via fibroblast-like synoviocyte pyroptosis. *Oxid Med Cell Longev.* (2019) 2019:6326517. doi: 10.1155/2019/6326517
26. Robin X, Turck N, Hainard A, Tiberti N, Lisacek F, Sanchez JC, et al. pROC: an open-source package for R and S+ to analyze and compare ROC curves. *BMC Bioinformatics.* (2011) 12:77. doi: 10.1186/1471-2105-12-77
27. Parker HS, Leek JT, Favorov AV, Considine M, Xia X, Chavan S, et al. Preserving biological heterogeneity with a permuted surrogate variable analysis for genomics batch correction. *Bioinformatics.* (2014) 30:2757–63. doi: 10.1093/bioinformatics/btu375
28. Zecchin M, Merlo M, Pivetta A, Barbati G, Lutman C, Gregori D, et al. How can optimization of medical treatment avoid unnecessary implantable cardioverter-defibrillator implantations in patients with idiopathic dilated cardiomyopathy presenting with "SCD-HeFT criteria?" *Am J Cardiol.* (2012) 109:729–735. doi: 10.1016/j.amjcard.2011.10.033
29. Witt E, Hammer E, Dörr M, Weitmann K, Beug D, Lehnert K, et al. Correlation of gene expression and clinical parameters identifies a set of genes reflecting LV systolic dysfunction and morphological alterations. *Physiol Genomics.* (2019) 51:356–67. doi: 10.1152/physiolgenomics.001 11.2018
30. Zhang K, Wu M, Qin X, Wen P, Wu Y, Zhuang J. Asporin is a potential promising biomarker for common heart failure. *DNA Cell Biol.* (2021) 40:303–15. doi: 10.1089/dna.2020.5995
31. Zhai Z, Zou P, Liu F, Xia Z, Li J. Ferroptosis Is a Potential Novel Diagnostic and Therapeutic Target for Patients With Cardiomyopathy. *Front Cell Dev Biol.* (2021) 9:649045. doi: 10.3389/fcell.2021.649045
32. Rosenbaum AN, Agre KE, Pereira NL. Genetics of dilated cardiomyopathy: practical implications for heart failure management. *Nat Rev Cardiol.* (2020) 17:286–97. doi: 10.1038/s41569-019-0284-0
33. Zeng C, Duan F, Hu J, Luo B, Huang B, Lou X, et al. NLRP3 inflammasome-mediated pyroptosis contributes to the pathogenesis of non-ischemic dilated cardiomyopathy. *Redox Biol.* (2020) 34:101523. doi: 10.1016/j.redox.2020.101523

34. Wittchen F, Suckau L, Witt H, Skurk C, Lassner D, Fechner H, et al. Genomic expression profiling of human inflammatory cardiomyopathy (DCMi) suggests novel therapeutic targets. *J Mol Med (Berl)*. (2007) 85:257–71. doi: 10.1007/s00109-006-0122-9

35. Jordan E, Peterson L, Ai T, Asatryan B, Bronicki L, Brown E, et al. An Evidence-Based Assessment of Genes in Dilated Cardiomyopathy. *Circulation*. (2021) 144:7–19. doi: 10.1161/CIRCULATIONAHA.120.053033

36. Feng J, Perry G, Mori T, Hayashi T, Oparil S, Chen Y. Pressure-independent enhancement of cardiac hypertrophy in atrial natriuretic peptide-deficient mice. *Clin Exp Pharmacol Physiol*. (2003) 30:343–9. doi: 10.1046/j.1440-1681.2003.03836.x

37. Mihailovici AR, Deliu RC, Mărgăritescu C, Simionescu CE, Donoiu I, Istrătoaie O, Tudoraşcu DR, Târtea EA, Gheonea DI. Collagen I and III, MMP-1 and TIMP-1 immunoexpression in dilated cardiomyopathy. *Rom J Morphol Embryol*. (2017) 58:777–81.

38. Kuhn M. Molecular physiology of natriuretic peptide signalling. *Basic Res Cardiol*. (2004) 99:76–82. doi: 10.1007/s00395-004-0460-0

39. Verstreken S, Delrue L, Goethals M, Bartunek J, Vanderheyden M. Natriuretic peptide processing in patients with and without left ventricular dysfunction. *Int Heart J*. (2019) 60:115–20. doi: 10.1536/ihj.18-012

40. Lemaître AI, Picard F, Maurin V, Faure M, Dos SP, Girerd N. Clinical profile and midterm prognosis of left ventricular thrombus in heart failure. *ESC Heart Fail*. (2021) 8:1333–41. doi: 10.1002/ehf2.13211

41. Bengtsson E, Neame PJ, Heinegård D, Sommarin Y. The primary structure of a basic leucine-rich repeat protein, PRELP, found in connective tissues. *J Biol Chem*. (1995) 270:25639 44. doi: 10.1074/jbc.270.43.25639

42. Uhlén M, Fagerberg L, Hallström BM, Lindskog C, Oksvold P, Mardinoglu A, et al. Proteomics. Tissue-based map of the human proteome. *Science*. (2015) 347:1260419. doi: 10.1126/science.1260419

43. Hong R, Gu J, Niu G, Hu Z, Zhang X, Song T, et al. PRELP has prognostic value and regulates cell proliferation and migration in hepatocellular carcinoma. *J Cancer*. (2020) 11:6376–89. doi: 10.7150/jca.46309

44. Sinkeviciute D, Skovlund GS, Sun S, Manon JT, Aspberg A, Önnerfjord P, et al. A novel biomarker of MMP-cleaved prolargin is elevated in patients with psoriatic arthritis. *Sci Rep*. (2020) 10:13541. doi: 10.1038/s41598-020-70327-0

45. Mortimer L, Moreau F, MacDonald JA, Chadee K. NLRP3 inflammasome inhibition is disrupted in a group of auto-inflammatory disease CAPS mutations. *Nat Immunol*. (2016) 17:1176–86. doi: 10.1038/ni.3538

46. Taskén K, Aandahl EM. Localized effects of cAMP mediated by distinct routes of protein kinase A. *Physiol Rev*. (2004) 84:137–67. doi: 10.1152/physrev.00021.2003

47. Hsiao YT, Shimizu I, Wakasugi T, Yoshida Y, Ikegami R, Hayashi Y, et al. Cardiac mitofusin-1 is reduced in non-responding patients with idiopathic dilated cardiomyopathy. *Sci Rep*. (2021) 11:6722. doi: 10.1038/s41598-021-86209-y

48. Liu Y, Chen J, Fontes SK, Bautista EN, Cheng Z. Physiological and pathological roles of protein kinase A in the heart. *Cardiovasc Res*. (2021) cvab008. doi: 10.1093/cvr/cvab008

49. Kang R, Kroemer G, Tang D. The tumor suppressor protein p53 and the ferroptosis network. *Free Radic Biol Med*. (2019) 133:162–8. doi: 10.1016/j.freeradbiomed.2018.05.074

50. Caron M, Auclair M, Donadille B, Béréziat V, Guerci B, Laville M, et al. Human lipodystrophies linked to mutations in A-type lamins and to HIV protease inhibitor therapy are both associated with prelamin A accumulation, oxidative stress and premature cellular senescence. *Cell Death Differ*. (2007) 14:1759–67. doi: 10.1038/sj.cdd.4402197

51. Pérez SA, Toro R, Sarquella BG, de Gonzalo CD, Cesar S, Carro E, et al. Genetic basis of dilated cardiomyopathy. *Int J Cardiol*. (2016) 224:461–72. doi: 10.1016/j.ijcard.2016.09.068

52. Shah S, Henry A, Roselli C, Lin H, Sveinbjörnsson G, Fatemifar G, et al. Genome-wide association and Mendelian randomisation analysis provide insights into the pathogenesis of heart failure. *Nat Commun*. (2020) 11:163. doi: 10.1038/s41467-019-13690-5

53. Tashima T, Nagatoishi S, Sagara H, Ohnuma SI, Tsumoto K. Osteomodulin regulates diameter and alters shape of collagen fibrils. *Biochem Biophys Res Commun*. (2015) 463:292–6. doi: 10.1016/j.bbrc.2015.05.053

54. Tashima T, Nagatoishi S, Caaveiro JMM, Nakakido M, Sagara H, Kusano AO, et al. Molecular basis for governing the morphology of type-I collagen fibrils by Osteomodulin. *Commun Biol*. (2018) 1:33. doi: 10.1038/s42003-018-0038-2

55. Wiśniowska SS, Dziewiecka E, Holcman K, Wypasek E, Khachatryan L, Karabinowska A, et al. Kinetics of selected serum markers of fibrosis in patients with dilated cardiomyopathy and different grades of diastolic dysfunction of the left ventricle. *Cardiol J*. (2020) 27:726–34. doi: 10.5603/CJ.a2018.0143

56. Guo W, Feng W, Fan X, HuangJ, Ou C, Chen M. Osteomodulin is a potential genetic target for hypertrophic cardiomyopathy. *Biochem Genet*. (2021) 59:1185–202. doi: 10.1007/s10528-021-10050-1

57. Zhang M, Mou T, Zhao Z, Peng C, Ma Y, Fang W, et al. Synthesis and 18F-labeling of the analogues of Omecamtiv Mecarbil as a potential cardiac myosin imaging agent with PET. *Nucl Med Biol*. (2013) 40:689–96. doi: 10.1016/j.nucmedbio.2013.02.013

58. Benitez AA, Samouillan V, Jorge E, Dandurand J, Nasarre L, et al. Identification of new biophysical markers for pathological ventricular remodelling in tachycardia-induced dilated cardiomyopathy. *J Cell Mol Med*. (2018) 22:4197–208. doi: 10.1111/jcmm.13699

12

The Diagnostic Value of Soluble ST2 in Heart Failure

Chaojun Yang [1†], Zhixing Fan [1†], Jinchun Wu [2†], Jing Zhang [1], Wei Zhang [3], Jian Yang [4*†] and Jun Yang [1*]

[1] Central Laboratory, Department of Cardiology, The First College of Clinical Medical Science, China Three Gorges University and Yichang Central People's Hospital, Yichang, China, [2] Department of Cardiology, Qinghai Provincial People's Hospital, Xining, China, [3] Department of Cardiology, Renmin Hospital of Wuhan University, Wuhan, China, [4] Department of Cardiology, The People's Hospital of Three Gorges University and The First People's Hospital of Yichang, Yichang, China

*Correspondence:
Jian Yang
yangjian@ctgu.edu.cn
Jun Yang
yangjun@ctgu.edu.cn

†These authors have contributed equally to this work and share first authorship

Objective: The diagnostic performance of soluble suppression of tumorigenicity (sST2) in heart failure (HF) had been investigated in multiple studies, but the results were inconsistent. This meta-analysis evaluated the diagnostic value of sST2 in HF.

Methods: Pubmed, Web of Science, Embase, and Cochrane Library databases were searched until March 2021. Cohort studies or case-control studies relevant to the diagnostic value of sST2 in HF were screened, and true positive (TP), false positive (FP), false negative (FN), and true negative (TN) data were extracted for calculating sensitivity, specificity, positive likelihood ratio (PLR), negative likelihood ratio (NLR), diagnostic odds ratio (DOR), and area under the curve (AUC). The quality of the included studies was evaluated using the Quality Assessment of Diagnostic Accuracy Studies (QUADAS), the threshold effect was determined by calculating Spearman correlation coefficients and summary receiver operating characteristic (SROC) curve patterns, the heterogeneity was evaluated using the I^2 statistic and the Galbraith radial plot, and sensitivity analysis was also performed. Deeks' test was used to assess publication bias.

Results: A total of 11 studies from 10 articles were included in this meta-analysis. The Spearman correlation coefficient was 0.114, $p = 0.739$, and the SROC curve did not show a "shoulder-arm" shape, which suggests that there was no threshold effect, but study heterogeneity existed because of non-threshold effects. The combined sensitivity was 0.72 [95% confidence interval (CI): 0.65–0.78], specificity was 0.65 (95% CI: 0.45–0.81), PLR was 1.75 (95% CI: 1.33–2.31), NLR was 0.48 (95% CI: 0.37–0.63), DOR was 3.63 (95% CI: 2.29–5.74), and AUC was 0.75. The Deeks' test suggested no significant publication bias in the included studies ($P = 0.94$).

Conclusion: sST has some diagnostic value in HF, but this should be further evaluated in additional studies with rigorous design and high homogeneity.

Keywords: soluble suppression of tumorigenicity, heart failure, diagnostic value, sensitivity, specificity, meta-analysis

INTRODUCTION

Heart failure (HF) is a clinical syndrome of cardiac blood flow impairment caused by ventricular systolic or diastolic insufficiency. It is a global health concern with high morbidity and mortality and has seriously endangered human health (1). Currently, HF is diagnosed based on clinical symptoms, medical history, echocardiography, B-type natriuretic peptide (BNP), and N-terminal (NT)-proBNP (2). However, because of the atypical symptoms and signs of HF, the ancillary tests such as echocardiography and invasive hemodynamics are often limited by factors such as medical condition, and BNP or NT-proBNP levels are easily affected by age, sex, body size, and renal function, which makes the diagnosis and management of HF still a clinical challenge (3). Simple, sensitive, and specific techniques are required to assist in the diagnosis of HF, and HF-related biological markers are the current focus of HF diagnosis (4). Soluble suppression of tumorigenicity 2 (sST2), a marker associated with cardiomyocyte traction, is a potential pathophysiological mediator of myocardial hypertrophy and myocardial fibrosis and an important biomarker of HF (5). Several trials have now confirmed that sST2 levels are significantly elevated in patients with HF and that the elevated levels of sST2 correlate significantly with the degree of HF (6, 7). In recent years, more studies have been reported on the diagnosis of HF using sST2, but the results of these studies vary significantly. In this study, we intend to systematically evaluate the diagnostic value of sST2 in HF using meta-analysis.

DATA AND METHODS

Literature Search Strategy

For English databases Pubmed, Web of Science, Embase, and Cochrane Library, Heart failure, ST2, and diagnostic test were searched as the key words by the combination of medical subject headings (MeSH) and entry term. The literature search start date was not restricted, and the search end date was March 2021. The search language was only English. The following search strategy was used for pubmed and modified to suit other databases (the detailed retrieval strategy of other databases in **Supplementary Documents**):

#1 heart failure[MeSH Terms]
#2 (((((((((((((Cardiac Failure[Title/Abstract]) OR (Heart Decompensation[Title/Abstract])) OR (Decompensation, Heart[Title/Abstract])) OR (Heart Failure, Right-Sided[Title/Abstract])) OR (Heart Failure, Right Sided[Title/Abstract])) OR (Right-Sided Heart Failure[Title/Abstract])) OR (Right Sided Heart Failure[Title/Abstract])) OR (Myocardial Failure[Title/Abstract])) OR (Congestive Heart Failure[Title/Abstract])) OR (Heart Failure, Congestive[Title/Abstract])) OR (Heart Failure, Left-Sided[Title/Abstract])) OR (Heart Failure, Left Sided[Title/Abstract])) OR (Left-Sided Heart Failure[Title/Abstract])) OR (Left Sided Heart Failure[Title/Abstract]))) OR (HF)

#3 #1 OR #2
#4 ((((((Soluble suppression of tumorigenicity 2[Title/Abstract]) OR (Soluble suppression of tumorigenicity-2[Title/Abstract])) OR (suppression of tumorigenicity 2[Title/Abstract])) OR (suppression of tumorigenicity-2[Title/Abstract])) OR (sST2[Title/Abstract])) OR (ST2[Title/Abstract])) OR (soluble ST2[Title/Abstract])
#5 "sensitiv*"[Title/Abstract] OR "sensitivity and specificity"[MeSH Terms] OR ("predictive"[Title/Abstract] AND "value*"[Title/Abstract]) OR ("predictive value of tests"[MeSH Terms] OR ("predictive"[All Fields] AND "value"[All Fields] AND "tests"[All Fields]) OR "predictive value of tests"[All Fields]) OR "accuracy*"[Title/Abstract]
#6 #3 AND #4 AND #5.

Literature Inclusion and Exclusion Criteria

Literature inclusion criteria: (1) cohort studies or case-control studies investigating sST2 for the diagnosis of HF; (2) valid data available in the literature for the calculation of true positives (TPs), false positives (FPs), false negatives (FNs), and true negatives (TNs) to obtain information for a four-grid table; and (3) high quality studies using quality evaluation (see below). Exclusion criteria: (1) reviews, conference papers, and letters; (2) literature that cannot provide valid data for a four-grid table; (3) literature with duplicate data; (4) literature reporting results from animals or cellular models; (5) literature with too small a sample size ($n < 100$); (6) literature of low quality using quality evaluation. This systematic evaluation was performed by two authors who independently judged whether the retrieved literature could be included in the study, and the third author made an independent judgment whether to include it in case of disagreement.

Literature Quality Evaluation Criteria

The quality assessment of diagnostic accuracy studies (QUADAS) tool provided by the Cochrane Collaboration system was used to evaluate the quality of the literature. The QUADAS tool evaluates the four biases in terms of case selection, trials to be evaluated, gold standard, and flow, and it evaluates the quality of the literature by assessing 11 landmark questions and three types of clinical applicability questions. The 11 landmark issues were evaluated as "Yes" for clear fit, "Unclear" for unclear, and "No" for not meeting the conditions; the four biases were evaluated as "High risk" for clear bias, "Unclear" for unclear bias, and "Low risk" for no clear bias; and the three types of clinical applicability were evaluated as "High concern" for good matches, "Unclear" for unclear matches, and "Low concern" for poor matches. For each included study, two authors evaluated the quality independently, and the third author made an independent judgment in case of disagreement.

Data Extraction

The extracted information included the basic information of the study and the four-grid table information. The basic information included authors, year of publication, country, sample size, mean age, sST2 detection method, sST2 cut-off, HF diagnostic criteria, HF type, control population, and study type. TP, FP, TN, and

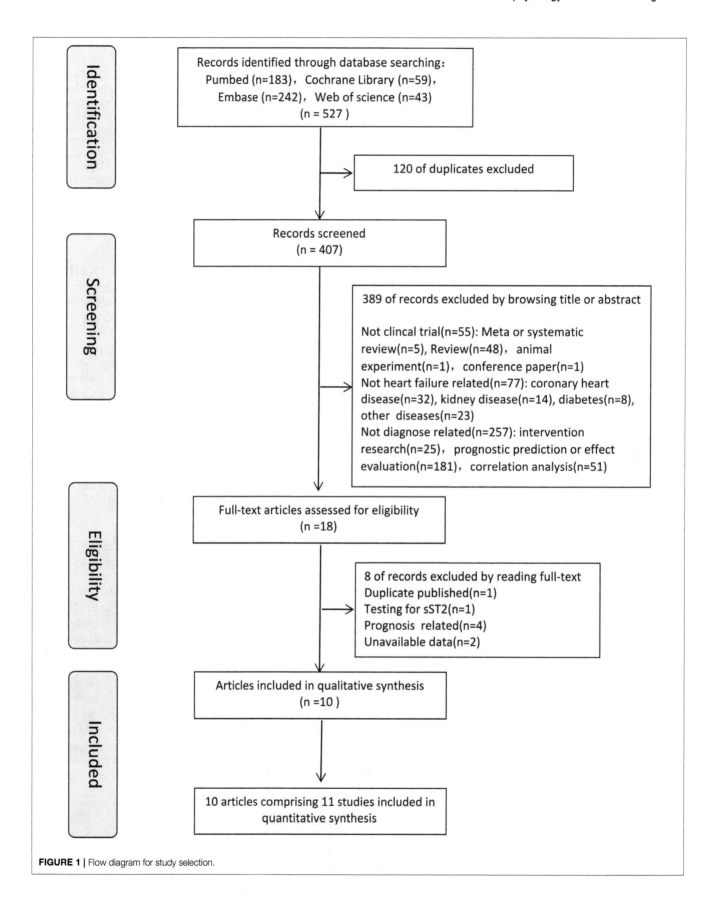

FIGURE 1 | Flow diagram for study selection.

TABLE 1 | Characteristics of the studies included in this meta-analysis.

No	References	Year	Country	Sample size	Male	Average age (year) HF/no HF	sST2 ELISAS kit source	Cut-off value	HF diagnostic criteria	Type of HF	Medical history of HF	Treatment history	Characteristics of controls	Type of research
1	Dieplinger et al. (8)	2009	Australia	251	234	72.82	MBL	121 ng/L	Framingham	HF	Arterial hypertension, diabetes mellitus	ACEI, ARB, calcium antagonist, β-blockers, digitalis, diuretics, amiodarone	ED patients with dyspnea	Cohort
2	Aldous et al. (9)	2012	New Zealand	995	591	66.00	-	34.3 U/mL	Chest radiograph evidence of pulmonary edema or symptoms of HF with raised BNP	HF	Ischemic heart disease, lung disease, stroke, Hypertension, dyslipidemia	-	ED patients with ischemic type pain	Cohort
3	Santhanakrishnan et al. (10)	2012	Singapore	100	52	66.00	Presage™	26.47 ng/mL	Framingham	HFPEF	Diabetes mellitus, hypertension, coronary artery disease, stroke	ACEI/ARB, Spironolactone, β-blocker, diuretics, digoxin, statin, aspirin,	Community adults	Case-Control
4	Santhanakrishnan et al. (10)	2012	Singapore	101	66	60.98	Presage™	30.32 ng/mL	Framingham	HFREF			Community adults	Case-Control
5	Wang et al. (11)	2013	Taiwan	107	57	65.08	R&D	13.5 ng/mL	Framingham	HFPEF	Diabetes, dyslipidemia, coronary artery disease, atrial fibrillation	Aspirin, nitrates, calcium channel blockers, ACEI/ARB, β-Blockers, diuretics, statins, antiarrythmic agents	Outpatients with hypertension	Cohort

(Continued)

TABLE 1 | Continued

No	References	Year	Country	Sample size	Male	Average age (year) HF/no HF	sST2 ELISAS kit source	Cut-off value	HF diagnostic criteria	Type of HF	Medical history of HF	Treatment history	Characteristics of controls	Type of research
6	Jakob et al. (12)	2016	Austria and UK	203		7.5	Presage™	44.4 pg/mL	Presence of HF symptoms and abnormal ventricular systolic function	HF	Dilated cardiomyopathy, functional single ventricle, pulmonary/right-sided obstruction, aortic/left-sided obstruction, ventricular septal defect, tetralogy of fallot, atrioventricular septal defect, patent arterial duct, hypertrophic cardiomyopathy, restrictive cardiomyopathy, atrial septal defect, mixed lesion/other	-	children without heart disease undergoing phlebotomy prior to an elective procedure	Case-Control
7	Mueller et al. (13)	2016	Austria	251	234	76/69	Presage™	26.5 ng/mL	Framingham	HF	Arterial hypertension, diabetes mellitus, atrial fibrillation, coronary artery disease	ACEI/ARB, calcium antagonists, β-blockers, digitalis, diuretics, amiodarone	dyspnoea attributed to other reasons	Cohort
8	Sinning et al. (14)	2016	Germany	4,972	2,526	67/55	Presage™	-	NYHA	HF	Diabetes, hypertension, dyslipidemi	-	Recruitment with no HF	Cohort

(Continued)

TABLE 1 | Continued

No	References	Year	Country	Sample size	Male	Average age (year) HF/no HF	sST2 ELISAS kit source	Cut-off value	HF diagnostic criteria	Type of HF	Medical history of HF	Treatment history	Characteristics of controls	Type of research
9	Jin et al. (15)	2017	China	303	200	61.89/60.31	Shanghai Research Institute for Enzyme-linked Biology	–	ESC Guidelines	HF	–	–	Healthy people	Case-Control
10	Luo et al. (16)	2017	China	876	460	67.49/65.93	–	0.159 µg/L	China Guidelines	HFPEF	Coronary heart disease, diabetes mellitus, hypertension, fatty liver, carotid plaque, gout	Antiplatelet drugs, ACEI/ARB, β-blockers, trimetazidine, diuretics, statins, digitalis	healthy individuals	Case-Control
11	Cui et al. (17)	2018	China	202	135	73/67	Shanghai Qiyi Biological Co.	68.6 pg/mL	ESC Guidelines	HFPEF	Hypertension, diabetes mellitus, coronary heart disease, Atrial fibrillation	β-blocker, ARB, dioxin, aldosterone antagonist, statin	Health examiner	Case-Control

TABLE 2 | Main findings of the included studies.

References	TP	FP	FN	TN	SEN	SPE
Dieplinger et al. (8)	123	89	14	25	0.90	0.22
Aldous et al. (9)	25	196	9	765	0.74	0.80
Santhanakrishnan et al. (10)	35	26	15	24	0.70	0.48
Santhanakrishnan et al. (10)	35	16	16	34	0.69	0.68
Wang et al. (11)	50	10	18	29	0.74	0.74
Jakob et al. (12)	65	39	49	50	0.57	0.56
Mueller et al. (13)	104	58	33	56	0.76	0.49
Sinning et al. (14)	81	2,882	27	1,982	0.75	0.41
Jin et al. (15)	154	0	43	106	0.78	1.00
Luo et al. (16)	267	166	109	334	0.71	0.67
Cui et al. (17)	83	13	89	17	0.48	0.57

TP, True positive; FP, False positive; FN, False negative; TN, True negative; SEN, Sensitivity; SPE, Specificity.

FN data were extracted from the included studies, and data that could not be extracted directly could be obtained by data transformation or by contacting the authors.

Statistical Methods

Statistical analysis of the data was performed using Stata 15 and Meta-Disc (version 14.0) software. First, threshold effects were determined using Spearman correlation coefficient and the pattern of the summary receiver operating characteristic cure (SROC) curve. Then, the combined effect indicators—sensitivity, specificity, positive likelihood ratio (PLR), negative likelihood ratio (NLR), diagnostic odds ratio (DOR), and area under the curve (AUC) of SROC—were calculated. Heterogeneity was tested with the chi-square test using the I^2 of Q statistic, and $I^2 < 50\%$ or $P > 0.05$ indicated no significant heterogeneity among studies, and the effect indicators were combined using the fixed effect model (FEM); $I^2 > 50\%$ or $P < 0.05$ indicated a significant heterogeneity among studies, so the effect indicators were combined using the randomized effect model (REM), and heterogeneity analysis and sensitivity analysis were conducted. The Deeks' test was used to assess publication bias. $P < 0.05$ was considered a statistically significant difference.

RESULTS

Literature Search Results

Five hundred and twenty-seven articles were obtained by searching with the proposed input, and a total of 407 articles were retrieved after removing duplicates. By reading the titles and abstracts, 389 articles were initially excluded (55 were not clincal trial; 77 were not heart failure related; 257 were not diagnose related) according to the inclusion and exclusion criteria. A total of 18 articles was investigated, and eight of them were excluded by reading full-text. For the eight excluded articles, one was duplicate publication, one was testing for sST2, four were prognosis related and two with no access to the four-grid table

information. Finally, 10 articles with 11 studies were included in the meta-analysis (8–17) (**Figure 1**).

Basic Characteristics of the Included Literature

A total of 11 studies were included. Santhanakrishnan et al. (9) divided HF patients into HF with preserved ejection fraction (HFPEF) and HF with reduced ejection fraction (HFREF) and studied them separately, and thus this literature was considered as two studies. The basic information of the included studies is shown in **Table 1**. The total sample size of 8,361 patients was included, involving cases from Australia, New Zealand, Singapore, the United Kingdom, Germany, and China. Ten studies investigated middle-aged and elderly populations, and one study focused on children. There were five cohort studies and six case-control studies. sST2 was detected using enzyme-linked immunosorbent assays (ELISAs), and sST2 kits were available from five manufacturers, including MBL, Presage™, and R&D. Regarding the type of HF, four studies included patients with HFPEF, one included patients with HFREF, and the other six studies did not distinguish between reduced and preserved ejection fractions. The control population included people with dyspnea unrelated to HF, children with hypertension unrelated to HF, healthy populations, and community populations. TP, FP, FN, and TN data were extracted from each study for the meta-analysis (**Table 2**), and the quality evaluation of the included studies is shown in **Figure 2**.

Threshold Effect Analysis

Meta-disc analysis showed that the Spearman correlation coefficient between the log of sensitivity and the log of (1-specificity) was 0.114, $P = 0.739$, and the SROC curve showed no "shoulder-arm" pattern, which suggests that there was no threshold effect in this study.

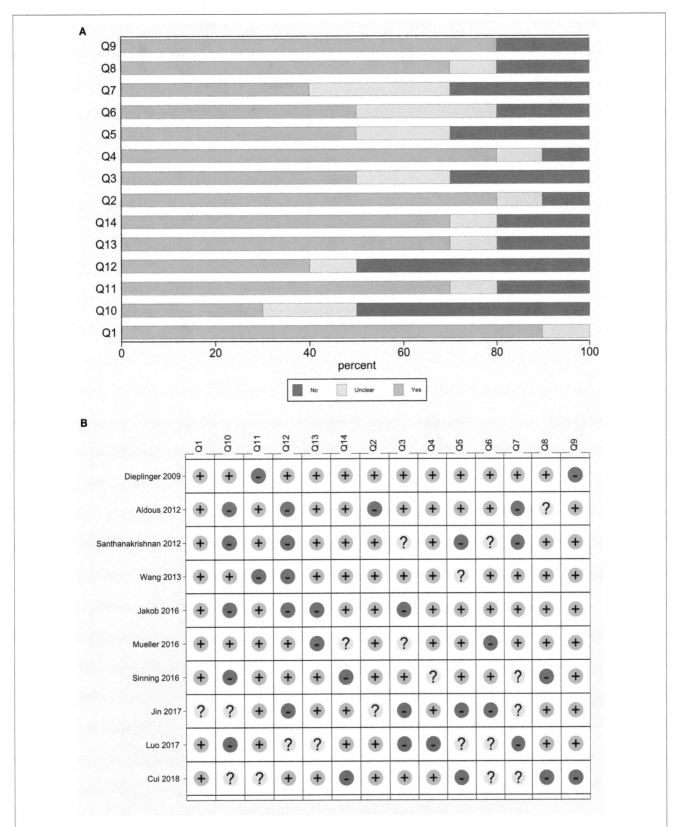

FIGURE 2 | Quality evaluation of the included studies. **(A)** Review authors' judgments presented as percentages for the included studies; **(B)** Review authors' judgements for each included study.

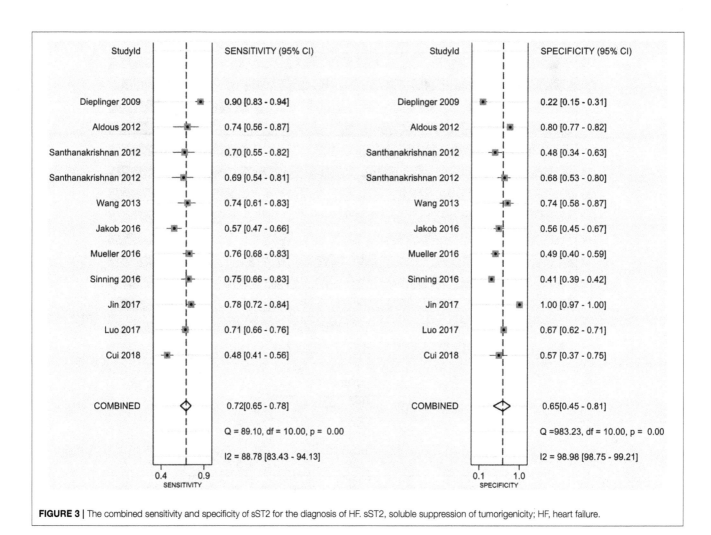

FIGURE 3 | The combined sensitivity and specificity of sST2 for the diagnosis of HF. sST2, soluble suppression of tumorigenicity; HF, heart failure.

Diagnostic Value of sST2 in Patients With HF

The combined sensitivity of sST2 for the diagnosis of HF was 0.72 (95% confidence interval (CI): 0.65–0.78) (**Figure 3**), the combined specificity was 0.65 (95% CI: 0.45–0.81) (**Figure 3**), the combined PLR was 1.75 (95% CI: 1.33–2.31) (**Figure 4A**), the combined NLR was 0.48 (95% CI: 0.37–0.63) (**Figure 4B**), and the combined DOR was 3.63 (95% CI: 2.29–5.74) (**Figure 4C**). The AUC of the SROC curve was 0.75 (**Figure 4D**).

Heterogeneity Analysis

Heterogeneity tests showed that $I^2 = 88.78\%$ ($P < 0.0001$) for sensitivity, $I^2 = 98.98\%$ ($P < 0.0001$) for specificity, $I^2 = 94.0\%$ ($P < 0.0001$) for PLR, $I^2 = 84.7\%$ ($P < 0.0001$) for NLR, and $I^2 = 82.2\%$ ($P < 0.0001$) for DOR, which suggests the presence of heterogeneity unrelated to threshold effects in this study, so the effect sizes were combined using a randomized effect model and the source of heterogeneity was analyzed. The Galbraith radial plot (**Figure 5**) showed that four studies conducted by Dieplinger et al., Santhanakrishnan et al., Jakob et al., and Cui et al. were the sources of the heterogeneity.

Sensitivity Analysis

Sensitivity analysis of the data from this study showed that the studies conducted by Santhanakrishnan et al. and Cui et al. had the most impact on the calculation of the results of this study (**Figure 6A**), while the other original studies had no impact on the calculation of the study results. Taken together, the results of this study were relatively stable. Sensitivity analysis of the impact of individual studies showed that the exclusion of the study conducted by Cui et al. had the most effect on the calculation of results in this meta-analysis (**Figure 6B**).

Publication Bias

The Deeks' test was performed using Stata software to assess publication bias (**Figure 7**); it showed a $P = 0.94$, which suggests that there was no significant publication bias in the included studies.

DISCUSSION

HF is a common outcome of multiple cardiovascular diseases. Cardiac overload and myocardial cell injury can lead to reduced cardiac function, which results in compensatory changes

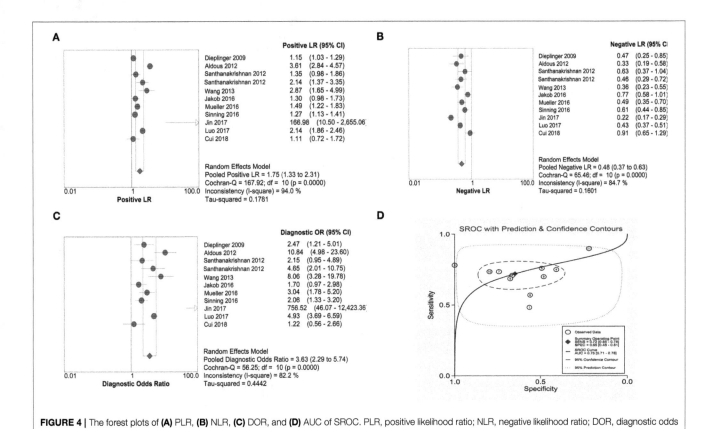

FIGURE 4 | The forest plots of **(A)** PLR, **(B)** NLR, **(C)** DOR, and **(D)** AUC of SROC. PLR, positive likelihood ratio; NLR, negative likelihood ratio; DOR, diagnostic odds ratio; AUC, area under curve; SROC, summary receiver operating characteristic.

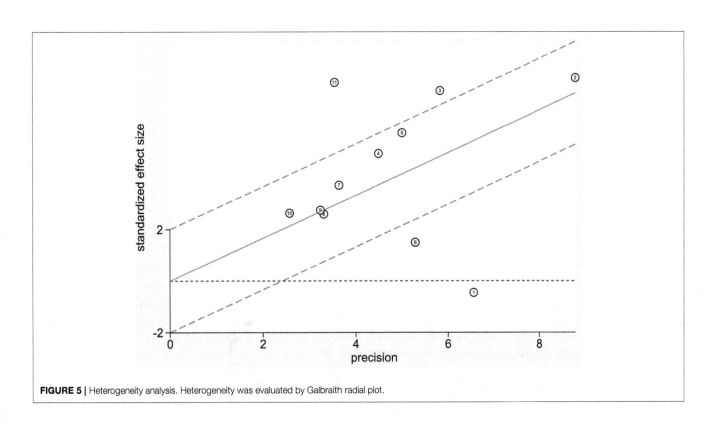

FIGURE 5 | Heterogeneity analysis. Heterogeneity was evaluated by Galbraith radial plot.

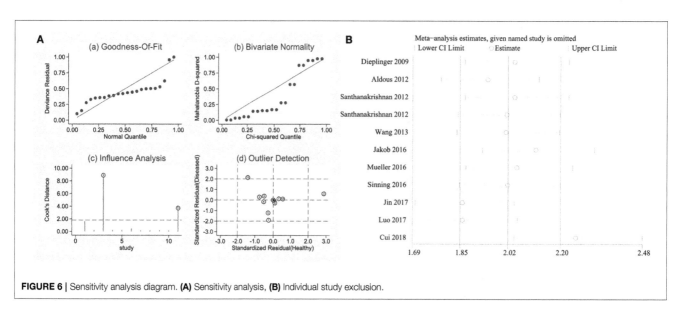

FIGURE 6 | Sensitivity analysis diagram. **(A)** Sensitivity analysis, **(B)** Individual study exclusion.

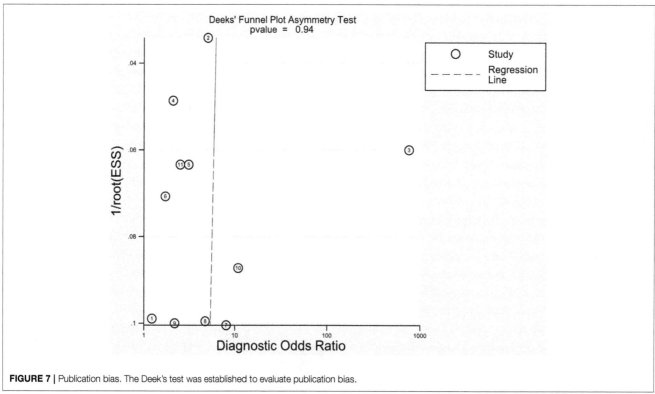

FIGURE 7 | Publication bias. The Deek's test was established to evaluate publication bias.

such as ventricular hypertrophy and chamber enlargement, as well as corresponding changes in cardiomyocytes, extracellular matrix, and collagen fiber networks followed by ventricular remodeling, leading to further deterioration of cardiac function (18). Multiple factors are involved in the progression of HF, such as myocardial necrosis, apoptosis, autophagy, fibrosis, oxidative stress, inflammatory response, and neurohumoral regulatory disorders, as well as changing

levels in a series of biomarkers (19). The American College of Cardiology/American Heart Association/Heart Failure Society of America (ACC/AHA/HFSA) guidelines released in 2017 stated that BNP and NT-proBNP provide clear diagnostic value in patients with chronic HF (20). BNP or NT-proBNP has been used clinically as a routine test for HF, but it is susceptible to various factors such as age, sex, and disease condition. Among these biomarkers, the myocardial fibrosis marker sST2 is not affected by factors like age, sex, renal function, and weight (21). Meanwhile, the 2017 ACC/AHA/HFSA guidelines recommend measuring sST2 for risk stratification of patients with chronic HF (20). This suggests that sST2 has some value in the diagnosis and prognosis of HF.

ST2 is a member of the interleukin-1 (IL-1) receptor superfamily, which is encoded by the *ST2* gene in cardiomyocytes during myocardial stretch and under mechanical stress. The *ST2* gene is located on human chromosome 2q12 and can encode two isoforms of sST2 and the transmembrane receptor form of ST2 (ST2L). Interleukin-33 (IL-33) is a functional ligand for ST2, and the ST2/IL-33 signaling pathway exerts cardioprotective effects by activating ST2L receptors to reduce myocardial fibrosis, inhibit cardiomyocyte hypertrophy, and improve cardiac function, which does not require the sST2 receptor (22). During HF, the increased cardiac load exposes the myocardium to excessive stretch stimulation, and the overproduced sST2 can compete with ST2L for binding IL-33, abrogating the cardioprotective effect of the ST2/IL-33 signaling pathway; this leads to apoptosis, hypertrophy and fibrosis of cardiomyocytes, and further deterioration of cardiac function, aggravating the HF process (23). This suggests that sST2 plays an important role in the development of HF. Clinical studies on the diagnostic value of sST2 in HF have gradually increased in recent years (24). In this study, the clinical diagnostic value of sST2 in HF was evaluated using meta-analysis.

Meta-analysis showed that the combined sensitivity was 0.72, specificity was 0.65, DOR was 3.63, and AUC was 0.75, which indicates that sST2 has a good diagnostic value for HF. The meta-analysis conducted by Huang et al. (24) included 10 original studies, all of which were conducted before 2014 and published in either Chinese or English, and their combined sensitivity was 0.84, specificity was 0.74, DOR was 8.49, and AUC was 0.81. Both the sensitivity and specificity in this study were about 10% lower than those in the Huang et al. (24), which may be related to the inclusion of recent literature and more stringent quality screening performed in this study, but both meta-analyses had a high degree of heterogeneity. Diagnostic studies are generally more heterogeneous than other types of clinical studies because of a possible bias in case selection, trials to be evaluated, gold standards, and flow. This study showed that four studies, those conducted by Dieplinger et al., Santhanakrishnan et al., Jakob et al., and Cui et al. may be the source of heterogeneity in this meta-analysis, and the study conducted by Cui et al. had the most impact on the results of the meta-analysis. The analysis revealed that Dieplinger et al. used a sST2 kit from MBL, Santhanakrishnan et al. conducted a case-control study, Jakob et al. focused on children, and Cui et al. performed a case-control study on patients with HFPEF using a sST2 kit from Shanghai Qiyi Biological Co.; thus, the above-mentioned differences may have contributed to the large heterogeneity observed in this study. In addition, the heterogeneity of this study may have also been caused by the disease typing (different degrees of HF in different studies), the composition of the disease spectrum (the patient group may be combined with other diseases, and the control group includes patients with various cardiovascular diseases without HF), the diagnostic thresholds (the thresholds were not uniform among studies), and differences in the sST2 detection methods. Moreover, there was also heterogeneity because of mixed bias caused by the HF type, control population, sST2 kit, HF diagnostic criteria, study type, and other biases.

Although this meta-analysis included a relatively comprehensive literature search, there were still some limitations. First, the heterogeneity of the included studies was high, and the potential sources include HF type, control population, sST2 kit, HF diagnostic criteria, and study type, with possible heterogeneity between subgroups and from other sources. Second, most of the included studies were case-control studies, which could cause selection bias in the selection of study subjects and increase diagnostic sensitivity. Third, the diagnostic cut-off values of sST2 were not uniform, and the diagnostic cut-off values of sST2 varied among the 11 included studies, which may have been related to factors such as kits, test conditions, and sample-handling methods.

In general, sST2 has some diagnostic value for HF, but factors such as HF type, control population, sST2 kits, HF diagnostic criteria, and study type in the original studies may have affected its diagnostic value. Therefore, we still need to design prospective cohort studies with high quality, large sample sizes, uniform study populations, uniform control populations, and uniform test methods to further explore and validate the reliability of the results of this analysis; we also need to establish an accurate cut-off value for sST2 to provide clinical guidance for the diagnosis of HF.

AUTHOR CONTRIBUTIONS

This study was designed by ZF and JuY. CY and JiY contributed data to the paper. Statistical analysis and interpretation of data were performed by JiY, JZ, WZ, and JW. All authors were involved in drafting and revision of the manuscript for important intellectual content and approved the final version to be published.

ACKNOWLEDGMENTS

We thank Mark Abramovitz, PhD, from Liwen Bianji, Edanz Group China (www.liwenbianji.cn/ac), for editing the English text of a draft of this manuscript.

SUPPLEMENTARY MATERIAL

Supplementary Document 1 | Literature searches and search strategy.

Supplementary Table 1 | Included and excluded reference.

REFERENCES

1. Agbor VN, Ntusi NAB, Noubiap JJ. An overview of heart failure in low- and middle-income countries. *Cardiovasc Diagn Ther.* (2020) 10:244–51. doi: 10.21037/cdt.2019.08.03

2. Shiraishi Y, Kawana M, Nakata J, Sato N, Fukuda K, Kohsaka S. Time-sensitive approach in the management of acute heart failure. *ESC Heart Fail.* (2021) 8:204–21. doi: 10.1002/ehf2.13139

3. Sabanayagam A, Cavus O, Williams J, Bradley E. Management of heart failure in adult congenital heart disease. *Heart Fail Clin.* (2018) 14:569–77. doi: 10.1016/j.hfc.2018.06.005

4. Sarhene M, Wang Y, Wei J, Huang Y, Li M, Li L, et al. Biomarkers in heart failure: the past, current and future. *Heart Fail Rev.* (2019) 24:867–903. doi: 10.1007/s10741-019-09807-z

5. Lotierzo M, Dupuy AM, Kalmanovich E, Roubille F, Cristol JP. sST2 as a value-added biomarker in heart failure. *Clin Chim Acta.* (2020) 501:120–30. doi: 10.1016/j.cca.2019.10.029

6. Sobieszek G, Powrózek T, Jaroszyński A, Skwarek-Dziekanowska A, Rahnama-Hezavah M, Małecka-Massalska T. Soluble ST2 proteins in male cachectic patients with chronic heart failure. *Nutr Metab Cardiovasc Dis.* (2021) 31:886–93. doi: 10.1016/j.numecd.2020.11.014

7. Crnko S, Printezi MI, Jansen TPJ, Leiteris L, van der Meer MG, Schutte H, et al. Prognostic biomarker soluble ST2 exhibits diurnal variation in chronic heart failure patients. *ESC Heart Fail.* (2020) 7:1224–33. doi: 10.1002/ehf2.12673

8. Dieplinger B, Gegenhuber A, Haltmayer M, Mueller T. Evaluation of novel biomarkers for the diagnosis of acute destabilised heart failure in patients with shortness of breath. *Heart.* (2009) 95:1508–13. doi: 10.1136/hrt.2009.170696

9. Aldous SJ, Richards AM, Troughton R, Than M. ST2 has diagnostic and prognostic utility for all-cause mortality and heart failure in patients presenting to the emergency department with chest pain. *J Card Fail.* (2012) 18:304–10. doi: 10.1016/j.cardfail.2012.01.008

10. Santhanakrishnan R, Chong JP, Ng TP, Ling LH, Sim D, Leong KT, et al. Growth differentiation factor 15, ST2, high-sensitivity troponin T, and N-terminal pro brain natriuretic peptide in heart failure with preserved vs. reduced ejection fraction. *Eur J Heart Fail.* (2012) 14:1338–47. doi: 10.1093/eurjhf/hfs130

11. Wang YC, Yu CC, Chiu FC, Tsai CT, Lai LP, Hwang JJ, et al. Soluble ST2 as a biomarker for detecting stable heart failure with a normal ejection fraction in hypertensive patients. *J Card Fail.* (2013) 19:163–8. doi: 10.1016/j.cardfail.2013.01.010

12. Hauser JA, Demyanets S, Rusai K, Goritschan C, Weber M, Panesar D, et al. Diagnostic performance and reference values of novel biomarkers of paediatric heart failure. *Heart.* (2016) 102:1633–9. doi: 10.1136/heartjnl-2016-309460

13. Mueller T, Gegenhuber A, Leitner I, Poelz W, Haltmayer M, Dieplinger B. Diagnostic and prognostic accuracy of galectin-3 and soluble ST2 for acute heart failure. *Clin Chim Acta.* (2016) 463:158–64. doi: 10.1016/j.cca.2016.10.034

14. Sinning C, Kempf T, Schwarzl M, Lanfermann S, Ojeda F, Schnabel RB, et al. Biomarkers for characterization of heart failure-Distinction of heart failure with preserved and reduced ejection fraction. *Int J Cardiol.* (2017) 227:272–7. doi: 10.1016/j.ijcard.2016.11.110

15. Jin XL, Huang N, Shang H, Zhou MC, Hong Y, Cai WZ, et al. Diagnosis of chronic heart failure by the soluble suppression of tumorigenicity 2 and N-terminal pro-brain natriuretic peptide. *J Clin Lab Anal.* (2018) 32:e22295. doi: 10.1002/jcla.22295

16. Luo NS, Zhang HF, Liu PM, Lin YQ, Huang TC, Yang Y, et al. Diagnostic value of combining serum soluble ST2 and interleukin-33 for heart failure patients with preserved left ventricular ejection fraction. *Zhonghua Xin Xue Guan Bing Za Zhi.* (2017) 45:198–203. doi: 10.3760/cma.j.issn.0253-3758.2017.03.006

17. Cui Y, Qi X, Huang A, Li J, Hou W, Liu K. Differential and predictive value of galectin-3 and soluble suppression of tumorigenicity-2 (sST2) in heart failure with preserved ejection fraction. *Med Sci Monit.* (2018) 24:5139–46. doi: 10.12659/MSM.908840

18. Hieda M, Sarma S, Hearon CM Jr, Dias KA, Martinez J, Samels M, et al. Increased myocardial stiffness in patients with high-risk left ventricular hypertrophy: the hallmark of stage-b heart failure with preserved ejection fraction. *Circulation.* (2020) 141:115–23. doi: 10.1161/CIRCULATIONAHA.119.040332

19. Mitic VT, Stojanovic DR, Deljanin Ilic MZ, Stojanovic MM, Petrovic DB, Ignjatovic AM, et al. Cardiac remodeling biomarkers as potential circulating markers of left ventricular hypertrophy in heart failure with preserved ejection fraction. *Tohoku J Exp Med.* (2020) 250:233–42. doi: 10.1620/tjem.250.233

20. Yancy CW, Jessup M, Bozkurt B, Butler J, Casey DE Jr, Colvin MM, et al. 2017 ACC/AHA/HFSA focused update of the 2013 ACCF/AHA guideline for the management of heart failure: a report of the American college of cardiology/american heart association task force on clinical practice guidelines and the heart failure society of America. *Circulation.* (2017) 136:e137–61. doi: 10.1161/CIR.0000000000000509

21. Homsak E, Gruson D. Soluble ST2: a complex and diverse role in several diseases. *Clin Chim Acta.* (2020) 507:75–87. doi: 10.1016/j.cca.2020.04.011

22. Weinberg EO, Shimpo M, De Keulenaer GW, MacGillivray C, Tominaga S, Solomon SD, et al. Expression and regulation of ST2, an interleukin-1 receptor family member, in cardiomyocytes and myocardial infarction. *Circulation.* (2002) 106:2961–6. doi: 10.1161/01.CIR.0000038705.69871.D9

23. Sanada S, Hakuno D, Higgins LJ, Schreiter ER, McKenzie AN, Lee RT. IL-33 and ST2 comprise a critical biomechanically induced and cardioprotective signaling system. *J Clin Invest.* (2007) 117:1538–49. doi: 10.1172/JCI30634

24. Huang DH, Sun H, Shi JP. Diagnostic value of soluble suppression of tumorigenicity-2 for heart failure. *Chin Med J.* (2016) 129:570–7. doi: 10.4103/0366-6999.177000

13

Development and Validation of a Random Forest Diagnostic Model of Acute Myocardial Infarction Based on Ferroptosis-Related Genes in Circulating Endothelial Cells

Chen Yifan[†‡], Shi Jianfeng[†] and Pu Jun[‡]*

State Key Laboratory for Oncogenes and Related Genes, Division of Cardiology, Renji Hospital, School of Medicine, Shanghai Jiao Tong University, Shanghai Cancer Institute, Shanghai, China

*Correspondence:
Pu Jun
pujun310@hotmail.com

[†] These authors have contributed equally to this work

The high incidence and mortality of acute myocardial infarction (MI) drastically threaten human life and health. In the past few decades, the rise of reperfusion therapy has significantly reduced the mortality rate, but the MI diagnosis is still by means of the identification of myocardial injury markers without highly specific biomarkers of microcirculation disorders. Ferroptosis is a novel reported type of programmed cell death, which plays an important role in cancer development. Maintaining iron homeostasis in cells is essential for heart function, and its role in the pathological process of ischemic organ damages remains unclear. Being quickly detected through blood tests, circulating endothelial cells (CECs) have the potential for early judgment of early microcirculation disorders. In order to explore the role of ferroptosis-related genes in the early diagnosis of acute MI, we relied on two data sets from the GEO database to first detect eight ferroptosis-related genes differentially expressed in CECs between the MI and healthy groups in this study. After comparing different supervised learning algorithms, we constructed a random forest diagnosis model for acute MI based on these ferroptosis-related genes with a compelling diagnostic performance in both the validation (AUC = 0.8550) and test set (AUC = 0.7308), respectively. These results suggest that the ferroptosis-related genes might play an important role in the early stage of MI and have the potential as specific diagnostic biomarkers for MI.

Keywords: ferroptosis, myocardial infarction, diagnostic model, random forest, supervised machine learning

INTRODUCTION

Myocardial infarction (MI), the most common and most precarious outcome of coronary heart disease, endangers the health of the majority (1). With the progress of interventional and reperfusion therapy in recent years, the mortality rate of acute MI has been significantly reduced. However, it cannot be ignored that there is still a lack of efficient tools and biomarkers for the early diagnosis of acute MI. Even in the early stage of acute MI, every hour of early diagnosis and timely treatment could increase the survival rate by about 15% (2, 3). Specific markers of myocardial injury, such as cardiac troponin T (cTnT) (4) and typical changes on an electrocardiogram (ECG) (5) take the top priority for MI diagnosis in recent clinical guidelines (6). However, such diagnostic strategy still faces a lot of challenges. The cTnT in myocardial cells lacks timeliness for the early diagnosis of acute MI because it only reflects myocardial damage and even rupture caused by ischemia, hypoxia, and other factors without characterizing the early myocardial perfusion abnormalities. Moreover, the half-life of cTnT in the blood is too long to identify the reinfarction (7). What is more, typical changes on ECG of MI are not always stable and could be interfered with by other cardiomyopathy. Hence, measures should be taken immediately to explore novel biomarkers for early diagnosis.

Circulating endothelial cells (CECs) are derived from the metabolism of the vascular endothelium (8), which directly reflects the contractile function of blood vessels, the perfusion of capillaries, and the state of ischemia and hypoxia earlier than cardiomyocytes (9). Meanwhile, ischemia and hypoxia directly lead to abnormal metabolism and programmed death of vascular endothelial cells, which could also be obtained from the state of circulating endothelial cells through direct blood tests.

Ferroptosis is a newly discovered type of programmed cell death in recent years. It is well-known for its iron-dependent phospholipid peroxidation process to cause cell membrane damage and even cell death (10). In fact, iron metabolism is tightly regulated in the organism, and excessive Fe^{2+} could induce the production of active reactive oxygen species (ROS), which would trigger the oxidative stress. Meanwhile, glutathione peroxidase (GPX4) could reverse lipid peroxidation and ferroptosis by consuming glutathione. Recent studies show that the regulation of ferroptosis is associated with autophagy in cancer (11). And $CD8^+$ T cells activated by immunotherapy can exert their antitumor effects by enhancing the ferroptosis of tumor cells. Although this evidence demonstrates the importance of ferroptosis in cancer, few studies focus on its role in ischemic disease. In the field of cerebrovascular disease, it is reported that activating the expression of GPX4 could protect neurons in the ischemic stroke model (12). However, the underlying regulation of ferroptosis is still in the veil in the field of cardiovascular disease, especially in MI (13).

Here, we screened the differentially expressed genes in CECs of acute MI patients from the GEO database. Then, the ferroptosis-related genes collected from the FerrDb database (http://zhounan.org/ferrdb) (14) and other previous literature (15–18) were utilized to identify the differential ferroptosis-related genes in acute MI. Finally, we established and evaluated a random forest diagnostic model based on these genes and verified it in another data set in GEO after comparing three different supervised machine learning algorithms.

METHODS AND MATERIALS

Original Gene Expression Profiles Acquisition and Data Preprocessing

Two related CEC databases, GSE66360 (19) and GSE48060 (20), were selected and downloaded from the GEO database (https://www.ncbi.nlm.nih.gov/GEO/). Both of these data sets were updated on March 25, 2019. Although these two databases shared the same supplementary microarray probe platform GPL570,

GSE66360 alone was selected as the training and validation sets. Meanwhile, GSE66360 is confirmed to be matched by both gender and age in the experimental and control groups (19). GSE48060 was treated as the test set to avoid the possible interference of a batch effect. Then, quality control and normalization of these two gene expression profiles were conducted through the scale function in R 4.0.3 software.

Differential Gene Expression

The latest version of the "stringr" and "limma" packages in R 4.0.3 software were used to perform differential expression analysis. The fold change (FC) was calculated based on the average gene expression of the acute MI and control groups, and the differentially expressed genes were defined by the cutoff values (FC > 1.5 and $P < 0.05$). Meanwhile, the gene probe IDs were matched with the "Gene Symbol" through "Gene ID Conversion" in the DAVID online database (http://david.ncifcrf.gov/) (21).

Functional Enrichment Analysis of Differential Genes

The DAVID online database was also adopted for the gene ontology (GO) enrichment analysis, including three aspects of biological process (BP), cell composition (CC), and molecular function (MF) for functional annotation (21). Meanwhile, the KEGG online database (http://genome.jp/kegg/pathway.html) (22) was used to analyze the KEGG signal pathway of those differentially expressed genes. In addition, hierarchical clustering of samples and differential genes were performed and visualized through the "heatmap" R package.

Collection of Ferroptosis-Related Genes

Ferroptosis-related genes were collected and retrieved from the FerrDb database (http://zhounan.org/ferrdb) (14), and other previous literature (15–18) was referenced for proofreading and completion. All the ferroptosis-related genes are provided in **Supplementary Table 1**.

Analysis of Differential Ferroptosis-Related Genes

The latest version of the "venneuler" package in R 4.0.3 software was applied to depict the intersection of differential and ferroptosis-related genes, and the "seaborn" library in Python 3.90 was used to visualize the expression of different ferroptosis-related genes between the MI and control groups, and Student's t-test was adopted as the statistical analysis by "scipy.stats" Python library. The P-value < 0.05 was considered statistically significant, and all P-values were two-tailed. Meanwhile, the STRING database (http://string-db.org/) (23) was used to perform a protein–protein interaction (PPI) network on the differentially expressed proteins of those ferroptosis-related genes. In addition, principal component analysis (PCA) was performed on the differentially expressed ferroptosis-related genes as a dimension-reduction strategy to distinguish the MI and control groups through the "sklearn" Python library.

Construction of Diagnostic Prediction Model Through Machine Learning

Differential expressions of ferroptosis-related genes were treated as independent variables to construct a prediction model for the diagnosis of acute MI based on CECs. In this study, we used the GSE66360 data set as the training and validation set (4:1), and the GSE48060 data set was treated as the test set. In order to prevent the overfitting phenomenon caused by the complex model, K-fold cross-validation with cv = 15 was adopted in this study to improve the generalization ability of the training set. Feature selection was implemented through the "sklearn.model_selection" Python library. Then, three different supervised machine learning algorithms were used to initially explore the diagnostic prediction model. The logistic regression, support vector classification, and random forest models were, respectively, built through the "sklearn.linear_model," "sklearn.svm," and "sklearn.ensemble" Python libraries. After comparing the performance of different models, the random forest algorithm was selected, and some parameters and structures were adjusted to optimize this algorithm. ROC curves were visualized through the "matplotlib" Python library. Then, the validation set was used to verify the prediction model, and the test set was applied to demonstrate the generalization ability of this diagnostic model.

RESULTS

Research Flow and the Collection of Ferroptosis-Related Genes

GSE66360, a CECs data set of acute MI with clinical information, was downloaded from the GEO database for further differential gene screening. This data set included 49 acute MI patients with strict diagnostic criteria and 50 healthy controls. Meanwhile, all the patient CECs were isolated from peripheral blood within 48 h of acute MI and identified with a $CD146^+$ specific antigen. Then, differential expression and functional enrichment analyses were performed after quality control and normalization of the gene expression matrix.

In addition, 259 ferroptosis-related genes were confirmed through the FerrDb database and other previous references after deduplication. Subsequently, the intersection of differentially expressed and ferroptosis-related genes were taken, and the expression differences of these genes were tested in the two groups. The PPI network of these differential ferroptosis-related genes was also built. Then, the GSE66360 data set was divided into the training and validation sets at a ratio of 4:1. Finally, a diagnostic prediction model of acute MI based on the random forest algorithm was constructed by those screened differential ferroptosis-related genes after K-fold cross-validation and algorithm comparison and verified on the test set GSE48060 including 26 acute MI patients with non-recurrent events and 21 normal controls (**Figure 1**).

Verification and Functional Analysis of Differentially Expressed Genes in Acute MI

The 99 samples in the MI and control groups of GSE66360 were normalized and the FC calculated through the "limma" R package. After setting the cutoff values (FC > 1.5 and $P < 0.05$), 256 differentially expressed genes of ECEs in the control and MI groups were screened, including 37 upregulated genes and 219 downregulated genes (**Figure 2A**). Meanwhile, the top five upregulated genes with huge significance were NR4A2, NLRP3, EFEMP1, CLEC7A, and CLEC4D in the MI group. The top five downregulated genes were XIST, TSIX, CTD-2528L19.6, LPAR5, and DAB1 in the MI group. Some of these genes were reported to be involved in various processes of the development of cardiovascular diseases, including hypoxia, autophagy, and oxidative stress (24–26).

In order to further explore the pathophysiology functions of these differentially expressed genes in acute MI, GO analysis according to the DAVID online database was adopted to cluster the BP, CC, and MF among them. The results were that most genes participated in the inflammatory response in BP, followed by extracellular space in CC and receptor activity in MF (**Figure 2B**).

In addition, the KEGG pathway analysis of these differentially expressed genes showed that the top three signal pathways with the largest number of enriched genes were the TNF signaling pathway, osteoclast differentiation, and Toll-like receptor signaling pathway (**Figure 2B**). All these pathway enrichments were also supported and echoed by corresponding literature (13, 27, 28).

What is more, hierarchical clustering was also applied to verify the reliability of these differential genes, and the two groups could be significantly distinguished according to a heat map (**Figure 2C**).

Expression and Functional Analysis of Differential Ferroptosis-Related Genes

By intersecting the collected ferroptosis-related genes with the differentially expressed genes described above, eight differentially expressed ferroptosis-related genes including C-X-C motif chemokine ligand 2 (CXCL2), endothelial PAS domain protein 1 (EPAS1), Jun dimerization protein 2 (JDP2), activating transcription factor 3 (ATF3), Toll-like receptor 4 (TLR4), ferritin heavy chain 1 (FTH1), AP-1 transcription factor subunit (JUN), and DNA damage-inducible transcript 3 (DDIT3) were obtained (**Figure 3A**). The relevant information of all these genes is demonstrated in **Table 1**. All these differentially expressed ferroptosis-related genes were shown to be significantly highly expressed in the acute MI group with P-values < 0.0001 (**Figure 3B**).

Although the specific mechanism of ferroptosis in cardiovascular disease was not clear, our results first confirmed the potential role of these ferroptosis-related genes in acute MI. CXCL2 occupied the most obvious difference in expression, which was thought to be associated with neutrophil-mediated inflammation (29). However, it is also gradually recognized as a key factor involved in cellular ferroptotic response in recent years. Meanwhile, it is also shown that CXCL2 is significantly highly expressed in the plaques and peripheral blood mononuclear cells of patients with coronary atherosclerosis, and it might be closely related to the prognosis (30). Another significant difference was shown on EPAS1, which played a critical role in ferroptosis through lipid peroxidation. It could

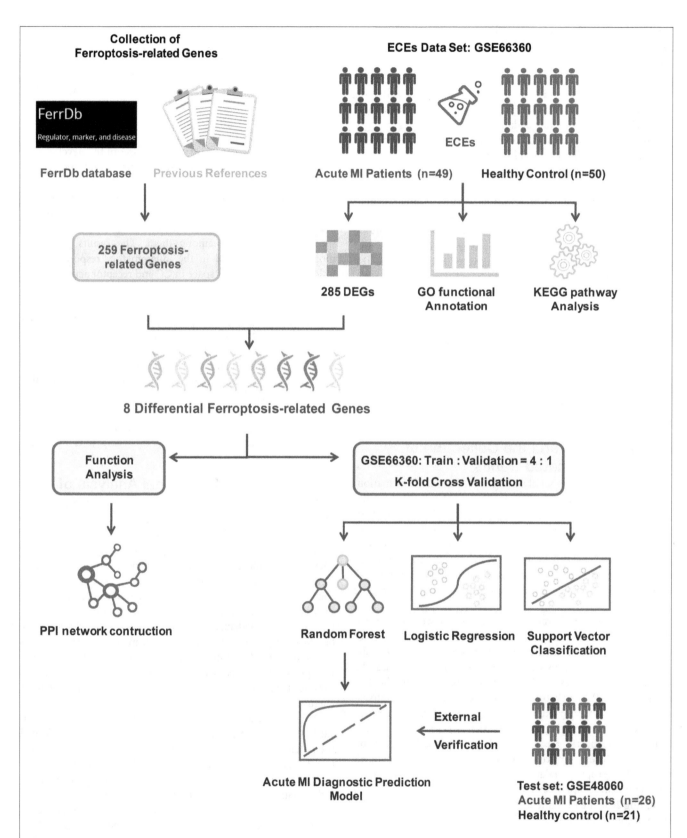

FIGURE 1 | Flow chart of research design and analysis. GSE66360 was applied to analyze differentially expressed genes (DEGs) between acute myocardial infarction (MI) and healthy controls. Ferroptosis-related genes were collected from the FerrDb database and other previous references. After checking the DEGs and the ferroptosis-related genes, eight differential ferroptosis-related genes were selected to perform functional analysis and construct a clinical diagnosis model. Compared with different supervised learning algorithms, including logistic regression and support vector classification, the random forest algorithm was determined to build the acute MI diagnostic model and was confirmed with the external verification of GSE48060.

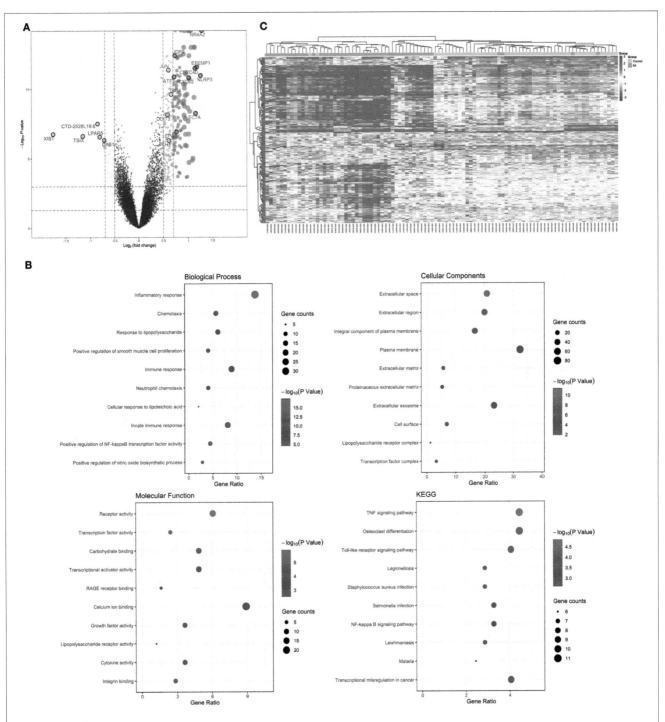

FIGURE 2 | Verification and functional analysis of differentially expressed genes (DEGs) in acute myocardial infarction (MI). **(A)** DEGs in acute MI and control group by the (FC > 1.5 and P < 0.05) cutoff value (top five upregulated genes are marked in red; top five downregulated genes are marked in green; the following differential ferroptosis-related genes are marked in purple); **(B)** gene ontology (GO) enrichment analysis among these DEGs, including biological process (BP), cell composition (CC), and molecular function (MF), and the KEGG pathway enriched by these DEGs; **(C)** the hierarchical clustering of all the DEGs and clinical status.

selectively enrich polyunsaturated lipids by upregulating hypoxia and lipid droplet-related protein. In some tumors, such as clear-cell carcinomas, EPAS1 may even promote the tumor-dependent ferroptotic death procession by recruiting some specific downstream factors (31). Another transcriptional regulator,

JDP2, could activate the expression of inflammatory genes and promote fibrosis, which has been shown as a prognostic marker for MI patients to develop heart failure (32). As a key effector of ferroptosis, TLR4 plays an important role in reducing cardiomyocyte death and improving left ventricular remodeling.

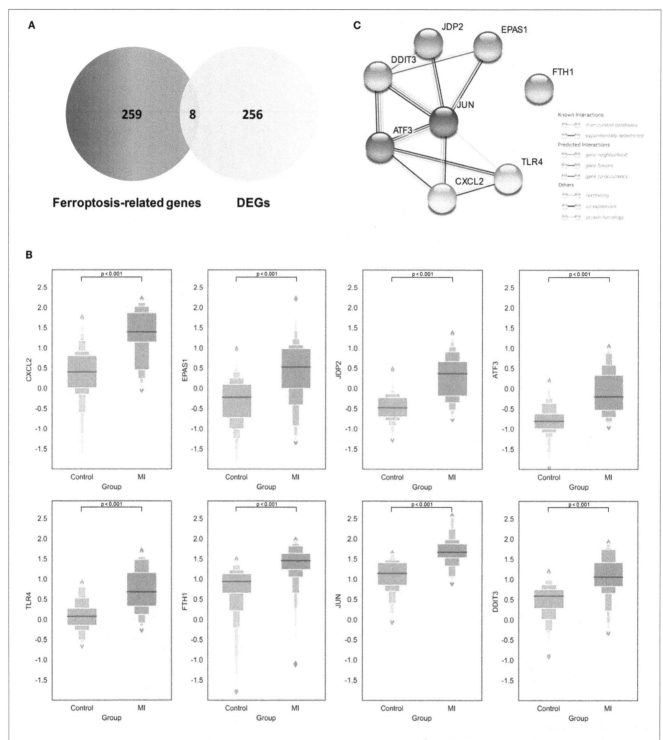

FIGURE 3 | Expression and functional analysis of differential Ferroptosis-related genes in acute myocardial infarction (MI). **(A)** The intersection between the collected ferroptosis-related genes and differentially expressed genes (DEGs) in acute MI; **(B)** the expression of different ferroptosis-related genes between the acute MI and control groups with the two-tailed Student's t-test ($P < 0.05$ as significance); **(C)** the protein–protein interaction (PPI) network on those ferroptosis-related genes.

After knocking down TLR4, autophagy and ferroptosis could be alleviated through the TLR4 and NADPH oxidase 4 (NOX4) pathway, which provides a potential treatment strategy for heart failure (33).

At the same time, the STRING database was used to construct the PPI interaction network of these differential ferroptosis-related proteins (**Figure 3C**). It was revealed that JUN might be the hub node in all eight differential ferroptosis-related

TABLE 1 | Summary of all these differential expressed ferroptosis-related genes in acute myocardial infarction (MI).

Gene	Full name	Role in Ferroptosis	logFC	P-value
CXCL2	C-X-C motif chemokine ligand 2	Marker	1.019	1.51×10^{-11}
EPAS1	Endothelial PAS domain protein 1	Driver	0.770	1.19×10^{-7}
JDP2	Jun dimerization protein 2	Marker	0.736	4.39×10^{-13}
ATF3	Activating transcription factor 3	Driver	0.722	1.33×10^{-11}
TLR4	Toll-like receptor 4	Driver	0.659	2.46×10^{-10}
FTH1	Ferritin heavy chain 1 (FTH1)	Marker	0.614	5×10^{-7}
JUN	AP-1 transcription factor subunit	Suppressor	0.606	4.27×10^{-12}
DDIT3	DNA damage-inducible transcript 3	Marker	0.588	7.1×10^{-9}

genes because it was related to almost all other genes except FTH1. In previous studies, Jun is shown to regulate the ferroptotic cell death with the help of hepatocyte nuclear factor 4 alpha (HNF4A) (16). Our results first report the potential role of Jun in acute MI by mediating abnormal ferroptosis. The following two key nodes are DDIT3 and ATF3, both of which are related to four other differential ferroptosis-related genes. The endoplasmic reticulum is an important organelle for maintaining cell homeostasis. As a key regulator of endoplasmic reticulum stress, DDIT3 is also reported to be involved in the ROS-dependent ferroptotic process (34), but its role in the pathological process of cardiovascular disease still remains unknown. In terms of ATF3, this famous common stress sensor could accelerate the progression of ferroptosis by inhibiting system Xc− (35). Some studies also show that suppressing the expression of ATF3 could improve the prognosis of cardiovascular and cerebrovascular diseases through reducing cell death (36). Meanwhile, the isolation of FTH1 did not make sense. As a regulatory element of cellular iron storage, FTH1 is critical for maintaining intracellular iron homeostasis. Knockout of FTH1 is shown to induce ferroptosis through erastin, sorafenib, and other pathways in various disease models (37) while overexpression of FTH1 could restrain ferritinophagy to reduce ferroptosis (38). Moreover, FTH1-mediated iron metabolism disorder is shown to exacerbate myocardial damage during MI and reduce heart function (39).

Establishment of the Diagnostic Model Based on Differential Ferroptosis-Related Genes

First, PCA was performed on the above differentially expressed ferroptosis-related genes as a dimension reduction strategy. The results demonstrate that the MI and the control groups could be distinguished accurately (Figure 4A), which means that these differential genes might be treated as independent feature parameters for the diagnosis of acute MI. Then, the GSE66360 data set including 49 acute MI patients with strict diagnostic criteria and 50 healthy controls was taken as the training and validation sets (4:1), and the GSE48060 data set including 26 acute MI patients with non-recurrent events and 21 normal controls was treated as the test set.

After utilizing the K-fold cross-validation with cv = 15, the generalization ability of the training set was improved to prevent overfitting. Then, three different supervised machine learning algorithms, including logistic regression, support vector classification, and random forest, were attempted to construct the diagnostic prediction model of acute MI. The evaluating results of all three algorithms is shown in Table 2. The Kolmogorov–Smirnov (KS) values reflect the power of the binary model to classify positive and negative samples. The random forest algorithm is shown to take the leading advantage of distinguishing the two groups with KS = 0.70 in this study, and the KS values of the other two algorithms was 0.60. Admittedly, we also found that the diagnostic accuracy of the random forest model (accuracy = 0.75) was not as good as the other two models (accuracy = 0.80). However, it was far from enough to rely on accuracy to evaluate the diagnostic power, which was easily affected by the bias caused by the imbalance of categories. In other words, the recall rate was another evaluation feature that could not be ignored for diagnosing acute MI. The recall rate of the random forest algorithm (recall = 0.90) was higher than the other two models (recall = 0.80). It was indicated that the random forest model could minimize the missed cases of acute MI, which might provide a sufficient treatment window and significantly improve the prognosis of patients.

In addition, the ROC curves of the validation set from GSE66360 also described that the area under the curve (AUC) of the random forest model was 0.8550, which was higher than AUC = 0.80 and 0.81 of the other two groups (Figure 4B). Hence, the random forest algorithm was selected to further construct the acute MI diagnostic model after comprehensively analyzing all these parameters.

Simultaneously, GSE48060 was used as a test set to externally verify the diagnostic model based on the random forest algorithm. Figure 4D shows the ROC curve verified by external data, and its AUC is 0.7308 (Figure 4C), demonstrating a compelling diagnostic performance. What's more, the confusion matrix was visualized to evaluate the classification model (Figure 4D). Twenty-six patients with MI were correctly classified, and three healthy volunteers were identified as the control group. There was no misidentification of patients with MI as healthy people, which meant that this method could effectively reduce the false negative rate. Admittedly, we also noticed that some healthy people were misclassified as MI (n = 18).

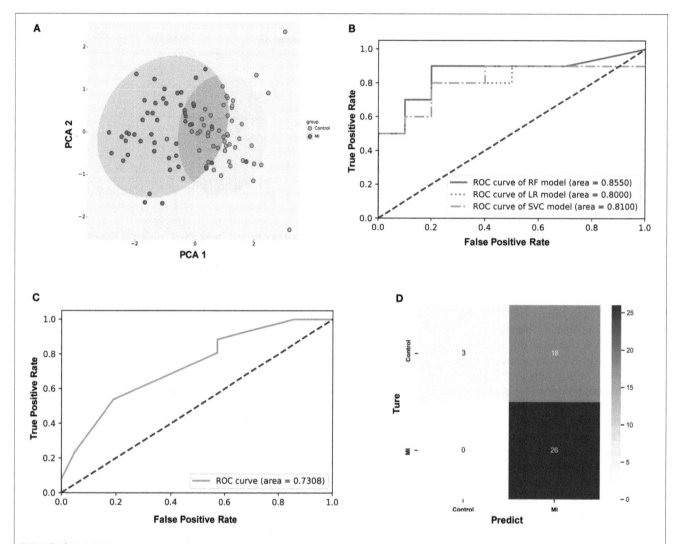

FIGURE 4 | Establishment of the random forest diagnostic model based on differential ferroptosis-related genes in acute myocardial infarction (MI). **(A)** Principal component analysis (PCA) of these differentially expressed ferroptosis-related genes as dimension reduction; **(B)** the comparison of three different supervised learning models (RF, random forest; LR, logistic regression; SVC, support vector classification); **(C)** the diagnostic performance of the predictive model in the test set; **(D)** the confusion matrix of the test set.

TABLE 2 | Comparison of the diagnostic efficacy of three different supervised learning models.

Model	Precision	Recall	F1-score	Accuracy	Error	KS
Random forest	0.69	0.90	0.78	0.75	0.25	0.70
Logistic regression	0.80	0.80	0.80	0.80	0.20	0.60
Support vector classification	0.80	0.80	0.80	0.80	0.20	0.60

CONCLUSION

In this study, we first identified eight differentially expressed ferroptosis-related genes in CECs of patients with acute MI and analyzed their potential functions by means of two GEO data sets. Compared with the performance of different supervised learning models, we established a random forest diagnostic models of MI based on these

ferroptosis-related genes in CECs (AUC = 0.8550) through K-fold cross-validation and verified it with another data set (AUC = 0.7308).

DISCUSSION

With the increase of global aging, how to deal with the medical challenges brought about by aging is a topic of general concern (40). Age-related diseases such as cardiovascular diseases, especially coronary artery diseases, continue to be a major threat to human health in the future. Advances in interventional technology and reperfusion therapy in recent years have effectively improved the prognosis of MI. However, there is still more attention that needs to be paid, and the early diagnosis of MI is still a key factor restricting mortality and prognosis.

As a kind of disease caused by insufficient myocardial perfusion, MI mainly contributes to coronary atherosclerosis. Although the current diagnostic methods are established on a series of biomarkers based on myocardial injury, which cannot give early warning when the myocardium has just appeared insufficient without yet being damaged. Not being a specific feature of MI, myocardial injury in many cardiomyopathies can also interfere with diagnosis in addition to the delayed diagnosis. Therefore, it is imperative to advance the diagnostic window of acute MI and develop diagnostic biomarkers that reflect myocardial hypoperfusion directly (9).

As a novel kind of iron-dependent programmed cell death, ferroptosis was first proposed in 2012 (41). The decrease in the activity of glutathione peroxidase (GPX4) and the depletion of glutathione interrupt the metabolic reaction of lipid oxides, which induces the Fe^{2+} to produce ROS, thereby promoting ferroptosis. Its sensitivity involves a large number of cellular metabolic processes, including amino acid, iron, and polyunsaturated fatty acid metabolism. Hence, the induction of ferroptosis leads to the increase of intracellular lipid ROS, and this regulating process could be inhibited by lipid antioxidants (17). As iron-rich and ROS production–based organelles, mitochondria are considered to be the critical place for ferroptosis with specific lipid precursors. Studies in recent years show that ferroptosis is associated with tumors (42), stroke (12), cerebral hemorrhage (43), and renal failure (44). However, the relationship between MI, especially the vascular endothelium and ferroptosis, still remains unknown.

Artificial intelligence and machine learning are important productivity tools in the twenty-first century (45). Different from traditional biomedical research, artificial intelligence, and machine learning are dedicated to learning natural laws from massive amounts of high-throughput data and then using the natural learned laws to predict unknown data, which are widely used in computer vision (46), natural language processing (47), biological features identification (48), and other fields. In the field of oncology research, a large number of machine learning diagnostic models based on gene expression have been widely developed and applied because samples of cancer can be obtained more conveniently through pathology. However, a majority of clinical prediction models are based on traditional risk factors and biomarkers for model fitting in non-tumor research fields. For example, a retrospective cohort study was used to construct a random forest model for atrial fibrillation diagnosis (49).

By means of machine learning and bioinformatics technology, our study first revealed the differential expression of ferroptosis genes in CECs of patients with acute MI. Meanwhile, all the results were verified in different data sets, which first implied that ferroptosis may be involved in regulating the metabolism

of CECs in acute MI. On one hand, the eight ferroptosis-related genes described in this article have been verified and functionally confirmed through different bioinformatics technologies (GO enrichment analysis, PPI interaction analysis). Among them, CXCL2 (30), JDP2 (32), TLR4 (33), ATF3 (36), and FTH1 (39) are reported to participate in the regulation of a variety of cardiovascular diseases through different pathways, and Jun and DDIT3 were first described to be related to acute MI. All these results provide the direction and cornerstone for subsequent basic experiments to explore the role of ferroptosis regulation mechanism in the pathogenesis of acute MI.

On the other hand, this study constructed a random forest diagnostic model of acute MI through the above eight differentially expressed ferroptosis-related genes in CECs. The AUC of some clinical prediction models is extremely high, and their external verification has unsatisfactory results due to the overfitting caused by the small sample data. In this study, the K-fold cross-validation with cv = 15 was utilized to improve the generalization power. Hence, the variability of AUC between our validation and test sets was small enough to be satisfying. Meanwhile, we compared the performance of three supervised machine learning algorithms, including logistic regression, support vector classification, and random forest. After comprehensively evaluating KS, accuracy, recall, and AUC of all these three algorithms, this random forest model showed good diagnostic performance (AUC = 0.8550) and was validated in different data sets (AUC = 0.7308), which provides new ideas and directions for finding new MI-specific biomarkers in advance of the diagnosis window. What is more, the results of a confusion matrix indicate that this model has a strong ability to eliminate false negative interference, which is critical for MI with a very high fatality rate. Changes of gene expression level are the first step in the occurrence and development of diseases. The application of machine learning to analyze different gene expression levels can help explain the original mechanism of the disease and can build the first line of defense for disease diagnosis and early warning at the same time, which plays a strong guiding role of diseases such as acute MI with rapid disease development, high fatality rate, and no obvious symptoms in the early stage.

Compared with the traditional diagnostic model based on the detection of myocardial injury markers, the new model in this article based on the ferroptosis-related genes of CECs focuses more on reflecting the damage of endothelial function and the non-invasive screening for high-risk populations. Vascular endothelial injury is the key factor and initiating link of atherosclerosis. Normally, the anti-inflammatory system composed of cytokines and endothelial progenitor cells in the body repairs damaged endothelium and blood vessels. However, when the endothelial anti-inflammatory self-repair system is exhausted, endothelial cells develop a series of dysfunctions, including aging, autophagy, apoptosis, ferroptosis, etc. (50, 51), which causes endothelial cells to leave the blood vessel wall and enter circulation, which, in turn, leads to a series of undesirable consequences, such as vascular plaque formation, vascular remodeling, inflammation, vasoconstriction, thrombosis formation, and even plaque rupture. In fact, changes in CECs are important predictors of cardiovascular events before the development of atherosclerotic morphological changes (52). At present, there have been a series of research on the evaluation of CEC functions (53, 54). So far, there is no reliable and recognized gold standard for the detection of functional changes of CECs (55). The identification and integrated analysis of ferroptosis-related genes in CECs in this model are helpful to reflect the early functional changes of CECs, which is ready for judging vascular endothelial function and predicting the occurrence of cardiovascular events, especially for early non-invasive detection of high-risk population screening.

It also cannot be ignored that coronary microcirculation dysfunction, an important independent prognostic factor for cardiovascular events, is inseparably related to functional changes in endothelial cells (56), which can lead to a decrease in coronary blood flow and myocardial perfusion. However, conventional coronary angiography cannot detect microcirculation cracks. At present, the methods for evaluating microcirculation disorders are mainly based on invasive methods, such as fractional flow reserve (FFR), and imaging detection, such as cardiovascular magnetic resonance (CMR). Studies suggest that microvascular occlusion (MVO) is inseparable from the swelling of capillary endothelial cells. The lack of endothelial integrity and functionality leads to the release of large amounts of cytokines, which, in turn, activates neutrophils and platelets, contributing to the formation of microthrombi. In this pathological process, the functional changes of CECs are considered to be an indispensable link. This model based on ferroptosis-related genes in CECs can directly reflect the regulation of ferroptosis-related networks in CECs, which may help determine whether the patient is in the process of MVO and the degree of MVO. In subsequent studies, the inclusion of more data related to MVO patients, such as FFR and CMR data collection, can help enhance the model's advantages in judging microcirculation lesions, which shows a large potential value in early non-invasive and accurate identification of patients with coronary microcirculation disorders.

Meanwhile, models based on CECs not only have important clinical significance for the diagnosis of endothelial function damage, but also play a crucial role in the risk stratification and prognosis of coronary heart disease. Early research on CECs focused on changes in their quantification, and the increase of CEC counts was shown to predict cardiovascular event risk to a large extent among patients with acute coronary syndrome (57), which suggests CECs would be applied for the judgment of long-term prognosis of MI. The development of more biomarker clusters with clinical application potential based on the internal genomics, transcriptomics, and secreted cytokines of CECs is still in its infancy, which is yet an unsolved mystery waiting for people to decipher. Due to the limitation of public data sets, data on patient severity is unfortunately not included in this model. However, according to the model constructed in this article and the support of the previous literature, it is very necessary in the subsequent cohort studies to associate the severity of coronary occlusion or the incidence of long-term cardiovascular events with ferroptosis-related genes in CECs to expand the scope of application of the model.

Of course, this study also has a few shortcomings. First, the biological functions of co-expressed genes have not been further explored through weighted gene co-expression network analysis and other technologies due to the small number of differentially expressed ferroptosis-related genes. Second, this model is not compared with some traditional clinical risk models because we cannot obtain individual specific clinical data from public data sets. This undoubtedly reduces the reliability of our results. However, every coin has two sides. Since the Framingham Study (58) proposed risk stratification for coronary heart disease, various risk scoring systems for coronary heart disease have been quickly built. The GRACE (59) and TIMI (60) risk scoring systems are two relatively representative scoring systems released in recent years. Several independent clinical predictive variables were screened out and applied to divide patients with different risk levels in these scoring systems through multivariate logistic regression analysis of large-scale clinical trials. However, most of the clinical predictive variables screened out rely on epidemiological evidence instead of the pathogenesis of the disease. Therefore, these traditional models can only perform macroscopic stratification without subtly reflecting the real endothelial function status of patients, not to mention achieving the purpose of precision medicine (61). In contrast, this diagnostic model based on ferroptosis-related genes has an irreplaceable advantage in reflecting the patient's immediate endothelial function status. It can provide diagnostic prediction models with pathological progress from the perspective of genetic and molecular pathology. In fact, these two kinds of diagnostic models are absolutely not opposite, and there is no sense comparing them in a single scale. On the contrary, they are complementary to pool their experiences. On one hand, the traditional model provides a macro-level risk assessment based on the past average body state of the patients. On the other hand, the novel gene–related score provides accurate evidence such as immediate and subtle molecular pathological changes for judging the pathological process of the patients. Under this cooperative consensus, future research directions should be to integrate traditional risk and novel gene–related scores and jointly develop a new model in order to help evaluate the patients and guide treatment in the mode of precision medicine. In addition, high-quality data determines the pros and cons of machine learning. The training and validation tests were built on the data set that was matched in both gender and age in the experimental and control groups so that the interference of potential confounding factors on our model could be eliminated. However, other data sources used in this study all come from the GEO database without additional clinical features. In future studies, traditional risk factors, such as age, gender, and hypertension in the cohort could be added to the existing models to construct new combined diagnostic model tools. Meanwhile, this diagnostic model can be further compared with myocardial markers such as cTnT, or a novel diagnostic model could be constructed by these ferroptosis-related genes in CECs combined with cTnT. What is more, there are different subtypes of acute MI (62), and different subtypes need different treatment measures. For example, acute ST-segment elevation MI (STEMI) requires immediate interventional treatment, and some non-ST-segment elevation MI (NSTEMI) could choose selective intervention. Whether ferroptosis-related genes are differentially expressed in these different subtypes of MI and play different regulatory roles remains to be revealed. As is known to all, cardiovascular disease is a complex pathological process involving multiple factors and multilevel biomarkers should be established for different types or stages of the same disease to precise classification and treatment through various machine learning algorithms. In fact, the method of constructing clinical prediction models based on differentially expressed genes related to tumor incidence, metastasis, and prognosis risk via gene chip screening has been widely used in the research of different tumors (63–65). However, a model based on gene-related score in the research of cardiovascular diseases is still in its infancy due to the lack of traditional pathological specimens. Because CECs stand for changes in endothelial cell function to a large extent, enrichment and detection of differential genes may be helpful for assessing vascular endothelial dysfunction, especially identifying the risk of early coronary heart disease. Meanwhile, whether the diagnostic model based on ferroptosis-related gene labels could be practically accessible in clinical practice is worthy of attention. At present, relatively mature CEC rapid enrichment schemes have been constructed (66), and a rapid test kit based on the eight ferroptosis-related genes included in this model could be designed and produced with available test results within 4–6 h. In the next study, the cohort can be expanded to optimize and improve the model, which might reduce the missed diagnosis of early coronary heart disease and acute MI due to the heterogeneity of myocardial enzyme spectrum and the limitations of invasive coronary angiography. It is believed that integrating diverse molecular tags through machine learning can guide clinicians to more reasonable management and treatment of acute coronary syndromes in the future.

There is no doubt that the precision medicine bring about a revolution in the medical world and change the whole clinical practice. With the continuous development of artificial intelligence and machine learning, the discovery and confirmation of biomarker groups becomes possible under the maturity of massive biological information data analysis technology. Fully discovering and verifying the biomarker groups of different types and stages of MI help to comprehensively improve the prediction risk power of cardiovascular and cerebrovascular diseases, thereby reducing the mortality rate and improving the prognosis of MI.

AUTHOR CONTRIBUTIONS

PJ and CY conceived the need for the article. CY finished the analysis and drafted the initial version. SJ helped revise the manuscript. PJ put forward many constructive comments for the final version. CY provided the production of the flowchart. All authors read and approved the manuscript.

REFERENCES

1. Mehta LS, Beckie TM, DeVon HA, Grines CL, Krumholz HM, Johnson MN, et al. Acute myocardial infarction in women: a scientific statement from the American Heart Association. *Circulation.* (2016) 133:916–47. doi: 10.1161/CIR.0000000000000351

2. Auer J, Berent R, Lassnig E, Eber B. C-reactive protein and coronary artery disease. *Jpn Heart J.* (2002) 43:607–19. doi: 10.1536/jhj.43.607

3. Boeddinghaus J, Nestelberger T, Koechlin L, Wussler D, Lopez-Ayala P, Walter JE, et al. Early diagnosis of myocardial infarction with point-of-care high-sensitivity cardiac troponin I. *J Am Coll Cardiol.* (2020) 75:1111–24. doi: 10.1016/j.jacc.2019.12.065

4. Odqvist M, Andersson PO, Tygesen H, Eggers KM, Holzmann MJ. High-sensitivity troponins and outcomes after myocardial infarction. *J Am Coll Cardiol.* (2018) 71:2616–24. doi: 10.1016/j.jacc.2018.03.515

5. Thygesen K, Alpert JS, White HD. Universal definition of myocardial infarction. *J Am Coll Cardiol.* (2007) 50:2173–95. doi: 10.1016/j.jacc.2007.09.011

6. Collet JP, Thiele H, Barbato E, Barthelemy O, Bauersachs J, Bhatt DL, et al. 2020 ESC Guidelines for the management of acute coronary syndromes in patients presenting without persistent ST-segment elevation. *Eur Heart J.* (2020) 42:1289–367. doi: 10.1016/j.rec.2021.05.002

7. White HD, Chew DP. Acute myocardial infarction. *Lancet.* (2008) 372:570–84. doi: 10.1016/S0140-6736(08)61237-4

8. Rakic M, Persic V, Kehler T, Bastiancic AL, Rosovic I, Laskarin G, et al. Possible role of circulating endothelial cells in patients after acute myocardial infarction. *Med Hypotheses.* (2018) 117:42–6. doi: 10.1016/j.mehy.2018.06.005

9. Konijnenberg LSF, Damman P, Duncker DJ, Kloner RA, Nijveldt R, van Geuns RM, et al. Pathophysiology and diagnosis of coronary microvascular dysfunction in ST-elevation myocardial infarction. *Cardiovasc Res.* (2020) 116:787–805. doi: 10.1093/cvr/cvz301

10. Mou Y, Wang J, Wu J, He D, Zhang C, Duan C, et al. Ferroptosis, a new form of cell death: opportunities and challenges in cancer. *J Hematol Oncol.* (2019) 12:34. doi: 10.1186/s13045-019-0720-y

11. Song X, Zhu S, Chen P, Hou W, Wen Q, Liu J, et al. AMPK-mediated BECN1 phosphorylation promotes ferroptosis by directly blocking system Xc(-) activity. *Curr Biol.* (2018) 28:2388–99 e5. doi: 10.1016/j.cub.2018.05.094

12. Alim I, Caulfield JT, Chen Y, Swarup V, Geschwind DH, Ivanova E, et al. Selenium drives a transcriptional adaptive program to block ferroptosis and treat stroke. *Cell.* (2019) 177:1262–79 e25. doi: 10.1016/j.cell.2019.03.032

13. Yang Y, Yang J, Sui F, Huo P, Yang H. Identification of potential molecular mechanisms and candidate genes involved in the acute phase of myocardial infarction. *Cell J.* (2018) 20:435–42. doi: 10.22074/cellj.2018.5213

14. Zhou N, Bao J. FerrDb: a manually curated resource for regulators and markers of ferroptosis and ferroptosis-disease associations. *Database.* (2020) doi: 10.1093/database/baaa021

15. Hassannia B, Vandenabeele P, Vanden Berghe T. Targeting ferroptosis to iron out cancer. *Cancer Cell.* (2019) 35:830–49. doi: 10.1016/j.ccell.2019.04.002

16. Dai C, Chen X, Li J, Comish P, Kang R, Tang D. Transcription factors in ferroptotic cell death. *Cancer Gene Ther.* (2020) 27:645–56. doi: 10.1038/s41417-020-0170-2

17. Stockwell BR, Friedmann Angeli JP, Bayir H, Bush AI, Conrad M, Dixon SJ, et al. Ferroptosis: a regulated cell death nexus linking metabolism, redox biology, and disease. *Cell.* (2017) 171:273–85. doi: 10.1016/j.cell.2017.09.021

18. Bebber CM, Muller F, Prieto Clemente L, Weber J, von Karstedt S. Ferroptosis in cancer cell biology. *Cancers.* (2020) 12:164. doi: 10.3390/cancers12010164

19. Muse ED, Kramer ER, Wang H, Barrett P, Parviz F, Novotny MA, et al. A whole blood molecular signature for acute myocardial infarction. *Sci Rep.* (2017) 7:12268. doi: 10.1038/s41598-017-12166-0

20. Suresh R, Li X, Chiriac A, Goel K, Terzic A, Perez-Terzic C, et al. Transcriptome from circulating cells suggests dysregulated pathways associated with long-term recurrent events following first-time myocardial infarction. *J Mol Cell Cardiol.* (2014) 74:13–21. doi: 10.1016/j.yjmcc.2014.04.017

21. da Huang W, Sherman BT, Lempicki RA. Systematic and integrative analysis of large gene lists using DAVID bioinformatics resources. *Nat Protoc.* (2009) 4:44–57. doi: 10.1038/nprot.2008.211

22. Kanehisa M, Furumichi M, Tanabe M, Sato Y, Morishima K. KEGG: new perspectives on genomes, pathways, diseases and drugs. *Nucleic Acids Res.* (2017) 45:D353–61. doi: 10.1093/nar/gkw1092

23. Szklarczyk D, Franceschini A, Wyder S, Forslund K, Heller D, Huerta-Cepas J, et al. STRING v10: protein-protein interaction networks, integrated over the tree of life. *Nucleic Acids Res.* (2015) 43:D447–52. doi: 10.1093/nar/gku1003

24. Peng H, Luo Y, Ying Y. lncRNA XIST attenuates hypoxia-induced H9c2 cardiomyocyte injury by targeting the miR-122-5p/FOXP2 axis. *Mol Cell Probes.* (2020) 50:101500. doi: 10.1016/j.mcp.2019.101500

25. Li Z, Zhang Y, Ding N, Zhao Y, Ye Z, Shen L, et al. Inhibition of lncRNA XIST improves myocardial I/R injury by targeting mir-133a through inhibition of autophagy and regulation of SOCS2. *Mol Ther Nucleic Acids.* (2019) 18:764–73. doi: 10.1016/j.omtn.2019.10.004

26. Xiao L, Gu Y, Sun Y, Chen J, Wang X, Zhang Y, et al. The long noncoding RNA XIST regulates cardiac hypertrophy by targeting miR-101. *J Cell Physiol.* (2019) 234:13680–92. doi: 10.1002/jcp.28047

27. Aluganti Narasimhulu C, Singla DK. The role of bone morphogenetic protein 7 (BMP-7) in inflammation in heart diseases. *Cells.* (2020) 9:280. doi: 10.3390/cells9020280

28. Li Y, Chen B, Yang X, Zhang C, Jiao Y, Li P, et al. S100a8/a9 signaling causes mitochondrial dysfunction and cardiomyocyte death in response to ischemic/reperfusion injury. *Circulation.* (2019) 140:751–64. doi: 10.1161/CIRCULATIONAHA.118.039262

29. Girbl T, Lenn T, Perez L, Rolas L, Barkaway A, Thiriot A, et al. Distinct compartmentalization of the chemokines CXCL1 and CXCL2 and the atypical receptor ACKR1 determine discrete stages of neutrophil diapedesis. *Immunity.* (2018) 49:1062–76 e6. doi: 10.1016/j.immuni.2018.09.018

30. Yang J, Liu H, Cao Q, Zhong W. Characteristics of CXCL2 expression in coronary atherosclerosis and negative regulation by microRNA-421. *J Int Med Res.* (2020) 48:300060519896150. doi: 10.1177/0300060519896150

31. Zou Y, Palte MJ, Deik AA, Li H, Eaton JK, Wang W, et al. A GPX4-dependent cancer cell state underlies the clear-cell morphology and confers sensitivity to ferroptosis. *Nat Commun.* (2019) 10:1617. doi: 10.1038/s41467-019-09277-9

32. Heger J, Bornbaum J, Wurfel A, Hill C, Brockmann N, Gaspar R, et al. JDP2 overexpression provokes cardiac dysfunction in mice. *Sci Rep.* (2018) 8:7647. doi: 10.1038/s41598-018-26052-w

33. Chen X, Xu S, Zhao C, Liu B. Role of TLR4/NADPH oxidase 4 pathway in promoting cell death through autophagy and ferroptosis during heart failure. *Biochem Biophys Res Commun.* (2019) 516:37–43. doi: 10.1016/j.bbrc.2019.06.015

34. Lee YS, Lee DH, Choudry HA, Bartlett DL, Lee YJ. Ferroptosis-induced endoplasmic reticulum stress: cross-talk between ferroptosis and apoptosis. *Mol Cancer Res.* (2018) 16:1073–76. doi: 10.1158/1541-7786.MCR-18-0055

35. Wang L, Liu Y, Du T, Yang H, Lei L, Guo M, et al. ATF3 promotes erastin-induced ferroptosis by suppressing system Xc(-). *Cell Death Differ.* (2020) 27:662–75. doi: 10.1038/s41418-019-0380-z

36. Huang CY, Chen JJ, Wu JS, Tsai HD, Lin H, Yan YT, et al. Novel link of anti-apoptotic ATF3 with pro-apoptotic CTMP in the ischemic brain. *Mol Neurobiol.* (2015) 51:543–57. doi: 10.1007/s12035-014-8710-0

37. Sun X, Ou Z, Chen R, Niu X, Chen D, Kang R, et al. Activation of the p62-Keap1-NRF2 pathway protects against ferroptosis in hepatocellular carcinoma cells. *Hepatology.* (2016) 63:173–84. doi: 10.1002/hep.28251

38. Tian Y, Lu J, Hao X, Li H, Zhang G, Liu X, et al. FTH1 inhibits ferroptosis through ferritinophagy in the 6-OHDA model of Parkinson's disease. *Neurotherapeutics.* (2020) 17:1796–812. doi: 10.1007/s13311-020-00929-z

39. Nishizawa H, Matsumoto M, Shindo T, Saigusa D, Kato H, Suzuki K, et al. Ferroptosis is controlled by the coordinated transcriptional regulation of glutathione and labile iron metabolism by the transcription factor BACH1. *J Biol Chem.* (2020) 295:69–82. doi: 10.1074/jbc.RA119.009548

40. Yifan C, Jun P. Understanding the clinical features of coronavirus disease 2019 from the perspective of aging: a systematic review and meta-analysis. *Front Endocrinol.* (2020) 11:557333. doi: 10.3389/fendo.2020.557333

41. Dixon SJ, Lemberg KM, Lamprecht MR, Skouta R, Zaitsev EM, Gleason CE, et al. Ferroptosis: an iron-dependent form of nonapoptotic cell death. *Cell.* (2012) 149:1060–72. doi: 10.1016/j.cell.2012.03.042

42. Liang C, Zhang X, Yang M, Dong X. Recent progress in ferroptosis inducers for cancer therapy. *Adv Mater.* (2019) 31:e1904197. doi: 10.1002/adma.201904197

43. Wan J, Ren H, Wang J. Iron toxicity, lipid peroxidation and ferroptosis after intracerebral haemorrhage. *Stroke Vasc Neurol.* (2019) 4:93–5. doi: 10.1136/svn-2018-000205

44. Friedmann Angeli JP, Schneider M, Proneth B, Tyurina YY, Tyurin VA, Hammond VJ, et al. Inactivation of the ferroptosis regulator Gpx4 triggers acute renal failure in mice. *Nat Cell Biol.* (2014) 16:1180–91. doi: 10.1038/ncb3064

45. Goecks J, Jalili V, Heiser LM, Gray JW. How machine learning will transform biomedicine. *Cell.* (2020) 181:92–101. doi: 10.1016/j.cell.2020.03.022

46. Murphy RR. Computer vision and machine learning in science fiction. *Sci Robot.* (2019) 4:eaax7421. doi: 10.1126/scirobotics.aax7421

47. Esteva A, Robicquet A, Ramsundar B, Kuleshov V, DePristo M, Chou K, et al. A guide to deep learning in healthcare. *Nat Med.* (2019) 25:24–9. doi: 10.1038/s41591-018-0316-z

48. Captur G, Heywood WE, Coats C, Rosmini S, Patel V, Lopes LR, et al. Identification of a multiplex biomarker panel for hypertrophic cardiomyopathy using quantitative proteomics and machine learning. *Mol Cell Proteomics.* (2020) 19:114–27. doi: 10.1074/mcp.RA119.001586

49. Hu WS, Hsieh MH, Lin CL. A novel atrial fibrillation prediction model for Chinese subjects: a nationwide cohort investigation of 682 237 study participants with random forest model. *Europace.* (2019) 21:1307–12. doi: 10.1093/europace/euz036

50. Damani S, Bacconi A, Libiger O, Chourasia AH, Serry R, Gollapudi R, et al. Characterization of circulating endothelial cells in acute myocardial infarction. *Sci Transl Med.* (2012) 4:126ra33. doi: 10.1126/scitranslmed.3003451

51. Boos CJ, Balakrishnan B, Blann AD, Lip GY. The relationship of circulating endothelial cells to plasma indices of endothelial damage/dysfunction and apoptosis in acute coronary syndromes: implications for prognosis. *J Thromb Haemost.* (2008) 6:1841–50. doi: 10.1111/j.1538-7836.2008.03148.x

52. Erdbruegger U, Dhaygude A, Haubitz M, Woywodt A. Circulating endothelial cells: markers and mediators of vascular damage. *Curr Stem Cell Res Ther.* (2010) 5:294–302. doi: 10.2174/157488810793351721

53. Chen S, Sun Y, Neoh KH, Chen A, Li W, Yang X, et al. Microfluidic assay of circulating endothelial cells in coronary artery disease patients with angina pectoris. *PLoS ONE.* (2017) 12:e0181249. doi: 10.1371/journal.pone.0181249

54. Budzyn M, Gryszczynka B, Boruczkowski M, Kaczmarek M, Begier-Krasinska B, Osinska A, et al. The potential role of circulating endothelial cells and endothelial progenitor cells in the prediction of left ventricular hypertrophy in hypertensive patients. *Front Physiol.* (2019) 10:1005. doi: 10.3389/fphys.2019.01005

55. Lanuti P, Simeone P, Rotta G, Almici C, Avvisati G, Azzaro R, et al. A standardized flow cytometry network study for the assessment of circulating endothelial cell physiological ranges. *Sci Rep.* (2018) 8:5823. doi: 10.1038/s41598-018-24234-0

56. Bekkers SC, Yazdani SK, Virmani R, Waltenberger J. Microvascular obstruction: underlying pathophysiology and clinical diagnosis. *J Am Coll Cardiol.* (2010) 55:1649–60. doi: 10.1016/j.jacc.2009.12.037

57. Boos CJ, Soor SK, Kang D, Lip GY. Relationship between circulating endothelial cells and the predicted risk of cardiovascular events in acute coronary syndromes. *Eur Heart J.* (2007) 28:1092–1. doi: 10.1093/eurheartj/ehm070

58. Sheridan S, Pignone M, Mulrow C. Framingham-based tools to calculate the global risk of coronary heart disease: a systematic review of tools for clinicians. *J Gen Intern Med.* (2003) 18:1039–52. doi: 10.1111/j.1525-1497.2003.30107.x

59. Granger CB, Goldberg RJ, Dabbous O, Pieper KS, Eagle KA, Cannon CP, et al. Global registry of acute coronary events, Predictors of hospital mortality in the global registry of acute coronary events. *Arch Intern Med.* (2003) 163:2345–53. doi: 10.1001/archinte.163.19.2345

60. Antman EM, Cohen M, Bernink PJ, McCabe CH, Horacek T, Papuchis G, et al. The TIMI risk score for unstable angina/non-ST elevation MI: a method for prognostication and therapeutic decision making. *JAMA.* (2000) 284:835–42. doi: 10.1001/jama.284.7.835

61. Yan AT, Jong P, Yan RT, Tan M, Fitchett D, Chow CM, et al. Canadian Acute Coronary Syndromes registry, Clinical trial–derived risk model may not

generalize to real-world patients with acute coronary syndrome. *Am Heart J* (2004) 148:1020–7. doi: 10.1016/j.ahj.2004.02.014

62. Sandoval Y, Jaffe AS. Type 2 myocardial infarction: JACC review topic of the week. *J Am Coll Cardiol.* (2019) 73:1846–60. doi: 10.1016/j.jacc.2019.02.018

63. Wang J, Chen X, Tian Y, Zhu G, Qin Y, Chen X, et al. Six-gene signature for predicting survival in patients with head and neck squamous cell carcinoma. *Aging.* (2020) 12:767–83. doi: 10.18632/aging.102655

64. Yang H, Liu H, Lin HC, Gan D, Jin W, Cui C, et al. Association of a novel seven-gene expression signature with the disease prognosis in colon cancer patients. *Aging.* (2019) 11:8710–27. doi: 10.18632/aging.102365

65. Chen L, Lu D, Sun K, Xu Y, Hu P, Li X, et al. Identification of biomarkers associated with diagnosis and prognosis of colorectal cancer patients based on integrated bioinformatics analysis. *Gene.* (2019) 692:119–25. doi: 10.1016/j.gene.2019.01.001

66. Bethel K, Luttgen MS, Damani S, Kolatkar A, Lamy R, Sabouri-Ghomi M, et al. Fluid phase biopsy for detection and characterization of circulating endothelial cells in myocardial infarction. *Phys Biol.* (2014) 11:016002. doi: 10.1088/1478-3975/11/1/016002

14

Circulating Vascular Adhesion Protein-1 Level Predicts the Risk of Cardiovascular Events and Mortality in Hemodialysis Patients

Dae Kyu Kim [1†], Yu Ho Lee [2†], Jin Sug Kim [3], Yang Gyun Kim [3], So-Young Lee [2], Shin Young Ahn [4], Dong-Young Lee [5], Kyung Hwan Jeong [3], Sang-Ho Lee [3], Hyeon Seok Hwang [3*] and Ju-Young Moon [3*]

[1] Department of Medicine, Graduate School, Kyung Hee University, Seoul, South Korea, [2] Division of Nephrology, Department of Internal Medicine, CHA Bundang Medical Center, CHA University, Seongnam, South Korea, [3] Division of Nephrology, Department of Internal Medicine, Kyung Hee University, Seoul, South Korea, [4] Division of Nephrology, Department of Internal Medicine, Korea University College of Medicine, Seoul, South Korea, [5] Division of Nephrology, Department of Internal Medicine, Veterans Health Service Medical Center, Seoul, South Korea

*Correspondence:
Hyeon Seok Hwang
hwanghsne@gmail.com
Ju-Young Moon
jymoon@khu.ac.kr

[†] These authors have contributed equally to this work and share first authorship

Background: Vascular adhesion protein-1 (VAP-1) is an oxidative enzyme of primary amines that facilitates the transmigration of inflammatory cells. Its oxidative and inflammatory effects are prominently increased in pathological conditions, such as metabolic, atherosclerotic, and cardiac diseases. However, the clinical significance of circulating VAP-1 levels in hemodialysis (HD) patients is unclear.

Methods: A total of 434 HD patients were enrolled in a prospective multicenter cohort study between June 2016 and April 2019. Plasma VAP-1 levels were measured at the time of data entry, and the primary endpoint was defined as a composite of cardiovascular (CV) and cardiac events.

Results: Circulating VAP-1 levels were positively correlated with plasma levels of cardiac remodeling markers, including brain natriuretic peptide, galectin-3, and matrix metalloproteinase-2. Multivariable logistic regression analysis revealed that patients with higher circulating VAP-1 levels were more likely to have left ventricular diastolic dysfunction [odds ratio, 1.40; 95% confidence interval [CI], 1.04–1.88]. The cumulative event rate of the composite of CV events was significantly greater in VAP-1 tertile 3 than in VAP-1 tertiles 1 and 2 ($P = 0.009$). Patients in tertile 3 were also associated with an increased cumulative event rate of cardiac events ($P = 0.015$), with a 2.06-fold higher risk each for CV (95% CI, 1.10–3.85) and cardiac (95% CI, 1.03–4.12) events after adjusting for multiple variables.

Conclusions: Plasma VAP-1 levels were positively associated with left ventricular diastolic dysfunction and the risk of incident CV and cardiac events in HD patients. Our results indicate that VAP-1 may aid clinicians in identifying HD patients at a high risk of CV events.

Keywords: vascular adhesion protein-1, hemodialysis, cardiovascular disease, endothelial dysfunction, diastolic dysfunction

INTRODUCTION

Patients receiving hemodialysis (HD) have substantial retention of uremic toxins, which lead to a number of adverse metabolic processes (1). Oxidative stress and inflammation are representative pathophysiologic processes of uremic complications and are major contributors of cardiovascular (CV) complications in HD patient (2–5), by promoting myocardial stiffening and left ventricular (LV) hypertrophy and inducing endothelial dysfunction and progression of atherosclerosis (5–7). These conditions severely increase the risk of CV complications, which have become leading causes of death in HD patients (8).

Vascular adhesion protein-1 (VAP-1) is a semicarbazide-sensitive amine oxidase that catalyzes the oxidative deamination of primary amines, which generates free radicals and causes oxidative stress (9, 10). It also facilitates the transmigration of inflammatory cells and worsens injuries in inflamed tissues (9, 11). These deleterious roles are prominently enhanced in pathological conditions. Circulating VAP-1 levels are increased in septic, metabolic, and autoimmune diseases, and higher VAP-1 levels increase the risk of atherosclerotic events and CV mortality (12–14). In patients with impaired renal function, excessive concentrations and abundant substrates of VAP-1 were observed, the latter of which undergo uncontrolled deamination and oxidative stress (14, 15). Furthermore, VAP-1 is suggested to play a pivotal role in HD patients because many dialysis-specific factors upregulate inflammatory processes (15, 16). Therefore, VAP-1 may be critically involved in the occurrence of adverse CV events in HD patients through oxidative stress and inflammation.

However, the clinical significance of VAP-1 has rarely been evaluated in HD patients, and no reports have investigated the prognostic significance of VAP-1. In this study, we investigated the association between circulating VAP-1 levels and risk of incident adverse CV events in HD patients, along with the relationship of echocardiographic parameters and circulating cardiac biomarkers with VAP-1 levels.

MATERIALS AND METHODS

Study Population

All data in this study were obtained from the K-cohort registry, which is a multicenter, internet-based, prospective cohort of HD patients in Korea designed to investigate the prognostic markers of CV complications and mortality. Patients from six general hospitals were enrolled if they were aged >18 years and received regular 4-h HD prescriptions per session that occurred thrice a week for at least 3 months. The exclusion criteria were as follows: pregnancy, hematological malignancy, presence of a solid tumor, and a life expectancy of <6 months. A total of 637 patients were recruited between June 2016 and April 2019, and 434 patients with whole plasma samples at the time of enrollment were included. The study protocol was approved by the local ethics committee (KHNMC 2016-04-039), and the study was conducted in accordance with the principles of the Declaration of Helsinki. All involved participants signed written informed consent forms before enrollment.

The patients were classified into three groups based on the circulating VAP-1 levels as follows: tertile 1, <343.2 ng/mL; tertile 2, 343.2–<438.2 ng/mL; and tertile 3, ≥438.2 ng/mL. All patients were prospectively followed up for specific clinical events after baseline assessments. Patient follow-up was censored at the time of transfer to peritoneal dialysis, kidney transplantation, loss of follow-up, or patient consent withdrawal.

Data Collection and Outcome Measures

Information on baseline demographic factors, laboratory data, dialysis, and concomitant medications were collected from medical records and interviews. Information on comorbidities were investigated and used to calculate the Charlson comorbidity index score (17). Fasting blood samples for laboratory data and enzymatic measurements were collected before the start of HD in a midweek session.

The primary endpoint was a composite of incident CV events and mortality, which included cardiac events such as coronary artery disease requiring coronary artery bypass surgery or percutaneous intervention, myocardial infarction, heart failure, ventricular arrhythmia, cardiac arrest, and sudden death, as well as cerebral infarction, cerebral hemorrhage, and peripheral vascular occlusive diseases requiring revascularization or surgical intervention. All-cause mortality events were recorded. The secondary endpoints were the correlation of VAP-1 levels with LV diastolic dysfunction, which was defined as peak early diastolic flow velocity (E)/peak early diastolic tissue velocity (E') of >15 on echocardiography, and levels of circulating cardiac markers.

Echocardiographic Measurements

Among the enrolled patients, 214 (49.3%) underwent echocardiography [61 (42.4%) in tertile 1, 75 (51.7%) in tertile 2, and 78 (53.8%) in tertile 3]. Cardiologists and trained sonographers examined two-dimensional and M-mode echocardiographs based on the recommendations of the American Society of Echocardiography (18). LV end-diastolic diameter (LVDd), LV end-systolic diameter, LV posterior wall thickness, and interventricular septal thickness were measured in the M-mode echocardiogram. LV mass was estimated using the Devereux formula, with the body surface area as the index. LV end-diastolic and LV end-systolic volumes, LV ejection fraction, and left atrial dimensions were determined in apical two- and four-chamber views. E and peak late diastolic flow velocity (A) was determined from the mitral valve inflow velocity curve using pulsed-wave Doppler ultrasonography. E' was measured from the septal aspect of the mitral annulus using tissue Doppler. The E/A and E/E' ratios were calculated.

Measurements of Circulating Cardiac Markers and VAP-1 Levels

Baseline plasma samples for the measurement of N-terminal pro-B-type natriuretic peptide (NT-proBNP), brain natriuretic peptide (BNP), matrix metalloproteinase-2 (MMP-2), and VAP-1 were collected using ethylenediaminetetraacetic acid-treated tubes. After centrifugation for 15 min at 1,000 × g at room temperature, the samples were stored at 80°C until use. Enzyme-linked immunosorbent assay was performed using Magnetic

Luminex® Screening Assay multiplex kits (R&D Systems, Inc., Minneapolis, MN, USA).

Statistical Analysis

Data are expressed as means ± standard deviations (SDs) or medians (interquartile ranges). Differences among the three groups were identified using analysis of variance or Kruskal-Wallis test. Tukey *post-hoc* test and Mann-Whitney *U*-test with Bonferroni correction were used to identify intergroup differences. Chi-square test or Fisher's exact test was used to compare the categorical variables. Log-transformed high-sensitivity C-reactive protein (hsCRP) values were used because of the skewed data distribution. Correlation between the VAP-1 levels and continuous variables was evaluated using Spearman's analyses. Binary logistic regression analysis was used to assess the association between the VAP-1 levels and LV diastolic dysfunction. A Cox proportional hazards model was constructed to identify independent variables related to CV and cardiac events and all-cause mortality. Parameters significantly associated with weight in the univariable analysis and clinically fundamental parameters were included in the multivariable models. Formal tests for the interaction between VAP-1 levels and predefined subgroups were conducted in addition to the main effects of the fully adjusted models. We modeled the association between VAP-1 levels and the hazard ratio to predict CV events. We used three knots and restricted cubic spline transformations to continuous measures. We calculated the sample size using standard formulas based on the number of patients to obtain the adequate statistical power for the primary endpoint and show a different composite event-free survival rate with an α-level of 0.05, β error of 0.20, and hazard ratio of 1.5. The minimum required sample size in each group was 98 patients. Statistical significance was set at $P < 0.05$. Statistical analyses were performed using the SPSS software (version 22.0; SPSS, IBM Corp., Armonk, NY, USA) and R software (version 3.6.2).

RESULTS

Baseline Demographic Characteristics and Laboratory Data

The mean VAP-1 level was 386.0 (range, 318.1–484.6) ng/mL, with mean VAP-1 levels in tertiles 1, 2, and 3 of 281.8 ng/mL (range, 242.6–318.5 ng/mL), 385.5 ng/mL (range, 365.6–411.0 ng/mL), and 523.6 ng/mL (range, 484.6–601.4 ng/mL), respectively. The baseline clinical characteristics, demographics, and laboratory results are shown in **Table 1**. Patients in tertile 3 had a shorter HD history, higher prevalence of diabetes mellitus, higher Charlson comorbidity index, higher pre-dialysis systolic blood pressure (SBP), and lower intact parathyroid hormone (i-PTH) than those in tertile 1. Regarding the circulating cardiac markers, patients in tertile 3 showed the highest BNP and MMP-2 levels. Plasma MMP-2 levels were moderately correlated with plasma VAP-1 levels, whereas BNP and galectin-3 showed weak positive correlations (**Supplementary Table S1**). In contrast, hsCRP levels demonstrated a weak negative correlation with circulating VAP-1 levels.

Relationship Between Plasma VAP-1 Levels and LV Diastolic Dysfunction in Hemodialysis Patients

Baseline echocardiographic measurements are presented in **Supplementary Table S2**. LVDd was significantly different among the tertiles, with the highest E wave and E/A and E/E' ratios observed in patients in VAP-1 tertile 3. We constructed univariable and multivariable binary logistic regression models to determine the association between VAP-1 and LV diastolic dysfunction (**Table 2**). In the univariable analysis, circulating VAP-1 level increment per SD [dds ratio [OR], 1.51; 95% confidence interval [CI], 1.15–2.00; $P = 0.004$] and Charlson comorbidity index (OR, 1.32; 95% CI, 1.08–1.62; $P = 0.006$) were significantly associated with an increased risk of LV diastolic dysfunction. Age, male sex, pre-dialysis SBP, and NT-proBNP increments per SD showed a borderline significant association with LV diastolic dysfunction. In the multivariable binary logistic regression model, the Charlson comorbidity index (OR, 1.24; 95% CI, 1.01–1.53; $P = 0.045$) and serum VAP-1 level (OR, 1.40; 95% CI, 1.04–1.88; $P = 0.028$) remained statistically significant as independent determinants of LV diastolic dysfunction in HD patients.

Prognostic Utility of the VAP-1 Level in Hemodialysis Patients

During a mean follow-up of 30.3 months, 61 deaths (14.1%) and 77 adverse CV events (17.7%) occurred. Regarding CV events, coronary artery disease occurred in 36 patients, heart failure in 7, ventricular arrhythmia in 1, cardiac arrest in 9, sudden death in 9, CV events in 9, and peripheral vascular occlusive diseases in 6. VAP-1 tertile 3 had the highest cumulative CV event rate ($P = 0.009$; **Figure 1A**) and a greater cumulative rate of cardiac events ($P = 0.015$; **Figure 1B**). The cumulative event rate of patient mortality did not differ among VAP-1 tertiles ($P = 0.747$).

Univariable Cox regression analysis revealed that VAP-1 tertile 3 was significantly associated with an increased risk of the composite of CV events [hazard ratio [HR], 2.51; 95% CI, 1.39–4.54; $P = 0.002$] (**Table 3**). In the multivariable Cox regression analysis, VAP-1 tertile 3 was significantly associated with a 2.06-fold higher risk of CV events (95% CI, 1.10–3.85; $P = 0.025$) and VAP-1 increment per SD was significantly associated with a 1.31-fold higher risk of CV events (95% CI, 1.05–1.64; $P = 0.019$). The risk of cardiac events and patient mortality was further investigated. Patients in VAP-1 tertile 3 had a 2.06-fold higher risk of cardiac disease after adjustment for multiple variables (95% CI, 1.03–4.12; $P = 0.041$). VAP-1 increment per SD was also significantly associated with the risk of cardiac events (HR, 1.29; 95% CI, 1.01–1.64; $P = 0.038$). However, among patients in VAP-1 tertile 3, VAP-1 levels were not significantly associated with the risk of mortality. To evaluate potential linear associations, we evaluated the association between VAP-1 and the risk of composite of CV events and cardiac events during follow-up. The restricted cubic spline model after multiple adjustments showed gradually increasing HRs for both CV and cardiac events with increasing VAP-1 levels (**Figure 2**).

TABLE 1 | Baseline demographic and laboratory data of the study population.

	Tertiles of circulating VAP-1 levels			
	Tertile 1 (<343.2 ng/mL)	Tertile 2 (343.2–438.2 ng/mL)	Tertile 3 (≥438.2 ng/mL)	P-value
Age (years)	60.5 ± 14.9	63.0 ± 12.1	61.6 ± 11.2	0.262
Males, n (%)	93 (64.6)	102 (70.3)	96 (66.2)	0.561
Body mass index (kg/m^2)	23.3 ± 4.1	23.1 ± 3.7	23.5 ± 4.5	0.725
HD duration (years)	4.4 ± 5.8	4.1 ± 5.6	2.7 ± 4.1[a,b]	0.014
History of CV events, n (%)	81 (84)	20 (86)	18 (87)	0.747
Diabetes mellitus, n (%)	45 (31.7)	82 (56.6)[a]	120 (82.8)[a,b]	< 0.001
Charlson comorbidity index	3.6 ± 1.6	4.2 ± 1.6[a]	4.5 ± 1.2[a]	< 0.001
Pre-dialysis SBP (mm Hg)	138.7 ± 20.8	142.0 ± 19.0	147.0 ± 20.1[a]	0.002
Hemoglobin (g/dL)	10.4 ± 1.4	10.6 ± 1.1	10.3 ± 1.1	0.338
Glucose (mg/dL)	139.3 ± 57.9	150.1 ± 61.9	172.6 ± 66.5[a,b]	< 0.001
Albumin (g/dL)	3.8 ± 0.4	3.8 ± 0.3	3.8 ± 0.3	0.515
LDL-C (mg/dL)	79.0 ± 26.9	75.4 ± 26.5	74.3 ± 23.7	0.276
hsCRP (mg/dL)	1.4 (0.2–5.5)	0.8 (0.2–2.9)	0.9 (0.2–2.7)	0.062
i-PTH (pg/mL)	287.0 ± 244.1	292.5 ± 232.3	233.9 ± 165.0[a,b]	0.040
spKt/V	1.6 ± 0.5	1.6 ± 0.3	1.5 ± 0.3	0.219
Catheter as vascular access, n (%)	8 (5.6)	5 (3.4)	7 (4.8)	0.679
Follow-up years	30.8 ± 14.8	29.9 ± 14.4	29.9 ± 14.0	0.823
NT-proBNP (pg/mL)	286 (165–466)	311 (207–431)	335 (226–508)	0.076
BNP (pg/mL)	33.4 (7.6–68.4)	33.4 (6.7–88.3)	55.6 (13.4–108.2)[a]	0.015
Galectin-3 (ng/mL)	16.8 (15.0–20.0)	17.8 (15.1–20.6)	18.2 (15.3–21.4)	0.057
MMP-2 (ng/mL)	577 (478–678)	665 (568–763)	746 (626–897)[a,b]	< 0.001

Data are expressed as means ± standard deviations or medians (interquartile ranges), unless otherwise specified. VAP, vascular adhesion protein; HD, hemodialysis; CV, cardiovascular; LDL-C, low-density lipoprotein cholesterol; i-PTH, intact parathyroid hormone; hsCRP, high-sensitivity C-reactive protein; SBP, systolic blood pressure; NT-proBNP, N-terminal pro-B-type natriuretic peptide; BNP, brain natriuretic peptide; MMP, matrix metalloproteinase.
[a]P < 0.05 vs. tertile 1.
[b]P < 0.05 vs. tertile 2.

The relationship between VAP-1 levels and the composite of incident CV events was further investigated in subgroups stratified by the presence of diabetes mellitus and NT-proBNP levels, with cut-offs defined as median values in each parameter (>386.5 ng/mL for VAP-1 and >313.3 pg/mL for NT-proBNP, respectively; **Table 4**). Multivariable analysis showed that higher VAP-1 levels were associated with an increased risk of CV events both in patients with (HR, 2.39; 95% CI, 1.14–5.03; $P = 0.022$) and without (HR, 2.57; 95% CI, 1.05–6.30; $P = 0.039$) diabetes mellitus. There was a significant interaction between higher VAP-1 levels and diabetes mellitus in association with CV events (HR, 0.51; 95% CI, 0.29–0.90; P for interaction = 0.02). Compared to those with low NT-proBNP levels, patients with high VAP-1 and NT-proBNP levels showed an increased risk of CV events (HR, 1.99; 95% CI, 1.01–3.89; $P = 0.046$), whereas those with isolated high NT-proBNP levels did not show this association. There was no significant interaction between VAP-1 and NT-proBNP levels (HR, 1.57; 95% CI, 0.59–4.18; P for interaction = 0.36).

DISCUSSION

In this prospective cohort study, we investigated the associations of plasma VAP-1 levels with cardiac dysfunction and CV outcomes in HD patients. Plasma VAP-1 levels were positively associated with circulating cardiac biomarker levels and LV diastolic dysfunction. Patients in VAP-1 tertile 3 had the greatest risk of a higher composite of CV events, and this association remained significant after adjusting for established CV risk factors. Taken together, our findings suggest that plasma VAP-1 may be a novel biomarker of incident CV events in HD patients.

High blood pressure and hyperglycemia were representative metabolic disorders that increased plasma VAP-1 levels in individuals without renal impairment (13, 19–23). In the present study, serum glucose level and pre-dialysis SBP were the highest among patients in VAP-1 tertile 3, suggesting that the relationship among blood pressure, serum glucose, and VAP-1 levels is consistent in HD patients. Because VAP-1 promoted the inflammatory process, the positive correlation between plasma VAP-1 levels and hsCRP was expected. However, we showed that the correlation between VAP-1 and hsCRP was negative and the correlation power was highly weak, implying that higher plasma VAP-1 levels may not merely be a secondary reflection of systemic inflammation in HD patients.

LV diastolic dysfunction is commonly identified in HD patients and is associated with high CV mortality (24–28). In this study, the E/E' ratio was used as a criterion for LV diastolic dysfunction because an E/E' ratio of >15 has been reported as a strong predictor of CV events in HD patients (29, 30). We found

TABLE 2 | Relationship between vascular adhesion protein-1 levels and left ventricle diastolic dysfunction.

	Univariable analysis		Multivariable analysis	
	OR (95% CI)	P-value	OR (95% CI)	P-value
Age	1.02 (1.00–1.04)	0.057	1.02 (1.00–1.05)	0.078
Male sex	0.59 (0.33–1.04)	0.066	0.58 (0.32–1.07)	0.083
BMI	1.01 (0.94–1.07)	0.880	–	–
Hemodialysis duration	1.04 (0.96–1.19)	0.362	–	–
Charlson comorbidity index	1.32 (1.08–1.62)	0.006	1.24 (1.01–1.53)	0.045
Pre-dialysis SBP	1.01 (1.00–1.03)	0.063	1.01 (0.99–1.02)	0.327
Hemoglobin	1.08 (0.85–1.37)	0.544	–	–
Albumin	0.62 (0.26–1.48)	0.281	–	–
LDL-C	1.00 (0.99–1.01)	0.365	–	–
hsCRP	1.05 (0.75–1.48)	0.765	–	–
NT-proBNP per SD	1.28 (0.95–1.73)	0.109	1.15 (0.83–1.60)	0.393
VAP-1 per SD	1.51 (1.15–2.00)	0.004	1.40 (1.04–1.88)	0.028

OR, odds ratio; CI, confidence interval; BMI, body mass index; LDL-C, low-density lipoprotein cholesterol; hsCRP, high-sensitivity C-reactive protein; NT-proBNP, N-terminal pro-B-type natriuretic peptide; SD, standard deviation; VAP, vascular adhesion protein.

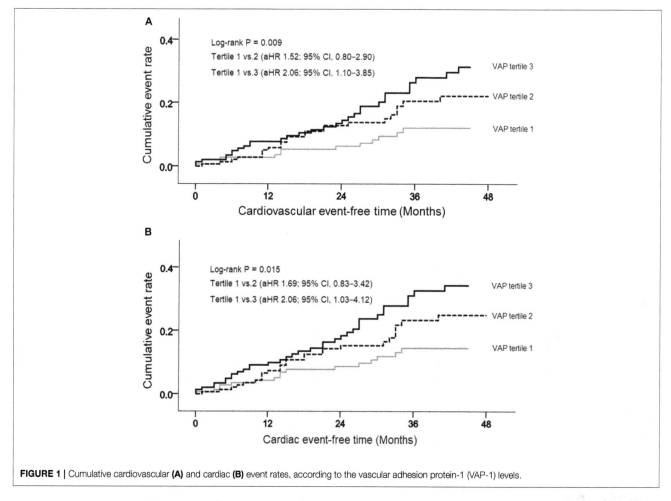

FIGURE 1 | Cumulative cardiovascular **(A)** and cardiac **(B)** event rates, according to the vascular adhesion protein-1 (VAP-1) levels.

that a higher VAP-1 level was independently associated with an increased risk of LV diastolic dysfunction. In addition, higher VAP-1 levels were correlated with an increased risk of cardiac events after adjusting for multiple confounders, indicating that

VAP-1 levels may reflect structural changes in cardiac pathology and that VAP-1 could be a potential biomarker of incident cardiac events in HD patients. Furthermore, we found a significant correlation between plasma VAP-1 and MMP-2, one of the main

TABLE 3 | Hazard ratios of plasma vascular adhesion protein-1 levels for cardiovascular events, cardiac events, and mortality.

	Number of events (%)	Univariable analysis HR (95% CI)	Multivariable analysis HR (95% CI)
Composite of CV events			
VAP-1 tertile 1	16 (11.1)	Reference	
VAP-1 tertile 2	26 (17.9)	1.74 (0.93–3.24)	1.52 (0.80–2.90)
VAP-1 tertile 3	35 (24.1)	2.51 (1.39–4.54)	2.06 (1.10–3.85)
VAP-1 per SD	–	1.40 (1.14–1.71)	1.31 (1.05–1.64)
Cardiac events			
VAP-1 tertile 1	13 (9.0)	Reference	
VAP-1 tertile 2	23 (15.9)	1.90 (0.96–3.75)	1.69 (0.83–3.42)
VAP-1 tertile 3	30 (20.7)	2.66 (1.38–5.10)	2.06 (1.03–4.12)
VAP-1 per SD	–	1.42 (1.14–1.77)	1.29 (1.01–1.64)
Patient deaths			
VAP-1 tertile 1	23 (16.0)	Reference	
VAP-1 tertile 2	20 (13.8)	0.90 (0.50–1.64)	0.85 (0.44–1.65)
VAP-1 tertile 3	18 (12.4)	0.81 (0.44–1.50)	0.86 (0.43–1.72)
VAP-1 per SD	–	0.96 (0.74–1.26)	0.98 (0.72–1.33)

HR, hazard ratio; CI, confidence interval; CV, cardiovascular; SD, standard deviation; VAP, vascular adhesion protein. All analyses were adjusted for the following covariates: age, sex, body mass index, hemodialysis duration, Charlson comorbidity index, pre-dialysis systolic blood pressure, hemoglobin, low-density lipoprotein cholesterol, high-sensitivity C-reactive protein, spKt/V, catheter use, and N-terminal pro-B-type natriuretic peptide.

mediators of pathologic extracellular matrix remodeling and fibrosis in several cardiac diseases (31–33). Previous studies have reported that MMP-2 is involved in LV diastolic dysfunction because circulating MMP-2 levels were correlated with the E/E' ratio (32, 33).

Patients in VAP-1 tertile 3 had a higher cumulative incidence of the composite of CV events than those in VAP-1 tertile 1. In addition, Cox regression analysis showed that high plasma VAP-1 levels were independently associated with a significantly increased risk of CV events, even after adjustments for possible confounders, including SBP and the Charlson comorbidity index. These findings suggest that VAP-1 may be a useful indicator for screening HD patients at a high risk of CV events. Positive correlations of plasma VAP-1 with traditional risk factors, including glucose levels, pre-dialysis SBP, and LV diastolic dysfunction, further support its usefulness in predicting CV outcomes. Notably, plasma VAP-1 levels did not predict all-cause mortality, despite their significant association with CV events. A possible explanation for this discrepancy might be that more than two-third (65.6%) of mortalities in this study were not attributed to CV events.

Subgroup analysis showed that higher plasma VAP-1 levels were associated with an increased risk of CV events in both patients with and without diabetes mellitus. However, the HR of higher VAP-1 levels was lower in HD patients with diabetes mellitus than in HD patients without diabetes mellitus (*P* for interaction = 0.02), indicating that the predictive power of VAP-1 may differ based on the presence of diabetes mellitus. Considering that more HD patients are developing diabetes

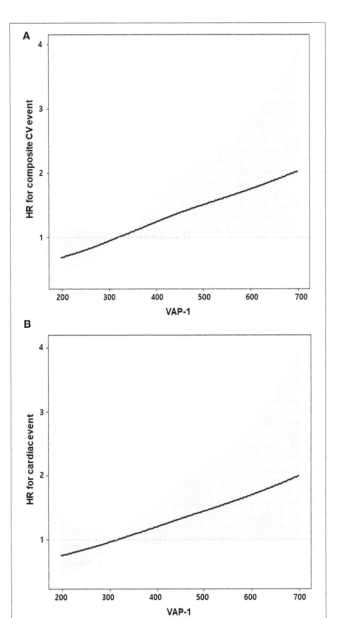

FIGURE 2 | Linear associations of VAP-1 and adjusted risks of the composite of cardiovascular (**A**) and cardiac (**B**) events. Gray shaded areas represent 95% confidence intervals. The adjusted multiple variables were age, sex, body mass index, hemodialysis duration, Charlson comorbidity index, pre-dialysis systolic blood pressure, hemoglobin, low-density lipoprotein cholesterol, high-sensitivity C-reactive protein, spKt/V, catheter use, and N-terminal pro-B-type natriuretic peptide.

mellitus (34, 35), a lower predictive power of plasma VAP-1 levels in this subpopulation could be a disadvantage as a prognostic biomarker of CV events. Although the underlying mechanism of this phenomenon could not be assessed in this study, we speculate that hyperglycemia-induced upregulation of unfavorable molecules, such as plasma proinflammatory cytokines and advanced glycation end products, reduce the relative contributions of plasma VAP-1 to the incidence of CV events (36, 37).

TABLE 4 | Hazard ratios of plasma vascular adhesion protein-1 levels for the composite of cardiovascular events according to predefined subgroups.

	Number of CV events (%)	Univariable analysis HR (95% CI)	Multivariable analysis HR (95% CI)	P for interaction
Diabetes mellitus				0.02
Low VAP-1, without DM	11 (8.1)	Reference		
High VAP-1, without DM	9 (17.6)	2.34 (0.97–5.66)	2.57 (1.05–6.30)	
Low VAP-1, with DM	15 (18.5)	2.45 (1.13–5.34)	1.68 (0.73–3.84)	
High VAP-1, with DM	42 (25.3)	3.67 (1.89–7.14)	2.39 (1.14–5.03)	
NT-proBNP				0.36
Low VAP-1, low NT-proBNP	14 (12.7)	Reference		
High VAP-1, low NT-proBNP	19 (17.8)	1.66 (0.83–3.30)	1.43 (0.71–2.89)	
Low VAP-1, high NT-proBNP	12 (11.2)	0.97 (0.45–2.09)	0.88 (0.40–1.96)	
High VAP-1, high NT-proNBP	32 (29.1)	2.64 (1.41–4.95)	1.99 (1.01–3.89)	

CV, cardiovascular; HR, hazard ratio; CI, confidence interval; VAP, vascular adhesion protein; DM, diabetes mellitus; NT-proBNP, N-terminal pro-B-type natriuretic peptide. High VAP-1 was defined as median value > 386.5 ng/mL, and criteria for predefined subgroups were also based on medians; high NT-proBNP > 313.3 pg/mL. All analyses were adjusted for the following covariates (except for the variable used to define the subgroup in each case): age, sex, body mass index, hemodialysis duration, Charlson comorbidity index, pre-dialysis systolic blood pressure, hemoglobin, low-density lipoprotein cholesterol, high-sensitivity C-reactive protein, spKt/V, catheter use, and N-terminal pro-B-type natriuretic peptide.

The clinical utility of NT-proBNP as a cardiac biomarker in HD patients had been inconclusive, partly because of intra-patient variations and different cut-off values used across studies (38–40). An observational study also reported that elevated NT-proBNP levels are likely caused by intravascular volume expansion rather than cardiac dysfunction in stable HD patients, further complicating the interpretations of its clinical value in HD patients with hypervolemia (41). Our subgroup analysis showed that increased VAP-1 and NT-proBNP levels were associated with a significantly higher risk of composite CV events, whereas isolated NT-proBNP levels were not (**Table 4**). These findings indicate that plasma VAP-1 levels can help differentiate those at a high risk of adverse CV outcomes among HD patients exhibiting increased baseline NT-proBNP levels.

Our study had some limitations. Analyses for individual CV events could not be performed because of the limited number of events and short follow-up period. Echocardiographic data were obtained in a small proportion of enrolled patients (49.3%), although the analysis of available data revealed an evident association between high plasma VAP-1 levels and LV diastolic dysfunction. Moreover, multivariable analysis might not have controlled all relevant confounding factors, and thus these were not thoroughly assessed in this study.

In conclusion, our study demonstrated that plasma VAP-1 levels were associated with circulating markers of cardiac remodeling, as well as a greater risk of LV diastolic dysfunction. In addition, higher plasma VAP-1 levels were correlated with an increased risk of future CV events in HD patients. Our results indicate that VAP-1 might help overcome the limitations of traditional risk factors in the setting of end-stage renal disease and help clinicians identify HD patients at a high risk of CV events.

AUTHOR CONTRIBUTIONS

DKK, YHL, and HSH constructed the research questions and designed the analysis. JSK, YGK, S-YL, SYA, D-YL, KHJ, S-HL, and J-YM conducted the data collection. DKK, YHL, J-YM, and HSH drafted the manuscript. All authors reviewed the results, commented on the manuscript, read, and approved the final manuscript.

ACKNOWLEDGMENTS

All authors acknowledge the support from Patient-Centered Clinical Research Coordinating Center funded by the Ministry of Health and Welfare, Republic of Korea (H19C0481 and HC19C0041).

REFERENCES

1. Rysz J, Franczyk B, Lawinski J, Gluba-Brzozka A. Oxidative stress in ESRD patients on dialysis and the risk of cardiovascular diseases. *Antioxidants.* (2020) 9:1079. doi: 10.3390/antiox9111079

2. Russa D, Pellegrino D, Montesanto A, Gigliotti P, Perri A, Russa A, et al. Oxidative balance and inflammation in hemodialysis patients: biomarkers of cardiovascular risk? *Oxid Med Cell Longev.* (2019) 2019:8567275. doi: 10.1155/2019/8567275

3. Hwang HS, Kim JS, Kim YG, Lee SY, Ahn SY, Lee HJ, et al. Circulating PCSK9 level and risk of cardiovascular events and death in hemodialysis patients. *J Clin Med.* (2020) 9:244. doi: 10.3390/jcm9010244

4. Verma S, Singh P, Khurana S, Ganguly NK, Kukreti R, Saso L, et al. Implications of oxidative stress in chronic kidney disease: a review

on current concepts and therapies. *Kidney Res Clin Pract.* (2021) 40:183–93. doi: 10.23876/j.krcp.20.163

5. Sasaki K, Shoji T, Kabata D, Shintani A, Okute Y, Tsuchikura S, et al. Oxidative stress and inflammation as predictors of mortality and cardiovascular events in hemodialysis patients: the DREAM cohort. *J Atheroscler Thromb.* (2021) 28:249–60. doi: 10.5551/jat.56069

6. Ren H, Zhou X, Luan Z, Luo X, Han S, Cai Q, et al. The relationship between carotid atherosclerosis, inflammatory cytokines, and oxidative stress in middle-aged and elderly hemodialysis patients. *Int J Nephrol.* (2013) 2013:835465. doi: 10.1155/2013/835465

7. Hwang HS, Kim JS, Kim YG, Lee YH, Lee DY, Ahn SY, et al. Circulating neprilysin level predicts the risk of cardiovascular events in hemodialysis patients. *Front Cardiovasc Med.* (2021) 8:684297. doi: 10.3389/fcvm.2021.684297

8. Cozzolino M, Mangano M, Stucchi A, Ciceri P, Conte F, Galassi A. Cardiovascular disease in dialysis patients. *Nephrol Dial Transplant.* (2018) 33:iii28–34. doi: 10.1093/ndt/gfy174

9. Noonan T, Lukas S, Peet GW, Pelletier J, Panzenbeck M, Hanidu A, et al. The oxidase activity of vascular adhesion protein-1 (VAP-1) is essential for function. *Am J Clin Exp Immunol.* (2013) 2:172–85.

10. Salmi M, Jalkanen S. VAP-1: an adhesin and an enzyme. *Trends Immunol.* (2001) 22:211–6. doi: 10.1016/S1471-4906(01)01870-1

11. Salmi M, Jalkanen S. Vascular adhesion protein-1: a cell surface amine oxidase in translation. *Antioxid Redox Signal.* (2019) 30:314–32. doi: 10.1089/ars.2017.7418

12. Aalto K, Havulinna AS, Jalkanen S, Salomaa V, Salmi M. Soluble vascular adhesion protein-1 predicts incident major adverse cardiovascular events and improves reclassification in a finnish prospective cohort study. *Circ Cardiovasc Genet.* (2014) 7:529–35. doi: 10.1161/CIRCGENETICS.113.000543

13. Boomsma F, de Kam PJ, Tjeersma G, van den Meiracker AH, van Veldhuisen DJ. Plasma semicarbazide-sensitive amine oxidase (SSAO) is an independent prognostic marker for mortality in chronic heart failure. *Eur Heart J.* (2000) 21:1859–63. doi: 10.1053/euhj.2000.2176

14. Pannecoeck R, Serruys D, Benmeridja L, Delanghe JR, van Geel N, Speeckaert R, et al. Vascular adhesion protein-1: role in human pathology and application as a biomarker. *Crit Rev Clin Lab Sci.* (2015) 52:284–300. doi: 10.3109/10408363.2015.1050714

15. Wong MY, Saad S, Pollock C, Wong MG. Semicarbazide-sensitive amine oxidase and kidney disease. *Am J Physiol Renal Physiol.* (2013) 305:F1637–44. doi: 10.1152/ajprenal.00416.2013

16. Nemcsik J, Szoko E, Soltesz Z, Fodor E, Toth L, Egresits J, et al. Alteration of serum semicarbazide-sensitive amine oxidase activity in chronic renal failure. *J Neural Transm.* (2007) 114:841–3. doi: 10.1007/s00702-007-0698-4

17. Charlson ME, Pompei P, Ales KL, MacKenzie CR. A new method of classifying prognostic comorbidity in longitudinal studies: development and validation. *J Chronic Dis.* (1987) 40:373–83. doi: 10.1016/0021-9681(87)90171-8

18. Lang RM, Badano LP, Mor-Avi V, Afilalo J, Armstrong A, Ernande L, et al. Recommendations for cardiac chamber quantification by echocardiography in adults: an update from the American Society of Echocardiography and the European Association of Cardiovascular Imaging. *J Am Soc Echocardiogr.* (2015) 28:1–39.e14. doi: 10.1016/j.echo.2014.10.003

19. Aalto K, Maksimow M, Juonala M, Viikari J, Jula A, Kahonen M, et al. Soluble vascular adhesion protein-1 correlates with cardiovascular risk factors and early atherosclerotic manifestations. *Arterioscler Thromb Vasc Biol.* (2012) 32:523–32. doi: 10.1161/ATVBAHA.111.238030

20. Boomsma F, van den Meiracker AH, Winkel S, Aanstoot HJ, Batstra MR, Man in 't Veld AJ, et al. Circulating semicarbazide-sensitive amine oxidase is raised both in type I (insulin-dependent), in type II (non-insulin-dependent) diabetes mellitus and even in childhood type I diabetes at first clinical diagnosis. *Diabetologia.* (1999) 42:233–7. doi: 10.1007/s001250051143

21. Boomsma F, van Veldhuisen DJ, de Kam PJ, Man in't Veld AJ, Mosterd A, Lie KI, et al. Plasma semicarbazide-sensitive amine oxidase is elevated in patients with congestive heart failure. *Cardiovasc Res.* (1997) 33:387–91. doi: 10.1016/S0008-6363(96)00209-X

22. Koc-Zorawska E, Malyszko J, Zbroch E, Malyszko J, Mysliwiec M. Vascular adhesion protein-1 and renalase in regard to diabetes in hemodialysis patients. *Arch Med Sci.* (2012) 8:1048–52. doi: 10.5114/aoms.2012.32413

23. Maciorkowska D, Zbroch E, Malyszko J. Circulating renalase, catecholamines, and vascular adhesion protein 1 in hypertensive patients. *J Am Soc Hypertens.* (2015) 9:855–64. doi: 10.1016/j.jash.2015.08.002

24. Antlanger M, Aschauer S, Kopecky C, Hecking M, Kovarik JJ, Werzowa J, et al. Heart failure with preserved and reduced ejection fraction in hemodialysis patients: prevalence, disease prediction and prognosis. *Kidney Blood Press Res.* (2017) 42:165–76. doi: 10.1159/000473868

25. Unger ED, Dubin RF, Deo R, Daruwalla V, Friedman JL, Medina C, et al. Association of chronic kidney disease with abnormal cardiac mechanics and adverse outcomes in patients with heart failure and preserved ejection fraction. *Eur J Heart Fail.* (2016) 18:103–12. doi: 10.1002/ejhf.445

26. Han JH, Han JS, Kim EJ, Doh FM, Koo HM, Kim CH, et al. Diastolic dysfunction is an independent predictor of cardiovascular events in incident dialysis patients with preserved systolic function. *PLoS ONE.* (2015) 10:e0118694. doi: 10.1371/journal.pone.0118694

27. Smith DH, Thorp ML, Gurwitz JH, McManus DD, Goldberg RJ, Allen LA, et al. Chronic kidney disease and outcomes in heart failure with preserved versus reduced ejection fraction: the Cardiovascular Research Network PRESERVE Study. *Circ Cardiovasc Qual Outcomes.* (2013) 6:333–42. doi: 10.1161/CIRCOUTCOMES.113.000221

28. Hillege HL, Nitsch D, Pfeffer MA, Swedberg K, McMurrayJJ, Yusuf S, et al. Renal function as a predictor of outcome in a broad spectrum of patients with heart failure. *Circulation.* (2006) 113:671–8. doi: 10.1161/CIRCULATIONAHA.105.580506

29. Nagueh SF, Smiseth OA, Appleton CP, Byrd BF III, Dokainish H, Edvardsen T, et al. Recommendations for the evaluation of left ventricular diastolic function by echocardiography: an update from the american society of echocardiography and the european association of cardiovascular imaging. *J Am Soc Echocardiogr.* (2016) 29:277–314. doi: 10.1016/j.echo.2016.01.011

30. Han SS, Cho GY, Park YS, Baek SH, Ahn SY, Kim S, et al. Predictive value of echocardiographic parameters for clinical events in patients starting hemodialysis. *J Korean Med Sci.* (2015) 30:44–53. doi: 10.3346/jkms.2015.30.1.44

31. Ahmed SH, Clark LL, Pennington WR, Webb CS, Bonnema DD, Leonardi AH, et al. Matrix metalloproteinases/tissue inhibitors of metalloproteinases: relationship between changes in proteolytic determinants of matrix composition and structural, functional, and clinical manifestations of hypertensive heart disease. *Circulation.* (2006) 113:2089–96. doi: 10.1161/CIRCULATIONAHA.105.573865

32. Zile MR, Jhund PS, Baicu CF, Claggett BL, Pieske B, Voors AA, et al. Plasma biomarkers reflecting profibrotic processes in heart failure with a preserved ejection fraction: data from the prospective comparison of ARNI with ARB on management of heart failure with preserved ejection fraction study. *Circ Heart Fail.* (2016) 9:e002551 doi: 10.1161/CIRCHEARTFAILURE.115.002551

33. Kobusiak-Prokopowicz M, Krzysztofik J, Kaaz K, Jolda-Mydlowska B, Mysiak A. MMP-2 and TIMP-2 in patients with heart failure and chronic kidney disease. *Open Med.* (2018) 13:237–46. doi: 10.1515/med-2018-0037

34. Oh KH, Kang M, Kang E, Ryu H, Han SH, Yoo TH, et al. The KNOW-CKD study: what we have learned about chronic kidney diseases. *Kidney Res Clin Pract.* (2020) 39:121–35. doi: 10.23876/j.krcp.20.042

35. Jeon HJ, Bae HJ, Ham YR, Choi DE, Na KR, Ahn MS, et al. Outcomes of end-stage renal disease patients on the waiting list for deceased donor kidney transplantation: a single-center study. *Kidney Res Clin Pract.* (2019) 38:116–23. doi: 10.23876/j.krcp.18.0068

36. Schottker B, Herder C, Rothenbacher D, Roden M, Kolb H, Muller H, et al. Proinflammatory cytokines, adiponectin, and increased risk of primary cardiovascular events in diabetic patients with or without renal dysfunction: results from the ESTHER study. *Diabetes Care.* (2013) 36:1703–11. doi: 10.2337/dc12-1416

37. Hegab Z, Gibbons S, Neyses L, Mamas MA. Role of advanced glycation end products in cardiovascular disease. *World J Cardiol.* (2012) 4:90–102. doi: 10.4330/wjc.v4.i4.90

38. Fahim MA, Hayen A, Horvath AR, Dimeski G, Coburn A, Johnson DW, et al. N-terminal pro-B-type natriuretic peptide variability in stable dialysis patients. *Clin J Am Soc Nephrol.* (2015) 10:620–9. doi: 10.2215/CJN.09060914

39. Madsen LH, Ladefoged S, Corell P, Schou M, Hildebrandt PR, Atar D. N-terminal pro brain natriuretic peptide predicts mortality in patients with end-stage renal disease in hemodialysis. *Kidney Int.* (2007) 71:548–54. doi: 10.1038/sj.ki.5002087

40. Vickery S, Price CP, John RI, Abbas NA, Webb MC, Kempson ME, et al. B-type natriuretic peptide (BNP) and amino-terminal proBNP in patients with CKD: relationship to renal function and left ventricular hypertrophy. *Am J Kidney Dis.* (2005) 46:610–20. doi: 10.1053/j.ajkd.2005.06.017

41. Booth J, Pinney J, Davenport A. N-terminal proBNP-marker of cardiac dysfunction, fluid overload, or malnutrition in hemodialysis patients? *Clin J Am Soc Nephrol.* (2010) 5:1036–40. doi: 10.2215/CJN.09001209

15

High Serum Carbohydrate Antigen (CA) 125 Level is Associated with Poor Prognosis in Patients with Light-Chain Cardiac Amyloidosis

Muzheng Li[1†], Zhijian Wu[1†], Ilyas Tudahun[1], Na Liu[1], Qiuzhen Lin[1], Jiang Liu[2], Yingmin Wang[1], Mingxian Chen[1], Yaqin Chen[1], Nenghua Qi[1], Qingyi Zhu[1], JunLi Li[3], Wei Li[4], Jianjun Tang[1] and Qiming Liu[1*]*

[1] Department of Cardiovascular Medicine, The Second Xiangya Hospital of Central South University, Changsha, China,
[2] Department of Cardiovascular Surgery, The Second Xiangya Hospital of Central South University, Changsha, China,
[3] Department of Radiology, The Second Xiangya Hospital of Central South University, Changsha, China, [4] Department of Cardiology, Huaihua Hospital of Traditional Chinese Medicine, Huaihua, China

Correspondence:
Jianjun Tang
tom200210@csu.edu.cn
Qiming Liu
qimingliu@csu.edu.cn

[†] *These authors have contributed equally to this work*

Background and Aims: Patients with light-chain cardiac amyloidosis (AL-CA) are characterized by high levels of serum carbohydrate antigen 125 (CA 125). However, studies have not explored the correlation between CA 125 and AL-CA. The aim of this study was to explore the clinical implications of an increase in CA 125 in patients with AL-CA.

Methods and Results: A total of 95 patients diagnosed with AL-CA at the Second Xiangya Hospital were enrolled in this study. Out of the 95 patients with AL-CA, 57 (60%) patients had elevated serum CA 125 levels. The mean age was 59.7 ± 10.0 years with 44 (77.2%) men in the high serum CA 125 group, and 61.8 ± 9.6 years with 28 (73.7%) men in the normal group. Patients with high CA 125 showed higher rates of polyserositis (79.3% vs. 60.5%, $p = 0.03$), higher levels of hemoglobin (117.4 ± 21.9 g/L vs. 106.08 ± 25.1 g/L, $p = 0.03$), serum potassium (4.11 ± 0.47 mmol/L vs. 3.97 ± 0.40 mmol/L, $p = 0.049$), low-density lipoprotein-cholesterol (3.0 ± 1.6 mmol/L vs. 2.3 ± 1.10 mmol/L, $p = 0.01$), and cardiac troponin T (96.0 pg/mL vs. 91.9 pg/mL, $p = 0.005$). The median overall survival times for patients with high or normal serum CA 125 were 5 and 25 months, respectively ($p = 0.045$). Multivariate Cox hazard analysis showed that treatment without chemotherapy (HR 1.694, 95% CI 1.121–2.562, $p = 0.012$) and CA 125 (HR 1.002, 95% CI 1.000–1.004, $p = 0.020$) was correlated with high all-cause mortality. The time-dependent receiver operating characteristic (t-ROC) curve showed that the prediction accuracy of CA 125 was not inferior to that of cardiac troponin T, N-terminal pro-B-type natriuretic peptide (NT-proBNP), and lactate dehydrogenase (LDH) based on the area under the curve.

Conclusions: CA 125 is a novel prognostic predictor. High serum CA 125 values are correlated with low overall survival, and the accuracy of predicting prognosis is similar to that of traditional biomarkers in AL-CA.

Keywords: light-chain cardiac amyloidosis, CA 125, prognostic predictor, overall survival, biomarkers

INTRODUCTION

Cardiac amyloidosis is a condition of systemic amyloidosis with myocardial involvement. It is caused by the deposition of amyloid proteins derived from misfolded transthyretin or immunoglobulin light-chain in the myocardial interstitium, small vessels, and conduction system. These changes lead to increased ventricular wall thickness, diastolic dysfunction, and arrhythmia. Although more than 30 types of amyloids have been characterized, there are three main types of cardiac amyloidosis, including, acquired monoclonal immunoglobulin light-chain cardiac amyloidosis (AL-CA), wild-type transthyretin amyloidosis (wtTTR-CA), and hereditary transthyretin amyloidosis (hTTR-CA) (1–3). The natural course, treatment, and prognosis of different types of cardiac amyloidosis are different and the diagnosis is performed in late stages and maybe missed (4, 5). Despite the advance in diagnostic and treatment approaches, the exact pathophysiological mechanism of AL-CA has not been elucidated, and the prognosis is extremely poor. Therefore, studies should explore the pathophysiology and clinical aspects of AL-CA.

Previous studies indicated that several biomarkers have a demonstrated diagnostic and/or prognostic value in patients with AL-CA such as cardiac troponin T (6, 7), N-terminal pro-B-type natriuretic peptide (NT-proBNP) (7), D-dimer (8), and lactate dehydrogenase (LDH) (9). However, these biomarkers are easily affected by other conditions such as end-stage liver disease and renal failure. Moreover, the biomarkers staging system cannot accurately stratify the risk of subjects. Therefore, a better prediction biomarker is needed to evaluate the condition of patients and predict the prognosis in clinical practice.

Carbohydrate antigen 125 (CA 125) is a tumor marker associated with ovarian cancer, which is a high-molecular-weight soluble glycoprotein produced by serosal epithelium (10, 11). Increased serum CA 125 levels have also been reported in other malignancies, such as hematological malignant tumors like leukemia and non-Hodgkin's lymphoma, breast and lung cancers, melanoma, and gastrointestinal carcinoma, as well as non-malignant conditions including abdominal surgery, bacterial peritonitis, and tuberculosis (12). Previous studies (13–16) reported that elevated serum CA 125 values are associated with the clinical severity, hemodynamic status, and short-term prognosis of patients with heart failure (HF).

Patients with AL-CA are characterized by a high level of CA125. Currently, the prevalence and implications of increased CA 125 levels in AL-CA are unknown. Therefore, the present study sought to explore the associations between serum CA 125 levels and AL-CA, and systematically evaluated the clinical implications of CA 125 elevation in patients with AL-CA.

PATIENTS AND METHODS

A retrospective analysis was conducted on 170 patients diagnosed with AL-CA in the Second Xiangya Hospital of Central South University, from June 2012 to September 2020. The diagnostic criteria for suspected cardiac amyloidosis are symptoms of HF; echocardiography that indicated the interventricular septum and/or the posterior thickness of left ventricular ≥ 12 mm without any other causes of left ventricular hypertrophy; electrocardiogram that showed low voltage in the limb leads; and positive serum free light chain or blood/urine Bence Jones protein. If the suspected criteria are met, cardiac magnetic resonance (CMR) or tissue biopsies will be performed to confirm the diagnosis. The diagnosis of AL-CA was confirmed based on previous literature reports (5) and described as below: (1) positive serum free light chain or blood/urine Bence Jones protein; (2) the presence of apple-green appearance viewed under cross-polarized light with Congo red staining and tissue typing by immunohistochemistry on tissue biopsies from endocardial myocardial tissue or at least one clinically involved organ, including abdominal fat tissue, bone marrow, kidney, and intestinal mucosa; (3) a typical diffuse subendocardial or transmural late gadolinium enhancement pattern on CMR. The compliance of patients with 1+2 or 1+3 was included in this study. The CA 125 test was completed in 102 patients, and four patients with cancer history (except multiple myeloma [MM]), and three patients with incomplete information were excluded. The demographic and clinical characteristics, comorbidities, baseline data of laboratory tests, electrocardiogram and echocardiography data, and treatment of 95 patients with AL-CA were included as the test group (**Figure 1**). To explore the levels of CA 125 in other diseases, 52 patients with chronic HF (CHF) in the same period were included as one group. AL amyloidosis and MM are plasma cell diseases, and AL amyloidosis is mostly associated with MM (5), therefore, 48 patients who had been diagnosed with MM in the corresponding period were included as another group. Patients with non-cardiac amyloidosis in the two groups, who had a history of cancer diseases and missed CA 125 level data, were excluded. Consequently, the population of the final two groups consisted of 41 and 39 patients.

The study protocol was performed following the ethical guidelines of the Declaration of Helsinki (17). The study was approved by the human research committee of the Second Xiangya Hospital of Central South University.

All patients have undergone venous blood samples for serum levels of CA 125 on the day of admission. Serum CA 125 levels were determined by using electrochemiluminescence (Relia Biotechnology [Jiangsu, China] Co., Ltd), and the cutoff value was set at 35 KU/L.

Follow-up started at the time of diagnosis of AL-CA. The primary endpoint for this study was death from any cause. The survival time (months) was defined as the duration between the diagnosis to the date of death. If the survival time was more than 15 days and <30 days, it would be calculated as 1 month. Data were obtained from medical records or from telephone interviews with patients or relatives by four trained physicians. The last date of follow-up was November 16, 2020. Patients were censored if they were still alive at the end of the research period or were lost to follow-up, on which occasion their last clinic visit or correspondence time was used.

Normally distributed parameters were expressed as mean ± SD, whereas non-normally distributed parameters were expressed as median with interquartile range (Q3-Q1).

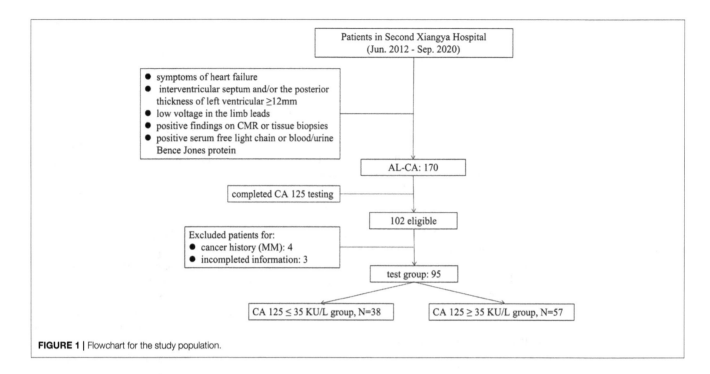

FIGURE 1 | Flowchart for the study population.

Categorical values were presented as numbers (percentages). Categorical variables were compared either with Chi-squared or Fisher's exact test. Comparison of continuous variables between two independent groups was performed using unpaired Student's t-test (if normally distributed) or Mann–Whitney U-test (non-normally distributed variables). One-way ANOVA or Kruskal-Wallis test was used for comparison of more than two groups. Prognostic factors with p-values < 0.05 after univariate Cox regression analysis were subjected to multivariate regression analysis to determine the independent factors of predicting survival according to the forward likelihood ratio method. The overall survival was evaluated with Kaplan-Meier curves, and the log-rank test was used to assess the significance of differences between groups. Time-dependent receiver operating characteristic (t-ROC) was used to reflect the accuracy of different biomarkers in predicting the overall survival at various time points based on the area under the curve (AUC). All tests were two-tailed and a p-value of <0.05 was considered to be statistically significant. Statistical analysis was performed using Statistical Product and Service Solutions (SPSS) 26.0 (IBM Software Inc), Empower Stats 3.0 software, and R (version 3.3.2) software.

RESULTS

Baseline and Characteristics of Patients With AL-CA

The characteristics of 95 patients in the test group were presented in **Table 1**. Out of the 95 patients, 57 (60%) and 38 (40%) patients were placed into high (CA 125 > 35 KU/L) and normal (CA 125 ≤ 35 KU/L) serum CA 125 groups, respectively. The mean age was 59.7 ± 10.0 years with 44 (77.2%) men in the

high serum CA 125 group, and 61.8 ± 9.6 years with 28 (73.7%) men in the normal group. Among all patients with elevated CA 125, 14 (24.5%) patients belonged to New York Heart Association (NYHA) class I-II, whereas 43 (75.5%) patients were at class III-IV. Analysis showed no significant difference in New York Heart Association classification compared with the normal serum CA 125 group ($p = 0.156$). Polyserositis was observed in 46 (80.7%) patients with high serum CA 125 group, compared with 20 (52.6%) patients in the normal CA 125 group ($p = 0.004$). Use of aspirin and furosemide was significantly different between normal and high serum CA 125 groups (28.9% vs. 10.5%, $p = 0.022$; 81.6% vs. 94.7%, $p = 0.041$, respectively). Patients with high serum CA 125 were more likely to present with higher median levels of hemoglobin (117.4 ± 21.9 g/L vs. 106.8 ± 25.1 g/L, $p = 0.032$), serum potassium (4.11 ± 0.47 mmol/L vs. 3.97 ± 0.40 mmol/L, $p = 0.049$), low-density lipoprotein-cholesterol (3.0 ± 1.6 mmol/L vs. 2.3 ± 1.1 mmol/L, $p = 0.031$), cardiac troponin T [96.0 pg/mL (83.3–144.8) vs. 91.6 pg/mL (41.7–96.0), $p = 0.008$], and serum CA 125 [165.4 (114.5–265.9) KU/L vs. 17.9 (11.8–27.3) KU/L, $p < 0.001$] compared with patients with normal serum CA 125. Analysis showed no statistically significant difference in the diameter of atriums and ventricles, the thickness of the ventricular wall, and the ejection fraction. Analysis of ECG showed that patients with elevated CA 125 had lower limb voltage compared with normal CA 125 (76.4% vs. 52.6%, $p = 0.017$).

Level of Serum CA 125 in Different Groups

The level of serum CA 125 in the polyserositis group was higher compared with that in the non-polyserositis group (150.2 ± 150.6 vs. 100.0 ± 140.4, $p = 0.015$). In the palliative care group, the CA 125 level was higher than the chemotherapy group

TABLE 1 | Characteristics of 95 patients with AL-cardiac amyloidosis.

	CA 125 ≤ 35 KU/L N = 38	CA 125 > 35 KU/L N = 57	P-value
Age, years	61.8 (9.6)	59.7 (10.0)	0.329
Male, n (%)	28 (73.7%)	44 (77.2%)	0.696
SBP, mmHg	119.2 (27.7)	109.4 (23.5)	0.067
DBP, mmHg	73.7 (14.0)	69.8 (13.0)	0.179
NYHA, n (%)			0.156
Class I-II	13 (34.2%)	14 (24.5%)	-
Class III-IV	25 (65.8%)	43 (75.5%)	-
Mayo AL 2004 stage, n (%)			0.097
I	2 (5.3%)	0 (0.0%)	-
II	13 (34.2%)	14 (24.6%)	-
IIIa	12 (31.6%)	14 (24.6%)	-
IIIb	11 (28.9%)	29 (50.98%)	-
Comorbidities, n (%)			
Multiple myeloma	15 (39.5%)	14 (24.6%)	0.122
Hypertension	15 (39.5%)	16 (28.1%)	0.246
Hyperlipidaemia	9 (23.7%)	15 (26.3%)	0.772
Polyserositis	20 (52.6%)	46 (80.7%)	**0.004**
T2DM	4 (10.5%)	9 (15.8%)	0.465
Medications, n (%)			
Pacemaker	4 (10.5%)	2 (3.5%)	0.168
Aspirin	11 (28.9%)	6 (10.5%)	**0.022**
Statins	17 (44.7%)	15 (26.3%)	0.063
ACEI or ARB	11 (28.9%)	16 (28.1%)	0.926
Furosemide	31 (81.6%)	54 (94.7%)	**0.041**
Digitalis	7 (18.4%)	12 (21.1%)	0.753
Chemotherapy regimens, n (%)			
Thalidomide	18 (47.4%)	16 (28.1%)	**0.055**
Prednisone or dexamethasone	19 (50.0%)	16 (28.1%)	**0.030**
Bortezomib-based	13 (34.2%)	9 (15.8%)	**0.037**
Melphalan-based	1 (2.6%)	4 (7.0%)	0.348
Palliative care, n (%)	18 (47.4%)	39 (68.4%)	**0.043**
Laboratory results			
Hemoglobin, g/L	106.8 (25.1)	117.4 (21.9)	**0.032**
ALB, g/L	29.7 (6.6)	28.5 (7.1)	0.402
LDH, U/L	261.8 (225.7–317.3)	255.3 (216.8–331.5)	0.258
Potassium, mmol/L	3.97 (0.40)	4.11 (0.47)	**0.049**
Calcium, mmol/L	2.1 (0.2)	2.0 (0.2)	0.064
LDL-C, mmol/L	2.3 (1.1)	3.0 (1.6)	**0.031**
TC, mmol/L	3.8 (1.6)	4.5 (2.5)	0.115
CRP, mg/L	18.6 (25.5)	25.6 (36.9)	0.480
ESR, mm/h	57.7 (39.6)	35.8 (30.8)	**0.011**
Cardiac troponin T, pg/mL	91.9 (41.7–96.0)	96.0 (83.3–144.8)	**0.008**
NT-proBNP, pg/mL	5618.6 (3309.0–10309.5)	8987.0 (4970.3–11649.0)	0.164
D-Dimer, ug/mL	1.52 (1.92)	2.13 (2.40)	0.221
CA 125, KU/L	17.9 (11.8–27.3)	165.4 (114.5–265.9)	**<0.001**
eGFR, mL/(min × 1.73 m^2)	62.8 (35.5)	58.6 (31.8)	0.567
24-h urine protein ≥ 1.0 g/24 h	26 (68.4%)	36 (63.2%)	0.598
Echocardiography			
LVEDd, mm	45.5 (7.2)	43.5 (6.4)	0.160

(Continued)

TABLE 1 | Continued

	CA 125 ≤ 35 KU/L N = 38	CA 125 > 35 KU/L N = 57	P-value
RVEDd, mm	32.6 (5.7)	32.9 (5.1)	0.560
LAESd, mm	40.6 (8.1)	41.2 (9.0)	0.759
RAESd, mm	37.9 (9.1)	39.3 (10.6)	0.514
IVS, mm	13.2 (3.1)	14.1 (3.8)	0.213
LVPW, mm	12.8 (2.9)	13.6 (3.3)	0.238
LVEF (%)	54.9 (8.1)	53.0 (10.2)	0.338
Electrocardiogram			
Atrial fibrillation, n (%)	6 (15.8%)	11 (20.0%)	0.606
Low limb voltage, n (%)	20 (52.6%)	42 (76.4%)	**0.017**
PRWP, n (%)	29 (76.3%)	47 (85.5%)	0.262

Data are (N) Mean (SD) or (N) n (%), Median (Q3–Q1), where N is the total number of patients with available data.
ACEI, Angiotensin-Converting Enzyme Inhibitor; AL-CA, Light-Chain amyloidosis; ALB, Albumin; ARB, Angiotensin Receptor Blocker; ThD/LeD, Thalidomide/Lenalidomide; CA 125, Carbohydrate Antigen 125; T2DM, Type 2 Diabetes Mellitus; ESR, Erythrocyte Sedimentation Rate; CRP, C-Reactive Protein; DBP, Diastolic Blood Pressure; eGFR, estimated Glomerular Filtration Rate; ESR, Erythrocyte Sedimentation Rate; IVS, Interventricular Septum; LAESd, Left Atrium End Systolic diameter; LDH, Lactate Dehydrogenase; LDL-C, Low Density Lipoprotein-Cholesterol; LVEDd, Left Ventricular End Diastolic diameter; LVEF, Left Ventricular Ejection Fraction; LVPW, Left Ventricular Posterior Wall; NT-proBNP, N-terminal pro–B-type Natriuretic Peptide; NYHA, New York Heart Association; PCT, Procalcitoin; PRWP, Poor R-wave progression; RAESd, Right Atrium End Systolic diameter; RVEDd, Right Ventricular End Diastolic diameter; SBP, Systolic Blood Pressure; TC, Total Cholesterol. Bold values are statistical significance p < 0.05.

$(150.8 \pm 153.7$ vs. 109.9 ± 138.7, $p = 0.053)$ as well. CA 125 levels varied among different Mayo AL 2004 stages and were statistically different, with higher Mayo stage associated with higher CA 125 levels [I (6.5 ± 2.6), II (117.1 ± 134.4), IIIa (84.4 ± 77.7), IIIb (185.3 ± 178.0)]. Serum CA 125 levels were not statistically different among different NYHA classifications [I (169.6 ± 175.6), II (134.2 ± 151.5), III (150.6 ± 202.5), IV (119.1 ± 92.2); **Figure 2**].

Further, the levels of CA 125 in different diseases were explored. Clinical characteristics of the test group and the other three groups were shown in **Supplementary Table 1**. Elevated serum CA 125 values were observed in 57 (60.0%) patients in the AL-CA group, with a mean value of 134.9 ± 148.6 KU/L, in 6 (54.5%) patients in the TTR-CA group, with a mean value of 112.4 ± 134.7 KU/L, in 16 (39.0%) patients in the CHF group with a mean value of 45.7 ± 44.9 KU/L and in 3 (7.7%) patients in the MM group with a mean value of 18.9 ± 20.9 KU/L ($p < 0.01$), **Supplementary Figure 1**.

Univariate and Multivariate Predictors of All-Cause Mortality

Prognostic factors for all-cause mortality were explored using univariate and multivariate Cox hazard analyses (**Table 2**). Univariate analysis showed that systolic blood pressure (HR 0.988, 95% CI 0.976–0.997, $p = 0.010$), diastolic blood pressure (HR 0.981, 95% CI 0.965–0.998, $p = 0.025$), palliative care (HR 2.259, 95% CI 1.309–3.898, $p = 0.003$), low-density lipoprotein-cholesterol (HR 1.232, 95% CI 1.039–1.461, $p = 0.017$), total cholesterol (HR 1.163, 95% CI 1.033–1.310, $p = 0.013$), CA 125 (HR 1.002, 95% CI 1.001-1.004, $p = 0.001$), interventricular septum (HR 1.049, 95% CI 1.000–1.136, $p = 0.048$), and left ventricular posterior wall (HR 1.085, 95% CI 1.004–1.174, $p = 0.040$) were statistically significant predictors of overall survival. However, multivariate analysis showed that the only independent predictors were palliative care (HR 2.613, 95% CI 1.300–5.251, $p = 0.007$) and CA 125 (HR 1.002, 95% CI 1.000–1.004, $p = 0.033$).

Kaplan–Meier Analyses of Overall Survival

Patients with high levels of CA 125 were followed up for a median period of 7 months (IQR 1.0–10.2) and those with normal levels were followed-up for a period of 9 months (IQR 1.5–19.0, $p = 0.10$). Forty-six (80.7%) patients died in elevated CA 125 group and 22 (57.9%) patients died in patients with normal CA 125 ($p = 0.016$) during the follow-up period. The median overall survival in patients with high level CA 125 was 5 months (95% CI 3.881–6.119) and 25 months (95% CI 0.602–39.398) in patients with normal CA 125 levels ($p = 0.012$, **Figure 3A**). Patients with palliative care had a median overall survival of only 5 months (95% CI 4.823–7.177). The overall survival was significantly shorter for patients with palliative care compared with 13 months (95% CI 2.103–23.897) in patients receiving chemotherapy ($p = 0.035$, **Figure 3B**).

Biomarkers for Predicting Overall Survival Using t-ROC Analysis

The accuracy of the four biomarkers for predicting overall survival was explored by t-ROC analysis. The AUC of 3-months, 6-months, 12-months, and 24-months overall survival for CA 125 were 0.60, 0.75, 0.75, and 0.77, respectively (**Figure 4A**), compared with NT-proBNP (**Figure 4B**), cardiac troponin T (**Figure 4C**), and LDH (**Figure 4D**).

DISCUSSIONS

AL-CA is the most common type of infiltrative cardiomyopathy. It is characterized by various clinical manifestations such as congestive HF, arrhythmia, orthostatic hypotension, syncope, or

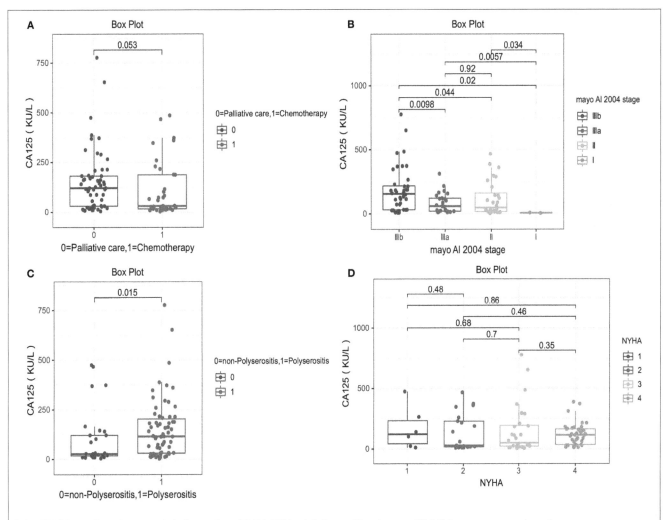

FIGURE 2 | Comparison of serum carbohydrate antigen 125 (CA 125) levels between different groups. **(A)** Palliative care group vs. chemotherapy group (150.8 ± 153.7 vs. 109.9 ± 138.7). **(B)** Mayo AL 2004 stage I (6.5 ± 2.6), II (117.1 ± 134.4), IIIa (84.4 ± 77.7), IIIb (185.3 ± 178.0). **(C)** Polyserositis group vs. non-Polyserositis group (150.2 ± 150.6 vs. 100.0 ± 140.4). **(D)** NHYA I (169.6 ± 175.6), II (134.2 ± 151.5), III (150.6 ± 202.5), IV (119.1 ± 92.2).

even other system expressions like gastrointestinal symptoms, albuminuria, and carpal tunnel syndrome leading to a high rate of missed diagnosis (1). In the present study, we analyzed serum CA 125 levels in 95 consecutive patients with AL-CA at an expertise center in China. To the best of our knowledge, this is the first study to explore the prevalence and evaluate the clinical significance of increased CA 125 levels in patients with AL-CA. The principal results of this study were as follows: (1) serum CA 125 levels were elevated in more than half of patients with AL-CA, compared with those with normal CA 125 levels. Patients who exhibited high serum CA 125 showed higher levels of hemoglobin, LDL-C, TC, and cardiac troponin T, and showed higher rates of polyserositis and low limb voltage compared with those with normal levels of CA 125; (2) patients with polyserositis or those who treated with palliative care seemed to express higher CA 125 levels in AL-CA, and higher Mayo stage was associated with higher CA 125 levels; (3) the values of CA 125 in patients with AL-CA were significantly higher compared with those in patients with CHF and MM; (4) CA 125

was a significant independent predictor of survival, with higher levels independently correlated with lower overall survival; (5) the prediction accuracy of CA 125 was not inferior to that of cardiac troponin T, NT-proBNP, and LDH based on the AUC. In addition, CA 125 seemed to be not affected by the estimated Glomerular Filtration Rate (eGFR) status of patients.

Serum CA 125 values are used for diagnosis and follow-up of patients with ovarian cancer and to evaluate the response to therapy (18, 19). An increase in serum CA 125 has also been observed in other malignancies (20–24) and non-malignant diseases (25–28). The first study on the relationship between CA 125 and the cardiovascular system investigated the association between serum CA 125 levels and pericardial effusion in 1993 (29). Following this, Nägele et al. (16) first revealed that CA 125 may be a valuable tool for monitoring the status and clinical course of patients with HF. A previous study (15) demonstrated that only CA 125 levels were correlated with baseline clinical status in CHF compared with CA 19-9, CA 15-3, carcinoembryonic antigen (CEA), and alpha-fetoprotein

TABLE 2 | Univariate and multivariate Cox hazard analyses of predictors for all-cause mortality.

Variables	Univariate			Multivariate		
	HR	95% CI	*p*-value	HR	95% CI	*p*-value
Male	0.797	0.452–1.407	0.435	-	-	-
Age	1.008	0.986–1.031	0.473	-	-	-
NYHA	1.210	0.941–1.580	0.295	-	-	-
SBP	0.988	0.976–0.997	**0.010**	0.988	0.964–1.011	0.302
DBP	0.981	0.965–0.998	**0.025**	0.995	0.953–1.038	0.995
MM	1.352	0.796–2.298	0.265	-	-	-
Hyperlipidemia	1.650	0.931–2.277	0.105	-	-	-
Polyserositis	1.060	0.633–1.776	0.824	-	-	-
Hemoglobin	1.008	0.999–1.018	0.464	-	-	-
ALB	0.973	0.999–1.019	0.078	-	-	-
Calcium	0.987	0.326–2.985	0.981	-	-	-
eGFR	0.998	0.991–1.006	0.672	-	-	-
Palliative care	2.259	1.309–3.898	**0.003**	2.613	1.300–5.251	**0.007**
LDL-C	1.232	1.039–1.461	**0.017**	0.822	0.439–1.539	0.539
TC	1.163	1.033–1.310	**0.013**	1.365	0.894–2.085	0.149
D-Dimer	1.097	0.989–1.216	0.079	-	-	-
CA 125	1.002	1.001–1.004	**0.001**	1.002	1.000–1.004	**0.033**
IVS	1.049	1.000–1.136	**0.048**	1.033	0.834–1.280	0.767
LVPW	1.085	1.004–1.171	**0.040**	1.029	0.804–1.316	0.820
LVEF	0.979	0.958–1.012	0.280	-	-	-
Low voltage	0.681	0.404–1.148	0.150	-	-	-
PRWP	0.687	0.339–1.392	0.297	-	-	-

HR, hazard ratio; CI, Confidence Interval.
*For other abbreviations, see **Table 1**. Bold values are statistical significance p < 0.05.*

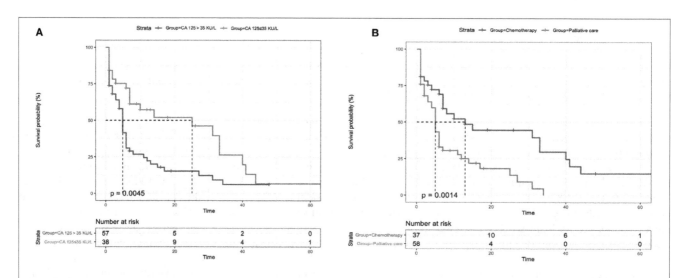

FIGURE 3 | Kaplan-Meier analysis for patients with light-chain cardiac amyloidosis (AL-CA) classified according to serum levels of CA 125 **(A)** and treatment with/without chemotherapy **(B)**. The median overall survival in elevated and normal CA 125 values were 5 months and 25 months, respectively (log rank, *p* = 0.0045). Patients with palliative care had a median overall survival of 5 months while the patients receiving chemotherapy had a median overall survival of 13 months (log-rank, *p* = 0.0014).

(AFP), and the serum CA 125 levels of patients with CHF were significantly higher in NYHA class III/IV compared with those in NYHA class I/II. In addition to CHF, elevated CA 125 values were observed in acute HF (AHF) and have been used to assess 6-months risk stratification in patients admitted with AHF (30). Studies have confirmed that cardiac troponin T and NT-proBNP have significant clinical values in determining the prognosis for newly diagnosed patients with AL-CA. Therefore,

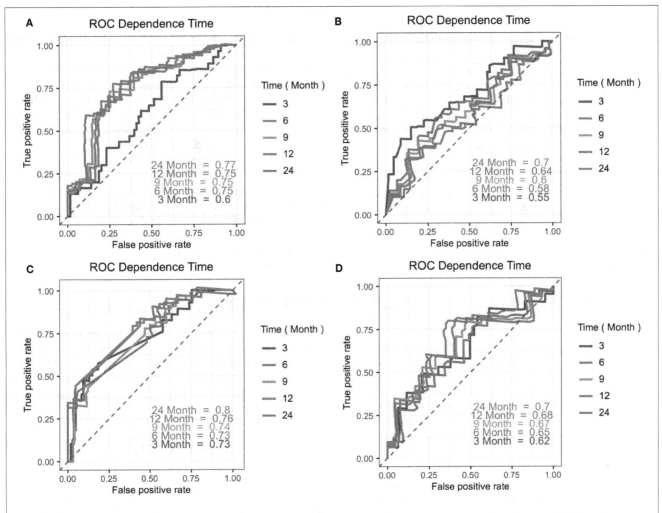

FIGURE 4 | Time-dependent ROC (t-ROC) curves for CA 125 **(A)**, N-terminal pro-B-type natriuretic peptide (NT-proBNP) **(B)**, cardiac troponin T **(C)**, and lactate dehydrogenase (LDH) **(D)** models. The area under the curve (AUC) presented the accuracy of predicting overall survival time (from diagnosis confirmed) for each biomarker at various time points.

the Mayo Clinic established a staging system using the two biomarkers (as well as free light chain) to predict patient outcomes (31, 32). This risk stratification system is also the most commonly used in clinical practice. However, the Mayo AL-stage is tremendously affected by renal function. The values of troponin and NT-proBNP in patients with decreased eGFR are severely overestimated, which leads to the conclusion that this system does not truly reflect the prognosis of patients with AL-CA, and novel prognostic biomarkers need to be continuously explored in clinical practice.

The potential mechanism of serum CA 125 levels elevation in AL-CA remains unclear. Seo et al. (29) reported that among 57 patients with different etiologies of pericardial effusion, 65% of the patients had significantly higher serum CA 125 levels compared with normal patients. Moreover, the levels of CA 125 decreased or normalized with the reduction or disappearance of effusion. In addition, the study used anti-CA 125 antibodies to stain the pericardial tissue obtained through autopsy of 17 patients and showed higher serum CA 125 levels in the

CA 125-positive-stained pericardium compared with those in negative-stained for CA 125. Except for pericardial effusion, elevated serum CA 25 levels have been reported in pleural and peritoneal effusions with non-malignant diseases and reported that CA 125 may be produced from the mesothelial cells of pleura and peritoneum (33–35). These findings were consistent with findings from our study that polyserositis was observed in 80.7% of 57 patients with AL-CA with elevated CA 125 levels, and we also found that patients with polyserositis were more likely to show higher CA 125 values ($p = 0.015$). Studies reported that blood levels of cytokines and/or their receptors, including Interleukin (IL)-6, IL-10, and tumor necrosis factor (TNF)-α, were more likely to be increased in patients with HF, and cytokine network activation is one of the main factors for serum CA 125 elevation in patients with CHF dependent on inflammation (36–38). Serum CA 125 levels with AL-CA were significantly higher in our study compared with those of patients with CHF ($p < 0.01$), although the blood mean levels of CA 125 in CHF were above normal. Analysis showed that only three patients with MM had a mild elevated serum CA 125 levels ($p < 0.01$). Therefore, the effect of plasma cell diseases on CA 125 was excluded. Previous findings and findings from the current study showed that the reasons for the elevation of serum CA 125 levels in AL-CA may be as follows: (1) abnormal deposition of amyloid in the serosal tissue and increased chronic right ventricular filling pressure caused by CHF leading to tissue stretching and stimulation of secretion by mesothelial cells; (2) amyloid activates the cytokine network by inflammation excitation and stimulates the mesothelial cells to produce and secrete CA 125. However, the underlying mechanism linked between CA 125, cytokines, CA 125-producing cells, and AL-CA should be explored further.

Our study revealed that the levels of cardiac troponin T were associated with the serum CA 125 levels. Higher cardiac troponin T levels were observed in the high serum CA 125 group compared with the level in the normal CA 125 group. Patients with elevated serum CA 125 may have more fluid accumulation leading to increased left ventricular filling pressure and polyserositis, thus causing increased wall stress due to diastolic dysfunction and compressed myocardial capillaries, inducing deficient myocardial blood supply and myocardial ischemia (6). In addition, patients with high serum CA 125 values had higher levels of hemoglobin, potassium, LDL-C, and TC. These findings imply that in most of the patients with AL-CA with elevated CA 125 levels, the kidney is involved, and combined with nephrotic syndrome (39), resulting in entry of body fluid to the interstitial space or serous cavity, leading to blood concentration and dyslipidemia. The significant difference between the serum CA 125 levels of low limb voltage can be attributed to serous effusion. However, the pathophysiological mechanisms should be explored in subsequent studies.

CA 125 was significantly correlated with prognosis after adjusting for systolic blood pressure, diastolic blood pressure, treatment without chemotherapy, low-density lipoprotein-cholesterol, total cholesterol, interventricular septum, and left ventricular posterior wall. The median overall survival of high levels of patients with CA 125 was only 5 months, whereas the median overall survival in normal CA 125 levels was 25 months. This finding implies that high levels of serum CA 125 are independently correlated with high mortality in patients with AL-CA. The accuracy of CA 125 in predicting the overall survival was not inferior compared with the classical prognostic biomarkers including cardiac troponin T, NT-proBNP, and LDH. The possible advantages of CA 125 compared with these biomarkers include being easy to obtain, repeatable, no preparations required, and inexpensive cost (<4 dollars per determination in China compared with more than 40 dollars for NT-proBNP). Notably, CA 125-guided therapy (keeping CA 125 levels at 35 KU/L or less by optimizing the use of a diuretic, enforcing the use of statins, and increasing the frequency of monitoring visits) is superior compared with the standard of care for AHF by reducing the risk of 1-year death and the rate of rehospitalization (40). Further studies should adjust the treatment strategy for patients with AL-CA to reduce the myocardial injury, improve the clinical condition of patients, assist chemotherapy, and decrease the rate of mortality and readmission based on serum CA 125 values.

LIMITATIONS

Several limitations of the study need to be addressed. First, the small sample size and information bias may affect the results of our study. Further research should be conducted with a larger sample size and minimize the information bias for more reliable results. Second, the effect of therapies including chemotherapy and palliative care on serum CA 125 levels was not explored, which may have a crucial influence on the evaluation of treatment outcome and short-term prognosis. Third, although analysis showed no significant difference in eGFR between different serum CA 125 levels groups, CA 125 levels were not evaluated in different renal function stages of patients with AL-CA. Notably, a nephrotic syndrome caused by renal involvement of AL-CA leads to fluid retention and polyserositis and may have caused increased serum CA 125. Therefore, further studies should explore the relationship between CA 125 and nephrotic syndrome.

CONCLUSION

The prevalence of elevated serum CA 125 levels is more than 50% in patients with AL-CA. CA 125 is a novel independent prognostic predictor. High serum CA 125 values are correlated with low overall survival and the accuracy of predicting prognosis was not inferior compared with conventional biomarkers.

AUTHOR CONTRIBUTIONS

QLiu and JT designed this study and performed quality control of data authenticity. ML drafted the manuscript. ZW and ML collected and analyzed these data. ML, ZW, IT, and NQ performed follow-up visits. JLi, WL, and QZ provided study guidance and revised the paper. QLin, JLiu, NL, YW, MC, YC, QLiu, and JT revised the paper and all authors approved the final version.

ACKNOWLEDGMENTS

We would like to thank the Home for the research editorial team (www.home-for-researchers.com) provided language emollient assistance during the writing of the manuscript.

SUPPLEMENTARY MATERIAL

Supplementary Figure 1 | Comparison of serum CA 125 levels between different groups. CHF, Chronic Heart Failure; AL-CA, Light-chain Cardiac Amyloidosis; TTR-CA, Transthyretin Amyloidosis; CA 125, Carbohydrate Antigen 125; MM, Multiple Myeloma.

Supplementary Table 1 | Clinical characteristics of several control groups.

REFERENCES

1. Banypersad SM, Moon JC, Whelan C, Hawkins PN, Wechalekar AD. Updates in cardiac amyloidosis: a review. *J Am Heart Assoc.* (2012) 1:e364. doi: 10.1161/JAHA.111.000364

2. Wechalekar AD, Gillmore JD, Hawkins PN. Systemic amyloidosis. *Lancet (London, England).* (2016) 387:2641–54. doi: 10.1016/S0140-6736(15)01274-X

3. Rapezzi C, Merlini G, Quarta CC, Riva L, Longhi S, Leone O, et al. Systemic cardiac amyloidoses: disease profiles and clinical courses of the 3 main types. *Circulation.* (2009) 120:1203–12. doi: 10.1161/CIRCULATIONAHA.108.843334

4. Ruberg FL, Grogan M, Hanna M, Kelly JW, Maurer MS. Transthyretin amyloid cardiomyopathy: JACC state-of-the-art review. *J Am Coll Cardiol.* (2019) 73:2872–91. doi: 10.1016/j.jacc.2019.04.003

5. Falk RH, Alexander KM, Liao R, Dorbala S. AL (Light-Chain) cardiac amyloidosis: a review of diagnosis and therapy. *J Am Coll Cardiol.* (2016) 68:1323–41. doi: 10.1016/j.jacc.2016.06.053

6. Takashio S, Yamamuro M, Izumiya Y, Hirakawa K, Marume K, Yamamoto M, et al. Diagnostic utility of cardiac troponin T level in patients with cardiac amyloidosis. *ESC Heart Failure.* (2018) 5:27–35. doi: 10.1002/ehf2.12203

7. Pregenzer-Wenzler A, Abraham J, Barrell K, Kovacsovics T, Nativi-Nicolau J. Utility of biomarkers in cardiac amyloidosis. JACC. *Heart Fail.* (2020). 8:701–11. doi: 10.1016/j.jchf.2020.03.007

8. Pudusseri A, Sanchorawala V, Sloan JM, Bever KM, Doros G, Kataria S, et al. Prevalence and prognostic value of D-dimer elevation in patients with AL amyloidosis. *Am J Hematol.* (2019) 94:1098–103. doi: 10.1002/ajh.25576

9. He H, Liu J, Jiang H, Du J, Li L, Lu J, et al. High serum lactate dehydrogenase adds prognostic value to cardiac biomarker staging system for light chain amyloidosis. *J Cancer.* (2019) 10:5622–7. doi: 10.7150/jca.30345

10. Kenemans P, Yedema CA, Bon GG, von Mensdorff-Pouilly S. CA 125 in gynecological pathology—a review. *Eur J Obstet Gynecol Reprod Biol.* (1993) 49:115–24. doi: 10.1016/0028-2243(93)90135-Y

11. Högberg T, Kågedal B. Long-term follow-up of ovarian cancer with monthly determinations of serum CA 125. *Gynecol Oncol.* (1992) 46:191–8. doi: 10.1016/0090-8258(92)90254-G

12. Kouris NT, Zacharos ID, Kontogianni DD, Goranitou GS, Sifaki MD, Grassos HE, et al. The significance of CA125 levels in patients with chronic congestive heart failure. Correlation with clinical and echocardiographic parameters. *Eur J Heart Fail.* (2005) 7:199–203. doi: 10.1016/j.ejheart.2004.07.015

13. Duman D, Palit F, Simsek E, Bilgehan K. Serum carbohydrate antigen 125 levels in advanced heart failure: relation to B-type natriuretic peptide and left atrial volume. *Eur J Heart Fail.* (2008) 10:556–9. doi: 10.1016/j.ejheart.2008.04.012

14. D'Aloia A, Faggiano P, Aurigemma G, Bontempi L, Ruggeri G, Metra M, et al. Serum levels of carbohydrate antigen 125 in patients with chronic heart failure: relation to clinical severity, hemodynamic and Doppler echocardiographic abnormalities, and short-term prognosis. *J Am Coll Cardiol.* (2003) 41:1805–11. doi: 10.1016/S0735-1097(03)00311-5

15. Varol E, Ozaydin M, Dogan A, Kosar F. Tumour marker levels in patients with chronic heart failure. *Eur J Heart Fail.* (2005) 7:840–3. doi: 10.1016/j.ejheart.2004.12.008

16. Nägele H, Bahlo M, Klapdor R, Schaeperkoetter D, Rödiger W. CA 125 and its relation to cardiac function. *Am Heart J.* (1999) 137:1044–9. doi: 10.1016/S0002-8703(99)70360-1

17. World Medical Association declaration of Helsinki. Recommendations guiding physicians in biomedical research involving human subjects. *JAMA.* (1997) 277:925–6. doi: 10.1001/jama.277.11.925

18. Canney PA, Moore M, Wilkinson PM, James RD. Ovarian cancer antigen CA125: a prospective clinical assessment of its role as a tumour marker. *Br J Cancer.* (1984) 50:765–9. doi: 10.1038/bjc.1984.254

19. Bates SE. Clinical applications of serum tumor markers. *Ann Intern Med.* (1991) 115:623–38. doi: 10.7326/0003-4819-115-8-623

20. Camera A, Villa MR, Rocco S, De Novellis T, Costantini S, Pezzullo L, et al. Increased CA 125 serum levels in patients with advanced acute leukemia with serosal involvement. *Cancer Am Cancer Soc.* (2000) 88:75–8. doi: 10.1002/(sici)1097-0142(20000101)88:1<75::aid-cncr11>3.0.co;2-#

21. Wu JZ, Tian T, Huang Y, Liang JH, Miao Y, Wang L, et al. Serum carbohydrate antigen 125 concentration as a superior predictor for serosal effusion at diagnosis and a prognostic factor in diffuse large B-cell lymphoma. *Cancer Biomark Sect A Dis Mark.* (2016) 17:205–12. doi: 10.3233/CBM-160632

22. Sakamoto K, Haga Y, Yoshimura R, Egami H, Yokoyama Y, Akagi M. Comparative effectiveness of the tumour diagnostics, CA 19-9, CA 125 and carcinoembryonic antigen in patients with diseases of the digestive system. *GUT.* (1987) 28:323–9. doi: 10.1136/gut.28.3.323

23. Lei Y, Zang R, Lu Z, Zhang G, Huang J, Liu C, et al. ERO1L promotes IL6/sIL6R signaling and regulates MUC16 expression to promote CA125 secretion and the metastasis of lung cancer cells. *Cell Death Dis.* (2020) 11:853. doi: 10.1038/s41419-020-03067-8

24. Yerushalmi R, Tyldesley S, Kennecke H, Speers C, Woods R, Knight B, et al. Tumor markers in metastatic breast cancer subtypes: frequency of elevation and correlation with outcome. *Ann Oncol Off J Eur Soc Med Oncol.* (2012) 23:338–45. doi: 10.1093/annonc/mdr154

25. Talbot RW, Jacobsen DJ, Nagorney DM, Malkasian GD, Ritts RE. Temporary elevation of CA 125 after abdominal surgical treatment for benign disease and cancer. *Surg Gynecol Obstet.* (1989) 168:407–412.

26. Devarbhavi H, Kaese D, Williams AW, Rakela J, Klee GG, Kamath PS. Cancer antigen 125 in patients with chronic liver disease. *Mayo Clin Proc.* (2002) 77:538–41. doi: 10.4065/77.6.538

27. Halila H, Stenman UH, Seppälä M. Ovarian cancer antigen CA 125 levels in pelvic inflammatory disease and pregnancy. *Cancer Am Cancer Soc.* (1986) 57:1327–9.

28. Shin HP, Lee JI, Seo HM, Lim SJ, Jung SW, Cha JM, et al. Laparoscopic appearance in a case of peritoneal tuberculosis with elevated cancer antigen 125 levels. *Gastrointest Endosc.* (2009) 69:180–2. doi: 10.1016/j.gie.2008.03.1079

29. Seo T, Ikeda Y, Onaka H, Hayashi T, Kawaguchi K, Kotake C, et al. Usefulness of serum CA125 measurement for monitoring pericardial effusion. *Jpn Circ J.* (1993) 57:489–94. doi: 10.1253/jcj.57.489

30. Núñez J, Sanchis J, Bodí V, Fonarow GC, Núñez E, Bertomeu-González V, et al. Improvement in risk stratification with the combination of the tumour marker antigen carbohydrate 125 and brain natriuretic peptide in patients with acute heart failure. *Eur Heart J.* (2010) 31:1752–63. doi: 10.1093/eurheartj/ehq142

31. Kumar S, Dispenzieri A, Lacy MQ, Hayman SR, Buadi FK, Colby C, et al. Revised prognostic staging system for light chain amyloidosis incorporating cardiac biomarkers and serum free light chain measurements. *J Clin Oncol Off J Am Soc Clin Oncol.* (2012) 30:989–95. doi: 10.1200/JCO.2011.38.5724

32. Lilleness B, Ruberg FL, Mussinelli R, Doros G, Sanchorawala V. Development and validation of a survival staging system incorporating BNP in patients with light chain amyloidosis. *Blood.* (2019) 133:215–23. doi: 10.1182/blood-2018-06-858951

33. Bergmann JF, Bidart JM, George M, Beaugrand M, Levy VG, Bohuon C. Elevation of CA 125 in patients with benign and malignant ascites. *Cancer Am Cancer Soc.* (1987) 59:213–7.

34. Epiney M, Bertossa C, Weil A, Campana A, Bischof P. CA125 production by the peritoneum: *in-vitro* and in-vivo studies. *Hum Reprod (Oxford, England).* (2000) 15:1261–5. doi: 10.1093/humrep/15.6.1261

35. Sevinc A, Buyukberber S, Sari R, Kiroglu Y, Turk HM, Ates M. Elevated serum CA-125 levels in hemodialysis patients with peritoneal, pleural, or pericardial fluids. *Gynecol Oncol.* (2000) 77:254–7. doi: 10.1006/gyno.2000.5776

36. Deswal A, Petersen NJ, Feldman AM, Young JB, White BG, Mann DL. Cytokines and cytokine receptors in advanced heart failure: an analysis of the cytokine database from the Vesnarinone trial (VEST). *Circulation.* (2001) 103:2055–9. doi: 10.1161/01.CIR.103.16.2055

37. Kosar F, Aksoy Y, Ozguntekin G, Ozerol I, Varol E. Relationship between cytokines and tumour markers in patients with chronic heart failure. *Eur J Heart Fail.* (2006) 8:270–4. doi: 10.1016/j.ejheart.2005.09.002

38. Stanciu AE, Stanciu MM, Vatasescu RG. NT-proBNP and CA 125 levels are associated with increased pro-inflammatory cytokines in coronary sinus serum of patients with chronic heart failure. *Cytokine.* (2018) 111:13–9. doi: 10.1016/j.cyto.2018.07.037

39. Sevinc A, Buyukberber S, Sari R, Turk HM, Ates M. Elevated serum CA-125 levels in patients with nephrotic syndrome-induced ascites. *Anticancer Res.* (2000) 20:1201–3. doi: 10.1006/gyno.1999.5670

16

Identification of CALU and PALLD as Potential Biomarkers Associated with Immune Infiltration in Heart Failure

Xing Liu [1†], Shiyue Xu [2†], Ying Li [3†], Qian Chen [1], Yuanyuan Zhang [1*] and Long Peng [1*]

[1] Department of Cardiovascular Medicine, The Third Affiliated Hospital, Sun Yat-sen University, Guangzhou, China,
[2] Department of Hypertension and Vascular Disease, The First Affiliated Hospital, Sun Yat-sen University, Guangzhou, China,
[3] Department of Dermatology, Guangzhou Eighth People's Hospital, Guangzhou Medical University, Guangzhou, China

*Correspondence:
Yuanyuan Zhang
zhangyy67@mail.sysu.edu.cn
Long Peng
pengl5@mail.sysu.edu.cn

[†] These authors have contributed equally to this work

Background: Inflammatory activation and immune infiltration play important roles in the pathologic process of heart failure (HF). The current study is designed to investigate the immune infiltration and identify related biomarkers in heart failure patients due to ischemic cardiomyopathy.

Methods: Expression data of HF due to ischemic cardiomyopathy (CM) samples and non-heart failure (NF) samples were downloaded from gene expression omnibus (GEO) database. Differentially expressed genes (DEGs) between CM and NF samples were identified. Single sample gene set enrichment analysis (ssGSEA) was performed to explore the landscape of immune infiltration. Weighted gene co-expression network analysis (WGCNA) was applied to screen the most relevant module associated with immune infiltration. The diagnostic values of candidate genes were evaluated by receiver operating curves (ROC) curves. The mRNA levels of potential biomarkers in the peripheral blood mononuclear cells (PBMCs) isolated from 10 CM patients and 10 NF patients were analyzed to further assess their diagnostic values.

Results: A total of 224 DEGs were identified between CM and NF samples in GSE5406, which are mainly enriched in the protein processing and extracellular matrix related biological processes and pathways. The result of ssGSEA showed that the abundance of dendritic cells (DC), mast cells, natural killer (NK) CD56dim cells, T cells, T follicular helper cells (Tfh), gammadelta T cells (Tgd) and T helper 2 (Th2) cells were significantly higher, while the infiltration of eosinophils and central memory T cells (Tcm) were lower in CM samples compared to NF ones. Correlation analysis revealed that Calumenin (CALU) and palladin (PALLD) were negatively correlated with the abundance of DC, NK CD56dim cells, T cells, Tfh, Tgd and Th2 cells, but positively correlated with the level of Tcm. More importantly, CALU and PALLD were significantly lower in PBMCs from CM patients compared to NF ones.

Conclusion: Our study revealed that CALU and PALLD are potential biomarkers associated with immune infiltration in heart failure due to ischemic cardiomyopathy.

Keywords: heart failure, ischemic cardiomyopathy, inflammatory activation, biomarker, diagnosis

INTRODUCTION

Heart failure refers to the complex clinical syndrome and the end-stage manifestations of cardiovascular disease (1, 2). Large-scale epidemiological analysis shows that the global prevalence of HF is on the rise due to the aging of the population and the progress in the diagnosis and treatment of cardiovascular diseases. In developed countries, the prevalence of HF is 1.5–2.2% (3). The latest report in China shows that the prevalence of HF among residents ≥35 years old is 1.3%, that is, there are ~13.7 million patients (3).Therefore, HF has always been a hot spot in the field of cardiovascular research.

HF is caused by the complicated interaction of myocardial damage, neurohormonal activation, inflammatory response, and renal dysfunction (4–6). During the process, the cytoskeletal and membrane associated proteins are increased and disorganized, while the contractile myofilaments and sarcomeric proteins are decreased in the heart (7). In addition, cardiomyocytes in the failing heart display impaired excitation-contraction coupling due to the decreased calcium transients, enhanced diastolic sarcoplasmic reticulum (SR) calcium leak and diminished SR calcium sequestration (8). Although the pathogenesis of HF is still perplexing, the persistent inflammation and immune abnormalities are believed to participate in the pathogenesis across the spectrum of HF (9). Elevated and long-lasting leukocyte recruitment mediated by G protein-coupled receptor kinase 5 (GRK5) in the injured heart is reported to be associated with chronic cardiac inflammation and heart failure (10). Moreover, evidence indicates that transcriptome changes in immune cells could affect the prognosis of HF. DNA methyltransferase 3 alpha (DNMT3A) mutations in monocytes significantly increase the expression of inflammatory genes and are correlated with the aggravation of chronic HF (11). Metabolically active genes such as fatty acid binding protein 5 (FABP5) are highly enriched in classical monocytes from heart failure patients, whereas b-catenin expression was significantly higher in another functionally distinct monocyte subset ($CD14^{++}CD16^{+}$ intermediate monocytes) (12). These studies suggest that further understanding of the inflammatory response and immune cell infiltration in HF is of great significance for optimizing the diagnosis and treatment of heart failure.

In recent years, microarray technology and integrated bioinformatics analyses have been performed to identify novel genes related to various diseases that might act as diagnostic and prognostic biomarkers (13–15). However, the diagnostic value of genes associated with immune infiltration in heart failure remains unclear. Thus, in the current study, we downloaded two microarray datasets of HF from the GEO database and used bioinformatic methods to screen for immune infiltration related biomarkers in heart failure, and to provide a theoretical basis for the diagnosis and treatment of HF patients.

MATERIALS AND METHODS

Ethics Statement

This study was approved by the institutional review board of the Third Affiliated Hospital, Sun Yat-sen University (IRB: 202102-201-01).

Data Source

In the current study, gene expression profiles of 16 non-failure controls (NF) and 108 heart failure samples caused by ischemic cardiomyopathy (CM) in GSE5406 dataset and 14 NF and 13 CM samples in GSE116250 dataset were downloaded from GEO database.

Identification and Functional Enrichment Analysis of DEGs

Limma R package was used to identify DEGs between NF and CM samples with |log2FC| >0.5 and adjusted $p < 0.05$ in GSE5406 datasets. ClusterProfiler R package was applied for GO and KEGG pathway enrichment analyses of DEGs. Biological process (BP), molecular function (MF) and cellular component (CC) were included in the GO analysis.

ssGSEA

ssGSEA was performed by Gene Set Variation Analysis (GSVA) R package to analyze the infiltraion of 24 immune cells in NF and CM samples (16). The 24 immune cells were TFH, Th2 cells, B cells, T cells, Tgd, NK CD56dim cells, Tem, macrophages, neutrophils, Th1 cells, mast cells, cytotoxic cells, DC, iDC, eosinophils, T helper cells, aDC, TReg, pDC, NK CD56bright cells, NK cells, Th17 cells, CD8 T cells, and Tcm.

WGCNA Analysis

A sample clustering tree map was first constructed to detect and eliminate outliers. Then, WGCNA was performed based on the gene expression profiles from GSE5406 dataset and sample traits (differentially infiltrated immune cells between NF and CM samples). The pick Soft Threshold function of WGCNA was used to calculate β from 1 to 20 in order to select the best soft threshold. Based on the selected soft threshold, the adjacency matrix was converted to topological overlap matrix to construct the network, and the gene dendrogram and module color were established by using the degree of dissimilarity. We further divided the initial module by dynamic tree cutting and merged similar modules. The Pearson correlation coefficient between the module eigengenes and sample traits were calculated to find out the most relevant module (hub module) associated with sample traits.

Identification of Biomarkers in CM

First, DEGs were intersected with genes from the hub module in WGCNA analysis to obtain immune infiltration related candidate genes. Next, gene signature was selected by least absolute shrinkage and selection operator (LASSO) algorithm using glmnet R package (17) and support vector machine-recursive feature elimination (SVM-RFE) method using e1071 package (18), respectively. Robust gene signature was identified by overlapping gene signature obtained from LASSO and SVM-RFE. The diagnostic values of gene signature were evaluated by receiver operating curves (ROC) curves. Then, the external validation dataset GSE116250 was used to verify the expressions and diagnostic values of gene signature identified in GSE5406. Validated gene signature was identified as robust diagnostic biomarkers in heart failure.

Functional Analysis of Biomarkers in CM

To investigate the potential mechanisms of diagnostic biomarkers in regulating heart failure, 108 patients in GSE5406 were divided into high- and low-expression groups based on the median expression of each diagnostic biomarker. Moreover, to explore the relationship between diagnostic biomarkers and immune infiltration, the correlations between the expressions of diagnostic biomarkers and the abundance of differentially infiltrated immune cells were calculated.

Subject Characteristics and Realtime-PCR

Patients aged 18 and older, diagnosed with CHD by coronary computed tomography angiography or coronary angiography, with ejection fraction of 40% or less were enrolled into CM group. Age-matched CHD patients without heart failure (ejection fraction of 50% or above) were enrolled into NF control group. Patients with a history of malignancy, acute coronary syndrome, pulmonary embolism, renal failure [Glomerular filtration rate <60 ml/(min·1.73 m^2)] were excluded. The characteristics of CM and NF patients were shown in **Supplementary Table 3**.

RNA of PBMCs from CM ($n = 10$, 7 male and 3 female) and NF ($n = 10$, 8 male and 2 female) patients were extracted using Nuclezol LS RNA Isolation Reagent (ABP Biosciences Inc.) according to manufacturer's instructions. Collected RNA was diluted using nuclease-free water and electrophoresed on a denaturing formaldehyde agarose gel to visualize rRNA and ensure overall sample quality. RNA concentrations and purity were detected on ultraviolet spectrophotometer (Jinghua, Shanghai, China). Reverse transcription was performed on 1 μg total RNA from each sample using the SureScript-First-strand-cDNA-synthesis-kit (GeneCopoeia) according to manufacturer's instructions, and a CFX96 Real-time PCR System (Bio-Rad) was utilized to conduct the real time quantitative PCR (qPCR) reactions. BlazeTaq^{TM} SYBR$^®$ Green qPCR Mix 2.0 (GeneCopoeia) was used for qPCR reactions, using 4 μL cDNA and appropriate volumes of specific primers in a final 10 μL volume. Triplicate reactions were performed to ensure accuracy. Glyceraldehyde-3-phosphate dehydrogenase (GAPDH) was used

TABLE 1 | Primers sequence.

Genes	Forward	Reverse
CALU	GTTTCTTATGTGCCTGTCCCT	TTCCTTGCTCTCTTCTGGTGT
PALLD	GCCTACTTTCCTCCTGTTTTT	AGTGGTCATTGTTGGATTCTC
GAPDH	CGCTGAGTACGTCGTGGAGTC	GCTGATGATCTTGAGGCTGTTGTC

as the reference gene, and the relative gene expression was quantified by the $2^{-\Delta\Delta CT}$ method (19). The primer sequences were given in **Table 1**.

Statistical Analysis

All data were analyzed by R software (version 4.0.0). Wilcoxon test was used to compare the data between two groups, and significant difference was considered as $p < 0.05$ unless specified.

RESULTS

Transcriptome Profile Analyses of NF and CM Samples

A total of 224 DEGs were identified in GSE5406, including 93 up-regulated and 131 down-regulated genes in CM group compared to NF group (**Figure 1A**). The expression profile of top 50 up-regulated DEGs and top 50 down-regulated DEGs were shown in the heatmap (**Figure 1B**). To investigate the biological function of DEGs, we performed GO and KEGG pathway analysis. A total of 217 BP, 42 CC, 37 MF, and 16 KEGG pathways were significantly enriched (**Supplementary Tables 1, 2**). As shown in **Figure 1C**, DEGs were mainly enriched into protein processing and extracellular matrix (ECM) related BPs, including response to topologically incorrect protein, response to unfolded protein (UPR), "de novo" protein folding, protein folding, chaperone-mediated protein folding, extracellular matrix organization, extracellular structure organization, "de novo" posttranslational protein folding, chaperone cofactor-dependent protein refolding, response to mechanical stimulus. Consistent with the results of GO analysis, protein processing and ECM related pathways were significantly enriched, including protein processing in endoplasmic reticulum, ECM-receptor interaction, and focal adhesion. In addition, estrogen signaling and MAPK signaling pathways showed to have close relationship with heart failure (**Figure 1D**).

Identification of Immune Infiltration Pattern in CM

Mounting evidence suggest that immune cells play important roles in heart failure (14–16). Thus, we explored the profile of immune cell infiltration in CM and NF samples by ssGSEA. Twenty-four subpopulations of infiltrated immune cells in CM and NF samples were identified and presented in the heatmap (**Figure 2A**). Interestingly, we found that the abundance of DC, mast cells, NK CD56dim cells, T cells, Tfh, Tgd, and Th2 cells were significantly higher, while the infiltration of eosinophils and Tcm were significantly

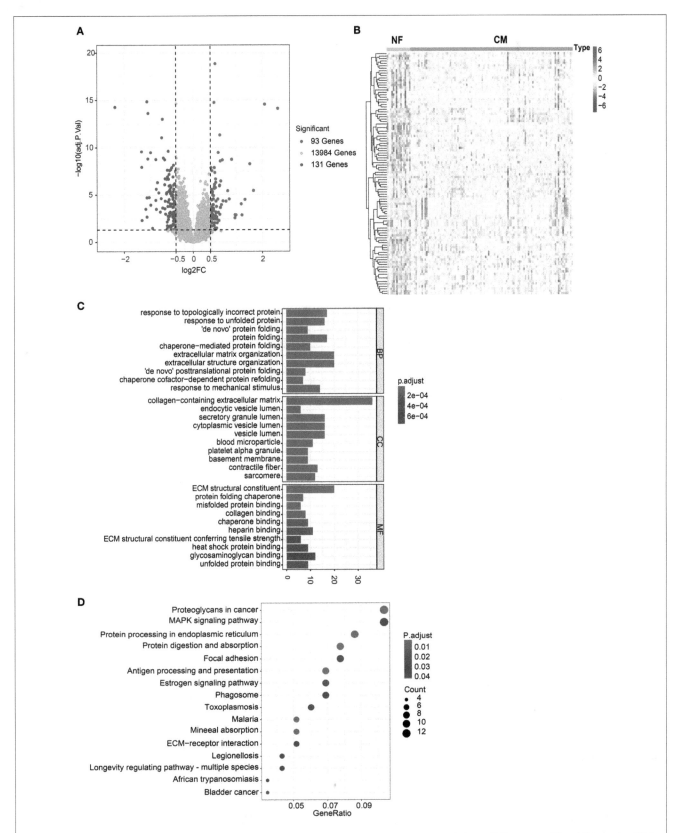

FIGURE 1 | Comprehensive analyses of the transcriptome profiles of NF and CM samples. **(A)** Volcano plot of significant DEGs between NF and CM samples. **(B)** A heatmap of the top 50 significantly upregulated or downregulated DEGs. **(C)** Bar plot of top 10 enriched GO terms of DEGs in each category. BP, biological process; CC, cellular components; MF, molecular functions. **(D)** Bubble plot of significantly enriched KEGG pathways of DEGs.

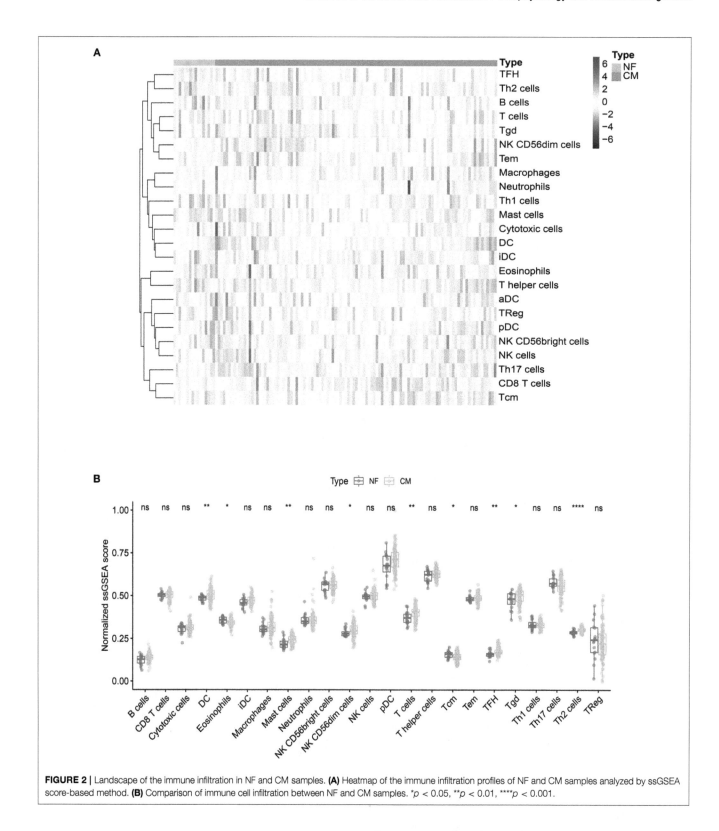

FIGURE 2 | Landscape of the immune infiltration in NF and CM samples. **(A)** Heatmap of the immune infiltration profiles of NF and CM samples analyzed by ssGSEA score-based method. **(B)** Comparison of immune cell infiltration between NF and CM samples. *$p < 0.05$, **$p < 0.01$, ****$p < 0.001$.

lower in CM samples compared to NF ones (**Figure 2B**). These results indicate that the inflammatory response of these immune cells may be critical for the etiology of heart failure.

Screening for Gene Signature of Immune Infiltration in CM

To further explore the genes mostly correlated with the inflammatory response in CM, we performed WGCNA

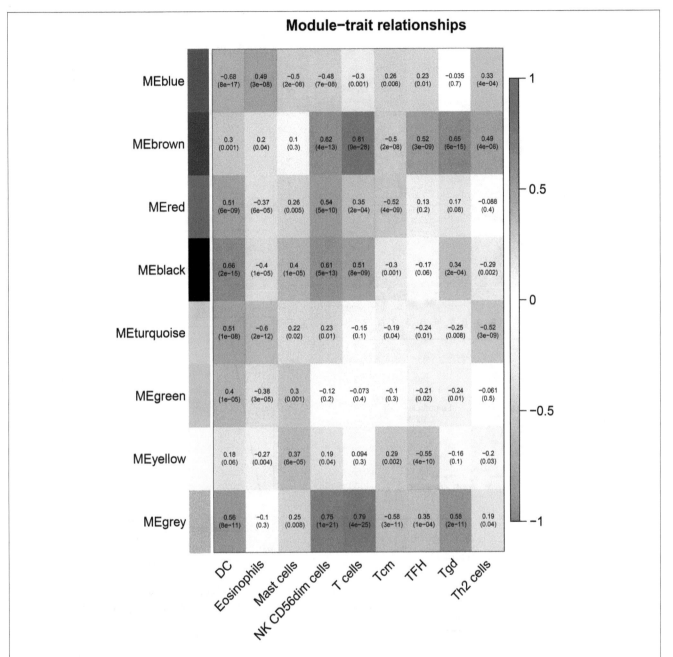

FIGURE 3 | Screening of the hub module associated with immune infiltration in CM. Heatmap of the correlation between module eigengene and differentially infiltrated immune cells. Each row represents a color-coded module eigengene, each column represents a type of infiltrated immune cells. The number in each cell means the correlation coefficient and p-value.

to screen for the hub module associated with above infiltrated immune cells. After eliminating the outlier samples (**Supplementary Figure 1**), we built the sample dendrogram and trait heatmap (**Supplementary Figure 2**). By using the pick Soft Threshold function of WGCNA, we found the optimal soft threshold power was 9, in which R^2 was 0.85 (**Supplementary Figure 3A**). After merging similar modules, eight modules from the co-expression network were identified (**Supplementary Figure 3B**). According to the module-trait

relationships in **Figure 3**, we found that the MEbrown module was the most relevant module associated with DC (Cor = 0.3, $p < 0.01$), NK CD56dim cells (Cor = 0.62, $p < 0.01$), T cells (Cor = 0.81, $p < 0.01$), Tcm (Cor = −0.5, $p < 0.01$), TFH (Cor = 0.52, $p < 0.01$), Tgd (Cor = 0.65, $p < 0.01$) and Th2 cells (Cor =0.49, $p < 0.01$). Thus, MEbrown module was selected for downstream analysis.

Next, we overlapped DEGs with genes in the MEbrown module and obtained 10 candidate genes (**Figure 4A**). Ten

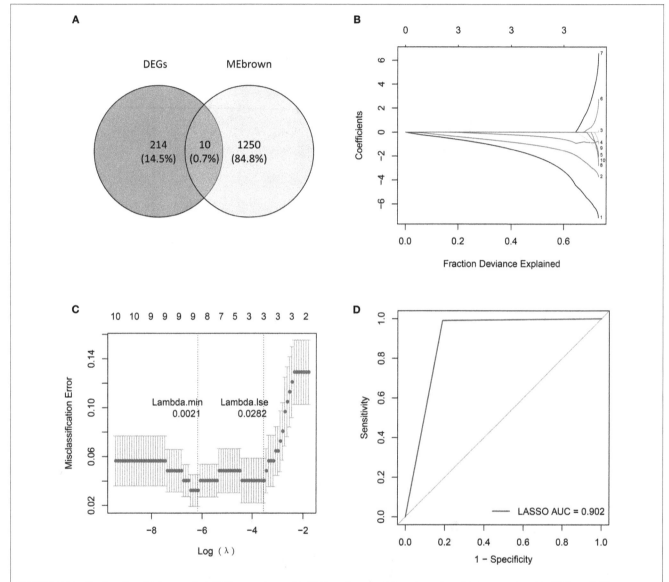

FIGURE 4 | Identification of candidate genes by LASSO regression model. **(A)** Venn diagram of 10 overlapped candidate genes shared by DEGs and MEbrown module. **(B)** LASSO coefficient profiles of candidate genes. **(C)** Cross-validation to select the optimal tuning parameter log (Lambda) in LASSO regression analysis. **(D)** ROC curve evaluation of LASSO regression analysis.

candidate genes were input into LASSO and SVM-RFE to identify gene signature, respectively. LASSO identified nine gene signatures under lambda.min = 0.0021, including PALLD, DexD-box helicase 39A (DDX39A), stress induced phosphoprotein 1 (STIP1), solute carrier family 38 member 2 (SLC38A2), CALU, CD164 molecule (CD164), selenoprotein T (SELT), four and a half LIM domain 1 (FHL1) and claudin domain containing 1 (CLDND1) (**Figures 4B,C**). The accuracy of LASSO was evaluated by ROC curve that the area under the ROC curve (AUC) was 0.902 (**Figure 4D**). Meanwhile, we identified 7 gene signatures by SVM-RFE, including PALLD, DDX39A, CD164, CLDND1, SLC38A2, CALU, and heat shock protein family D member 1 (HSPD1) with the accuracy of 0.962 (**Figures 5A,B**). To get the robust gene signature in heart failure, we overlapped

genes from LASSO and SVM-RFE and got six gene signatures (**Figure 5C**), including PALLD, DDX39A, CD164, CLDND1, SLC38A2, and CALU. The expression levels of PALLD, DDX39A, CD164, CLDND1, SLC38A2, and CALU were all significantly higher in NF samples compared to CM ones in GSE5406 (**Figure 5D**).

Verification of the Potential Biomarkers for CM

We further evaluated the diagnostic values of PALLD, DDX39A, CD164, CLDND1, SLC38A2, and CALU in GSE5406 by ROC curves. We found that they all had high accuracy with AUC >0.7 (**Figure 6A**). To verify the diagnostic values of the

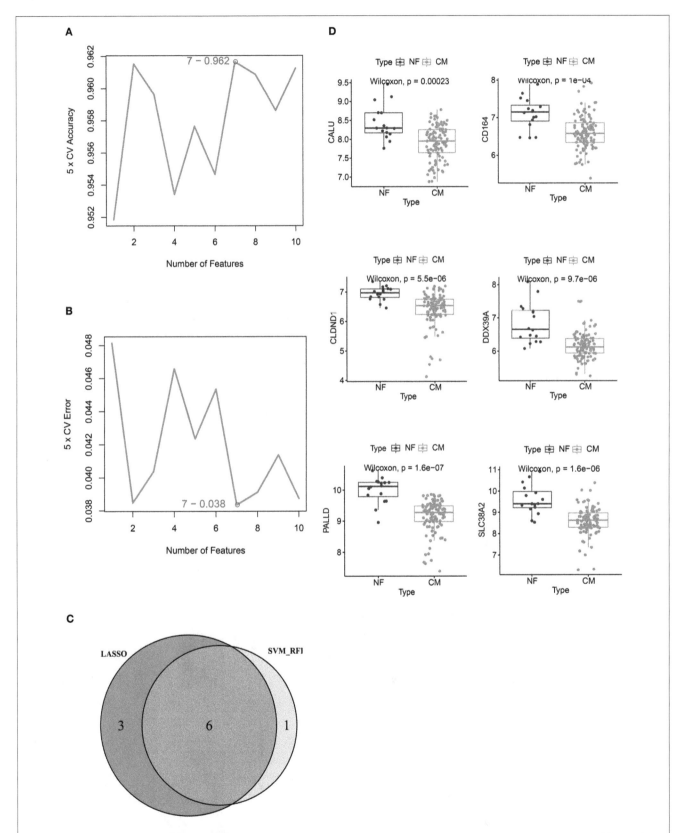

FIGURE 5 | Identification of candidate genes by SVM-RFE. **(A)** 7 gene signatures are identified by SVM-RFE analysis with the accuracy of 0.962 and **(B)** error of 0.038. **(C)** Venn diagram of six overlapped candidate genes shared by the LASSO and SVM-RFE algorithms. **(D)** The expressions of candidate diagnostic biomarkers in the NF and CM samples from GSE5406 dataset.

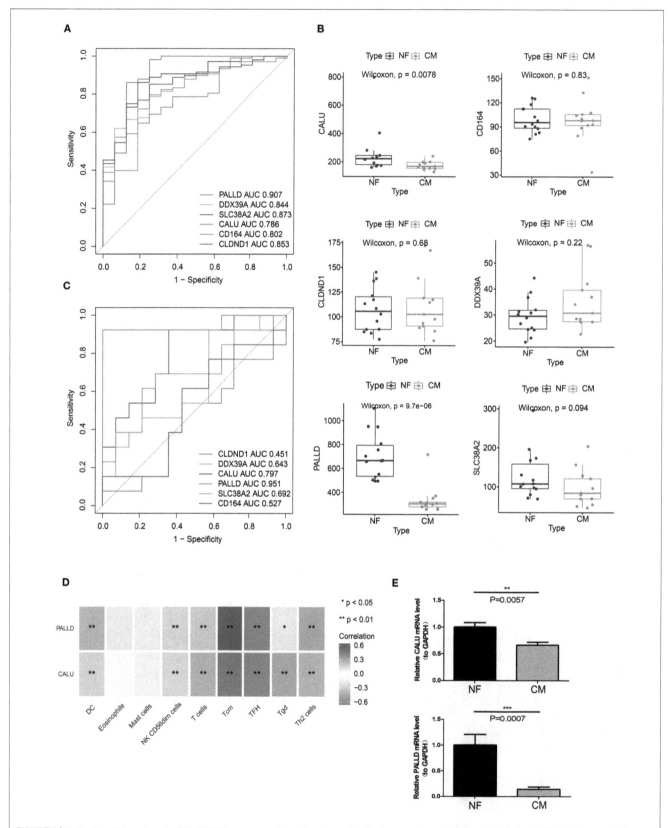

FIGURE 6 | Verification of biomarkers for CM. **(A)** ROC curve evaluation of the diagnostic effectiveness of candidate biomarkers using GSE5406 dataset. **(B)** The expressions of candidate diagnostic biomarkers in the GSE116250 dataset. **(C)** ROC curve evaluation of the diagnostic effectiveness of candidate biomarkers using GSE116250 dataset. **(D)** Heatmap of correlations between PALLD, CALU and differentially infiltrated immune cells. **(E)** Real-time PCR analyses of the expression levels of PALLD and CALU in PBMCs isolated from CM and NF patients *p < 0.05, **p < 0.01, ***p <0.001

candidate biomarkers, we examined their expressions in an external validation dataset GSE116250 to get robust diagnostic biomarkers. We found that the expression trends of CALU and PALLD in GSE116250 were consistent with those in GSE5406 (**Figure 6B**), and that CALU and PALLD also had high accuracy in classifying heart failure samples, as evidenced by AUC >0.7 (**Figure 6C**). Moreover, we found that the expressions of CALU and PALLD were significantly negative correlated with DC, NK CD56dim cells, T cells, Tfh, Tgd, and Th2 cells, and positive correlated with Tcm (**Figure 6D**).

To further evaluate the value of CALU and PALLD as biomarkers, the levels of CALU and PALLD were assessed in PBMCs isolated from CM and NF patients. In agreement with the results in GSE116250 and GSE5406, the levels of CALU and PALLD were also significantly lower in PBMCs collected from CM patients compared to NF ones (**Figure 6E**) Collectively, these results suggest that CALU and PALLD may be potential diagnostic biomarkers for heart failure due to ischemic cardiomyopathy.

DISCUSSION

The prevalence of HF is increasing worldwide and has reached epidemic proportions. Although significant progress has been made in the medications and interventions for HF, the mortality and hospitalization rates remain high (20). Recently, immune cell infiltration has been confirmed to play a vital role in the occurrence and development of cardiovascular diseases (10, 13). Cardiac inflammation and subsequent tissue damage are orchestrated by the infiltration and activation of various immune cells in the myocardium which result in heart failure eventually (20). Thus, it is essential to comprehensively investigate the contributions of infiltrated immune cells in HF. In this study, we analyzed the immune infiltration profiles of CM and NF samples, and identified CALU and PALLD as potential diagnostic biomarkers for heart failure due to ischemic cardiomyopathy by using integrated bioinformatics analyses.

Consistent with a previous report (21), we found that DEGs between NF and CM were mainly enriched into biological processes and pathways related to protein processing and ECM. Structural changes occur in the level of ER and UPR components in cardiomyocytes of patients with HF (22). When maladaptive UPR fails to restore ER homeostasis, it might induce risk factors for HF including increased reactive oxygen species (ROS) production, inflammation and apoptosis which further aggravate HF (22). In addition, numerous studies have explored the relationship between ECM and heart diseases (23, 24). Alterations in the architecture, composition, and distribution of interstitial ECM play a major role in pathological myocardial structural remodeling and left ventricular diastolic dysfunction (25, 26). Myocardial fibrosis is characterized by accumulation of collagen-rich ECM, such as collagen type I and III fibers, results from the predominance of fiber formation and deposition over its degradation and removal (27). ECM dyshomeostasis is also postulated to occur during the development and progression of HF, including changes in the synthesis, processing, degradation, and turnover of proteins such as fibrillar collagen (28). Therefore, those DEGs we found may regulate HF through protein processing and ECM.

Increasing evidence show that immune cell infiltration in the myocardium has adverse effect on heart function (29–31). Single-cell sequencing analyses reveal that the immune cell profiles are remarkably different in healthy and diseased hearts (15, 32, 33). In this study, we found that the abundance of DC, mast cells, NK CD56dim cells, T cells, Tfh, Tgd, and Th2 cells were higher, while the infiltration of eosinophils and Tcm were lower in HF samples, indicating their important roles in the etiology of HF. Consistent with our findings, Patella V et al. and Abdolmaleki F et al. found an increase in numbers of mast cells and T cells in HF, respectively (34, 35). Mast cells initiate adverse myocardial remodeling by activating matrix metalloproteinase (MMP) and fibrosis in the heart (36). Moreover, the profibrotic and antiangiogenic functions of Th17, Th2, and dysfunctional Treg cells are indispensable for the progression to ischemic heart failure (37, 38). On the contrary, inducible depletion of eosinophils exacerbates cardiac dysfunction, cell death, and fibrosis, by producing IL-4 and cationic protein mEar1, fibroblast activation, and neutrophil adhesion (39). Studies from our and other groups suggest a critical role of immune infiltration in the development of heart failure, and further understandings of the effect of each type of infiltrated immune cells may provide us clues for developing novel therapeutic strategies for heart failure.

PALLD encodes a cytoskeleton protein involved in actin reorganization (40), which plays an important role in heart development (41). PALLD was reported to be related to vein graft stenosis after coronary artery bypass grafting. A single-nucleotide polymorphism (SNP) in the PALLD has been reported to be associated with coronary heart disease (CHD) (42). CALU produces a Ca^{2+}-binding protein that is localized in the endoplasmic reticulum (ER) (43). During the excitation-contraction coupling process, CALU regulates Ca^{2+} uptake and plays an important role in maintaining normal heart function (44). Our analyses show that the expressions of CALU and PALLD were significantly negative correlated with the abundances of DC, NK CD56dim cells, T cells, Tfh, Tgd and Th2 cells, and Tcm, suggesting that CALU and PALLD may regulate HF via immune-related pathways mediated by the infiltration of these immune cells. More importantly, we confirmed that the expression levels of CALU and PALLD were markedly lower in PBMCs from CM patients compared with NF ones. Collectively, these findings indicate that CALU and PALLD are potential biomarkers for the diagnosis of HF.

Several limitations of the present study should be noted. Firstly, the study was retrospective, further prospective studies are needed to assess the diagnostic and prognostic value of CALU and PALLD in HF. Secondly, the relationships between the biomarkers and immune regulation in heart failure were only verified by assessing their levels in PBMCs from CM and NF patients. Further *in vitro* and *in vivo* experiments are required to explore the detailed mechanisms through which CALU and PALLD regulate inflammatory responses in HF. Taken together, our analyses delineate the potential etiology of HF due to CM and identified immune infiltration related biomarkers in HF, which may provide guidance for diagnosis and treatment of patients with HF.

AUTHOR CONTRIBUTIONS

YZ and LP contributed to the study concepts and study design and helped in revising the manuscript. XL, SX, and YL drafted the

manuscript, performed data management, and bioinformatics analysis. QC were responsible for clinical sample collection. All authors were involved in reporting the results of this study and approved the final version of the submitted manuscript.

REFERENCES

1. Ponikowski P, Voors AA, Anker SD, Bueno H, Cleland JGF, Coats AJS, et al. 2016 ESC Guidelines for the diagnosis treatment of acute chronic heart failure: The Task Force for the diagnosis treatment of acute chronic heart failure of the European Society of Cardiology (ESC)Developed with the special contribution of the Heart Failure Association (HFA) of the ESC. Eur Heart J. (2016) 37:2129–200. doi: 10.1093/eurheartj/ehw128

2. Yancy CW, Jessup M, Bozkurt B, Butler J, Casey DE, Colvin MM, et al. 2017 ACC/AHA/HFSA Focused Update of the 2013 ACCF/AHA guideline for the management of heart failure: a report of the American College of Cardiology/American heart association task force on clinical practice guidelines and the heart failure society of America. Circulation. (2017) 136:e137–61. doi: 10.1161/CIR.0000000000000509

3. Cunningham JW, Claggett BL, O'Meara E, Prescott MF, Pfeffer MA, Shah SJ, et al. Effect of sacubitril/valsartan on biomarkers of extracellular matrix regulation in patients with HFpEF. J Am Coll Cardiol. (2020) 76:503–14. doi: 10.1016/j.jacc.2020.05.072

4. Mann DL. Inflammatory mediators and the failing heart: past, present, and the foreseeable future. Circ Res. (2002) 91:988–98. doi: 10.1161/01.RES.0000043825.01705.1B

5. Zimmet JM, Hare JM. Nitroso-redox interactions in the cardiovascular system. Circulation. (2006) 114:1531–44. doi: 10.1161/CIRCULATIONAHA.105.605519

6. Braunwald E. Biomarkers in heart failure. N Engl J Med. (2008) 358:2148–59. doi: 10.1056/NEJMra0800239

7. Hein S, Kostin S, Heling A, Maeno Y, Schaper J. The role of the cytoskeleton in heart failure. Cardiovasc Res. (2000) 45:273–8. doi: 10.1016/S0008-6363(99)00268-0

8. Luo M, Anderson ME. Mechanisms of altered Ca(2)(+) handling in heart failure. Circ Res. (2013) 113:690–708. doi: 10.1161/CIRCRESAHA.113.301651

9. Dick SA, Epelman S. Chronic heart failure and inflammation what do we really know? Circul Res. (2016) 119:159–76. doi: 10.1161/CIRCRESAHA.116.308030

10. de Lucia C, Grisanti LA, Borghetti G, Piedepalumbo M, Ibetti J, Maria Lucchese A, et al. GRK5 contributes to impaired cardiac function and immune cell recruitment in post-ischemic heart failure. Cardiovasc Res. (2021) 9:cvab044. doi: 10.1093/cvr/cvab044

11. Abplanalp WT, Cremer S, John D, Hoffmann J, Schuhmacher B, Merten M, et al. Clonal hematopoiesis-driver DNMT3A mutations alter immune cells in heart failure. Circ Res. (2021) 128:216–28. doi: 10.1161/CIRCRESAHA.120.317104

12. Abplanalp WT, John D, Cremer S, Assmus B, Dorsheimer L, Hoffmann J, et al. Single-cell RNA-sequencing reveals profound changes in circulating immune cells in patients with heart failure. Cardiovasc Res. (2021) 117:484–94. doi: 10.1093/cvr/cvaa101

13. Zhao E, Xie H, Zhang Y. Predicting diagnostic gene biomarkers associated with immune infiltration in patients with acute myocardial infarction. Front Cardiovasc Med. (2020) 7:586871. doi: 10.3389/fcvm.2020.586871

14. Cao Y, Tang W, Tang W. Immune cell infiltration characteristics and related core genes in lupus nephritis: results from bioinformatic analysis. BMC Immunol. (2019) 20:37. doi: 10.1186/s12865-019-0316-x

15. Martini E, Kunderfranco P, Peano C, Carullo P, Cremonesi M, Schorn T, et al. Single-cell sequencing of mouse heart immune infiltrate in pressure overload-driven heart failure reveals extent of immune activation. Circulation. (2019) 140:2089–107. doi: 10.1161/CIRCULATIONAHA.119.041694

16. Hanzelmann S, Castelo R, Guinney J. GSVA: gene set variation analysis for microarray and RNA-seq data. BMC Bioinformatics. (2013) 14:7. doi: 10.1186/1471-2105-14-7

17. Vasquez MM, Hu CC, Roe DJ, Chen Z, Halonen M, Guerra S. Least absolute shrinkage and selection operator type methods for the identification of serum biomarkers of overweight and obesity: simulation and application. Bmc Med Res Methodol. (2016) 16:254. doi: 10.1186/s12874-016-0254-8

18. Noble WS. What is a support vector machine? Nat Biotechnol. (2006) 24:1565–7. doi: 10.1038/nbt1206-1565

19. Schmittgen TD, Livak KJ. Analyzing real-time PCR data by the comparative C-T method. Nat Protoc. (2008) 3:1101–8. doi: 10.1038/nprot.2008.73

20. Strassheim D, Dempsey EC, Gerasimovskaya E, Stenmark K, Karoor V. Role of inflammatory cell subtypes in heart failure. J Immunol Res. (2019) 2019:2164017. doi: 10.1155/2019/2164017

21. Ren J, Bi YG, Sowers JR, Hetz C, Zhang YM. Endoplasmic reticulum stress and unfolded protein response in cardiovascular diseases. Nat Rev Cardiol. (2021) 18:499–521. doi: 10.1038/s41569-021-00511-w

22. Glembotski CC. Endoplasmic reticulum stress in the heart. Circ Res. (2007) 101:975–84. doi: 10.1161/CIRCRESAHA.107.161273

23. Frangogiannis NG. The extracellular matrix in ischemic and nonischemic heart failure. Circul Res. (2019) 125:117–46. doi: 10.1161/CIRCRESAHA.119.311148

24. Guo Y, Gupte M, Umbarkar P, Singh AP, Sui JY, Force T, et al. Entanglement of GSK-3beta, beta-catenin and TGF-beta1 signaling network to regulate myocardial fibrosis. J Mol Cell Cardiol. (2017) 110:109–20. doi: 10.1016/j.yjmcc.2017.07.011

25. Kasner M, Westermann D, Lopez B, Gaub R, Escher F, Kuhl U, et al. Diastolic tissue Doppler indexes correlate with the degree of collagen expression and cross-linking in heart failure and normal ejection fraction. J Am Coll Cardiol. (2011) 57:977–85. doi: 10.1016/j.jacc.2010.10.024

26. Zile MR, Baicu CF, Ikonomidis JS, Stroud RE, Nietert PJ, Bradshaw AD, et al. Myocardial stiffness in patients with heart failure and a preserved ejection fraction: contributions of collagen and titin. Circulation. (2015) 131:1247–59. doi: 10.1161/CIRCULATIONAHA.114.013215

27. Lopez B, Ravassa S, Gonzalez A, Zubillaga E, Bonavila C, Berges M, et al. Myocardial collagen cross-linking is associated with heart failure hospitalization in patients with hypertensive heart failure. J Am College Cardiol. (2016) 67:251–60. doi: 10.1016/j.jacc.2015.10.063

28. Gonzalez A, Schelbert EB, Diez J, Butler J. Myocardial interstitial fibrosis in heart failure: biological and translational perspectives. J Am Coll Cardiol. (2018) 71:1696–706. doi: 10.1016/j.jacc.2018.02.021

29. Carrillo-Salinas FJ, Ngwenyama N, Anastasiou M, Kaur K, Alcaide P. Heart inflammation immune cell roles and roads to the heart. Am J Pathol. (2019) 189:1482–94. doi: 10.1016/j.ajpath.2019.04.009

30. Lafuse WP, Wozniak DJ, Rajaram MVS. Role of cardiac macrophages on cardiac inflammation, fibrosis and tissue repair. Cells. (2020) 10:51. doi: 10.3390/cells10010051

31. Kawada J, Takeuchi S, Imai H, Okumura T, Horiba K, Suzuki T, et al. Immune cell infiltration landscapes in pediatric acute myocarditis analyzed by CIBERSORT. J Cardiol. (2021) 77:174–8. doi: 10.1016/j.jjcc.2020.08.004

32. Farbehi N, Patrick R, Dorison A, Xaymardan M, Janbandhu V, Wystub-Lis K, et al. Single-cell expression profiling reveals dynamic flux of cardiac stromal, vascular and immune cells in health and injury. Elife. (2019) 8:43882. doi: 10.7554/eLife.43882

33. Suryawanshi H, Clancy R, Morozov P, Halushka MK, Buyon JP, Tuschl T. Cell atlas of the foetal human heart and implications for autoimmune-mediated congenital heart block. Cardiovasc Res. (2020) 116:1446–57. doi: 10.1093/cvr/cvz257

34. Patella V, Marino I, Arbustini E, Lamparter-Schummert B, Verga L, Adt M, et al. Stem cell factor in mast cells and increased mast cell density

in idiopathic and ischemic cardiomyopathy. *Circulation*. (1998) 97:971–8. doi: 10.1161/01.CIR.97.10.971

35. Abdolmaleki F, Gheibi Hayat SM, Bianconi V, Johnston TP, Sahebkar A. Atherosclerosis and immunity: A perspective. *Trends Cardiovasc Med*. (2019) 29:363–71. doi: 10.1016/j.tcm.2018.09.017

36. Ngkelo A, Richart A, Kirk JA, Bonnin P, Vilar J, Lemitre M, et al. Mast cells regulate myofilament calcium sensitization and heart function after myocardial infarction. *J Exp Med*. (2016) 213:1353–74. doi: 10.1084/jem.20160081

37. Bansal SS, Ismahil MA, Goel M, Patel B, Hamid T, Rokosh G, et al. Activated T lymphocytes are essential drivers of pathological remodeling in ischemic heart failure. *Circ-Heart Fail*. (2017) 10:3688. doi: 10.1161/CIRCHEARTFAILURE.116.003688

38. Bansal SS, Ismahil MA, Goel M, Zhou GH, Rokosh G, Hamid T, et al. Dysfunctional and proinflammatory regulatory T-lymphocytes are essential for adverse cardiac remodeling in ischemic cardiomyopathy. *Circulation*. (2019) 139:206–21. doi: 10.1161/CIRCULATIONAHA.118.036065

39. Liu J, Yang CZ, Liu TX, Deng ZY, Fang WQ, Zhang X, et al. Eosinophils improve cardiac function after myocardial infarction. *Nat Commun*. (2020) 11:5. doi: 10.1038/s41467-020-19297-5

40. Mykkanen OM, Gronholm M, Ronty M, Lalowski M, Salmikangas P, Suila H, et al. Characterization of human palladin, a microfilament-associated protein. *Mol Biol Cell*. (2001) 12:3060–73. doi: 10.1091/mbc.12.10.3060

41. Mori M, Nakagami H, Koibuchi N, Miura K, Takami Y, Koriyama H, et al. Zyxin mediates actin fiber reorganization in epithelial-mesenchymal transition and contributes to endocardial morphogenesis. *Mol Biol Cell*. (2009) 20:3115–24. doi: 10.1091/mbc.e09-01-0046

42. Bare LA, Morrison AC, Rowland CM, Shiffman D, Luke MM, Iakoubova OA, et al. Five common gene variants identify elevated genetic risk for coronary heart disease. *Genet Med*. (2007) 9:682–9. doi: 10.1097/GIM.0b013e318156fb62

43. Sahoo SK, Kim DH. Characterization of calumenin in mouse heart. *BMB Rep*. (2010) 43:158–63. doi: 10.5483/BMBRep.2010.43.3.158

44. Sahoo SK, Kim DH. Calumenin interacts with SERCA2 in rat cardiac sarcoplasmic reticulum. *Mol Cells*. (2008) 26:265–9. doi: 10.1186/1476-4598-7-74

17

Renocardiovascular Biomarkers: From the Perspective of Managing Chronic Kidney Disease and Cardiovascular Disease

Shinichiro Niizuma[1†], Yoshitaka Iwanaga[2*†], Takaharu Yahata[3] and Shunichi Miyazaki[2]

[1] Department of Cardiology, Nihon University Hospital, Tokyo, Japan, [2] Division of Cardiology, Kindai University Faculty of Medicine, Osakasayama, Japan, [3] Department of Cardiology, Yokohama Chuo Hospital, Yokohama, Japan

*Correspondence:
Yoshitaka Iwanaga
yiwanaga@med.kindai.ac.jp

†These authors have contributed equally to this work.

Mortality among the patients with chronic kidney disease (CKD) and end-stage renal disease (ESRD) remains high because of the very high incidence of cardiovascular disease (CVD) such as coronary artery disease, cardiac hypertrophy, and heart failure. Identifying CVD in patients with CKD/ESRD remains a significant hurdle and the early diagnosis and therapy for CVD is crucial in these patients. Therefore, it is necessary for the better management to identify and utilize cardiovascular (CV) biomarkers in profiling CVD risk and enabling stratification of early mortality. This review summarizes current evidence about renocardiovascular biomarkers: CV biomarkers in patients with CKD as well as with ESRD, emphasizing on the emerging biomarkers: B-type natriuretic peptide, cardiac troponins, copeptin, the biomarker of renal injury (neutrophil gelatinase-associated lipocalin), and the mineral and bone disorder hormone/marker (fibroblast growth factor-23). Furthermore, it discusses their potential roles especially in ESRD and in future diagnostic and therapeutic strategies for CVD in the context of managing cardiorenal syndrome.

Keywords: biomarker, cardiovascular disease, cardiorenal syndrome, chronic kidney disease, end-stage renal disease

CARDIOVASCULAR (CV) DISEASES IN CHRONIC KIDNEY DISEASE (CKD)/END-STAGE RENAL DISEASE (ESRD)

Chronic kidney disease is frequently associated with a progressive decrease in glomerular filtration rate (GFR), which leads to ESRD. The number of patients with CKD as well as ESRD is increasing markedly worldwide, with poor outcomes and high cost. Cardiovascular disease (CVD) is closely associated with CKD and ESRD and is well shown as the leading cause of morbidity and mortality in the patients with CKD, most notably those on ESRD or dialysis (1). The prevalence of concomitant coronary artery disease (CAD), left ventricular hypertrophy (LVH), congestive heart failure (CHF), cardiac arrhythmia (most commonly atrial fibrillation), and valvular/vascular calcification are increased in CKD patients. Recently, the term, cardiorenal syndrome (CRS) has been introduced in an attempt to emphasize the interaction between the CV and renal systems in acute or chronic disease setting (2). CRS is a pathophysiological condition in which combined cardiac and renal dysfunction amplifies the progression of failure of the individual organs and has an extremely bad prognosis. It is more than simultaneous cardiac and renal disease. It is now necessary for us to expand our knowledge regarding its pathogenesis, prevention, and potential treatment.

RENOCARDIOVASCULAR BIOMARKERS

A number of biomarkers have been evaluated in CVD or CKD/ESRD, and biomarkers pertinent to the CV and renal interface are defined as renocardiovascular biomarkers (3). From the perspective of pathophysiology, they are classified into (I) neurohormones (4–9), (II) metabolic hormones/peptides (10–13), (III) cardiac injury markers (14, 15), (IV) oxidative stress markers (16–21), (V) matrix-related markers (22–27), (VI) inflammatory markers (28–31), (VII) renal markers (32), and (VIII) mineral and bone disorder hormones/markers (33–41), as summarized in **Table 1**.

EMERGING RENOCARDIOVASCULAR BIOMARKERS

Among the biomarkers listed in **Table 1**, the critical biomarkers in the context of managing CRS are discussed in detail, first briefly describing their pathological associations and then the evidence for their usefulness in relation to important clinical endpoints (**Figure 1**).

A: B-Type Natriuretic Peptide (BNP) and Its Amino-Terminal Fragment (NT-proBNP)

Upon ventricular myocyte stretch, preproBNP is enzymatically cleaved to proBNP and released in the form of the active hormone BNP (amino acids 79–108) or an inactive fragment, NT-proBNP (amino acids 1–76, released in a1:1 ratio). The hemodynamic

TABLE 1 | Potential renocardiovascular biomarkers.

Biomarkers		Reference
(I) Neurohormones		
Natriuretic peptides (ANP, B-type natriuretic peptide (BNP), CNP, and related peptides)	BNP and its amino-terminal fragment (NT-proBNP) have become established as the most ideal markers of HF so far available	(4)
Endothelin and C-terminal-pro-endothelin-1 (CT-proET-1)	CT-proET-1 increases in CKD and may be potentially useful biomarkers of renal injury	(5)
Arginine vasopressin (AVP) and copeptin	Copeptin which is released with AVP, emerges to be a more reliable marker for HF and is also released into the circulation early after MI onset and may aid in rapid diagnosis	(6, 7)
Adrenomedullin (ADM) and mid-regional proadrenomedullin (MR-proADM)	MR-proADM, which is relatively more stable than ADM, is used to explore the prognostic power for HF related deaths, suggesting better predictability than the natriuretic peptides	(8, 9)
(II) Metabolic hormones/peptides		
Triiodothyronine, adrenocorticotropic hormone and cortisol	Hormonal derangements at the level of the hypothalamic-pituitary axis are often seen with the CKD or CVD	(10)
Adiponectin	Although hyperadiponectinemia is a common phenomenon in CKD and is considered to have similar beneficial effects on metabolic risk in this patient group, many recent studies have unexpectedly shown that high, rather than low, concentrations predict mortality	(11)
Leptin	Hyperleptinemia, frequently observed in CKD patients, may play a key role in the pathogenesis of complications associated with CKD such as cachexia, protein energy wasting, chronic inflammation, insulin resistance, cardiovascular (CV) damages, and bone complications. Leptin may be also involved in the progression of renal disease through its pro-fibrotic and pro-hypertensive actions	(12, 13)
(III) Cardiac injury markers		
Cardiac troponins (cTns)	There are accumulating evidences of the usefulness of cTns in conditions other than ACS, including HF	(14)
Heart-type fatty acid-binding protein (H-FABP)	H-FABP as well as cTns is influenced by renal function and the utilities may be somewhat limited in CKD patients	(15)
(IV) Oxidative stress markers		
Malondialdehyde, 8-hydroxy-2'-deoxyguanosine, oxidized low-density lipoproteins	A number of biological markers of oxidative stress have been evaluated for CVD as well as CKD, since oxidative stress is a common mediator in pathophysiology of risk factors for the both diseases	(16)
Uric acid	Although at present, there are no definite data whether uric acid is causal, compensatory, coincidental, or it is only an epiphenomenon in CKD patients, hyperuricemia may contribute to the development and progression of CKD and also be linked to CVD	(17, 18)
Advanced glycation endproduct (AGE)	Chronic overstimulation of the AGE-receptor for AGE pathway is likely one of major contributors involved in the pathophysiology of CVD in patients with CKD	(19)
Asymmetric dimethylarginine (ADMA)	ADMA level is a marker and mediator of oxidative stress as well as endothelial dysfunction/atherosclerosis. It is accumulated in plasma during CKD and a strong predictor for the progression of CKD and CVD in CKD patients. Also in patients with HD, plasma ADMA is a strong and independent predictor of overall mortality and CV outcome	(20, 21)

(Continued)

TABLE 1 | Continued

Biomarkers		Reference
(V) Matrix-related markers		
Matrix metalloproteinases and tissue inhibitors of MMPs	They have been increasingly linked to both normal physiology and abnormal pathology in the kidney as well as heart. However, their roles in the pathophysiology of CRS are extremely complex	(22)
Galectin-3	Galectin-3 has been associated with increased risk for morbidity and mortality in patients with HF. Also, it may be causally involved in mechanisms of tubulointerstitial fibrosis and CKD progression	(23–25)
ST2	ST2 is reflective of fibrosis and cardiac remodeling and strongly related to HF outcomes. Also, cross-sectionally, higher ST2 concentrations appear to be associated with worse kidney function in patients with CVD	(26, 27)
(VI) Inflammatory markers		
High-sensitive C-reactive protein (hs-CRP), cytokines and related receptors [Interleukin (IL)-1, -2, -6, -8, -18, TNF-α]	Among CKD patients, inflammatory biomarkers including hs-CRP and IL-6 correlate with known CVD and provide prognostic information, which suggests inflammation and oxidative stress may contribute to CV risk in CKD patients	(28)
Pentraxin-3 (PTX3)	Elevated systemic PTX3 levels appear to be a powerful marker of inflammatory status and a superior outcome predictor in patients with CKD. It may also provide more information on development and progression of atherosclerosis than other less specific markers such as CRP	(29)
Growth differentiation factor-15 (GDF-15)	Measurement of circulating GDF-15 provides incremental improvement in mortality risk prediction in addition to traditional risk factors as well as cTns and BNP in healthy individuals as well in patients with a spectrum of CVD including AMI and HF. Higher circulating GDF-15 is associated with incident renal outcomes and improves risk prediction of incident CKD	(30, 31)
(VII) Renal markers		
Neutrophil gelatinase-associated lipocalin (NGAL), kidney injury molecule-1, liver-type fatty acid-binding protein, cystatin C	In AKI and CKD, these renal biomarkers have become useful for assessment and prognostication both in plasma and in urine. They are expected to be useful in early diagnosis of renal involvement in CVD such as HF, and contrast nephropathy, and to suggest the timing of treatment initiation and its likely effectiveness	(32)
(VIII) Mineral and bone disorder hormones/markers		
Vitamin D/parathyroid hormone (PTH)	Serum markers such as calcium, phosphate, vitamin D and PTH are already in use in clinical practice, and increased calcium, increased phosphate, decreased (active) vitamin D, or increased PTH are reported to be associated with CVD in CKD/ESRD patients by epidemiologic data. However, the relationship between these markers and CVD in CKD patients is complex and may lack causality	(33–37)
Osteoprotegerin (OPG)	Elevated OPG levels have been associated with aortic stiffness and markers of CV dysfunction such as raised serum troponin T levels	(38)
Fetuin-A	Decreased fetuin-A levels are observed in CKD patients, especially in ESRD and are associated with the development of vascular calcification	(39)
Fibroblast growth factor-23 (FGF-23)	FGF-23 levels among CKD patients are higher than in the general population and are further elevated in the dialysis population. It may cause not only rapid progression of renal functional decline, but also the development of LVH and HF	(40, 41)

ACS, acute coronary syndromes; AKI, acute kidney injury; CKD, chronic kidney disease; CRS, cardio-renal syndrome; CVD, cardiovascular disease; ESRD, end-stage renal disease; HD, hemodialysis; HF, heart failure; LVH, left ventricular hypertrophy; MI, myocardial infarction.

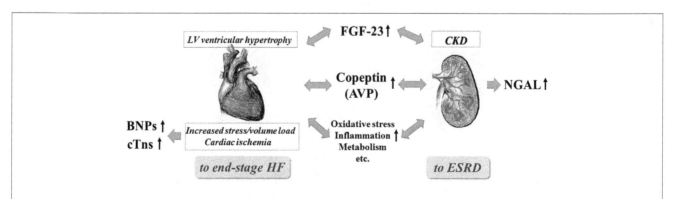

FIGURE 1 | Interrelationships and pivotal roles of the five emerging biomarkers in cardiorenal syndrome. AVP, arginine vasopressin; BNPs, B-type natriuretic peptides (BNP and NT-proBNP), CKD, chronic kidney disease; cTns, cardiac troponins (troponin I and T); CVD, cardiovascular disease; ESRD, end-stage renal disease; FGF-23, fibroblast growth factor-23; and NGAL, neutrophil gelatinase-associated lipocalin.

load (i.e., myocardial stretch) is the most important stimulus for BNP and NT-proBNP secretion, based on the results of both basic and clinical studies. Iwanaga et al. have demonstrated an excellent correlation between BNP and LV end-diastolic wall stress (EDWS) ($r^2 = 0.89$, $P < 0.001$) in HF patients with normal creatinine levels, and they found that this relationship was more robust than any other parameter previously reported (42). Currently, both BNP and NT-proBNP are widely used as markers for a variety of CVD. However, there are differences between the two assays; NT-proBNP has a longer half-life and thus, its levels may be more stable (less sensitive to acute stress). In addition, NT-proBNP might be more dependent on renal clearance than BNP. To date, most studies have demonstrated that both are equally useful for diagnosis, management and prognosis, even in CKD and hemodialysis (HD) patients.

BNP/NT-proBNP vs. Renal Function

The relationship between BNP/NT-proBNP levels and renal dysfunction is complex. Any change in value may be influenced by renal dysfunction due to change in clearance. When renal dysfunction causes cardiac damage/stress, directly or indirectly, this will cause increased BNP/NT-proBNP values. It remains unclear whether, in patients with CKD and ESRD, increased plasma BNP levels might be due to more hemodynamic stimuli or might result from other factors such as anemia, obesity, and cachexia or impaired renal clearance of natriuretic peptide, despite similar hemodynamic stimuli. Multiple studies have shown an inverse moderate, but significant, correlation between estimated glomerular filtration ratio (eGFR) and BNP or NT-proBNP concentrations. Niizuma et al. have recently shown that renal dysfunction (reduced eGFR) may contribute to increased BNP levels (inverse correlation) independent of EDWS (a critical hemodynamic determinant of BNP), anemia, HF type, and BMI in a wide spectrum of HF patients with both CKD and ESRD (43). Some reports suggest that NT-proBNP is more strongly influenced with the severity of renal dysfunction than BNP, whereas others show that they are equally dependent on the renal function for their clearance. van Kimmenade et al. showed BNP and NT-proBNP had nearly identical correlations to eGFR ($r = -0.35$ and $r = -0.3$, respectively; $P < 0.001$ for both) in 165 hypertensive subjects (44). They went a step further by measuring renal fractional extraction (FE) [(renal artery concentration − renal vein concentration)/renal artery concentration] of these NPs and found that, across a range of eGFR as low as 9 mL/min/1.73 m^2, FE for BNP and NT-proBNP diminished only modestly and correlated minimally with eGFR ($r = 0.20$–0.26). Furthermore, they found in a multivariate regression analysis that cardio-related factors such as blood pressure, LV mass, and eGFR, but not FE, were significantly associated with NPs concentrations.

BNP and NT-proBNP Elevations in ESRD

Among patients with HD or peritoneal dialysis (PD), considerable heterogeneity in BNP and NT-proBNP levels has been recognized and seems to increase exponentially, which may have caused some confusion in interpreting results. In ESRD or dialysis patients, the question of whether increased plasma NP levels are due to cardiac

hemodynamic stimuli, accompanying comorbidities or impaired renal clearance of NPs is also a matter of controversy. Recent reports in ESRD patients suggest that the NT-proBNP/BNP ratio increases even further in patients receiving HD (45). In dialysis patients, the parameters related to the dialysis treatment itself may influence BNP and NT-proBNP concentrations, like the type of dialysis membrane and a patient's volume status or change (46, 47). Certainly, the very high prevalence of LV structural and functional abnormalities in ESRD patients may account for the remarkable elevations. Zoccali et al. demonstrated that ANP/BNP levels were only slightly elevated in dialysis patients who had normal cardiac function and no LVH on echocardiography (48).

Diagnostic and Prognostic Utility of BNP and NT-proBNP in ESRD

The best cut-off values for detecting HF may need to be raised when the eGFR is less than 60 mL/min. It should be noted that the diagnostic accuracy of plasma BNP and NT-proBNP for HF is reduced in this setting, and natriuretic peptide testing for HF should be discouraged in patients especially on dialysis. Recently, Mishra et al. reported in the large CKD cohort without HF that NT-proBNP had strong associations with prevalent LVH and LV systolic dysfunction (49). Also, some studies demonstrated a close association between BNP or NT-proBNP levels and LV mass and systolic function in the ESRD population. Experimental studies suggested myocardial ischemia apart from an increased mechanical stress, upregulated BNP gene expression, and release from ventricular myocardium (50). Recently, Niizuma et al. used CAG for a thorough evaluation of disease severity and assessed the relationship between BNP and CAD in 125 patients with long-term HD (51). Plasma BNP levels showed a predictive value for CAD and were closely correlated with disease severity, and similar findings were observed also in the studies of patients with CKD. Thus, the measurement of plasma BNP levels in combination with other non-invasive investigations might help in assessing CAD involvement and aggressive management in this high-risk population. In addition to their roles in detecting LV abnormality or ischemic status, a number of studies suggest BNP testing as promising cardiac biomarkers for mortality prediction and CV risk stratification also in dialysis patients (48). The largest study by Apple et al. examined the predialysis NT-proBNP levels in 399 HD patients and showed that NT-proBNP was significantly predictive of mortality, and the area under the receiver operating characteristic curve in relation to mortality was higher with NT-proBNP than with cTnT or High-sensitive C-reactive protein (52). Also in the largest study in the PD population, patients in the highest quartile of NT-proBNP had significantly greater risk of mortality, CV death, and events after a median follow-up of 36 months (53). All of these data suggest the prognostic importance of BNP or NT-proBNP level at a single time point, irrespective of whether the measurement was taken before dialysis, after dialysis, or midweek between dialysis. In addition to CV outcomes, several studies suggested that increased BNP and NT-proBNP concentrations were associated with an increased risk for accelerated progression of CKD to ESRD (54). The mechanism may be complex and cardiac abnormalities or other comorbidities in addition to the decreased clearance may attribute to the results. In any case, it strongly suggests a dynamic interplay between the heart and the kidney as CRS.

B: Troponins

After myocardial cell damage, cardiac troponin (cTn) T and I are released from the myocytes and their levels are detectable 3–12 h after the injury and mean time to peak cTn level is approximately 12–48 h. The concentration returns to the normal range after 5–14 days, which is four times longer than for the creatine kinase myocardial band isoenzyme (CK-MB) fraction. The increasing sensitivity of cTn assays has had a dramatic impact on the use of cTn testing, which is now an essential component of the diagnostic workup and management of acute coronary syndromes (ACS). More importantly, the test has prognostic value because it identifies ACS patients who are at substantially increased risk of death or recurrent MI (15). Also, the elevated cTn in asymptomatic individuals in the community is associated with a tripling of risk of all-cause and CV mortality as shown by a recent systematic review (55).

cTns in CKD/ESRD

Elevated cTns may be detected in conditions other than ACS, including HF, cardiomyopathies, myocarditis, tachyarrhythmia, and pulmonary embolism, and even after strenuous exercise in healthy individuals (14). Levels of cTns are frequently elevated in the absence of ACS among patients with renal dysfunction, specifically in 30–75% of ESRD patients. In general, the use of more sensitive cTn assays likely shows that the presence of cTn elevations in ESRD patients might be even more frequent than previously thought. Jacobs et al. found that by using a more sensitive cTnT assay, 94% of patients had cTnT elevations above the 99th percentile (56). At one time, it was considered that an elevation of the cTns in a setting of decreased creatinine clearance was not of substantial diagnostic or prognostic importance. However, the GUSTO IV trial, which included 7,033 patients with suspected ACS, indicated that an elevated cTnT level was strongly predictive of poor short-term prognosis, regardless of creatinine clearance (57). Although the important limitations were the very small number of patients with severe CKD or ESRD and its confinement to symptomatic patients, cTnT elevation had even greater prognostic importance among patients with a mild to moderate degree of CKD. Stacy et al. have showed that cTns can identify those with a poor prognosis in patients with CKD and suspected ACS by a systemic review (58). In addition, they found that cTns levels can be helpful but that their diagnostic utility is limited by varying estimates of sensitivity and specificity. In the clinical setting, serial measurements should be performed in patients CKD and suspected ACS because an exact cut-off point cannot yet be specified. Moreover, over the past decade, data have emerged to suggest that elevated levels of cTns may predict death among ESRD patients without symptoms of ACS. A recent research by Michos and colleagues have reviewed 98 studies systematically and showed the association of elevated cTns with worse prognosis in CKD patients (receiving or not receiving dialysis) without suspected ACS (59). Although the precise mechanism of death is unknown, several studies suggest that the prevalence of increased levels of cTns may correlate with increased risk of

CAD. deFillippi et al. found that a high level (>median) vs. a low level of cTnT remained an independent predictor of multivessel disease (prevalence ratio, 3.7 fold) after adjustment for age and history of clinical CAD in stable patients undergoing long-term HD (60). They also suggested the potential complementary role of serum CRP, which is elevated in more than 70% of HD patients, for predicting all-cause mortality. Routine measurement of cTns may be prognostically valuable and may help frame therapeutic decisions. However, the pathophysiologic mechanisms causing random increases in cTn concentrations in patients with renal dysfunction or dialysis are still unclear. Elevation of cTn levels in ESRD patients is unlikely to be the result of decreased clearance by the failing kidney, and cTn elevation might reflect cardiac damage in non-ischemic cardiomyopathy or microvascular disease in the setting of LV hypertrophy. There is also an evidence that dialysis can affect cTn levels (cTnT is increased after HD, whereas cTnI is decreased). It should be noted again that cTn testing does not provide any insight into the mechanism of cardiac injury and that a broad differential diagnosis including renal failure, pulmonary embolism and HF is routinely considered when cTn concentration is elevated in the absence of ACS. In the recent guideline (61), measurement of cTns is recommended for the evaluation of ACS in patients with ESRD (level of evidence A). A dynamic change in cTns of ≥20% after presentation should be used to define ACS (level of evidence B). Baseline cTns can aid in defining mortality and CV risk for patients with ESRD and provide baseline levels for the subsequent comparison (level of evidence B).

cTns in HF

In the context of HF, evidence for a role of cTns continues to accumulate, particularly for use in risk stratification. Evidence of myocyte cell death in human myocardium has been suggested by histologic information of biopsies and more recently by the measurement of the serum cTns, which may be able to identify subclinical injury to the myocardium. Not only in ischemic HF but also in non-ischemic HF, cTns could identify a subgroup of patients with severe HF. In patients with acute decompensated HF, 6.2% were positive for cTn testing and they showed higher in-hospital mortality than those with negative test (62). During routine clinical follow-up of ambulatory patients, elevations in cTns, particularly frequently or persistently, could be associated with an increased risk of events. In addition, Sundström et al. reported that the elevated serum level of cTnI was an independent contributor to the development of HF in a community-based sample of 1,089 70-year-old men (63). Clinical significance of increased cTns concentrations in CKD patients with HF as well as those with ACS or stable CAD is unclear. Chen et al. reported the association of an elevated cTnI with HF in 293 non-ACS patients with CKD, where Stage 5 CKD did not modify it (64). Bansal et al. reported that cTnT level was strongly associated with incident HF in a prospective cohort of 3,483 people with mild to severe CKD (65). They also showed not only cTnT but also NT-proBNP was independently associated with HF. In patients with dialysis, elevated cTnT may be a more important risk factor than LV systolic dysfunction alone and adds value when used in combination with LV mass index and ejection fraction in predicting circulatory congestion. Recently, Tsutamoto et al. reported that decreased clearance *via* the kidney might contribute to the elevated cTnT in HF patients with CKD by measuring the difference of TnT concentration between coronary sinus and aortic root (66). However, it is a controversial issue and further large studies will be needed to clarify whether renal dysfunction itself or additional myocyte damage might impact the clinical outcome in HF patients with CKD in the context of CRS. Interestingly, recent studies suggest that cTnT and NT-proBNP levels independently predicted ESRD risk in the general population or patients with diabetic nephropathy and anemia (67). These results may support a link between cardiac injury and the development of ESRD. To date, the data support the concept that structural markers of myocardial damage or strain are perhaps the best prognostic markers in high-risk patients with CVD.

C: Copeptin

The effects of arginine vasopressin (AVP) are mediated by three receptor types: V1aR, V1bR, and V2R. V1aR-dependent vasoconstriction that increases afterload, ventricular stress, and cardiac hypertrophy may result in systemic vascular resistance and a decrease in cardiac output and contractility while V2R is the receptor that governs water retention by activating the aquaporin-2 channel on the apical plasma membrane of the collecting duct cells (6). Despite its suggested importance in the pathogenesis of CVD, the evaluation of AVP secretion has been difficult because of the considerable technical issues related to AVP measurement and AVP's short plasma half-life or instability (68). Copeptin, a glycosylated 39-amino acid long peptide, is the C-terminal part of pro-AVP and is cosecreted in equimolar amounts with together with AVP during precursor processing (7). In contrast to AVP, copeptin has a longer plasma half-life, is very stable at room temperature and easy and robust to measure. Studies in healthy subjects have shown plasma copeptin and AVP concentrations to correlate strongly over a wide range of osmolality. For these reasons, copeptin is now considered as a robust surrogate for AVP, overcoming the technical problems related to AVP dosage.

During the last few years, plasma copeptin concentration has been measured in a number of clinical investigations. Significant associations have been found between baseline copeptin level and the incidence or progression of various pathological situations such as HF, diabetes, and CKD, suggesting that AVP may play causal roles. Other studies have shown that plasma copeptin may be a useful diagnostic marker in patients with AMI, sepsis, or unexplained hyponatremia. Furthermore, the prognostic values of copeptin have already been shown in patients with HF, CAD, and with acute stroke. It should be noted that most findings as the diagnostic and prognostic marker of CVD were from subjects without renal dysfunction.

Copeptin in CKD/ESRD

In CKD, a few data exist evaluating copeptin concentrations, which found copeptin to be associated with renal function (69). It might be because AVP causes renal function decline, subjects with low renal function are less sensitive to the actions of AVP or increased copeptin may result from reduced renal elimination. Increased AVP concentrations in CKD have already been

reported and are associated with biologic activity. A number of contributive factors such as LV dysfunction (or HF), endothelial stress, V2 receptor resistance, and diabetes might be related with its elevation. However, a recent study in a normal population showed that the close relationship between copeptin and AVP was distorted in CKD, suggesting that the peptide clearances might differ when the renal function is impaired (70). It is not conclusive and further studies are necessary. Meijer et al. examined the role of copeptin baseline values and the change in renal function in a cohort of 548 renal transplant recipients (71). Elevated copeptin concentration was associated with an accelerated renal function decline in patients with renal transplant, as seen by a decrease in GFR during a median follow-up of 3.6 years. A recent cross-sectional study describes the association of plasma copeptin levels with eGFR, urinary albumin excretion, kidney length, and renal simple cysts in a large, multicentric population-based cohort (72). There are a few studies investigating associations between plasma copeptin and CVD in CKD/ESRD. Fenske et al. have reported an increased incidence of CV events in a subgroup of ESRD patients who had elevated levels of copeptin (73), and Engelbertz et al. showed elevated copeptin as a prognostic factor, independent of serum creatinine (SCr) in patients with both CAD and CKD (74). Whether increased AVP (copeptin) secretion is prognostic or causative for CVD especially in CKD patients and copeptin may serve as a biomarker to identify CVD high-risk patients with CKD needs to be evaluated in future studies (75).

D: Neutrophil Gelatinase-Associated Lipocalin (NGAL)

Although acute kidney injury (AKI) and CKD are conditions that substantially increase morbidity and mortality, the both diagnosis is still made with surrogate markers of GFR, such as SCr, urine output, and creatinine based estimating equations. The creatinine-base equations are an unreliable indicator during acute and chronic changes in kidney function, and new biomarkers should have the potential to identify earlier patients with AKI and CKD and in the future potentially intervene to modify outcomes. Among them, NGAL is considered one of excellent biomarkers in urine and plasma for the early prediction of AKI as well as CKD detection (32, 76).

NGAL in AKI/CKD

Neutrophil gelatinase-associated lipocalin (NGAL), also known as lipocalin-2, is a 25-kDa secretary glycoprotein and a member of lipocalin superfamily of proteins and has been shown to be induced rapidly in renal tubules in response to acute injury. NGAL seems to be one of the earliest kidney markers of ischemic or nephrotoxic injury in animal models and is detected in the blood and urine of humans soon after AKI. A meta-analysis by Haase et al. demonstrated that NGAL was an early predictor of subclinical AKI, with early elevations in plasma NGAL levels compared to SCr (77). Moreover, in-patient mortality was highest in those patients with elevated NGAL levels, with or without elevated SCr. In a prospective observational cohort study of 158 patients with Stage 3 or 4 CKD, it is suggested that urinary NGAL in addition to conventional established CV and renal risk factors may improve the prediction of progression to ESRD requiring renal replacement therapy (78). The role of NGAL has also been studied in the setting of post-cardiac surgery, cardiac catheterization, hemolytic uremic syndrome, and kidney transplantation.

NGAL in CVD

Aghel et al. recently reported that elevated admission serum NGAL levels was associated with heightened risk of subsequent development of worsening renal function (WRF) in 91 patients who admitted with acute HF (79). NGAL could be useful as an earlier marker of impending WRF during the treatment of acute HF. In patients with chronic HF, Damman et al. suggested that renal impairment is not only characterized by decreased eGFR and increased urinary albumin excretion but also by increased urinary NGAL concentration (80). Poniatowski et al. reported that predictors of serum NGAL in 150 patients with chronic HF were NYHA class, cystatin C, and eGFR in multiple regression analysis (81). NGAL might be investigated as a potential early and sensitive marker of kidney dysfunction/injury in order to select the appropriate strategy for reducing the risk in the setting of CRS.

However, recent evidence demonstrates a diversity of expression and function of NGAL. NGAL in plasma is also generated by a systemic inflammation, which induces NGAL synthesis by extrarenal tissues and the release of NGAL from neutrophils. It has been implicated not only as a marker of renal function but also as that of neutrophil activation, a protective factor against apoptosis and oxidative stress. Recent reports have suggested that NGAL could be a biomarker of atherosclerosis or CVD as well as in AKI and CKD progression (82). Increased NGAL expression in atherosclerotic plaques has been demonstrated and serum NGAL levels were significantly higher in the presence of CAD and were correlated with the severity of the disease. Also, in HF, increased myocardial expression of NGAL might be one of mechanisms for its prognostic value, independent on the coexisting renal injury. A recent study by Daniels et al. showed that plasma NGAL was a significant predictor of mortality and CVD in community-dwelling older adults, independent of traditional risk factors and kidney function, and adds incremental value to NT-proBNP and CRP (83).

Recently, among patients with CKD, urine levels of NGAL, were reported to be associated independently with future ischemic atherosclerotic events, but not with HF events or deaths (84). Higher urine NGAL may reflect a heavier burden of vascular diseases including subclinical inflammation and endothelial damage in the kidney as well as other organs. Clinical studies on the role of NGAL in ESRD patients are few. However, recent one study has showed that serum levels of NGAL in HD patients with CVD were significantly higher than those without CVD, and serum NGAL levels were independent risk factors in multivariate logistic regression analysis (85). Also in HD patients, increased serum NGAL might reflect the CV inflammation and damages. Further basic and clinical studies are warranted to elucidate the true pathogenic role of increased NGAL and to confirm the use as a biomarker for CRS.

E: Fibroblast Growth Factor (FGF)-23

Fibroblast growth factor-23 (FGF-23) is a recently discovered member of the FGF family, involved in the regulation of the body's calcium-phosphate metabolism (40). It increases renal phosphate excretion by reducing the expression of Na/Pi IIa cotransporter and decreases circulating calcitriol [1,25(OH)2D3] levels, leading to increased parathyroid hormone levels resulting in secondary hyperparathyroidism. FGF-23 levels gradually increase with declining renal function, starting at the very earliest stages of CKD, increasing by many orders of magnitude in ESRD. Some studies suggested that most circulating FGF-23 may be functionally intact, indicating a mechanism involving increased FGF-23 secretion as the cause of elevated FGF-23 levels. Oversecretion of FGF-23 may allow the body to maintain phosphate levels within a "physiological" range (~2.5–4.5 mg/dl) until very advanced CKD stages.

FGF-23 and Mortality

Elevated FGF-23 levels are associated with an increased risk of adverse outcomes, including all-cause mortality, CV events, and progression of CKD (86). Isakova et al. evaluated FGF-23 as a risk factor for adverse outcomes in a prospective 5-year study of 3,879 participants with CKD stages 2–4. They have shown that elevated FGF-23 was an independent risk factor for ESRD in patients with relatively preserved kidney function and for mortality across the spectrum of CKD (41). In a nested case–control sample of 200 subjects who died and 200 who survived during the first year taken from a prospective cohort of 10,044 incident HD patients, Gutiérrez et al. also showed that increased FGF-23 levels appear to be independently associated with mortality (87). Interestingly, some studies have described an association of FGF-23 with CV events and mortality in patients without CKD in whom the typical constellation of abnormal bone-mineral metabolism seen in CKD and ESRD is not present (88). Thus, FGF-23 may be a novel marker of CVD in patients with CKD and ESRD as well as in normal renal function, although these associations appear to be stronger in patients with CKD/ESRD. Also, they are independent of serum phosphate levels, and FGF-23 levels are a significant independent predictor among various parameters of calcium-phosphate metabolism.

FGF-23 and CVD

In cross-sectional studies, increased FGF-23 levels in patients with CKD were found to be associated not only with therapy-resistant secondary hyperparathyroidism but were also independently related to LVH and endothelial dysfunction after adjustment for traditional markers of calcium–phosphate metabolism. In a large study of 3,939 CKD patients, Faul et al. showed that FGF-23 was independently associated with LVH, which is an important mechanism of CVD in patients with CKD (89). In basic studies, this may be *via* the FGF receptor–dependent activation of the calcineurin-NFAT-signaling pathway independent of klotho (the co-receptor of FGF-23 only expressed in kidney and parathyroid glands). Treatment with an FGF receptor blocker is also reported to attenuate LVH. In contrast, observational studies reported conflicting results on the association of FGF-23 with arterial calcification, which is another prominent pattern of CV injury in CKD. In the largest study to date, FGF-23 was not independently associated with coronary artery calcification in patients with CKD stages 2–4 (90). These data suggest that direct effects of FGF-23 on cardiac remodeling, rather than the arterial vasculature, may underlie its association with mortality. Recently, Scialla et al. reported that higher FGF-23 level was independently associated with greater risk of CV events, particularly CHF, in a prospective cohort of 3,860 participants with CKD stages 2–4 (91). They demonstrated that elevated FGF-23 was associated more strongly with CHF than with atherosclerotic events ($P = 0.02$), and uniformly was associated with greater risk of CHF events across subgroups stratified by eGFR, proteinuria, prior heart disease, diabetes, BP control, anemia, LV mass index, and ejection fraction. Their findings suggest that FGF-23 could represent a novel mechanism of CHF that mediates at least a portion of excess CVD risk attributable to CKD. Recently, additional analysis in their study showed the association of FGF-23 with atrial fibrillation in CKD, which is frequently observed and has clinical impact in patients with CKD (92). Thus, in light of the high CV morbidity in CKD patients, as well as the failure of traditional therapeutic concepts (e.g., cholesterol-lowering or angiotensin-converting enzyme inhibitor therapy) and of non-traditional approaches (e.g., normalization of hemoglobin levels, increasing dialysis dose, and use of high-flux dialyzer), the option of pharmacological lowering of high circulating FGF-23 levels is expected to be a promising therapeutic pathway for reducing CVD in CKD and ESRD.

CONCLUSION AND FUTURE PERSPECTIVES

Of great importance is recognizing the presence of CRS and appreciating the impact it can play on treatment options and survival. However, our understanding of the pathophysiology of CRS or CVD in CKD/ESRD remains relatively poor. Reliable renocardiovascular biomarkers are nowadays necessary for evaluating accurately the complex interactions that are the basis of CRS and for early diagnosis and staging of CVD and CKD/ESRD, which lead to more accurate and efficient patient management and the development of strategies for CV risk stratification and prevention in this condition. On the contrary, it is neces-

sary for clinicians and investigators to consider the pathologic mechanisms linking heart and kidney for the interpretation and utilization in such biomarkers and to look beyond just biomarkers measured at presentation and statistical tests of association. From such an integrating viewpoint, further studies into the biomarkers will facilitate our knowledge of CRS and improve the clinical managements.

Recently, the aberrant profiles of circulating microRNAs (miRNAs) have been evaluated as emerging biomarkers for CV or renal disease. For example, miR-21 is associated with organ fibrosis and the measurement may be useful in the detection of renal or myocardial fibrosis (93, 94). Several studies have started to clarify the prognostic roles of various miRNAs in large cohorts (95). However, available data are limited especially in the context of CRS, and more studies and validation in large cohorts are necessary for establishing the clinical utility of circulating and urinary miRNAs. In addition, a multi-biomarker approach for targeting several organs or pathophysiologies is quite reasonable in this situation since CRS is a very complex disorder not of a single organ but of multi-organs including heart, vasculatures and kidney (52, 65). More integrated assessments of a multi-biomarker approach will be performed and shed light on the clinical management in CKD and ESRD patients. Another advance may be in "biomarker-guided monitoring of therapy". An individual patient meta-analysis suggested that BNP-guided monitoring of HF therapy is associated with a significant reduction in all-cause mortality in 11 studies randomizing 2,000 patients (96). Currently, the impact of renal insufficiency on the treatment effect by BNP guiding remains uncertain. However, such trials using BNP as well as other renocardiovascular biomarkers in CKD patients will be performed not only on HF, but also on CAD or LVH.

AUTHOR CONTRIBUTIONS

The contribution of each author on this work was as follows: SN and YI, the primary investigator; TY, the secondary investigator (data analysis); and SM, the consultant and supervisor.

REFERENCES

1. Herzog CA, Asinger RW, Berger AK, Charytan DM, Díez J, Hart RG, et al. Cardiovascular disease in chronic kidney disease. A clinical update from kidney disease: improving global outcomes (KDIGO). Kidney Int (2011) 80:572–86. doi:10.1038/ki.2011.223
2. Ronco C, McCullough P, Anker SD, Anand I, Aspromonte N, Bagshaw SM, et al. Cardio-renal syndromes: report from the consensus conference of the acute dialysis quality initiative. Eur Heart J (2010) 31:703–11. doi:10.1093/eurheartj/ehp507
3. Iwanaga Y, Miyazaki S. Heart failure, chronic kidney disease, and biomarkers – an integrated viewpoint. Circ J (2010) 74:1274–82. doi:10.1253/circj.CJ-10-0444
4. Tang WH, Francis GS, Morrow DA, Newby LK, Cannon CP, Jesse RL, et al. National Academy of Clinical Biochemistry Laboratory Medicine

practice guideline: clinical utilization of cardiac biomarker testing in heart failure. Circulation (2007) 116:e99–109. doi:10.1161/CIRCULATIONAHA.107.185267
5. Dhaun N, Yuzugulen J, Kimmitt RA, Wood EG, Chariyavilaskul P, MacIntyre IM, et al. Plasma pro-endothelin-1 peptide concentrations rise in chronic kidney disease and following selective endothelin A receptor antagonism. J Am Heart Assoc (2015) 4:e001624. doi:10.1161/JAHA.114.001624
6. Niizuma S, Iwanaga Y. Revisiting vasopressin and heart failure. Expert Rev Cardiovasc Ther (2013) 11:1451–4. doi:10.1586/14779072.2013.839203
7. Yalta K, Yalta T, Sivri N, Yetkin E. Copeptin and cardiovascular disease: a review of a novel neurohormone. Int J Cardiol (2013) 167:1750–9. doi:10.1016/j.ijcard.2012.12.039
8. Shah RV, Truong QA, Gaggin HK, Pfannkuche J, Hartmann O, Januzzi JL Jr. Mid-regional pro-atrial natriuretic peptide and pro-adrenomedullin testing for the diagnostic and prognostic evaluation of patients with

acute dyspnoea. *Eur Heart J* (2012) 33:2197–205. doi:10.1093/eurheartj/ehs136

9. Bosselmann H, Egstrup M, Rossing K, Gustafsson I, Gustafsson F, Tonder N, et al. Prognostic significance of cardiovascular biomarkers and renal dysfunction in outpatients with systolic heart failure: a long term follow-up study. *Int J Cardiol* (2013) 170:202–7. doi:10.1016/j.ijcard.2013.10.064

10. Meuwese CL, Carrero JJ. Chronic kidney disease and hypothalamic-pituitary axis dysfunction: the chicken or the egg? *Arch Med Res* (2013) 44:591–600. doi:10.1016/j.arcmed.2013.10.009

11. Stenvinkel P. Adiponectin in chronic kidney disease: a complex and context sensitive clinical situation. *J Ren Nutr* (2011) 21:82–6. doi:10.1053/j.jrn.2010.10.019

12. Dong M, Ren J. What fans the fire: insights into mechanisms of leptin in metabolic syndrome-associated heart diseases. *Curr Pharm Des* (2014) 20:652–8. doi:10.2174/1381612820041402131160930

13. Alix PM, Guebre-Egziabher F, Soulage CO. Leptin as a uremic toxin: deleterious role of leptin in chronic kidney disease. *Biochimie* (2014) 105:12–21. doi:10.1016/j.biochi.2014.06.024

14. De Gennaro L, Brunetti ND, Cuculo A, Pellegrino PL, Izzo P, Roma F, et al. Increased troponin levels in nonischemic cardiac conditions and noncardiac diseases. *J Interv Cardiol* (2008) 21:129–39. doi:10.1111/j.1540-8183.2007.00336.x

15. Kehl DW, Iqbal N, Fard A, Kipper BA, De La Parra Landa A, Maisel AS. Biomarkers in acute myocardial injury. *Transl Res* (2014) 159:252–64. doi:10.1016/j.trsl.2011.11.002

16. Sedeek M, Nasrallah R, Touyz RM, Hébert RL. NADPH oxidases, reactive oxygen species, and the kidney: friend and foe. *J Am Soc Nephrol* (2013) 24:1512–8. doi:10.1681/ASN.2012111112

17. Jalal DI, Chonchol M, Chen W, Targher G. Uric acid as a target of therapy in CKD. *Am J Kidney Dis* (2013) 61:134–46. doi:10.1053/j.ajkd.2012.07.021

18. Okazaki H, Shirakabe A, Kobayashi N, Hata N, Shinada T, Matsushita M, et al. The prognostic impact of uric acid in patients with severely decompensated acute heart failure. *J Cardiol* (2016) 68:384–91. doi:10.1016/j.jjcc.2016.04.013

19. Leurs P, Lindholm B. The AGE-RAGE pathway and its relation to cardiovascular disease in patients with chronic kidney disease. *Arch Med Res* (2013) 44:601–10. doi:10.1016/j.arcmed.2013.11.002

20. Sibal L, Agarwal SC, Home PD, Boger RH. The role of asymmetric dimethylarginine (ADMA) in endothelial dysfunction and cardiovascular disease. *Curr Cardiol Rev* (2010) 6:82–90. doi:10.2174/157340310791162659

21. Zoccali C, Bode-Böger S, Mallamaci F, Benedetto F, Tripepi G, Malatino L, et al. Plasma concentration of asymmetrical dimethylarginine and mortality in patients with end-stage renal disease: a prospective study. *Lancet* (2001) 358:2113–7. doi:10.1016/S0140-6736(01)07217-8

22. Tan RJ, Liu Y. Matrix metalloproteinases in kidney homeostasis and diseases. *Am J Physiol Renal Physiol* (2012) 302:F1351–61. doi:10.1152/ajprenal.00037.2012

23. van der Velde AR, Gullestad L, Ueland T, Aukrust P, Guo Y, Adourian A, et al. Prognostic value of changes in galectin-3 levels over time in patients with heart failure: data from CORONA and COACH. *Circ Heart Fail* (2013) 6:219–26. doi:10.1161/CIRCHEARTFAILURE.112.000129

24. O'Seaghdha CM, Hwang SJ, Ho JE, Vasan RS, Levy D, Fox CS. Elevated galectin-3 recedes the development of CKD. *J Am Soc Nephrol* (2013) 24:1470–7. doi:10.1681/ASN.2012090909

25. Gopal DM, Kommineni M, Ayalon N, Koelbl C, Ayalon R, Biolo A, et al. Relationship of plasma galectin-3 to renal function in patients with heart failure: effects of clinical status, pathophysiology of heart failure, and presence or absence of heart failure. *J Am Heart Assoc* (2012) 1:e000760. doi:10.1161/JAHA.112.000760

26. Bayes-Genis A, de Antonio M, Vila J, Peñafiel J, Galán A, Barallat J, et al. Head-to-head comparison of 2 myocardial fibrosis biomarkers for long-term heart failure risk stratification: ST2 versus galectin-3. *J Am Coll Cardiol* (2014) 63:158–66. doi:10.1016/j.jacc.2013.07.087

27. Januzzi JL Jr, Peacock WF, Maisel AS, Chae CU, Jesse RL, Baggish AL, et al. Measurement of the interleukin family member ST2 in patients with acute dyspnea: results from the PRIDE (Pro-Brain Natriuretic Peptide Investigation of Dyspnea in the Emergency Department) study. *J Am Coll Cardiol* (2007) 50:607–13. doi:10.1016/j.jacc.2007.05.014

28. Cottone S, Lorito MC, Riccobene R, Nardi E, Mulè G, Buscemi S, et al. Oxidative stress, inflammation and cardiovascular disease in chronic renal failure. *J Nephrol* (2008) 21:175–9.

29. Kume N, Mitsuoka H, Hayashida K, Tanaka M. Pentraxin 3 as a biomarker for acute coronary syndrome: comparison with biomarkers for cardiac damage. *J Cardiol* (2011) 58:38–45. doi:10.1016/j.jjcc.2011.03.006

30. Kempf T, von Haehling S, Peter T, Allhoff T, Cicoira M, Doehner W, et al. Prognostic utility of growth differentiation factor-15 in patients with chronic heart failure. *J Am Coll Cardiol* (2007) 2007(50):1054–60. doi:10.1016/j.jacc.2007.04.091

31. Ho JE, Hwang SJ, Wollert KC, Larson MG, Cheng S, Kempf T, et al. Biomarkers of cardiovascular stress and incident chronic kidney disease. *Clin Chem* (2013) 59:1613–20. doi:10.1373/clinchem.2013.205716

32. Taub PR, Borden KC, Fard A, Maisel A. Role of biomarkers in the diagnosis and prognosis of acute kidney injury in patients with cardiorenal syndrome. *Expert Rev Cardiovasc Ther* (2012) 10:657–67. doi:10.1586/erc.12.26

33. Bover J, Cozzolino M. Mineral and bone disorders in chronic kidney disease and end-stage renal disease patients: new insights into vitamin D receptor activation. *Kidney Int* (2011) 1:122–9. doi:10.1038/kisup.2011.28

34. Nitta K. Vascular calcification in patients with chronic kidney disease. *Ther Apher Dial* (2011) 15:513–21. doi:10.1111/j.1744-9987.2011.00979.x

35. Slinin Y, Foley RN, Collins AJ. Calcium, phosphorus, parathyroid hormone, and cardiovascular disease in hemodialysis patients: the USRDS waves 1, 3, and 4 study. *J Am Soc Nephrol* (2005) 16:1788–93. doi:10.1681/ASN.2004040275

36. Rostand SG, Drüeke TB. Parathyroid hormone, vitamin D, and cardiovascular disease in chronic renal failure. *Kidney Int* (1999) 56:383–92. doi:10.1046/j.1523-1755.1999.00575.x

37. Stenvinkel P, Carrero JJ, Axelsson J, Lindholm B, Heimbürger O, Massy Z. Emerging biomarkers for evaluating cardiovascular risk in the chronic kidney disease patient: how do new pieces fit into the uremic puzzle? *Clin J Am Soc Nephrol* (2008) 3:505–21. doi:10.2215/CJN.03670807

38. Moe SM, Reslerova M, Ketteler M, O'neill K, Duan D, Koczman J, et al. Role of calcification inhibitors in the pathogenesis of vascular calcification in chronic kidney disease (CKD). *Kidney Int* (2005) 67:2295–304. doi:10.1111/j.1523-1755.2005.00333.x

39. Zheng S, de Las Fuentes L, Bierhals A, Ash-Bernal R, Spence K, Slatopolsky E, et al. Relation of serum fetuin-A levels to coronary artery calcium in African-American patients on chronic hemodialysis. *Am J Cardiol* (2009) 103:46–9. doi:10.1016/j.amjcard.2008.08.032

40. Jüppner H. Phosphate and FGF-23. *Kidney Int* (2011) 79:S24–7. doi:10.1038/ki.2011.27

41. Isakova T, Xie H, Yang W, Xie D, Anderson AH, Scialla J, et al. Fibroblast growth factor 23 and risks of mortality and end-stage renal disease in patients with chronic kidney disease. *JAMA* (2011) 305:2432–9. doi:10.1001/jama.2011.826

42. Iwanaga Y, Nishi I, Furuichi S, Noguchi T, Sase K, Kihara Y, et al. B-type natriuretic peptide strongly reflects diastolic wall stress in patients with chronic heart failure: comparison between systolic and diastolic heart failure. *J Am Coll Cardiol* (2006) 47:742–8. doi:10.1016/j.jacc.2005.11.030

43. Niizuma S, Iwanaga Y, Yahata T, Tamaki Y, Goto Y, Nakahama H, et al. Impact of left ventricular end-diastolic wall stress on plasmaB-type natriuretic peptide in heart failure with chronic kidney disease and end-stage renal disease. *Clin Chem* (2009) 255:1347–53. doi:10.1373/clinchem.2008.121236

44. van Kimmenade RR, Januzzi JL Jr, Bakker JA, Houben AJ, Rennenberg R, Kroon AA, et al. Renal clearance of B-type natriuretic peptide and amino terminal pro-B-type natriuretic peptide a mechanistic study in hypertensive subjects. *J Am Coll Cardiol* (2009) 53:884–90. doi:10.1016/j.jacc.2008.11.032

45. Jacobs LH, Mingels AM, Wodzig WK, van Dieijen-Visser MP, Kooman JP. Renal dysfunction, hemodialysis, and the NT-proBNP/BNP ratio. *Am J Clin Pathol* (2010) 134:516–7. doi:10.1309/AJCPIZHTDSR2OGGX

46. Booth J, Pinney J, Davenport A. N-terminal proBNP – marker of cardiac dysfunction, fluid overload, or malnutrition in hemodialysis patients? *Clin J Am Soc Nephrol* (2010) 5:1036–40. doi:10.2215/CJN.09001209

47. Jacobs LH, van de Kerkhof JJ, Mingels AM, Passos VL, Kleijnen VW, Mazairac AH, et al. Inflammation, overhydration and cardiac biomarkers in

haemodialysis patients: a longitudinal study. *Nephrol Dial Transplant* (2010) 25:243–8. doi:10.1093/ndt/gfp417

48. Zoccali C, Mallamaci F, Benedetto FA, Tripepi G, Parlongo S, Cataliotti A, et al. Cardiac natriuretic peptides are related to left ventricular mass and function and predict mortality in dialysis patients. *J Am Soc Nephrol* (2001) 12:1508–15.

49. Mishra RK, Li Y, Ricardo AC, Yang W, Keane M, Cuevas M, et al. Association of N-terminal pro-B-type natriuretic peptide with left ventricular structure and function in chronic kidney disease (from the Chronic Renal Insufficiency Cohort [CRIC]). *Am J Cardiol* (2013) 111:432–8. doi:10.1016/j.amjcard.2012.10.019

50. Möllmann H, Nef HM, Kostin S, Dragu A, Maack C, Weber M, et al. Ischemia triggers BNP expression in the human myocardium independent from mechanical stress. *Int J Cardiol* (2010) 143:289–97. doi:10.1016/j.ijcard.2009.03.012

51. Niizuma S, Iwanaga Y, Yahata T, Goto Y, Kita T, Miyazaki S, et al. Plasma B-type natriuretic peptide levels reflect the presence and severity of stable coronary artery disease in chronic haemodialysis patients. *Nephrol Dial Transplant* (2009) 24:597–603. doi:10.1093/ndt/gfn491

52. Apple FS, Murakami MM, Pearce LA, Herzog CA. Multi-biomarker risk stratification of N-terminal pro-B-type natriuretic peptide, high-sensitivity C-reactive protein, and cardiac troponin T and I in end-stage renal disease for all-cause death. *Clin Chem* (2004) 50:2279–85. doi:10.1373/clinchem.2004.035741

53. Wang AY, Lam CW, Yu CM, Wang M, Chan IH, Zhang Y, et al. N-Terminal pro-brain natriuretic peptide: an independent risk predictor of cardiovascular congestion, mortality, and adverse cardiovascular outcomes in chronic peritoneal dialysis patients. *J Am Soc Nephrol* (2007) 18:321–30. doi:10.1681/ASN.2005121299

54. Yasuda K, Kimura T, Sasaki K, Obi Y, Iio K, Yamato M, et al. Plasma B-type natriuretic peptide level predicts kidney prognosis in patients with predialysis chronic kidney disease. *Nephrol Dial Transplant* (2012) 27:3885–91. doi:10.1093/ndt/gfs365

55. Sze J, Mooney J, Barzi F, Hillis GS, Chow CK. Cardiac troponin and its relationship to cardiovascular outcomes in community populations – a systematic review and meta-analysis. *Heart Lung Circ* (2016) 25:217–28. doi:10.1016/j.hlc.2015.09.001

56. Jacobs LH, van de Kerkhof J, Mingels AM, Kleijnen VW, van der Sande FM, Wodzig WK, et al. Haemodialysis patients longitudinally assessed by highly sensitive cardiac troponin T and commercial cardiac troponin T and cardiac troponin I assays. *Ann Clin Biochem* (2009) 46:283–90. doi:10.1258/acb.2009.008197

57. Aviles RJ, Askari AT, Lindahl B, Wallentin L, Jia G, Ohman EM, et al. Troponin T levels in patients with acute coronary syndromes, with or without renal dysfunction. *N Engl J Med* (2002) 346:2047–52. doi:10.1056/NEJMoa013456

58. Stacy SR, Suarez-Cuervo C, Berger Z, Wilson LM, Yeh HC, Bass EB, et al. Role of troponin in patients with chronic kidney disease and suspected acute coronary syndrome: a systematic review. *Ann Intern Med* (2014) 161:502–12. doi:10.7326/M14-0746

59. Michos ED, Wilson LM, Yeh HC, Berger Z, Suarez-Cuervo C, Stacy SR, et al. Prognostic value of cardiac troponin in patients with chronic kidney disease without suspected acute coronary syndrome: a systematic review and meta-analysis. *Ann Intern Med* (2014) 161:491–501. doi:10.7326/M14-0743

60. deFilippi C, Wasserman S, Rosanio S, Tiblier E, Sperger H, Tocchi M, et al. Cardiac troponin T and C-reactive protein for predicting prognosis, coronary atherosclerosis, and cardiomyopathy in patients undergoing long-term hemodialysis. *JAMA* (2003) 290:353–9. doi:10.1001/jama.290.3.353

61. NACB Writing Group. National Academy of Clinical Biochemistry Laboratory medicine practice guidelines: use of cardiac troponin and B-type natriuretic peptide or N-terminal proB-type natriuretic peptide for etiologies other than acute coronary syndromes and heart failure. *Clin Chem* (2007) 53:2086–96. doi:10.1373/clinchem.2007.095679

62. Peacock WF IV, De Marco T, Fonarow GC, Diercks D, Wynne J, Apple FS, et al. Cardiac troponin and outcome in acute heart failure. *N Engl J Med* (2008) 358:2117–26. doi:10.1056/NEJMoa0706824

63. Sundström J, Ingelsson E, Berglund L, Zethelius B, Lind L, Venge P, et al. Cardiac troponin-I and risk of heart failure: a community-based cohort study. *Eur Heart J* (2009) 30:773–81. doi:10.1093/eurheartj/ehp047

64. Chen S, Huang C, Wu B, Lian X, Mei X, Wan J. Cardiac troponin I in non-acute coronary syndrome patients with chronic kidney disease. *PLoS One* (2013) 8:e82752. doi:10.1371/journal.pone.0082752

65. Bansal N, Hyre Anderson A, Yang W, Christenson RH, deFilippi CR, Deo R, et al. High-sensitivity troponin T and N-terminal pro-B-type natriuretic peptide (NT-proBNP) and risk of incident heart failure in patients with CKD: the chronic renal insufficiency cohort (CRIC) study. *J Am Soc Nephrol* (2015) 26:946–56. doi:10.1681/ASN.2014010108

66. Tsutamoto T, Kawahara C, Yamaji M, Nishiyama K, Fujii M, Yamamoto T, et al. Relationship between renal function and serum cardiac troponin T in patients with chronic heart failure. *Eur J Heart Fail* (2009) 11:653–8. doi:10.1093/eurjhf/hfp072

67. Desai AS, Toto R, Jarolim P, Uno H, Eckardt KU, Kewalramani R, et al. Association between cardiac biomarkers and the development of ESRD in patients with type 2 diabetes mellitus, anemia, and CKD. *Am J Kidney Dis* (2011) 58:717–28. doi:10.1053/j.ajkd.2011.05.020

68. Neuhold S, Huelsmann M, Strunk G, Struck J, Adlbrecht C, Gouya G, et al. Prognostic value of emerging neurohormones in chronic heart failure during optimization of heart failure-specific therapy. *Clin Chem* (2010) 56:121–6. doi:10.1373/clinchem.2009.125856

69. Velho G, Bouby N, Hadjadj S, Matallah N, Mohammedi K, Fumeron F, et al. Plasma copeptin and renal outcomes in patients with type 2 diabetes and albuminuria. *Diabetes Care* (2013) 36:3639–45. doi:10.2337/dc13-0683

70. Roussel R, Fezeu L, Marre M, Velho G, Fumeron F, Jungers P, et al. Comparison between copeptin and vasopressin in a population from the community and in people with chronic kidney disease. *J Clin Endocrinol Metab* (2014) 99:4656–63. doi:10.1210/jc.2014-2295

71. Meijer E, Bakker SJ, de Jong PE, Homan van der Heide JJ, van Son WJ, Struck J, et al. Copeptin, a surrogate marker of vasopressin, is associated with accelerated renal function decline in renal transplant recipients. *Transplantation* (2009) 88:561–7. doi:10.1097/TP.0b013e3181b11ae4

72. Ponte B, Pruijm M, Ackermann D, Vuistiner P, Guessous I, Ehret G, et al. Copeptin is associated with kidney length, renal function, and prevalence of simple cysts in a population-based study. *J Am Soc Nephrol* (2015) 26:1415–25. doi:10.1681/ASN.2014030260

73. Fenske W, Wanner C, Allolio B, Drechsler C, Blouin K, Lilienthal J, et al. Copeptin levels associate with cardiovascular events in patients with ESRD and type 2 diabetes mellitus. *J Am Soc Nephrol* (2011) 22:782–90. doi:10.1681/ASN.2010070691

74. Engelbertz C, Brand E, Fobker M, Fischer D, Pavenstädt H, Reinecke H. Elevated copeptin is a prognostic factor for mortality even in patients with renal dysfunction. *Int J Cardiol* (2016) 221:327–32. doi:10.1016/j.ijcard.2016.07.058

75. Dünser MW, Schmittinger CA, Torgersen C. Copeptin and the transplanted kidney: friends or foes? *Transplantation* (2009) 88:455–6. doi:10.1097/TP.0b013e3181b050a2

76. Wasung ME, Chawla LS, Madero M. Biomarkers of renal function, which and when? *Clin Chim Acta* (2015) 438:350–7. doi:10.1016/j.cca.2014.08.039

77. Haase M, Bellomo R, Devarajan P, Schlattmann P, Haase-Fielitz A; NGAL Meta-analysis Investigator Group. Accuracy of neutrophil gelatinase-associated lipocalin (NGAL) in diagnosis and prognosis in acute kidney injury: a systematic review and meta-analysis. *Am J Kidney Dis* (2009) 54:1012–24. doi:10.1053/j.ajkd.2009.07.020

78. Smith ER, Lee D, Cai MM, Tomlinson LA, Ford ML, McMahon LP, et al. Urinary neutrophil gelatinase-associated lipocalin may aid prediction of renal decline in patients with non-proteinuric Stages 3 and 4 chronic kidney disease (CKD). *Nephrol Dial Transplant* (2013) 28:1569–79. doi:10.1093/ndt/gfs586

79. Aghel A, Shrestha K, Mullens W, Borowski A, Tang WH. Serum neutrophil gelatinase-associated lipocalin (NGAL) in predicting worsening renal function in acute decompensated heart failure. *J Card Fail* (2010) 16:49–54. doi:10.1016/j.cardfail.2009.07.003

80. Damman K, van Veldhuisen DJ, Navis G, Voors AA, Hillege HL. Urinary neutrophil gelatinase associated lipocalin (NGAL), a marker of tubular damage, is increased in patients with chronic heart failure. *Eur J Heart Fail* (2008) 10:997–1000. doi:10.1016/j.ejheart.2008.07.001

81. Poniatowski B, Malyszko J, Bachorzewska-Gajewska H, Malyszko JS, Dobrzycki S. Serum neutrophil gelatinase-associated lipocalin as a marker

of renal function in patients with chronic heart failure and coronary artery disease. *Kidney Blood Press Res* (2009) 32:77–80. doi:10.1159/000208989

82. Bolignano D, Coppolino G, Lacquaniti A, Buemi M. From kidney to cardiovascular diseases: NGAL as a biomarker beyond the confines of nephrology. *Eur J Clin Invest* (2010) 40:273–6. doi:10.1111/j.1365-2362.2010.02258.x

83. Daniels LB, Barrett-Connor E, Clopton P, Laughlin GA, Ix JH, Maisel AS. Plasma neutrophil gelatinase-associated lipocalin is independently associated with cardiovascular disease and mortality in community-dwelling older adults: The Rancho Bernardo Study. *J Am Coll Cardiol* (2012) 59:1101–9. doi:10.1016/j.jacc.2011.11.046

84. Liu KD, Yang W, Go AS, Anderson AH, Feldman HI, Fischer MJ, et al. Urine neutrophil gelatinase-associated lipocalin and risk of cardiovascular disease and death in CKD: results from the chronic renal insufficiency cohort (CRIC) study. *Am J Kidney Dis* (2015) 65:267–74. doi:10.1053/j.ajkd.2014.07.025

85. Furuya F, Shimura H, Yokomichi H, Takahashi K, Akiyama D, Asakawa C, et al. Neutrophil gelatinase-associated lipocalin levels associated with cardiovascular disease in chronic kidney disease patients. *Clin Exp Nephrol* (2014) 18:778–83. doi:10.1007/s10157-013-0923-4

86. Parker BD, Schurgers LJ, Brandenburg VM, Christenson RH, Vermeer C, Ketteler M, et al. The associations of fibroblast growth factor 23 and uncarboxylated matrix Gla protein with mortality in coronary artery disease: the Heart and Soul Study. *Ann Intern Med* (2010) 152:640–8. doi:10.7326/0003-4819-152-10-201005180-00004

87. Gutiérrez OM, Mannstadt M, Isakova T, Rauh-Hain JA, Tamez H, Shah A, et al. Fibroblast growth factor 23 and mortality among patients undergoing hemodialysis. *N Engl J Med* (2008) 359:584–92. doi:10.1056/NEJMoa0706130

88. Ix JH, Katz R, Kestenbaum BR, de Boer IH, Chonchol M, Mukamal KJ, et al. Fibroblast growth factor-23 and death, heart failure, and cardiovascular events in community-living individuals: CHS (Cardiovascular Health Study). *J Am Coll Cardiol* (2012) 60:200–7. doi:10.1016/j.jacc.2012.03.040

89. Faul C, Amaral AP, Oskouei B, Hu MC, Sloan A, Isakova T, et al. FGF23 induces left ventricular hypertrophy. *J Clin Invest* (2011) 121:4393–408. doi:10.1172/JCI46122

90. Scialla JJ, Lau WL, Reilly MP, Isakova T, Yang HY, Crouthamel MH, et al. Fibroblast growth factor 23 is not associated with and does not induce arterial calcification. *Kidney Int* (2013) 83:1159–68. doi:10.1038/ki.2013.3

91. Scialla JJ, Xie H, Rahman M, Anderson AH, Isakova T, Ojo A, et al. Fibroblast growth factor-23 and cardiovascular events in CKD. *J Am Soc Nephrol* (2014) 2:349–60. doi:10.1681/ASN.2013050465

92. Mehta R, Cai X, Lee J, Scialla JJ, Bansal N, Sondheimer JH, et al. Association of fibroblast growth factor 23 with atrial fibrillation in chronic kidney disease, from the chronic renal insufficiency cohort study. *JAMA Cardiol* (2016) 1:548–56. doi:10.1001/jamacardio.2016.1445

93. Chung AC, Lan HY. MicroRNAs in renal fibrosis. *Front Physiol* (2015) 6:50. doi:10.3389/fphys.2015.00050

94. Villar AV, García R, Merino D, Llano M, Cobo M, Montalvo C, et al. Myocardial and circulating levels of microRNA-21 reflect left ventricular fibrosis in aortic stenosis patients. *Int J Cardiol* (2013) 167:2875–81. doi:10.1016/j.ijcard.2012.07.021

95. Jakob P, Kacprowski T, Briand-Schumacher S, Heg D, Klingenberg R, Stähli BE, et al. Profiling and validation of circulating microRNAs for cardiovascular events in patients presenting with ST-segment elevation myocardial infarction. *Eur Heart J* (2016). doi:10.1093/eurheartj/ehw563

96. Troughton RW, Frampton CM, Brunner-La Rocca HP, Pfisterer M, Eurlings LW, Erntell H, et al. Effect of B-type natriuretic peptide-guided treatment of chronic heart failure on total mortality and hospitalization: an individual patient meta-analysis. *Eur Heart J* (2014) 35:1559–67. doi:10.1093/eurheartj/ehu090

18

Epigenetic Biomarkers in Cardiovascular Diseases

Carolina Soler-Botija[1,2]*, Carolina Gálvez-Montón[1,2] and Antoni Bayés-Genís[1,2,3,4]

[1] Heart Failure and Cardiac Regeneration (ICREC) Research Program, Health Science Research Institute Germans Trias i Pujol (IGTP), Badalona, Spain, [2] CIBERCV, Instituto de Salud Carlos III, Madrid, Spain, [3] Cardiology Service, HUGTiP, Badalona, Spain, [4] Department of Medicine, Barcelona Autonomous University (UAB), Badalona, Spain

*Correspondence:
Carolina Soler-Botija
csoler@igtp.cat

Cardiovascular diseases are the number one cause of death worldwide and greatly impact quality of life and medical costs. Enormous effort has been made in research to obtain new tools for efficient and quick diagnosis and predicting the prognosis of these diseases. Discoveries of epigenetic mechanisms have related several pathologies, including cardiovascular diseases, to epigenetic dysregulation. This has implications on disease progression and is the basis for new preventive strategies. Advances in methodology and big data analysis have identified novel mechanisms and targets involved in numerous diseases, allowing more individualized epigenetic maps for personalized diagnosis and treatment. This paves the way for what is called pharmacoepigenetics, which predicts the drug response and develops a tailored therapy based on differences in the epigenetic basis of each patient. Similarly, epigenetic biomarkers have emerged as a promising instrument for the consistent diagnosis and prognosis of cardiovascular diseases. Their good accessibility and feasible methods of detection make them suitable for use in clinical practice. However, multicenter studies with a large sample population are required to determine with certainty which epigenetic biomarkers are reliable for clinical routine. Therefore, this review focuses on current discoveries regarding epigenetic biomarkers and its controversy aiming to improve the diagnosis, prognosis, and therapy in cardiovascular patients.

Keywords: epigenetics, biomarker, microRNA, cardiovascular diseases, myocardial infarction, heart failure, atherosclerosis, hypertension

INTRODUCTION

Cardiovascular diseases (CVDs) are one of the leading causes of mortality in developed countries. Cardiovascular diseases refer to disorders affecting the structures or function of the heart and blood vessels, including hypertension, atherosclerosis, myocardial infarction (MI), ischemia/reperfusion injury, stroke, and heart failure (HF), among others (Wang et al., 2016a; Thomas et al.,

Abbreviations: AMI, acute myocardial infarction; ApoE, apolipoprotein E; BNP B-type natriuretic peptide; CK, creatine kinase; cTnI, cardiac troponin I; cTnT, cardiac troponin T; DOT1L, disruptor of telomeric silencing-1; ENaC, epithelial sodium channel; EZH2, enhancer of zeste homolog 2; GEO, Gene Expression Omnibus; HDAC, histone deacetylase; HF, heart failure; HFrEF, heart failure with reduced ejection fraction; HFpEF, heart failure with preserved ejection fraction; hs-cTnT, high-sensitivity cardiac troponin T; hs-CRP, high-sensitivity C-reactive protein; lncRNAs, long noncoding RNAs; LV, left ventricular; MI, myocardial infarction; miRNAs, microRNAs; ncRNAs, noncoding RNAs; NSTEMI, non- ST-segment elevation myocardial infarction; STEMI, ST-segment elevation myocardial infarction; pmiRNAs, platelet miRNAs; piRNAs, p-element-induced wimpy testis (PIWI)-interacting RNAs; tRNA, transfer RNA; ZEB1, zinc finger E-box binding homeobox 1.

2018). Mechanisms underlying the complex pathophysiology that leads to CVDs are of great interest but still far from clear. Progress in the field of epigenetics have opened a new world for the comprehension and management of human diseases, including the prevalence of CVDs, based on the role of genetics and its environmental interaction in pathological conditions (Jaenisch and Bird, 2003). Significant evidence suggests that the environment and lifestyle can define epigenetic patterns throughout life. These epigenetic patterns are a cellular memory of further environmental exposure. Epigenetic modifications are reversible, different among cell types, and can potentially lead to disease susceptibility by producing long-term changes in gene transcription (Fraga et al., 2005; Beekman et al., 2010).

Epigenetic modifications include DNA methylation and posttranslational modifications of histone tails. However, in this review, posttranscriptional regulation of gene expression by noncoding RNAs (ncRNAs) is also considered a part of the epigenetic machinery. MicroRNAs (miRNAs) are small ncRNAs that contribute to regulation of the expression of different epigenetic regulators such as DNA methyltransferases (DNMTs) and histone deacetylases (HDACs), among others. Similarly, DNA methylation and histone modifications can regulate the expression of some miRNAs, forming a feedback loop. Thus, miRNAs and epigenetic regulators cooperate to modulate the expression of mutual targets. Therefore, although miRNAs

are not strictly considered epigenetic factors, they contribute to the modulation of gene expression through epigenetics. Disruption of this complex regulation may participate in the development of different diseases (Iorio et al., 2010; Hoareau-Aveilla and Meggetto, 2017; Moutinho and Esteller, 2017; Wang et al., 2017a) (**Figure 1**). DNA and histone proteins comprise the chromatin, which can be remodeled into a tightly condensed state (heterochromatin) or an open conformation (euchromatin) that would allow access to transcription factors or DNA binding proteins, allowing the regulation of gene expression (Kouzarides, 2007). Thus, epigenetics involves changes in gene expression due to chromatin adjustments that change the accessibility of DNA without changing its sequence, leading to silencing or downregulation/upregulation of gene expression (Baccarelli et al., 2010). Chromatin modifications, such as DNA methylation, consist of the transfer of a methyl group to carbon 5 of the cytosine residues [5-methylcytosine (5mC)] in CpG dinucleotides sites. CpG dinucleotides are localized throughout the genome but are more abundant in certain regions, such as gene promoters, forming so-called CpG islands. CpG methylation causes transcriptional repression by directly blocking transcription factor access to the DNA or indirectly *via* chromatin-modifying proteins (methyl-binding proteins) that recognize the methylated regions and recruit corepressors. DNA methyltransferases catalyze DNA methylation by recognizing

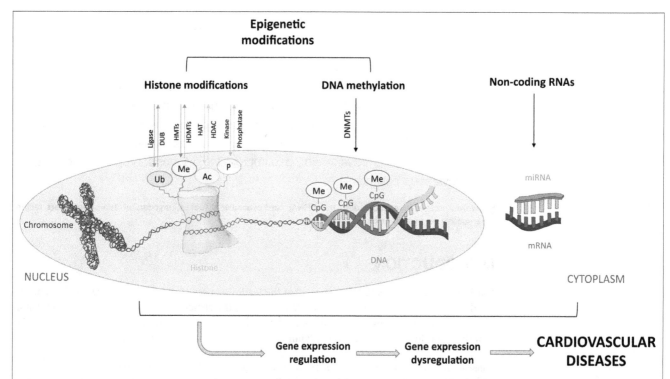

FIGURE 1 | Epigenetic regulatory mechanisms. Posttranslational modifications of histone tails by acetylation, deacetylation, ubiquitination, methylation, and phosphorylation. DNA methylation by DNA methyltransferases (DNMTs). Posttranscriptional regulation of gene expression by microRNAs. Epigenetic modifications involve silencing or downregulation/upregulation of gene expression. Dysregulation of the epigenetic machinery could lead to gene expression dysregulation and cardiovascular diseases. Ubiquitin (Ub), methionine (Me), acetyl group (Ac), phosphate (P), deubiquitinating enzyme (DUB), histone methyltransferase (HMTs), histone demethylase (HDMTs), histone acetyltransferase (HAT), histone deacetylase (HDAC), a cytosine followed by a guanine (CpG), microRNAs (miRNAs), and messenger RNA (mRNA).

and maintaining hypermethylated DNA during replication (DNMT1) or by *de novo* methylation (DNMT3a and DNMT3b). Moreover, gene bodies of actively transcribed genes normally show slightly higher DNA methylation levels as compared to gene bodies of nontranscribed genes. In contrast, hypomethylation is usually found in enhancer regions and promoters (Costantino et al., 2018). Posttranslational modification of histone tails is another epigenetic modification that regulates gene expression by chromatin remodeling. Histone acetylation, deacetylation, methylation, phosphorylation and ubiquitination change DNA accessibility, regulating gene transcription. The acetylation of histone tails is regulated by histone acetyltransferases (HATs) and HDACs. Histone acetyltransferase enzymes acetylate the lysine residues of the histones, whereas HDACs deacetylate them, promoting gene activation or silencing, respectively. Histone methylation is regulated by histone methyltransferases (HMTs) and histone demethylases (HDMT). Methylation occurs at the lysine or arginine residues and can activate or repress gene transcription depending on the degree of methylation and which residue is methylated (Li et al., 2017c; Sabia et al., 2017). The serine, threonine, and tyrosine residues of histone tails can also be phosphorylated and dephosphorylated by protein kinases and phosphatases, respectively. Histone tail phosphorylation modulates chromatin structure, taking part in transcription, DNA repair, and chromatin compaction in cell division and apoptosis (Rossetto et al., 2012). Lastly, histone tail ubiquitination is sequentially catalyzed by ligases enzymes, which attach ubiquitin to lysine residues. Ubiquitination and deubiquitination are involved in the activation of transcription and are usually associated with histone methylation. Their effect on repressing or activating transcription generally depends on what histone is modified (Cao and Yan, 2012). Finally, miRNAs regulate gene expression *via* degradation of the transcript or repression of translation when binding to the 3′-untranslated region of the target mRNA. Thus, miRNA represses mRNA translation without changing the DNA sequence of the gene. MicroRNA binding to mRNA is imperfect, so each miRNA has multiple targets. This allows the regulation of a great part of the human genome (Bartel, 2009). The miRNAs are 19-25 nucleotides in length, encoded in the genome and transcribed into primary miRNA (pri-miRNA). Pri-miRNAs derive into miRNAs precursors (pre-miRNA) by the nuclear RNase III called Dorsha and are transferred to the cytoplasm and processed by the endonuclease Dicer to generate a double-stranded miRNA duplex. This product is incorporated into an RNA-induced silencer complex (RISC)–loading complex. Then, one strand is removed from the complex, and the other strand forms a mature RISC, serving as a template for target mRNAs (Sato et al., 2011; Nishiguchi et al., 2015).

Due to this important function in gene regulation, epigenetic modifications and miRNA may play a crucial role in the development of pathological conditions, including CVDs. Understanding the epigenetic machinery underlying cardiac disorders and how these epigenetic mechanisms can be introduced into diagnostics (i.e., biomarkers) and therapies is fundamental to improving the quality of life of patients. In medicine, a biomarker is defined as a measurable characteristic that indicates a particular physiological or pathological state or a

response to a therapeutic treatment (Strimbu and Tavel, 2010). Ideally, biomarkers should have easy accessibility, predictable detection, and reliability (Sun et al., 2017). It is mandatory to present a specific measurable change that clearly associates with a diagnosis or a predictable outcome. Thus, biomarkers provide information to physicians when evaluating the probability of developing a disease, making a diagnosis, evaluating the severity of a disease and its progression; during therapeutic decision making; or when monitoring a patient's response and may result in significant cost reduction (Baccarelli et al., 2010). Their classification can be based on their application (predisposition, diagnosis, monitoring, safety, prognostic, or predictive biomarkers). Predisposition biomarkers determine how likely it is for a patient to develop a certain disease and are usually utilized when there is a personal or family history that indicates a disease risk, and the results can help guide medical care. Diagnostic biomarkers are used to detect or confirm the existence of a health disorder and may assist its early detection. Monitoring biomarkers evaluate the status of a disease or determine exposure to an environmental agent or medical product. Safety biomarkers indicate the probability, presence, or extent of toxicity of a certain medical product or environmental agent. Prognostic biomarkers indicate how a disease may progress in patients who already have the particular disease. These biomarkers do not predict the treatment response but can be useful when selecting patients for treatment. Predictive biomarkers identify patients who are most likely to have a favorable or unfavorable response to a specific treatment. Thus, they can predict treatment success or undesired side effects in a particular patient. A particular disease can have different biological mechanisms in different patients. Predictive biomarkers can be associated with the specific mechanism of a health disorder. This facilitates a targeted therapy, which uses drugs specific for a particular biological mechanism associated with a disease, increasing its effectiveness (FDA-NIH Biomarker Working Group, 2016). Specifically, epigenetic biomarkers belonging to most of these classifications are discussed in this review, with a focus on CVDs. Among the epigenetic biomarkers, miRNAs are the most attractive, as they can be detected in small sample volumes, are stable, and can be obtained from plasma, serum, saliva, and urine. Interestingly, they are highly conserved, and this allows a reliable comparison between patients and animal models of disease (Matsumoto et al., 2013). Therefore, although all epigenetic mechanisms are being intensively investigated, miRNAs are evaluated the most for their use as predictive biomarkers. This review presents an overview of current research on epigenetic biomarkers in CVDs and how this knowledge can benefit the diagnosis, prognosis, and therapy for cardiovascular patients.

EPIGENETIC BIOMARKERS IN CVDS

Over the last few years, numerous studies have linked cardiovascular risk factors to epigenetic modifications in human patients. Modification of the epigenetic environment alters cardiovascular homeostasis and impacts cardiovascular disorders. The function of epigenetic mechanisms in the regulation of gene expression is well known, although the role of epigenetic marks in CVDs is not clearly understood. Thus, the exploration of epigenetic biomarkers may lead to a deep comprehension of the molecular mechanisms and pathways associated with CVDs. In this section, we focus on major CVDs, such as hypertension, atherosclerosis, MI, and HF, and the epigenetic biomarkers associated with them.

Hypertension

Arterial hypertension is a multifactorial disease with several mechanisms and metabolic systems involved in its pathogenesis. Genetic factors and environmental background may lead to alterations in multiple pathways that can eventually trigger development of the disease (Franceschini and Le, 2014). Intrauterine alterations, such as malnutrition, starvation, obesity, alcohol, drugs, nicotine, or environmental toxins, are some of the environmental factors directly related to hypertension development in the progeny (Bogdarina et al., 2007; Nuyt and Alexander, 2009). In addition, individuals who have aerobic training present with lower blood pressure than nontrained individuals (Fagard, 2006). This has an important impact on CVD risk factor control and is a nonpharmacological way to treat patients. There are also epigenetic factors that can influence the appearance of hypertension in adults, such as hypermethylation of genes, including superoxide dismutase-2 (SOD2) or Granulysin, or increased levels of histone acetylation at the promoter of the endothelial oxide synthetase gene (eNOS) (Wang et al., 2018b). Environmental factors are important to determining an individual's predisposition to developing major cardiovascular risk factors by means of epigenetic modifications, and identification of the epigenetic mechanisms that participate in hypertension development may help generate new treatments. This is of great interest because hypertension is a key risk factor for CVDs, including MI, HF, stroke, and end-stage renal disease (**Table 1** and **Figure 2**).

Essential hypertension is a multifactorial disease with no identifiable cause that is affected by environmental and epigenetic factors. Environmental stressors cause acetylation of histone 3 in the neurons of the area postrema, leading to an increase in pressure that results in hypertension (Irmak and Sizlan, 2006). Low activity of the 11 beta-hydroxysteroid dehydrogenase 2 (HSD11B2) induces hypertension. In a study performed in patients with essential hypertension or glucocorticoid-induced hypertension, the HSD11B2 promoter was highly methylated. These changes may reflect a global status, with methylation of gene promoter being a potentially useful molecular biomarker to characterize hypertensive patients (Alikhani-Koopaei et al., 2004; Friso et al., 2008). Moreover, a polymorphism in the disruptor of telomeric silencing-1 gene (DOT1L), which encodes a methyltransferase that enhances methylation of histone 3 (H3K79) in the renal epithelial sodium channel gene (ENaC) promoter, is associated with blood pressure regulation (Duarte et al., 2012). It has also been reported that a DOT1A and ALL1 (fused gene from chromosome 9 [Af9]) interaction is associated with H3K79 hypermethylation of the ENaC promoter, suppressing its transcriptional activity. This interaction is

disrupted by aldosterone and causes hypomethylation of H3K79 at specific regions, disinhibiting the ENaC promoter and leading to hypertension. Thus, the Dot1a-Af9 pathway may also be involved in the control of genes implicated in hypertension (Zhang et al., 2009). Hypomethylation of the α-adducin gene (ADD1) promoter has been found to be connected to the risk of essential hypertension. However, differences between females and males have been found (Zhang et al., 2013a). Moreover, histone 3 (H3K4 or H3K9) demethylation is induced by lysine-specific demethylase-1 (LSD1), which modifies gene transcription. Hypermethylation of histone 3 has been associated with hypertension, increased vascular contraction, and decreased relaxation *via* the nitric oxide-cGMP (NO-cGMP) pathway in heterozygous LSD1 knockout mice fed a high-salt diet (Pojoga et al., 2011). Histone deacetylation is also important in the development of pulmonary arterial hypertension. HDAC1 and HDAC5 protein levels have been demonstrated to be elevated in the lungs of patients and hypoxic rats. Inhibition of these proteins by valproic acid and suberoylanilide hydroxamic acid diminished the development of hypoxia-induced pulmonary hypertension in rats. Thus, HDAC1 and HDAC5 levels could be useful predictive biomarkers for the treatment of pulmonary hypertension in patients (Zhao et al., 2012).

In a study evaluating alterations in the global DNA methylation status of patients with essential hypertension, the level of the epigenetic marker 5mC was lower in hypertensive patients than in healthy people (Smolarek et al., 2010). In an *in vivo* model of hypertension using Dahl salt-sensitive rats, the levels of 5mC and 5-hydroxymethylcytosine (5hmC) were evaluated in the outer renal medulla. In response to salt administration, the 5mC levels were significantly higher for genes with low transcription and 5hmC levels higher in genes with higher expression. This study revealed important features of 5mC and 5hmC for understanding the role of epigenetic modifications in the regulation of hypertension (Liu et al., 2014).

Rivière et al. (2011) analyzed the regulation of somatic angiotensin-converting enzyme gene (sACE) expression by promoter methylation. sACE regulates blood pressure by catalyzing the conversion of angiotensin I into angiotensin II, a potent vasopressor. Hypermethylation of sACE promoter in cultures of human endothelial cells and rats was associated with transcriptional repression, suggesting an epigenetic mechanism in hypertension regulation (Rivière et al., 2011). More recently, Fan et al. (2017) demonstrated opposite results in patients with essential hypertension. The authors indicated that hypermethylation of the ACE2 promoter may increase essential hypertension risk, with variabilities in CpG islands methylation in males and females (Fan et al., 2017).

Moreover, a genome-wide methylation study on essential hypertension revealed that changes in the DNA methylation of leukocytes are involved in the pathogenesis of hypertension. They found increased methylation in the gene encoding sulfatase 1 (SULF1), which is involved in apoptosis, and decreased methylation in the gene encoding prolylcarboxypeptidase (PRCP), a regulator of angiotensin II and III cleavage (Wang et al., 2013b). Another genome-wide study of blood pressure characteristics found new genetic variants that influence blood pressure and are

TABLE 1 | Epigenetic biomarkers in hypertension.

Epigenetic modification	Biomarker	Regulation in hypertension	Sample source	Study type	References
DNA methylation	HSD11B2 promoter	Highly methylated	Rat's urine and tissues and human cell lines	Experimental: in vitro and rat model	(Alikhani-Koopaei et al., 2004)
	SERPIN3 CpG island	Hypomethylation	Placental tissue	Clinical	(Chelbi et al., 2007)
	HSD11B2 promoter	Highly methylated	Blood and urine	Clinical	(Friso et al., 2008)
	5mC	Lower levels	Blood	Clinical	(Smolarek et al., 2010)
	NKCC1 promoter	Hypomethylation	Aorta, heart and kidney	Experimental: spontaneously hypertensive rodent model	(Lee et al., 2010; Cho et al., 2011)
	sACE promoter	Hypermethylation	Blood	Clinical and experimental: in vitro	(Rivière et al., 2011)
	ERα promoter	Methylation	Uterine arteries	Clinical	(Dasgupta et al., 2012)
	SULF1, PRCP	SULF1: hypermethylation; PRCP: hypomethylation	Blood	Clinical	(Wang et al., 2013b)
	ADD1 promoter	Hypomethylation	Plasma	Clinical	(Zhang et al., 2013a)
	5mC, 5hmC	Higher levels	Tissue	Experimental: Dahl salt-sensitive rats	(Liu et al., 2014)
	AGT promoter	Demethylation	H295R cells and visceral adipose tissue	Experimental: in vitro and rat model	(Wang et al., 2014a)
	DSCR3	Hypermethylation	Maternal blood and placental tissue	Clinical	(Kim et al., 2015)
	miRNA-34a gene promoter	Hypomethylation	Placental tissue	Clinical	(Rezaei et al., 2018)
	ACE2 promoter	Hypermethylation	Plasma	Clinical	(Fan et al., 2017)
	CBS promoter	Hypermethylation	Maternal blood and placental tissue	Clinical	(Kim et al., 2015)
	MTHFD1 promoter	Hypermethylation	Plasma	Clinical	(Xu et al., 2019)
Histone modifications	H3K79	Hypermethylation	NA	Clinical	(Rodriguez-Iturbe, 2006; Duarte et al., 2012)
	Histone 3	Acetylation	Germ cells	Review	(Irmak and Sizlan, 2006)
	H3K79	DNA methylation	Bibliography	Review	(Zhang et al., 2009)
	HDAC8	Inhibition	mDCT cells and tissues	Experimental: rat models of salt-sensitive hypertension	(Mu et al., 2011)
	H3K4 or H3K9	Hypermethylation	Tissue, plasma, and urine	Experimental: LSD1 knockout mice with a high-salt diet	(Pojoga et al., 2011)
	HDAC1, HDAC5	High levels	Lung tissue and adventitial fibroblasts	Clinical and experimental: in vitro and hypoxic rat	(Zhao et al., 2012)
miRNA	miR-18a, miR-210, miR-152, miR-363, miR-377, miR-411, miR-518b, miR-542-3p	miR-18a, miR-363, miR-377, miR-411, miR-542-3p: underexpression; miR-210, miR-152, miR-518b: overexpression	Placental tissue	Clinical	(Zhu et al., 2009)
	22 miRNAs	15 upregulated and 7 downregulated	Serum	Clinical	(Yang et al., 2011)
	let-7b, miR-302*, miR-104, miR-128a, miR-182*, miR-133b	Overexpression	Placental tissue	Clinical	(Noack et al., 2011)
	miR-92b, miR-197, miR-342-3p, miR-296-5p, miR-26b, miR-25, miR-296-3p, miR-26a, miR-198, miR-202, miR-191, miR-95, miR-204, miR-21, miR-223	miR-92b, miR-197, miR-342-3p, miR-296-5p, miR-26b, miR-25, miR-296-3p, miR-26a, miR-198, miR-202, miR-191, miR-95, miR-204: overexpression; miR-21, miR-223: underexpression	Placental tissue	Clinical	(Choi et al., 2013)
	miR-9, miR-126	Lower levels	Peripheral blood mononuclear cells	Clinical	(Kontaraki et al., 2014)
	miR1233	Higher levels	Serum	Clinical	(Ura et al., 2014)

(Continued)

TABLE 1 | Continued

Epigenetic modification	Biomarker	Regulation in hypertension	Sample source	Study type	References
	miR-18a, miR-19b1, miR-92a1, miR-210	miR-210: upregulation; miR-18a, miR-19b1, and miR-92a1: downregulation	Plasma and placental tissue	Clinical	(Xu et al., 2014)
	miR-505	Upregulation	Plasma	Clinical	(Yang et al., 2014)
	miR-106a, miR-18b, miR-20b, miR-19b-2, miR-92a-2, miR-363	Dysregulation	Placental tissue	Clinical	(Zhang et al., 2015a)
	miR-515-5p, miR-518b, miR-518f-5p, miR-519d, miR-520h	Downregulation	Placental tissue	Clinical	(Hromadnikova et al., 2015)
	miR-335, miR-584	Upregulation	Placental tissue and HTR8/Svneo cells	Clinical and experimental: in vitro	(Jiang F. et al., 2015)
	miR-125b	Overexpression	Plasma and placental tissue	Clinical	(Yang et al., 2016b)
	miR-215, miR-155, miR-650, miR-210, miR-21, miR-18a, miR-19b1	MiR-215, miR-155, miR-650, miR-210, miR-21: upregulation; miR-18a, miR-19b1: downregulation	Plasma	Clinical	(Jairajpuri et al., 2017)
	miR-204-5p	Higher levels	Serum	Clinical	(Mei et al., 2017)
	let-7b*, let-7f-1*, miR-1183, miR-23c, miR-425*	miR-1183: upregulation; let-7b*, miR-23c, miR-425*, let-7f-1*: downregulation	Plasma and placental tissue	Clinical	(Gunel et al., 2017)
	miR-145	Downregulation	Placental tissue	Clinical	(Han et al., 2017)
	miR-202-3p	Upregulation	Placental tissue	Clinical	(Singh et al., 2017)
	let-7	Higher	Plasma	Clinical	(Huang et al., 2017b)
	miRNA	Dysregulation	Bibliography: Maternal serum and placental tissue	Bibliography review	(Laganà et al., 2018)
	miR-19a	Upregulation	Plasma and lung tissue	Clinical	(Chen and Li, 2017)
	miR-21	Upregulation	Peripheral blood mononuclear cells	Clinical	(Parthenakis et al., 2017)
	miR-21	Upregulation	Bibliography review	Bibliography review	(Sekar et al., 2017)
	miR-510	Upregulation	Serum	Clinical	(Krishnan et al., 2017)
	miR-206	Lower levels	Serum	Clinical	(Jin et al., 2017)
	miR-424(322)	Upregulation	Plasma	Clinical	(Baptista et al., 2018)
	miR-199a-3p, miR-208a-3p, miR-122-5p, miR-223-3p	Downregulation	Serum	Clinical	(Zhang et al., 2018c)
	miR-431-5p	Upregulation	Tissue	Experimental: mice made hypertensive and in vitro	(Huo et al., 2019)
	miR-143, NR_034083, NR_104181,	miR-143: upregulation; NR_034083: downregulation and NR_104181 and	Peripheral blood leucocytes	Clinical	(Chen et al., 2018b)

NA, not available.

strongly associated with local CpG island methylation. This study demonstrated the role of DNA methylation in the regulation of blood pressure (Kato et al., 2015).

The pathogenesis of hypertension is affected by alterations in ion flux mechanisms. Hypomethylation of the Na/K/2Cl cotransporter 1 gene (*NKCC1*) promoter results in overexpression in a rodent model with spontaneous hypertension (Lee et al., 2010). DNA methyltransferase activity maintained hypomethylation in the *NKCC1* promoter, playing an important role in *NKCC1* upregulation during the course of the disease. This encourages evaluation of the *NKCC1* methylation status in hypertensive patients (Cho et al., 2011). Furthermore, WNK4 is a serine-threonine kinase that negatively

regulates the Na(+)-Cl(−)-cotransporter (NCC) and ENaC. This would affect the distal nephron, increasing the reabsorption of sodium. Stimulation of β(2)-adrenergic receptor (β(2)AR) in salt intake conditions would reduce *WNK4* transcription, resulting in inhibition of HDAC8 activity and increased histone acetylation. In the rat models of salt-sensitive hypertension, salt diet repressed renal WNK4 expression, activating the NCC and inducing salt-dependent hypertension. Thus, *WNK4* transcription is epigenetically modulated in the course of salt-sensitive hypertension, with the β(2)AR-WNK4 pathway as a potential therapeutic target for this disease (Mu et al., 2011).

Goyal et al. (2010) demonstrated that a low protein diet in pregnant mice leads to alterations in DNA methylation, miRNA,

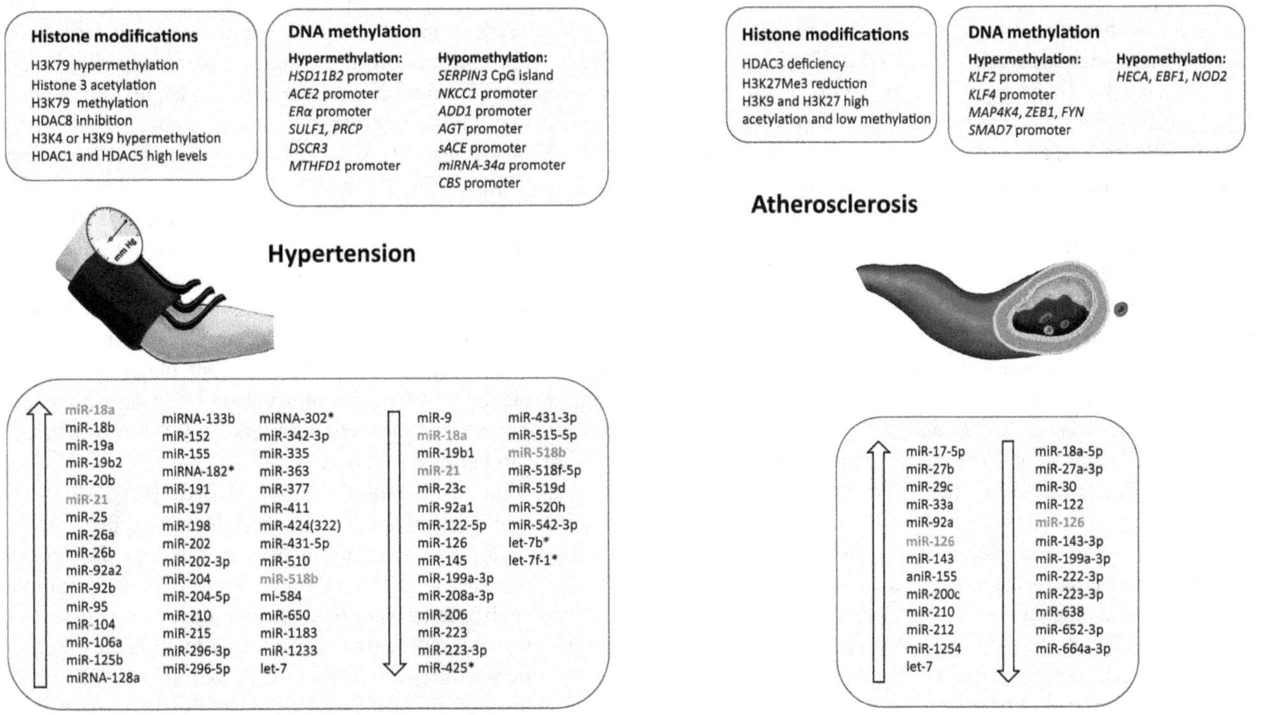

FIGURE 2 | Epigenetic modifications and microRNAs biomarkers dysregulated in atherosclerosis and hypertension. Ascending arrows indicate higher levels or upregulation, and descending arrows denote lower levels or downregulation, both compared to control conditions. Those miRNAs presenting opposite results are shown in orange.

and gene expression in the brain renin–angiotensin system, a key regulator of hypertension in adults (Goyal et al., 2010). Along the same lines, in a study carried out *in vitro* and in a rat model, DNA demethylation of the angiotensinogen gene (*AGT*) promoter activated its expression. AGT is an important substrate of the renin–angiotensin–aldosterone system and an important target in hypertension research. Elevated concentrations of circulating aldosterone and high consumption of salt stimulate the AGT gene expression in adipose-induced hypertension (Wang et al., 2014a). In addition, cystathionine β-synthase (CBS), an important enzyme in the metabolism of plasma homocysteine, is associated with hypertension and stroke. Hypermethylation of the *CBS* promoter has been demonstrated to increase the risk of both diseases, especially in male patients (Wang et al., 2019a). Similarly, hypermethylation of the methylenetetrahydrofolate dehydrogenase 1 gene (*MTHFD1*) promoter, which is also associated with homocysteine metabolism, was observed in hypertensive patients, and proposed as a potential diagnostic biomarker in patients with essential hypertension (Xu et al., 2019).

In addition to the previous classic epigenetic modifications, miRNAs often regulate hypertension and are attractive biomarkers for the disease. The miR-9 and miR-126 expression levels are significantly lower in hypertensive patients than healthy individuals and are related to hypertension prognosis and organ damage. Thus, miR-9 and miR-126 may be possible biomarkers in essential hypertension (Kontaraki et al., 2014). Moreover, ncRNAs, such as miR-143, miR-145, and NR_104181,

are significantly higher in essential hypertensive patients than controls, whereas NR_027032 and NR_034083 are significantly reduced. After evaluating cardiovascular risk factors, they concluded that lower expression levels of NR_034083 and higher expression levels of NR_104181 and miR-143 were risk factors for essential hypertension (Chen et al., 2018b). Another study evaluated the correlation between miRNA let-7 expression and subclinical atherosclerosis in untreated patients with newly diagnosed essential hypertension and found increased levels in hypertensive patients, suggesting that plasma let-7 could be an indicator for monitoring end-organ damage and a biomarker for atherosclerosis in these patients (Huang et al., 2017b). Similarly, upregulation of miR-505, miR-19a, miR-21, miR-510, or miR-424(322) in blood from hypertensive patients suggests a possible use for miR-510 as a diagnostic biomarker and therapeutic target (Yang et al., 2014; Chen and Li, 2017; Krishnan et al., 2017; Parthenakis et al., 2017; Sekar et al., 2017; Baptista et al., 2018). Lower levels of the combination of miR-199a-3p, miR-208a-3p, miR-122-5p, and miR-223-3p have also been shown to be suitable for diagnosis of hypertension (Zhang et al., 2018c). Decreased miR-206 levels might also be especially useful in the detection of pulmonary hypertension in patients with left heart disease (Jin et al., 2017). Furthermore, a study in hypertensive mice produced by infusion of angiotensin II concluded that miR-431-5p knockdown delays the increase in blood pressure induced by angiotensin II and reduces vascular injury. This demonstrates its potential as a target for the treatment of hypertension and vascular injury (Huo et al., 2019).

Preeclampsia is an important pregnancy-induced syndrome characterized by hypertension and proteinuria. Chronic hypoxia is a common pregnancy stress that increases the risk of preeclampsia and is associated with changes in methylation of the estrogen receptor α gene (ERα) promoter. ERα is involved in adjustments to the uterine blood flow, and promoter methylation results in gene repression in uterine arteries, increasing blood pressure (Dasgupta et al., 2012). Preeclampsia also modifies the expression profile of several serine protease inhibitors (SERPINs) in the placenta. Specifically, SERPIN3 CpG islands have a significantly low level of methylation in preeclampsia, providing a new potential marker for early diagnosis (Chelbi et al., 2007). Another study demonstrated a positive association between placenta global DNA methylation and hypertension in preeclampsia (Kulkarni et al., 2011). Next-generation sequencing technology and microarray assay analyses of the miRNA expression pattern in preeclamptic placentas versus healthy placentas have revealed that miRNAs expression is dysregulated in preeclampsia (Zhu et al., 2009; Noack et al., 2011; Yang et al., 2011; Choi et al., 2013; Xu et al., 2014; Hromadnikova et al., 2015; Zhang et al., 2015a; Gunel et al., 2017; Han et al., 2017). These results were in agreement with those found in the miRNA database from cell and tissue analyses. Thus, circulating miRNAs in the serum of pregnant women could be used as biomarkers for the diagnosis and prognosis of preeclampsia. To further demonstrate that miRNAs could be good predictors of preeclampsia, as well as its severity, circulating miRNA signatures were evaluated in women divided into groups based on preeclampsia severity. MiR-21, miR-29a, miR-125b, miR-155, miR-202-3p, miR-204-5p, miR-210, miR-215, miR-335, miR-518b, miR-584, miR-650, and miR-1233 were upregulated, whereas miR-15b, miR-18a, miR-19b1, and miR-144 were downregulated in women with severe preeclampsia compared to mild preeclampsia (Ura et al., 2014; Jiang et al., 2015; Yang et al., 2016b; Jairajpuri et al., 2017; Mei et al., 2017; Singh et al., 2017). In addition, a recent data recompilation supported a direct association between high or low expression of miRNAs in pregnancy serum and placenta in preeclamptic pregnancies (Laganà et al., 2018). Interestingly, an association has also been demonstrated between hypomethylation of the miR-34a promoter and preeclampsia severity (Rezaei et al., 2018). Another study analyzed the concentrations of Down syndrome critical region 3 (DSCR3), Ras association domain family 1 isoform A (RASSF1A), and sex-determining region Y (SRY) cell-free fetal DNA in maternal plasma from preeclamptic pregnancies and found that all of the markers significantly correlated with gestational age. The authors demonstrated that DSCR3 is a novel epigenetic biomarker and an alternative to RASSF1A for the prediction of early-onset preeclampsia (Kim et al., 2015). However, no association was found between the methylation status of the cortisol-controlling gene (HSD11B2), tumor suppressor gene (RUNX3), or long interspersed nucleotide element-1 gene (LINE-1) and hypertensive disorders of pregnancy when placental DNA methylation was analyzed (Majchrzak-Celińska et al., 2017).

Atherosclerosis

Atherosclerosis is a chronic inflammatory disease characterized by the accumulation of cholesterol in the walls of large- and medium-sized arteries, the accumulation of extracellular matrix and lipids, and smooth muscle cell proliferation. This process leads to the infiltration of immune cells (mostly macrophages) and endothelial dysfunction, forming a plaque, and eventually developing into acute cardiovascular events, such as MI, peripheral vascular disease, aneurysms, and stroke (Wissler, 1991). Proatherogenic stimuli, such as low-density lipoprotein (LDL) cholesterol and oxidized LDL, have been suggested to stimulate a long-term epigenetic reprogramming of innate immune system cells. This induces a constant activation, even after the removal of atherosclerotic stimuli (Bekkering et al., 2016). Emerging evidence supports epigenetic modifications being involved in the initiation and progression of atherosclerosis, playing an important role in plaque development and vulnerability, and highlighting the importance of epigenetic biomarkers as predictors of CVDs (**Table 2** and **Figure 2**) (Xu et al., 2018).

Regarding histone modifications, HDAC3 is reported to have a protective effect in apolipoprotein E deficient (apoE−/−) mice. HDAC3 maintains the endothelial integrity, and its deficiency results in atherosclerosis (Zampetaki et al., 2010). Similarly, increased histone acetylation has been proposed to play some role in the progression of atherogenesis by modulating the expressions of proatherogenic genes (Choi et al., 2005). Histone deacetylases are upregulated in aortic smooth muscle cells when they were stimulated with mitogens. In contrast, inhibition of HDACs reduces aortic smooth muscle cell proliferation by changing cell cycle genes expression. This suggests a protective effect against atherosclerosis (Findeisen et al., 2011). Investigations of the association between changes in lysine 27 trimethylation of histone 3 (H3K27Me3), and atherosclerotic plaque development revealed a reduction in global levels of H3K27Me3 modification in vessels with advanced atherosclerotic plaques. This does not correlate with a reduction in the corresponding HMT, enhancer of zeste homolog 2 (EZH2). There was a relationship between the repression of H3K27Me3 mark in the vessels with advanced atherosclerotic plaques and the dynamic differentiation and proliferation of smooth muscle cells associated with atherosclerotic disease (Wierda et al., 2015). Histone acetylation, methylation, and the expression of their corresponding transferases in the atherosclerotic plaques of patients with carotid artery stenosis have been analyzed. Greißel et al. (2016) analyzed the expression of HATs GCN5L, P300, MYST1, and MYST2 and HMTs MLL2/4, SET7/9, hSET1A, SUV39H1, SUV39H2, ESET/SETDB1, EHMT1, EZH2, and G9a and described an enhancement in histone acetylation on H3K9 and H3K27 in the smooth muscle cells from severe atherosclerotic lesions that correlated with plaque severity. In addition, H3K9 and H3K27 methylation were significantly lower in atherosclerotic plaques and significantly associated with disease severity (Greißel et al., 2016).

DNA methylation is also involved in atherosclerosis. To identify CpG methylation profiles in the progression of atherosclerosis in the human aorta, Valencia-Morales et al. (2015) performed DNA methylation microarray analyses. They detected a correlation between histological pathology and the differential methylation of numerous autosomal genes in vascular tissue, providing potential biomarkers of damage severity and

TABLE 2 | Epigenetic biomarkers in atherosclerosis.

Epigenetic modification	Biomarker	Regulation in atherosclerosis	Sample source	Study type	References
DNA methylation	*KLF2* promoter	Methylation	HUVEC cells	Experimental: *in vitro*	(Kumar et al., 2013)
	KLF4 promoter *HECA, EBF1, NOD2, MAP4K4, ZEB1, FYN*	Methylation *HECA, EBF1, NOD2:* Hypomethylated; *MAP4K4, ZEB1, FYN:* Hypermethylated	HAEC cells Human aortic intima and HEK293 cells	Experimental: *in vitro* Clinical and experimental: *in vitro*	(Jiang et al., 2014) (Yamada et al., 2014)
	TIMP1, ABCA1, ACAT1 promoters	Altered methylation status	Peripheral blood	Clinical	(Ma et al., 2016)
	SMAD7 promoter	Hypermethylation	Peripheral blood and atherosclerotic plaques	Clinical	(Wei et al., 2018)
	5mC, 5-hmC	Higher levels	Peripheral blood	Clinical	(Jiang et al., 2019)
Histone modifications	HDAC3	Deficiency	Aorta and HUVEC cells	Experimental: apoE–/– mice and *in vitro*	(Zampetaki et al., 2010)
	H3K27Me3	Reduction in H3K27Me3 modification	Perirenal aortic tissue patches	Clinical	(Wierda et al., 2015)
	H3K9, H3K27	Higher histone acetylation and lower histone methylation	Carotid tissue	Clinical	(Greißel et al., 2016)
miRNA	miR-130a, miR-27b, miR-210	Higher levels	Serum and intima tissue	Clinical	(Li et al., 2011)
	miR-17-5p	Higher levels	Plasma	Clinical	(Chen et al., 2015a)
	miR-143-3p, miR-222-3p	Lower levels	Microparticles	Clinical	(de Gonzalo-Calvo et al., 2016)
	miR-30	Lower levels	Plasma	Clinical	(Huang et al., 2016b)
	miR-92a	Higher levels	Plasma	Clinical	(Huang et al., 2017a)
	miR-18a-5p, miR-27a-3p, miR-199a-3p, miR-223-3p, miR-652-3p	Lower levels	Plasma	Clinical	(Vegter et al., 2017)
	miR-33a	Higher levels	Plasma	Clinical	(Kim et al., 2017)
	miR-126	Lower levels	Plasma	Experimental: apoE–/– mice	(Hao and Fan, 2017)
	miR-212	Overexpression	Serum	Clinical	(Jeong et al., 2017)
	miRNA let-7	Higher levels	Plasma	Clinical	(Huang et al., 2017b)
	miR-1254	Higher levels	Plasma	Clinical	(de Gonzalo-Calvo et al., 2018)
	miR-200c	Overexpression	Carotid plaques and plasma	Clinical	(Magenta et al., 2018)
	miR-29c	Higher levels	Plasma	Clinical	(Huang et al., 2018)
	miR-221, miR-222	Lower expression levels	Serum	Clinical	(Yilmaz et al., 2018)
	miR-638	Lower levels	Serum	Clinical	(Luque et al., 2018)
	miR-122	Higher levels	Serum	Clinical	(Wang and Yu, 2018)
	miR-221, miR-222	Higher levels in tissue samples and lower levels in whole blood	Coronary artery atherosclerotic plaques, and internal mammary arteries and whole blood	Clinical	(Bildirici et al., 2018)
	miR-664a-3p	Downregulation	Serum	Clinical	(Li et al., 2018b)
	miR-155	Higher levels	Serum	Clinical	(Qiu and Ma, 2018)
	miR-19A, miR-19B, miR-126, miR-155	Differential levels	GEO dataset	High throughput	(Mao et al., 2018)
	miR-126, miR-143	Higher levels	Plasma	Clinical	(Gao et al., 2019)

treatment targets (Valencia-Morales et al., 2015). Genes such as *Drosophila* headcase (*HECA*), early B-cell factor 1 (*EBF1*), and nucleotide-binding oligomerization domain containing 2 (*NOD2*) are significantly hypomethylated, whereas mitogen-activated protein kinase kinase kinase kinase 4 (*MAP4K4*), zinc finger E-box binding homeobox 1 (*ZEB1*), and proto-oncogene tyrosine-protein kinase (*FYN*) are hypermethylated in atheromatous plaque lesions compared to the plaque-free intima

(Yamada et al., 2014). Another study described differentially methylated regions in genes associated with atherosclerosis in swine aorta endothelial cells (Jiang et al., 2015). Low-density lipoprotein cholesterol risk factor upregulates DNMT1, which methylates and represses the Krüppel-like factor 2 gene (*KLF2*) promoter. KLF2 is a transcription factor essential for endothelium homeostasis, and its repression results in endothelial dysfunction (Kumar et al., 2013). Similarly, DNMT3a upregulation in human aortic endothelial cells exposed to disturbed flow induces the methylation and repression of the Krüppel-like factor 4 gene (*KLF4*) promoter, increasing regional atherosusceptibility (Jiang et al., 2014). In an attempt to determine biomarkers of atherosclerosis in the primary stages, the DNA methylation status was determined in a selection of gene promoters associated with the disease. They analyzed the promoter methylation of ATP binding cassette subfamily A member 1 (*ABCA1*), TIMP metallopeptidase inhibitor 1 (*TIMP1*), and acetyl-CoA acetyltransferase 1 (*ACAT1*) and observed significant alterations in the peripheral blood of atherosclerosis patients (Ma et al., 2016). A recent study found that *SMAD7* expression is decreased and its promoter highly methylated in atherosclerotic plaques compared to normal artery walls. There was also increased DNA methylation of the *SMAD7* promoter in the peripheral blood of atherosclerosis patients. Thus, the *SMAD7* promoter is hypermethylated in atherosclerosis patients and their atherosclerotic plaques, with a positive association with homocysteine levels (Wei et al., 2018). Moreover, increased 5mC and 5-hmC levels, which indicate DNA methylation and hydroxymethylation, respectively, have been demonstrated in peripheral blood mononuclear cells from elderly patients with coronary heart disease. These results positively correlate with the severity of coronary atherosclerosis (Jiang et al., 2019).

MicroRNAs have also been identified as attractive epigenetic biomarkers for atherosclerosis. Li et al. (2011) examined miRNA levels in serum samples and the intima of atherosclerosis obliterans patients and compared them to controls. They observed increased levels of miR-27b, miR-130a, and miR-210 in serum and sclerotic tissue from patients, proposing these miRNAs as epigenetic biomarkers for early stages of the disease (Li et al., 2011). Later, a study with a reduced number of patients suggested that elevated levels of circulating miR-17-5p may be a useful biomarker in the diagnosis of coronary atherosclerosis (Chen et al., 2015a).

Microparticles secreted by human coronary artery smooth muscle cells are a different source of cardiovascular biomarkers. These extracellular vesicles can contain miRNAs, such as miR-21-5p, miR-143-3p, miR-145-5p, miR-221-3p, and miR-222-3p. Lower levels of miR-143-3p and miR-222-3p have been found in microparticles derived from atherosclerotic plaque areas compared to nonatherosclerotic areas (de Gonzalo-Calvo et al., 2016).

Huang et al. (2016b) evaluated the expression of miR-30 in patients with essential hypertension compared to control individuals. They observed a reduction in miR-30 levels in the hypertensive patients and in the increased carotid intima-media thickness group. Thus, the authors suggested that circulating miR-30 may be a useful noninvasive atherosclerosis biomarker for patients with essential hypertension (Huang et al., 2016b). Later, the authors also identified higher levels of miR-92a as a possible biomarker of atherosclerosis in the same type of patients (Huang et al., 2017a). With the aim of investigating correlations between circulating miRNAs specific for HF and atherosclerosis in HF patients, Vegter et al. (2017) assessed miRNAs levels and related them to biomarkers associated with atherosclerotic disease and rehospitalizations of cardiovascular patients. They demonstrated

a consistent trend between a high number of atherosclerosis manifestations and lower levels of miR-18a-5p, miR-27a-3p, miR-199a-3p, miR-223-3p, and miR-652-3p. Thus, lower levels of circulating miRNAs in HF patients with atherosclerotic disease and an elevated probability of cardiovascular-related rehospitalization were described (Vegter et al., 2017). High levels of miR-33a have also been demonstrated to be a potential cause of cholesterol accumulation and to exacerbate vessel walls inflammation in atherosclerotic disease. Thus, plasma miR-33a has been proposed as a suitable biomarker in atherosclerosis (Kim et al., 2017).

In an attempt to identify more atherosclerosis biomarkers, Hao and Fan (2017) performed microarray analysis using the plasma from apoE−/− mice and discovered that a reduction in miR-126 levels is a good indicator of atherosclerotic disease. They also determined that miR-126 is involved in the mitogen-associated protein kinase (MAPK) signaling pathway, reducing cytokine release and progressing atherosclerotic pathogenesis (Hao and Fan, 2017). In contrast, Gao et al. (2019) determined that higher expression levels of miR-126 and miR-143 correlate with the presence and severity of cerebral atherosclerosis (Gao et al., 2019). In another study, the authors evaluated the synergy of circulating miRNAs with cardiovascular risk factors to estimate the presence of atherosclerosis in ischemic stroke patients. They identified miR-212 as a novel marker that enhances the estimation of atherosclerosis presence in combination with hemoglobin A_{1c}, high-density lipoprotein cholesterol, and lipoprotein(a) (Jeong et al., 2017). Another candidate biomarker for atherosclerosis is miR-200c. The authors analyzed plaque instability in the carotid arteries of patients undergoing carotid endarterectomy by examining the expression of miR-200c. Higher expression of miR-200c positively correlated with instability biomarkers, such as monocyte chemoattractant protein-1, cyclooxygenase-2, interleukin 6 (IL-6), metalloproteinases, and miR-33a/b, and negatively correlated with stability biomarkers, such as ZEB1, endothelial nitric oxide synthase, forkhead boxO1, and Sirtuin1. Thus, miR-200c could be a biomarker of atherosclerotic plaque progression and clinically useful for identifying patients at high embolic risk (Magenta et al., 2018). Along the same lines, lower serum levels of miR-638 may be a suitable biomarker of plaque vulnerability and ischemic stroke in individuals with high cardiovascular risk (Luque et al., 2018). With the intention to explore the role of miRNAs associated with carotid atherosclerosis, Mao et al. (2018) analyzed the genes differentially expressed between primary and advanced atherosclerotic plaques using two public datasets from the Gene Expression Omnibus (GEO) databases. The authors found a total of 23 miRNAs and focused on miR-19A, miR-19B, miR-126, and miR-155, which may be considered biomarkers of carotid atherosclerosis (Mao et al., 2018). In addition, Li et al. (2018b) identified downregulation of specific circulating miR-664a-3p as a biomarker of atherosclerosis in patients with obstructive sleep apnea and enlarged maximum carotid intima-media thickness (Li et al., 2018b).

Circulating miR-221 and miR-222 could also be suitable biomarkers for the diagnosis of atherosclerosis, as lower levels of these miRNAs correlate with the disease (Bildirici et al., 2018;

Yilmaz et al., 2018). However, higher levels have been found in samples from coronary atherosclerotic plaques and internal mammary arteries (Bildirici et al., 2018). On the other hand, higher circulating levels of miR-29c, miR-122, and miR-155 in coronary atherosclerosis patients might allow noninvasive detection of the disease and its severity (Huang et al., 2018; Qiu and Ma, 2018; Wang and Yu, 2018). In another interesting study that assessed whether atherosclerosis of different arterial territories, not including the coronary artery, is associated with specific circulating miRNAs, the investigators were able to identify specific miRNA profiles for each territory with atherosclerotic disease. These findings may provide a pathophysiological understanding and be useful for selecting potential biomarkers for clinical practice (Pereira-da-Silva et al., 2018).

Myocardial Infarction

Acute MI (AMI) is a threatening disease worldwide. Early and accurate differential diagnosis is critical for immediate medical intervention and improved prognosis (Reed et al., 2017). In particular, it is important to notice that patients with ST-segment elevation MI (STEMI) have different requirements than patients with non-STEMI (NSTEMI). For the first group, reperfusion therapy should be administered quickly to reduce infarct size and mortality (Authors/Task Force members et al., 2014). However, in NSTEMI patients, revascularization strategies are recommended based on individual clinical characteristics (Reed et al., 2017). Therefore, biomarkers with the capacity to diagnose and personalize a therapeutic schedule in AMI would be of great interest. Currently, the favored diagnostic biomarkers of AMI are cardiac troponin I (cTnI) and T (cTnT), both of which are released from necrotic cardiomyocytes within 2 to 4 h post-MI (Babuin and Jaffe, 2005), with maximum levels at 24 to 48 h and lasting for more than 1 week (Jaffe et al., 2006). For this reason, small repeat infarctions after the main infarction are difficult to detect. Thus, it is fundamental to identify biomarkers for very early diagnosis of STEMI and for monitoring the entire pathological process of AMI (**Table 3** and **Figure 3**).

Regarding methylation as an indicator of MI, Talens et al. (2012) investigated the association between MI and DNA methylation at six loci described to be sensitive to prenatal nutrition. As a result, the researchers demonstrated that the risk of MI in women is associated with DNA hypermethylation at *INS* and *GNASAS*-specific loci (Talens et al., 2012). Moreover, microarray analyses investigating whole-genome DNA methylation using cases from the EPICOR study and EPIC-NL cohort (Fiorito et al., 2014) identified a hypomethylated region in the zinc finger and BTB domain-containing protein 12 (*ZBTB12*) and *LINE-1*, concluding that it is possible to detect specific methylation profiles in white blood cells a few years before MI occurs. This provides a promising early biomarker of MI (Guarrera et al., 2015). Another example is the hypermethylation of the aldehyde dehydrogenase 2 gene (*ALDH2*) promoter, which is associated with myocardial injury after MI in rats. The hypermethylation downregulates *ALDH2*, inhibiting its cardioprotective role (Wang et al., 2015). Rask-Andersen et al. (2016) performed an epigenome-wide association study to identify disease-specific alterations

in DNA methylation. The authors observed differential DNA methylation at 211 CpG sites in individuals with MI, and some of these sites represented genes related to cardiac function, CVD, cardiogenesis, and recovery after ischemic injury. Their results highlight genes that might be important in the pathogenesis of MI or in recovery (Rask-Andersen et al., 2016). Along the same lines, a genome-wide DNA methylation and gene ontology analysis of white blood cells from a population-based study identified four differentially methylated sites in individuals who had a previous MI. Interestingly, they found a correlation between differences in DNA methylation in blood cells and the levels of growth differentiation factor 15 (GDF-15), which was overexpressed in the myocardium of MI patients (Ek et al., 2016). Later, a genome-wide DNA methylation study of whole blood samples from MI patients and controls identified two methylated regions in zinc finger homeobox 3 (*ZFHX3*) and SWI/SNF-related, matrix-associated, actin-dependent regulator of chromatin, subfamily a, member 4 (*SMARCA4*) that were independently related to MI (Nakatochi et al., 2017).

Histone modifications are also involved in the pathological process of MI. To investigate the role of the HAT p300 in adverse left ventricular (LV) remodeling, Miyamoto et al. (2006) generated transgenic mice overexpressing wild-type p300 or its mutant in the heart. They subjected these mice to surgical MI and demonstrated that cardiac overexpression of p300 stimulated adverse LV remodeling. They concluded that the HAT activity of p300 is fundamental for the pathological course of MI (Miyamoto et al., 2006). Moreover, the class III deacetylase sirtuin 1 (SIRT1) is well known to confer a cardioprotective effect and is downregulated after cardiac injury. To understand the underlying mechanism, primary rat neonatal ventricular myocytes were exposed to ischemic or oxidative stress, leading to upregulation of the histone H3K9 methyltransferase SUV39H and downregulation of *SIRT1*. In addition, inhibition of SUV39H activity by chaetocin in wild-type mice and *SUV39H*-knockout mice protected against induced MI. SUV39H and heterochromatin protein 1 gamma cooperate to methylate the *SIRT1* promoter and repress its transcription. Thus, the authors described a role for SUV39H linking SIRT1 repression to MI (Yang et al., 2017a). To examine the role of HDAC4 in the modulation of cardiac function after an MI, Zhang et al. (2018b) generated a myocyte-specific activated HDAC4-transgenic mouse. They found that HDAC4 overexpression increases myocardial fibrosis and hypertrophy, leading to cardiac dysfunction. Furthermore, the overexpression of activated HDAC4 aggravated cardiac dysfunction and increased adverse remodeling and apoptosis in the infarcted myocardium. Thus, HDAC4 is an indicator of heart injury (Zhang et al., 2018b). More recently, the role of HDAC6 in the development of HF following MI was investigated using a rat model. The authors found that the deacetylase activity of HDAC6 is increased after MI (Nagata et al., 2019).

Abundant research has focused on miRNAs as novel biomarkers for MI. MiR-1 levels have been analyzed in plasma from patients with AMI and found to be significantly elevated, but decreased to normal levels with medication (Ai et al., 2010; Long et al., 2012a). MiR-1, miR-126, and cTnI expression levels exhibited a similar tendency. Thus, circulating miR-1 and

TABLE 3 | Epigenetic biomarkers in myocardial infarction.

Epigenetic modification	Biomarker	Regulation in myocardial infarction	Sample source	Study type	References
DNA methylation	*INS, GNASAS*	Hypermethylation	Leukocytes	Clinical	(Talens et al., 2012)
	LINE-1, ZBTB12	Hypomethylation	White blood cells	Clinical	(Guarrera et al., 2015)
	ALDH2 promoter	Hypermethylation	Experimental: rat model of MI	Experimental: rat model of MI	(Wang et al., 2015)
	ZFHX3, SMARCA4	Methylation	Whole blood	Clinical	(Nakatochi et al., 2017)
Histone modifications	p300	Overexpression	Myocardium	Experimental: mouse model of MI in HATmut p300-Tg mice	(Miyamoto et al., 2006)
	SUV39H, SIRT1	SUV39H upregulation and SIRT1 downregulation	H9C2 cells primary rat neonatal ventricular myocytes	Experimental: mouse model of MI in SUV39H–/– mice	(Yang et al., 2017a)
	HDAC4	Overexpression	Myocardium	Experimental: mouse model of MI in MHC-HDAC4-Tg mice	(Zhang et al., 2018b)
	HDAC6	Higher levels	Myocardium	Experimental: rat model of MI	(Nagata et al., 2019)
miRNA	miR-1	Higher levels	Plasma	Clinical	(Ai et al., 2010)
	miR-31, miR-126, miR-214, miR-499-5p	miR-31, miR-214: upregulation; miR-126, miR-499-5p: downregulation	Myocardium	Experimental: rat model of MI	(Shi et al., 2010)
	miR-499	Higher levels	Tissues and plasma	Clinical	(Adachi et al., 2010)
	miR-1, miR-133a, miR-133b, miR-499-5p, miR-122, miR-375	miR-1, miR-133a, miR-133b, miR-499-5p: upregulation; miR-122, miR-375: downregulation	Plasma	Clinical and experimental: mouse model of MI	(D'Alessandra et al., 2010)
	miR-1, miR-126	miR-1: increased; miR-126: decreased	Plasma	Clinical	(Long et al., 2012a)
	miR-133a	Higher levels	Plasma	Clinical	(Eitel et al., 2012)
	miR-30a, miR-195, let-7b	miR-30a, miR-195: increased; let-7: decreased	Plasma	Clinical	(Long et al., 2012b)
	miR-499-5p	Higher levels	Plasma	Clinical	(Olivieri et al., 2013)
	miR-1, miR-133a, miR-208b, miR-499	Higher levels	Plasma	Clinical	(Li et al., 2013)
	miR-150	Downregulation	plasma	Clinical	(Devaux et al., 2013)
	miR-133a	Higher levels	Plasma	Clinical	(Wang et al., 2013a)
	miR-21-5p, miR-361-5p, miR-519e-5p	miR-21-5p, miR-361-5p: increased; miR-519e-5p: reduced	Plasma	Clinical	(Wang et al., 2014b)
	miR-208a, miR-499	Higher levels in serum; miR-499: lower levels in scar, miR-208a: unchanged in scar	Serum and heart tissues	Experimental: mouse model of MI	(Xiao et al., 2014)
	miR-208b, miR-34a	Higher levels	Plasma	Clinical	(Lv et al., 2014)
	miR-328, miR-134	Higher levels	Plasma	Clinical	(He et al., 2014)
	miR-133, miR-1291, miR-663b	Higher levels	Plasma	Clinical	(Peng et al., 2014)
	miR-497	Upregulation	Plasma	Clinical	(Li et al., 2014b)
	miR-1	Higher levels	Plasma	Clinical	(Li et al., 2014a)
	miR-19a	Higher levels	Plasma	Clinical	(Zhong et al., 2014)
	miR-486-3p, miR-150-3p, miR-126-3p, miR-26a-5p, and miR-191-5p	miR-486-3p, miR-150-3p: upregulation; miR-126-3p, miR-26a-5p, miR-191-5p: downregulation	Serum	Clinical	(Hsu et al., 2014)
	miR-145	Higher levels	Serum	Clinical	(Dong et al., 2015)

(Continued)

TABLE 3 | Continued

Epigenetic modification	Biomarker	Regulation in myocardial infarction	Sample source	Study type	References
	hsa-miR-493-5p, hsa-miR-369-3p, hsa-miR-495, hsa-miR-3615, hsa-miR-433, hsa-miR-877-3p, hsa-miR-1306-3p, hsv1-miR-H2, hsa-miR-3130-5p, hcmv-miR-UL22A	hsa-miR-493-5p, hsa-miR-369-3p, hsa-miR-495, hsa-miR-3615, hsa-miR-433: upregulation, hsa-miR-877-3p, hsa-miR-1306-3p, hsv1-miR-H2, hsa-miR-3130-5p, hcmv-miR-UL22A: downregulation	Plasma	Clinical	(Liang et al., 2015)
	miR-499	Higher levels	Plasma	Clinical	(Zhang et al., 2015b)
	miR-486, miR-150	Higher levels	Plasma	Clinical	(Zhang et al., 2015c)
	miR-499	Higher levels	Plasma	Clinical	(Chen et al., 2015b)
	miR-146a, miR-21	Higher levels	Plasma	Clinical	(Liu et al., 2015a)
	miR-1, miR-208, miR-499	Higher levels	Plasma	Clinical	(Liu et al., 2015b)
	miR-208a	Higher levels	Plasma	Clinical	(Białek et al., 2015)
	miR-208	Overexpression	Plasma	Clinical	(Han et al., 2015)
	miR-122-5p	Higher levels	Plasma	Clinical	(Yao et al., 2015)
	miR-21	Higher levels	Plasma	Clinical	(Zhang et al., 2016)
	miR-99a	Downregulation	Plasma	Clinical	(Yang et al., 2016a)
	miR-19b-3p, miR-134-5p and miR-186-5p	Higher levels	Plasma	Clinical	(Wang et al., 2016b)
	miR-106a-5p, miR-424-5p, let-7g-5p, miR-144-3p, miR-660-5p	Higher levels	Blood	Clinical	(Bye et al., 2016)
	miR-19b-3p, miR-134-5p and miR-186-5p	Overexpression	Plasma	Clinical	(Wang et al., 2016b)
	miR-125b-5p, miR-30d-5p	Overexpression	Plasma	Clinical	(Jia et al., 2016)
	miR-423-5p, miR-30d	Overexpression	Plasma	Clinical	(Eryilmaz et al., 2016)
	miR-221-3p	Overexpression	Plasma	Clinical	(Coskunpinar et al., 2016)
	miR-208a	Overexpression in myocardium and high levels in serum	Myocardium and serum	Experimental: rat model of MI	(Feng et al., 2016)
	miR-133b, miR-22-5p	Upregulation	Serum/plasma	Clinical	(Maciejak et al., 2016)
	miR-103a	Higher levels in plasma	Plasma and peripheral blood mononuclear cells	Clinical and experimental: in vitro	(Huang et al., 2016a)
	miR-122-5p/133b	High ratio	Serum	Clinical	(Cortez-Dias et al., 2016)
	miR499a-5p	Higher levels	Plasma	Clinical	(O'Sullivan et al., 2016)
	miR-181a	Higher levels	Plasma	Clinical	(Zhu et al., 2016)
	miR-145	Decreased	Plasma	Clinical	(Zhang et al., 2017b)
	miR-133a	Higher levels	Plasma	Clinical	(Yuan et al., 2016)
	miR-208b	Higher levels	Plasma	Clinical	(Liu et al., 2017)
	miR-1, miR-92a, miR-99a, miR-143, miR-223	miR-143: increased; miR-1, miR-92a, miR-99a, miR-223: decreased	Monocytes	Clinical	(Parahuleva et al., 2017)
	miR-92a	Higher levels	Plasma	Clinical	(Zhang et al., 2017c)
	miR-208b	Overexpression	Plasma	Clinical	(Zhang and Xie, 2017)
	miR-124	Higher levels	Peripheral blood	Clinical	(Guo et al., 2017)
	miR-1, miR-21, miR-29b and miR-92a	miR-1, miR-21, miR-29b: increased	Plasma	Clinical	(Grabmaier et al., 2017)
	miR-874-3p	Downregulation	Plasma	Clinical	(Yan et al., 2017)
	pmiR-126	Lower levels	Platelet	Clinical	(Li et al., 2017b)
	miR-133a	Lower levels	Serum/Plasma	Clinical	(Zhu et al., 2018)
	miR-21	Upregulation	Serum	Clinical	(Wang et al., 2017b)
	miR-4478	Higher levels	Serum	Clinical	(Gholikhani-Darbroud et al., 2017)
	miR-23b	Higher levels	Plasma	Clinical	(Zhang et al., 2018a)
	MiR-27a, miR-31, miR-1291, miR-139-5p, miR-204, miR-375	Higher levels	GEO database	High throughput	(Wu et al., 2018a)
	miR-1, miR-133a, miR-34a	Lower levels	Myocardium	Experimental: mouse model of MI	(Qipshidze Kelm et al., 2018)

(Continued)

TABLE 3 | Continued

Epigenetic modification	Biomarker	Regulation in myocardial infarction	Sample source	Study type	References
	miR-19b, miR-223, miR-483-5p	Higher levels	Plasma	Clinical	(Li et al., 2019)
	miR-17-5p, miR-126-5p, miR-145-3p	Higher levels	Plasma	Clinical	(Xue et al., 2019)
	miR-150	Lower levels	Serum	Clinical	(Lin et al., 2019)
	miR-208b, miR-499	Higher levels	Plasma	Clinical	(Devaux et al., 2012)

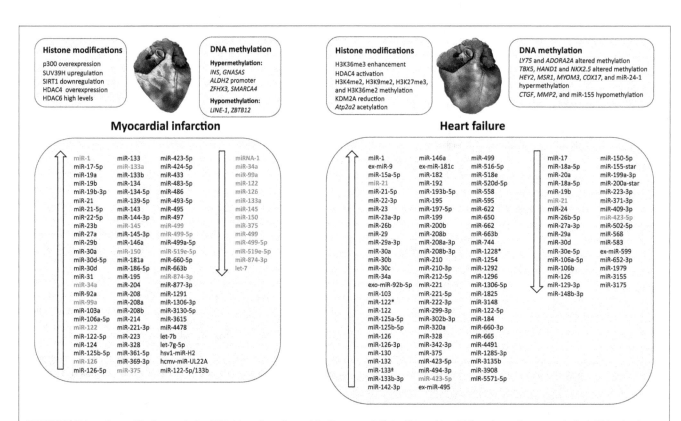

FIGURE 3 | Epigenetic modifications and microRNAs biomarkers dysregulated in myocardial infarction and heart failure. Ascending arrows indicate higher levels or upregulation, and descending arrows denote lower levels or downregulation, both compared to control conditions. Those miRNAs presenting opposite results are shown in orange.

miR-126 may be useful indicators of AMI (Long et al., 2012a). However, when miR-1 was compared to cTnT, the authors found that cTnT was more specific and sensitive than miR-1 (Li et al., 2014a). Experiments performed in a rat model of MI revealed dysregulation of several miRNAs in the myocardium. Specifically, miR-31, miR-208, and miR-214 were upregulated, and miR-126 and miR-499-5p were downregulated in infarcted rats compared to sham-operated animals (Ji et al., 2009; Shi et al., 2010). MiR-499 has been widely analyzed as a possible biomarker of MI. MiR-499 has been reported to be produced almost exclusively in the heart and plasma and is significantly increased in individuals with AMI (Adachi et al., 2010; Devaux et al., 2012). MiR-499 positively correlates with serum creatine kinase-MB (CK-MB) and cTnI increasing their diagnostic accuracy (Chen et al., 2015b; Zhang et al., 2015b). Thus, miR-499 might be a suitable

biomarker for MI and a predictor of myocardial ischemia risk (Adachi et al., 2010; Chen et al., 2015b; Zhang et al., 2015b). These results were confirmed in the mouse model of MI, with elevated serum miR-208a levels. However, the expression of miR-499 was significantly reduced in the MI region, whereas miR-208a remained unchanged in the same area. One explanation is that the damaged heart might release miR-499 into the circulation (Xiao et al., 2014). Other authors observed a high correlation between circulating miRNA-208a in STEMI patients and the levels of cTnI and CK-MB mass liberated from the infarcted zone (Białek et al., 2015). Thus, cardiac miR-208 and miR-499 seemed to be better biomarkers for predicting AMI than miR-1 (Liu et al., 2015b; Liu et al., 2018a). Another study analyzed the expression of miR-208a in the myocardium and serum of infarcted rats compared to control groups, as well as the expression of cAMP-PKA to evaluate the effect of this signaling pathway in the primary stages of MI; they found increased expression of miR-208a and cAMP-PKA. Moreover, the transfection of human myocardial cells with the miR-208a analog significantly increased the amount of cAMP-PKA protein. Thus, higher expression of miR-208a in the infarcted myocardium and serum may play a role in MI by affecting the cAMP-PKA signaling pathway (Feng et al., 2016).

D'Alessandra et al. (2010) investigated plasma levels of miRNAs in acute STEMI patients and infarcted mice and found higher levels of miR-1, miR-133a, miR-133b, and miR-499-5p compared to controls, whereas miR-122 and miR-375 levels were lower only in STEMI patients. Peak miR-1, miR-133a, and miR-133b expression correlated with cTnI levels in time, whereas the time course of miR-499-5p was slower (D'Alessandra et al., 2010). This was later confirmed in an exhaustive meta-analysis of relevant publications (Cheng et al., 2014). Similarly, geriatric patients with acute NSTEMI had greater miR-499-5p levels, exhibiting greater precision in diagnosis than cTnT in patients with mild ST elevation (Olivieri et al., 2013). On the other hand, increased levels of miR-1, miR-133a, miR-208b, and miR-499 in patients with AMI have been demonstrated to not be superior to cTnT (Li et al., 2013). The use of miR-133a as a biomarker in reperfused STEMI has been evaluated and compared to cardiovascular magnetic resonance imaging; high levels of miR-133a correlated with an increased infarct scar size, worse myocardial recovery, and prominent reperfusion injury. Nevertheless, miR-133a did not add further predictive information to cardiovascular magnetic resonance and conventional markers used in clinical practice in high-risk STEMI patients (Eitel et al., 2012). Moreover, the circulating levels of miR-133a were significantly enhanced in AMI patients compared to coronary heart disease and myocardial ischemia patients, presenting a similar trend as plasma cTnI concentration. Remarkably, we found a positive correlation between circulating miR-133a levels and the severity of coronary artery stenosis. Thus, circulating miR-133a may be a suitable tool for AMI diagnosis and predicting the presence and severity of coronary damage in coronary heart disease patients (Wang et al., 2013a). These results were later confirmed (Yuan et al., 2016; Zhu et al., 2018). Nevertheless, in another study analyzing miR-133a and miR-423-5p and their relationship with cardiac biomarkers, such as B-type natriuretic peptide (BNP), C-reactive protein, and cTnI in MI patients, an increase in circulating levels of both miRNAs was observed, but these changes were not associated with LV remodeling or BNP. The authors claimed that miR-133a and miR-423-5p are not useful biomarkers of LV remodeling after MI (Bauters et al., 2013). Another controversial pair of biomarkers is miR-423-5p and miR-30d, which were found to be higher in STEMI patients without a significant correlation with cTnI (Eryılmaz et al., 2016). In addition, the analysis of circulating miR-124a and miR-133 in STEMI and cardiogenic shock patients revealed a significant upregulation of both molecules. A negative correlation was found between miR-133 and MMP-9 levels, and a relationship between miR-124 and soluble ST2 levels, a marker associated with cardiac damage. Surprisingly, this study did not connect any of the miRNAs to the extent of the injury, disease progression, or the prognosis of patient outcomes. In this case, miRNAs would not bring any benefit compared to current

markers (Goldbergova et al., 2018). Moreover, elevated circulating miR-1254 was described as predicting adverse LV remodeling in STEMI patients when compared to magnetic resonance imaging. However, the diagnosis and prognosis values of miR-1254 require further research (de Gonzalo-Calvo et al., 2018). Other investigations have described miR-150-3p and miR-486-3p as being upregulated, whereas miR-26a-5p, miR-126-3p, and miR-191-5p were significantly downregulated in STEMI patients (Hsu et al., 2014). In the same manner, circulating miR-19b-3p, miR-134-5p, and miR-186-5p have been reported to be significantly elevated in the initial stages of AMI. The expression of miR-19b-3p and miR-134-5p in the plasma reached a maximum earlier than miR-186-5p. However, all three positively correlated with cTnI and achieved peak expression before cTnI, which was 8 h after admission. Interestingly, the expression of these circulating miRNAs was not altered by heparin and medications for AMI, and the combination of all three miRNAs increased their diagnostic efficacy (Wang et al., 2016b). Moreover, a higher miR-122-5p/133b ratio was found in serum from STEMI patients (Cortez-Dias et al., 2016). The NSTEMI patients presented higher serum levels of miR-4478, soluble leptin receptor, cTnI, CKMB, urea, creatinine, glucose, cholesterol, TG, and ALP but lower levels of ALT compared to healthy individuals (Gholikhani-Darbroud et al., 2017). Moreover, there was an increase in miR-143 expression in monocytes from STEMI patients, whereas miR-1, miR-92a, miR-99a, and miR-223 expression was significantly reduced. Also, monocytic expression of miR-143 positively correlated with high-sensitivity C-reactive protein (hs-CRP), but not cTnT. These findings demonstrated that circulating monocytes could also be suitable biomarkers (Parahuleva et al., 2017).

Interestingly, cell-specific miRNA patterns are able to distinguish STEMI and NSTEMI patients. A correlation was found between miRNA 30d-5p and plasma, platelets, and leukocytes in patients with STEMI and NSTEMI. Furthermore, miR-221-3p and miR-483-5p were associated with plasma and platelets, but only in NSTEMI patients (Ward et al., 2013).

High levels of plasma miR-134 and miR-328 are described as being possible AMI biomarkers, as they correlate with a superior risk of developing HF and mortality. However, the miRNA levels were not superior to high-sensitivity cTnT (hs-cTnT) concentrations (He et al., 2014). In addition, elevated levels of miR-19a, miR-22-5p, miR-27a, miR-30a, miR-30a-5p, miR-30d-5p, miR-31, miR-34a, miR-122-5p, miR-125b-5p, miR-133, miR-133b, miR-139-5p, miR-150, miR-181a, miR-195, miR-204, miR-208, miR-208b, miR-221-3p, miR-375, miR-486, miR-497, miR-499a-5p, miR-663b, miR-1291, and let-7b can be potential biomarkers for AMI, increased risk of mortality, or HF (Devaux et al., 2012; Long et al., 2012b; Devaux et al., 2013; Li et al., 2014b; Lv et al., 2014; Peng et al., 2014; Zhong et al., 2014; Han et al., 2015; Yao et al., 2015; Zhang et al., 2015c; Coskunpinar et al., 2016; Jia et al., 2016; Maciejak et al., 2016; O'Sullivan et al., 2016; Zhu et al., 2016; Liu et al., 2017; Zhang and Xie, 2017; Alavi-Moghaddam et al., 2018; Maciejak et al., 2018; Wu et al., 2018a; Wang et al., 2019b). Other potential biomarkers for AMI are downregulated in patients' plasma, such as miR-99a, miR-122-5p, and miR-874-3p (Yang et al., 2016a; Yan et al., 2017; Wang et al., 2019b). Interestingly, high levels of the combination of miR-21-5p, miR-361-5p, and miR-519e-5p or the reduction of miR-519e-5p correlates with cTnI concentrations, significantly increasing the diagnostic accuracy in AMI patients (Wang et al., 2014b; Liu et al., 2015a). Similarly, miR-21 and miR-124 have similar diagnostic ability compared to CK, CK-MB, and cTnI (Zhang et al., 2016; Guo et al., 2017).

In an attempt to predict HF and cardiovascular death after AMI, circulating miR-145, the N-terminal fragment of the precursor BNP, myocardial-band CK, and cTnI concentrations were analyzed for short- and long-term clinical outcomes. As a result, the authors concluded that miR-145 was a significant independent predictor of cardiac events, predicting long-term outcomes after AMI (Dong et al., 2015). Later, another group found that miR-145 levels were significantly lower in AMI patients and correlate with increased serum BNP and cTnT and decreased LV ejection fraction (Zhang et al., 2017b).

An miRNA array revealed differences in the miRNA expression patterns in patients with different phases of HF after MI. Specifically, human miR-369-3p, miR-433, miR-493-5p, miR-495, and miR-3615 were overexpressed, whereas miR-877-3p, miR-1306-3p, hsv1-miR-H2, miR-3130-5p, and hcmv-miR-UL22A were underexpressed in these patients. Thus, these circulating miRNAs are novel candidates as biomarkers of MI and HF (Liang et al., 2015).

An important aspect of circulating miRNAs as biomarkers is their temporal release, source, and transportation. Using the ischemia–reperfusion injury model, Deddens et al. (2016) showed that the ischemic myocardium releases extracellular vesicles. They also demonstrated that these extracellular vesicles transported specific miRNAs from the heart and muscle and were quickly detected in plasma. Interestingly, these vesicles had a high miRNAs content and rapid detection compared to traditional injury markers. This makes them a promising tool for the early detection of MI (Deddens et al., 2016). Along the same lines, microparticles and the expression levels of miR-92a were investigated in AMI and stable coronary artery disease patients and compared to cTnI. The number of microparticles and expression levels of miR-92a were higher in AMI patients than in the stable coronary artery disease patients and control groups, with a positive correlation between the levels of microparticles and cTnI. Thus, microparticles containing miR-92a may be suitable for MI diagnosis and possibly regulate dysfunctional endothelial tissue in AMI patients (Zhang et al., 2017c). However, according to Grabmaier et al. (2017), miR-92a seems to not be a good biomarker of adverse ventricular remodeling in post-AMI patients. The authors evaluated circulating miR-1, miR-21, miR-29b, and miR-92a from the SITAGRAMI trial population and found that miR-1, miR-21, and miR-29b expression was higher in AMI patients. The levels of miR-1 and miR-29b in plasma post-AMI correlated with variations in infarct volume, and the levels of miR-29b and changes in LV ejection fraction over time were also associated (Grabmaier et al., 2017).

Investigation of the expression of miR-103a in AMI patients with and without high blood pressure and the effect on endothelial cell function revealed increased levels of miR-103a in all patients but no changes in peripheral blood mononuclear cells. Moreover, miR-103a suppressed the expression of Piezo1

protein, which diminished the capacity to produce capillary tubes and the viability of human umbilical vein endothelial cells (HUVECs). Thus, miR-103a may take part in the development of high blood pressure and the initiation of AMI *via* regulation of Piezo1 expression (Huang et al., 2016a).

In a study based on samples from the HUNT study biobank, Bye et al. (2016) analyzed the utility of circulating miRNAs to predict future fatal AMI in healthy participants. MiR-424-5p and miR-26a-5p were associated exclusively with risk in men and women, respectively, suggesting a gender-specific association. They discovered that the best model for predicting future AMI consisted of miR-106a-5p, miR-424-5p, let-7g-5p, miR-144-3p, and miR-660-5p, and these miRNAs were proposed as a panel to enhance the prediction of AMI risk in healthy individuals (Bye et al., 2016).

Platelet activation is critical for AMI pathogenesis, but the role of platelet miRNAs (pmiRNAs) as biomarkers in AMI and their correlation with indices of platelet activity are unclear. Assessment of pmiR-126 expression in STEMI patients revealed reduced levels and a correlation with plasma cTnI. However, pmiR-126 expression did not correlate well with platelet activity indices, and its potential diagnostic utility is limited (Li et al., 2017b).

MiR-1, miR-133a, and miR-34a induce adverse structural remodeling to impair cardiac contractile function. Increased levels of all three miRNAs have been shown in the hearts of old MI mice compared to young MI mice, and the miR-1 increase was more prolonged and corresponded to LV wall thinning. This suggests that significantly increased levels of miR-1 in the aged post-MI heart could be a biomarker for high-risk prediction (Qipshidze Kelm et al., 2018). In addition, miRNA-21 has been reported to be overexpressed in the serum of ancient patients with AMI and to positively correlate with serum levels of CK-MB and cTnI. *In vitro* experiments with human cardiomyocytes transfected with the miR-21 mimic short hairpin RNA have shown that, following tumor necrosis factor α (TNF-α) induction, apoptosis rates are downregulated. The upregulation of miR-21 expression in the serum of elderly patients with AMI inhibited apoptosis induced by TNF-α in human cardiomyocytes *via* activation of the JNK/p38/caspase-3 signaling pathway (Wang et al., 2017b). Along the same lines, cardiomyocyte apoptosis and hypoxic reduction of cell growth can be promoted by miR-23b overexpression, suggesting that it could be a potential biomarker for STEMI (Zhang et al., 2018a).

A recent study explored the diagnostic use of circulating miRNAs in patients with acute chest pain in the emergency department. They found that higher circulating miR-19b, miR-223, and miR-483-5p levels may be clinically useful for AMI diagnosis in early phases (Li et al., 2019). Similarly, circulating miR-17-5p, miR-126-5p, and miR-145-3p levels are elevated in plasma from AMI patients. Combining these three miRNAs achieves a more precise AMI diagnosis (Xue et al., 2019). Interestingly, next-generation miRNA sequencing from whole blood samples has been useful for identifying new biomarkers of MI (Kanuri et al., 2018).

Heart Failure

Heart failure is a chronic and progressive condition that hampers the ability of the heart to pump enough blood to the body and fulfill its needs. Heart failure is caused by multiple disorders, such as hypertension, cardiomyopathy, MI, arrhythmias, or valvular diseases, among others (Khatibzadeh et al., 2013). Numerous scientific reports connect HF and epigenetic modifications (**Table 4** and **Figure 3**). High-density epigenome-wide mapping of DNA methylation in the myocardium and blood from dilated cardiomyopathy patients and healthy individuals has been analyzed. This technology has been used to find regions of epigenetic susceptibility and new biomarkers related to HF and heart dysfunction; they recognized different patterns of epigenetic methylation that were preserved through tissues—the CpGs regions identified as novel biomarkers of HF (Meder et al., 2017; Rau and Vondriska, 2017). Differentially methylated DNA regions were also identified in blood leukocytes from HF patients (Li et al., 2017a). Dilated cardiomyopathy is an important cause of HF. Genome-wide cardiac DNA methylation in idiopathic dilated cardiomyopathy patients revealed abnormal DNA methylation, which was related to important variations in the expression of lymphocyte antigen 75 (*LY75*) and adenosine receptor A2A (*ADORA2A*) mRNA (Haas et al., 2013). Similarly, genome-wide maps of DNA methylation and enrichment of histone 3 lysine-36 trimethylation (H3K36me3) in pathological and healthy hearts were analyzed. Differences in DNA methylation were found in promoter CpG islands, genes, intragenic CpG islands, and H3K36me3-rich regions of the genome. The promoters of upregulated genes had altered DNA methylation, but not the promoters of downregulated genes. In particular, an abundance of *DUX4* transcripts was associated with differences in DNA methylation and H3K36me3 enrichment. Although further studies need to be carried out, there is evidence that the expression of genes critical for the development of cardiomyopathies may be controlled by the epigenome (Movassagh et al., 2011). Moreover, in patients with dilated cardiomyopathy, there is an altered methylation pattern in the regulatory regions of cardiac development genes, such as T-box protein 5 (*TBX5*), heart and neural crest derivatives expressed 1 (*HAND1*), and NK2 homeobox 5 (*NKX2.5*) (Jo et al., 2016). Koczor et al. (2013) also studied the differential methylation patterns in patients with dilated cardiomyopathy, which is characterized by congestive HF. Computational analysis detected few differentially methylated gene promoters (*AURKB*, *BTNL9*, *CLDN5*, and *TK1*). This study provides relevant information on DNA methylation and altered expression in dilated cardiomyopathy that would help in treatment (Koczor et al., 2013).

Furthermore, epigenetic modifications have been proposed to play an important role in HF progression in the murine model of pressure overload. The researchers observed a reduction in sarcoplasmic reticulum Ca^{2+}ATPase (*Atp2a2*) levels and a significant induction of β-myosin-heavy chain (*Myh7*) mRNA levels. They also detected H3K4me2, H3K9me2, H3K27me3, and H3K36me2 and a reduction in the lysine-specific demethylase KDM2A after 8 weeks of transverse aortic constriction (Angrisano et al., 2014). *Atp2a2* is a determinant of cardiac function, and its reduced activity is a clear feature of HF. Gorski et al. (2019) investigated the role of lysine acetylation in *Atp2a2* function in HF patients and found that acetylation at lysine 492 is regulated by SIRT1 and HAT p300 and significantly reduced

the gene activity (Gorski et al., 2019). All of this knowledge would be fundamental to identifying potential biomarkers and new epigenetic drugs in HF therapy. Interestingly, an association has been reported between epigenetic remodeling in the atrial natriuretic peptide (*ANP*) and *BNP* promoters and reactivation of the fetal gene program in HF. Their reported upregulation in HF patients did not respond to an increase in histone acetylation but HDAC4, which is exported from the nucleus. In contrast, demethylation of H3K9 and dissociation of heterochromatin protein 1 from gene promoters were regulated by HDAC4. Thus, HDAC4 is fundamental to histone methylation in HF caused by increased cardiac load and a potential target for treatment (Hohl et al., 2013). More recently, Glezeva et al. (2019) performed targeted DNA methylation sequencing to detect DNA methylation alterations in coding and ncRNA in cardiac interventricular septal tissue from HF patients. They found hypermethylation in *HEY2*, *MSR1*, *MYOM3*, *COX17*, and miR-24-1 and hypomethylation in *CTGF*, *MMP2*, and miR-155. Therefore, they defended a unique cohort of loci useful as diagnostic and therapeutic targets in HF (Glezeva et al., 2019).

More than 10 years ago, few reports suggested that specific miRNAs are differentially regulated in the failing heart (Divakaran and Mann, 2008; Small and Olson, 2011). Since then, an extensive evidence base has been published in the literature regarding the use of miRNAs as possible biomarkers for HF diagnosis and prognosis. In evaluating whether miRNAs can differentiate clinical HF from healthy individuals and from non-HF dyspnea, miRNA arrays have revealed miR423-5p enrichment in the blood of HF patients (Tijsen et al., 2010). However, criticisms have been raised in this study regarding age differences between groups, reduced sample size, and statistics (Kumarswamy et al., 2010). Moreover, patients with HF of different etiologies presented with different expression levels of circulating miRNAs. Ischemic HF patients were found to have a positive transcoronary gradient for miR-423-5p, miR-423, and miR-34a, but the nonischemic HF group was positive only for miR-21-3p and miR-30a. The transcoronary concentration gradient suggests that the failing heart may selectively release the miRNAs into the coronary circulation. These miRNAs could be useful for discriminating different etiologies of HF (Goldraich et al., 2014; De Rosa et al., 2018).

Circulating miRNAs have been screened in an attempt to identify any that could be used for the prognosis of ischemic HF in post-AMI patients. Knowing that p53 has been involved in HF development in mice (Sano et al., 2007), the authors took great interest in p53-responsive miRNAs. The serum levels of miR-34a, miR-192, and miR-194 were significantly and coordinately upregulated in AMI patients with ischemic HF progression, and all three were p53-responsive. Interestingly, these miRNAs were contained in extracellular vesicles, suggesting that they are circulating regulators of HF. Furthermore, there was a significant correlation between the LV end-diastolic dimension 1 year after AMI and the miR-194 and miR-34a expression levels. Thus, although further investigations are needed, these results suggest the usefulness of miR-34a, miR-192, and miR-194 in predicting the risk of HF progression after AMI (Evans and Mann, 2013; Matsumoto et al., 2013; Klenke et al., 2018).

TABLE 4 | Epigenetic biomarkers in heart failure.

Epigenetic modification	Biomarker	Regulation in heart failure	Sample source	Study type	References
DNA methylation	*LY75* and *ADORA2A*	Aberrant DNA methylation	Left ventricle myocardium and zebrafish	Clinical and experimental: zebrafish	(Haas et al., 2013)
	TBX5, *HAND1*, and *NKX2.5* *HEY2*, *MSR1*, *MYOM3*, *COX17*, miR-24-1, *CTGF*, *MMP2*, miR-155	Altered DNA methylation *HEY2*, *MSR1*, *MYOM3*, *COX17*, and miR-24-1: hypermethylation; *CTGF*, *MMP2*, and miR-155: hypomethylation	Myocardium Myocardium	Clinical Clinical	(Jo et al., 2016) (Glezeva et al., 2019)
Histone modifications	H3K36me3	H3K36me3 enhancement	Myocardium	Clinical	(Movassagh et al., 2011)
	HDAC4	HDAC4 activation	Myocardium	Clinical and experimental: mouse model of pressure overload	(Hohl et al., 2013)
	H3K4me2, H3K9me2, H3K27me3, H3K36me2, KDM2A	H3K4me2, H3K9me2, H3K27me3, and H3K36me2 methylation and KDM2A reduction	Myocardium	Experimental: mouse model of pressure overload	(Angrisano et al., 2014)
	Atp2a2	*Atp2a2* acetylation	Ventricular myocytes and myocardium	Clinical and experimental: mouse model of pressure overload in *MHC-SIRT1−/−* Tg mice and swine model of MI	(Gorski et al., 2019)
miRNA	miR423-5p miR-192 miR-122*, miR-200b, miR-520d-5p, miR-622, miR-1228*, miR-558	Higher levels Upregulation miR-122*, miR-200b, miR-520d-5p, miR-622, miR-1228*: upregulation; miR-558: downregulation	Plasma Serum Whole peripheral blood	Clinical Clinical Clinical	(Tijsen et al., 2010) (Matsumoto et al., 2013) (Vogel et al., 2013)
	miR-103, miR-142-3p, miR-30b, miR-342-3p	Differentially expressed	Plasma	Clinical	(Ellis et al., 2013)
	miR-210, miR-30a miR-210	Upregulation Higher levels	Serum Plasma, mononuclear cells, and skeletal muscles	Clinical Clinical and experimental: Dahl salt-sensitive rats	(Zhao et al., 2013) (Endo et al., 2013)
	miR-1 miR-423-5p	Higher levels Positive transcoronary gradients	Plasma Transcoronary gradients	Clinical Clinical	(Zhang et al., 2013b) (Goldraich et al., 2014)
	miR-423-5p MiR-30c, miR-146a, miR-221, miR-328, miR-375	Lower levels Downregulation	Plasma Serum	Clinical Clinical	(Seronde et al., 2015) (Watson et al., 2015)
	miR-21, miR-650, miR-744, miR-516-5p, miR-1292, miR-182, miR-1228, miR-595, miR-663b, miR-1296, miR-1825, miR-299-3p, miR-662 miR-122, miR-3148, miR-518e, miR-129-3p, miR-3155, miR-3175, miR-583, miR-568, miR-30d, miR-200a-star, miR-1979, miR-371-3p, miR-155-star, miR-502-5p	miR-21, miR-650, miR-744, miR-516-5p, miR-1292, miR-182, miR-1228, miR-595, miR-663b, miR-1296, miR-1825, miR-299-3p, miR-662 miR-122, miR-3148, miR-518e: increased; miR-129-3p, miR-3155, miR-3175, miR-583, miR-568, miR-30d, miR-200a-star, miR-1979, miR-371-3p, miR-155-star, miR-502-5p: decreased	Serum	Clinical	(Cakmak et al., 2015)
	miR-1233, miR-671-5p, miR-183-3p, miR-190a, miR-193b-3p, miR-193b-5p, miR-211-5p, miR-494	miR-1233, miR-671-5p: Upregulation; miR-183-3p, miR-190a, miR-193b-3p, miR-193b-5p, miR-211-5p, miR-494: downregulation	Whole blood and plasma	Clinical	(Wong et al., 2015)

(Continued)

TABLE 4 | Continued

Epigenetic modification	Biomarker	Regulation in heart failure	Sample source	Study type	References
	miR-1, miR-21	miR-1: downregulation; miR-21: upregulation	Serum	Clinical	(Sygitowicz et al., 2015)
	miR-126	Downregulation	Serum	Clinical	(Wei et al., 2015)
	miR-1, miR-21, miR-23, miR-29, miR-130, miR-195, miR-199	Upregulation	Myocardial biopsy	Clinical	(Lai et al., 2015)
	miR-106a-5p, miR-223-3p, miR-652-3p, miR-199a-3p, miR-18a-5p	Downregulation	Plasma	Clinical	(Vegter et al., 2016)
	miR-148b-3p, miR-409-3p	Downregulation	Serum and left atrial tissue	Clinical	(Chen et al., 2016)
	miR-122-5p, miR-184	Upregulation	H9C2 cells and blood and myocardium	Experimental: in vitro and rat model of post-MI HF	(Liu et al., 2016)
	miR-660-3p, miR-665, miR-1285-3p, miR-4491	Upregulation	Plasma and heart	Clinical	(Li et al., 2016)
	miR-18a-5p, miR-26b-5p, miR-27a-3p, miR-30e-5p, miR-106a-5p, miR-199a-3p, miR-652-3p	Lower levels	Plasma	Clinical	(Ovchinnikova et al., 2016)
	miR-19b	Lower levels	Serum and myocardial	Clinical and experimental: in vitro	(Beaumont et al., 2017)
	miR-30d	Lower levels	Serum	Clinical	(Xiao et al., 2017)
	miR-195-3p	Higher levels	Plasma	Clinical	(He et al., 2017)
	miR-22-3p	Higher levels	Blood	Clinical	(van Boven et al., 2017)
	miR-150-5p	Downregulation	Blood	Clinical	(Scrutinio et al., 2017)
	miR-133b-3p, miR-208b-3p, miR-125a-5p, miR-125b-5p, miR-126-3p, miR-21-5p, miR-210-3p, miR-29a-3p, miR-320a, miR-494-3p	Upregulation	Blood	Experimental: sheep model of HF	(Wong et al., 2017)
	miR-146a	Upregulation	Exosomal and total plasma	Clinical and experimental: in vitro	(Beg et al., 2017)
	miR-9, miR-495, miR-599, miR-181c	ex-miR-9, ex-miR-181c, ex-miR-495: increased; ex-miR-599: decreased	Exosomal and total plasma	Experimental: dogs with myxomatous mitral valve disease, mitral valve prolapse	(Yang et al., 2017b)
	miR-21-5p, miR-23a-3p, miR-222-3p	Higher levels	Plasma	Clinical and experimental: rat model of post-MI HF	(Dubois-Deruy et al., 2017)
	miRNA-21	Higher levels	Serum	Clinical	(Zhang et al., 2017a)
	miR-132	Higher levels	Plasma	Clinical	(Masson et al., 2018)
	miR-1254, miR-1306-5p	Higher levels	Blood	Clinical	(Bayés-Genis et al., 2018)
	miR-423, miR-34a, miR-21-3p, miR-30a	miR-21-3p, miR-30a: Positive transcoronary gradient in non-ischemic HF; miR-423, miR-34a: Negative transcoronary gradient in ischemic HF	Transcoronary gradients	Clinical	(De Rosa et al., 2018)
	miR-3135b, miR-3908, miR-5571-5p	Upregulation	Plasma	Clinical	(Chen et al., 2018a)
	miR-302b-3p	Higher levels	Plasma	Clinical	(Li et al., 2018a)
	exo-miR-92b-5p	increased	Serum	Clinical	(Wu et al., 2018c)
	miR-26b, miR-208b, miR-499	Higher levels	Peripheral blood mononuclear cells	Clinical	(Marketou et al., 2018)
	miR-423-5p, miR-221-5p, miR-212-5p, miR-193b-5p, miR-15a-5p, miR-208a-3p	Upregulation	Plasma, mouse myocardium and NRVMs cells	Clinical and experimental: in vitro, and murine model of hypertrophy and HF	(Shah et al., 2018b)
	miR-192	Upregulation	Serum	Clinical	(Klenke et al., 2018)

(Continued)

TABLE 4 | Continued

Epigenetic modification	Biomarker	Regulation in heart failure	Sample source	Study type	References
	miR-34a, miR-208b, miR-126, miR-24, miR-29a	miR-34a, miR-208b, miR-126: upregulation; miR-24, miR-29a: downregulation	Serum	Clinical	(Lakhani et al., 2018)
	miR-17, miR-20a, miR-106b	Lower levels	Plasma	Clinical	(Shah et al., 2018a)
	miR-197-5p	Upregulation	Plasma	Clinical	(Liu et al., 2018b)
	miR-133a, miR-221	Higher levels	Plasma	Clinical	(Guo et al., 2018)
	exo-miR-92b-5p	Higher levels	Serum	Clinical	(Wu et al., 2018b; Wu et al., 2018c)

Vogel et al. (2013) assessed the genome-wide miRNA expression profiles in HF patients with reduced ejection fraction (HFrEF). They demonstrated that dysregulated levels of miRNAs, such as miR-122*, miR-200b, miR-520d-5p, miR-622, miR-1228* (upregulated), or miR-558 (downregulated) significantly correlate with disease severity, as indicated by LV ejection fraction (Vogel et al., 2013). Moreover, Ellis et al. (2013) tried to find differences between HF patients and non–HF-related breathlessness, and between HFrEF and HF with preserved ejection fraction (HFpEF); although they found a differential expression of miR-103, miR-142-3p, miR-30b, and miR-342-3p in HF and breathless patients, individually, classical biomarkers such as NT-proBNP and hs-cTnT exhibited greater sensitivity and specificity. However, the combination of miRNAs with NT-proBNP significantly improved prediction performance (Ellis et al., 2013). Similarly, elevated plasma levels of miR-210 were reported in congestive HF patients, although no significant correlation was observed with BNP. However, patients with an improved BNP profile presented with low plasma miR-210 levels. MiR-210 might reflect a mismatch between heart contraction and oxygen demand in the peripheral tissues (Endo et al., 2013). Interestingly, miR-210 and miR-30a expression is upregulated in HF patients, with a tendency toward fetal values (Zhao et al., 2013). Moreover, changes in myocardial miRNA in patients with stable and end-stage HF partially resemble the fetal myocardium. Target mRNA levels negatively correlate with changes in highly expressed miRNAs in HF and fetal hearts. The circulation is dominated by miRNAs, fragments of tRNAs, and small cytoplasmic RNAs. Heart- and muscle-specific circulating miRNAs (myomirs) are also increased in advanced HF, correlating with cTnI levels. These findings support miRNA-based therapies and the use of circulating miRNAs as biomarkers for heart injury (Akat et al., 2014). Cardiac fibroblast–derived miRNAs, such as miR-660-3p, miR-665, miR-1285-3p, and miR-4491, have also been found to be significantly upregulated in heart and plasma during HF, discriminating patients from controls (Li et al., 2016). However, miRNAs in the pericardial fluid are not related to cardiovascular pathologies or clinically assessed stages of HF. MicroRNAs may be paracrine signaling factors that intervene in cardiac cells crosstalk (Kuosmanen et al., 2015).

In another study performed in patients with chronic congestive HF, microarray profiling demonstrated increased expression of miR-21, miR-122, miR-182, miR-299-3p, miR-516-5p, miR-518e, miR-595, miR-650, miR-662, miR-663b, miR-744, miR-1228, miR-1292, miR-1296, miR-1825, and miR-3148 and decreased expression of miR-30d, miR-129-3p, and miR-502-5p, miR-155-star miR-200a-star, miR-371-3p, miR-583, miR-568, miR-1979, miR-3155, and miR-3175. Among these miRNAs, miR-182 seemed to have a better prognostic value than hs-CRP (Cakmak et al., 2015). Furthermore, miR-30c, miR-146a, miR-221, miR-328, and miR-375 had different expression levels in HFrEF and HFpEF. The combination of two or more miRNAs with BNP could significantly improve the discrimination of these pathological conditions compared to BNP alone (Watson et al., 2015). Additional miRNAs have been identified as promising biomarkers to discriminate HF from healthy individuals and to differentiate HFrEF from HFpEF: miR-125a-5p, miR-183-3p, miR-190a, miR-193b-3p, miR-193b-5p, miR-211-5p, miR-494, miR-545-5p, miR-550a-5p, miR-638, miR-671-5p, miR-1233, miR-3135b, miR-3908, and miR-5571-5p. The use of a combination of miRNAs and NT-proBNP increases its discernment capacity (Schulte et al., 2015; Wong et al., 2015; Chen et al., 2018a). Similarly, increased levels of miR-133a and miR-221 can be used as suitable HF diagnostic biomarkers in elderly HF patients, and the combination of NT-proBNP and miR-133a can improve the diagnostic accuracy (Guo et al., 2018). Serum levels of miR-1, miR-21, and miR-208a have also been analyzed in symptomatic HF patients. Expression of miR-1 is reduced in symptomatic HF patients, with decreasing levels correlating with increasing severity. In contrast, miR-21 has been shown to be overexpressed with no relation to HF severity. No circulating miR-208a has been observed in symptomatic HF patients. A negative correlation between miR-1 expression and NT-proBNP has been reported in HF patients, whereas miR-21 and galectin-3 have been positively correlated. Therefore, dysregulated levels of miR-1 and miR-21 may be fundamental for HF progression (Sygitowicz et al., 2015). An inverse correlation between miR-1 levels and ejection fraction has also been reported. Thus, elevated levels of miR-1 may inhibit cardiac function and be a predictor of the onset of HF secondary to AMI (Zhang et al., 2013b).

MiR-126 has also been studied in atrial fibrillation and/or HF patients, with downregulated expression in patients and positive correlation with LV ejection fraction but a negative association with the cardiothoracic ratio and NT-proBNP. Thus, the reduction in miR-126 expression is a potential indicator of severity in atrial fibrillation and HF (Wei et al., 2015). A significant negative correlation has also been found between several miRNAs and classical clinical biomarkers indicative of a worse clinical outcome in HF patients. MiR-16-5p has been correlated to CRP, miR-106a-5p to creatinine, miR-223-3p to growth differentiation factor 15, miR-652-3p to soluble ST-2, miR-199a-3p to procalcitonin and galectin-3, and miR-18a-5p to procalcitonin (Vegter et al., 2016). Furthermore, an analysis of myocyte and fibroblast-related miRNAs and mRNAs in myocardium samples from HF patients and control individuals revealed that miR-1, miR-21, miR-23, miR-29, miR-130, miR-195, and miR-199 are significantly upregulated in HF patients, whereas miR-30, miR-133, miR-208, and miR-320 do not significantly change. Related mRNAs, such as caspase 3, collagenase I, collagenase III, and transforming growth factor (TGF), are also upregulated in HF patients. MicroRNAs involved in apoptosis, hypertrophy, and fibrosis are upregulated in the myocardium of HF patients and may be suitable biomarkers in the early stages of chronic HF and future therapeutic targets (Lai et al., 2015).

Evaluation of miR-148b-3p and miR-409-3p in mitral regurgitation patients, asymptomatic mitral regurgitation patients, and controls revealed that circulating and tissue miR-148b-3p and circulating miR-409-3p are significantly downregulated in mitral regurgitation patients with HF, and miR-148b-3p is significantly downregulated only in the mitral regurgitation patients without HF. Notably, the mRNAs of target genes of both miRNAs have been shown to be upregulated in HF patients with mitral regurgitation. Thus, circulating miR-148b-3p may be used as a biomarker of HF and miR-409-3p for incident HF in mitral regurgitation patients (Chen et al., 2016).

Specific overexpression of miR-221 in the hearts of transgenic mice has been shown to induce cardiac dysfunction and HF by impairing autophagy. In addition, *in vitro* miR-221 upregulation inhibits autophagic vesicle formation. Thus, autophagy balance and cardiac remodeling are regulated by miR-221 levels through modulation of the p27/CDK2/mTOR axis, and miR-221 might be a therapeutic target in HF (Su et al., 2015). Furthermore, high-throughput sequencing has been used to determine the differential miRNA pattern in a rat model of post-MI HF. Upregulation of miR-122-5p and miR-184 was found in HF rats, describing a proapoptotic role of both miRNAs (Liu et al., 2016). In another study using the same model, the authors identified a significant increase in miR-21-5p, miR-23a-3p, and miR-222-3p and their target *SOD2* in the plasma and myocardium of HF rats. They showed a direct interaction between miR-222-3p and *SOD2*. An inhibition or increase in *SOD2* expression was found when human cardiomyocytes were transfected with miR-222-3p mimic or inhibitor, respectively (Dubois-Deruy et al., 2017).

Myocardial fibrosis–related miRNAs, such as miR-19b, are reduced in the myocardium and serum of HF patients with aortic stenosis. Inhibition of miR-19b in cultured human fibroblasts increases the expression of connective tissue growth factor protein and the enzyme lysyl oxidase (LOX). This could lead to excessive collagen fibril cross-linking and a subsequent increase in LV stiffness in aortic stenosis patients, particularly those with HF. Thus, miR-19b could be a biomarker of alterations in the myocardial collagen network (Beaumont et al., 2017).

Numerous studies have been performed to find miRNAs with a predictive value in HF patients. Increased levels of miR-1, miR-21, miR-21-5p, miR-22-3p, miR-29a-3p, miR30d, miR-125a-5p,

miR-125b-5p, miR-126-3p, miR-133b-3p, miR-195-3p, miR-197-5P, miR-208b-3p, miR-210-3p, miR-302b-3p, miR-320a, and miR-494-3p (Zhang et al., 2013b; He et al., 2017; van Boven et al., 2017; Wong et al., 2017; Xiao et al., 2017; Zhang et al., 2017a; Li et al., 2018a; Liu et al., 2018b;) or decreased levels of miR-17, miR-18a-5p, miR-20a, miR-150, miR-26b-5p, miR-27a-3p, miR-30e-5p, miR-106a-5p, miR-106b, miR-150-5p, miR-199a-3p, miR-423-5p, and miR-652-3p (Seronde et al., 2015; Ovchinnikova et al., 2016; Scrutinio et al., 2017; Shah et al., 2018a; Lin et al., 2019) have been described as potential biomarkers in HF patients. These discoveries may serve to develop miRNA-based therapies and to identify new pharmacological targets.

Beg et al. (2017) measured exosomal and total plasma miRNAs separately in HF patients to distinguish between the transfer of biological materials for signaling alteration in distant organs (exosomal) and the level of tissue damage (plasma). They found that the circulating exosomal miR-146a/miR-16 ratio was higher in HF patients, with miR-146a induced in response to inflammation. These results suggest circulating exosomal miR-146a as a biomarker of HF (Beg et al., 2017). Moreover, elevation of exosomal miRNA exo-miR-92b-5p has been suggested as a potential biomarker for the diagnosis of HF (Wu et al., 2018b; Wu et al., 2018c). In a preclinical study in dogs with myxomatous mitral valve disease, dysregulation of exosomal miR-9, miR-495, and miR-599 was observed as the dogs aged. In addition, levels of miR-9, miR-599, miR-181c, and miR-495 changed in myxomatous mitral valve disease. Thus, the exosomal miRNA expression level appears to be more specific to disease states than total plasma miRNA (Yang et al., 2017b). Furthermore, the downregulation of miR-425 and miR-744 in the plasma exosomes has been shown to induce cardiac fibrosis by suppressing TGFβ1 expression (Wang et al., 2018a).

Circulating miR-132 levels increased in chronic HF with disease severity, and lower levels improve risk prediction for HF readmission beyond traditional risk factors, but not for mortality. MiR-132 may be useful for finding strategies that would reduce rehospitalization in HF patients (Masson et al., 2018; Panico and Condorelli, 2018). Moreover, in an exhaustive analysis of two independent cohorts using a strict quality evaluation for miRNA testing, an association was found between high levels of miR-1254 and miR-1306-5p and mortality and HF hospitalization in HF patients. However, these two circulating miRNAs were not shown to improve standard predictors of prognostication, such as age, sex, hemoglobin, renal function, and NT-proBNP (Bayés-Genis et al., 2018).

MiR-26b, miR-208b, and miR-499 expression levels have been assessed in peripheral blood mononuclear cells from hypertensive HFpEF patients to evaluate their association with their exercise capacity. All three miRNAs were expressed at higher levels in the patients group, but miR-208b showed the strongest correlations with cardiopulmonary exercise test parameters, including oxygen uptake, exercise duration, and the minute ventilation–carbon dioxide production relationship (Marketou et al., 2018). In a study performed in patients and a mice model of hypertrophy and HF, miRNAs dysregulation was shown to occur during HF development in animals, with downregulation of target genes. These miRNAs were associated with adverse LV remodeling in humans, suggesting coordinated regulation of miRNA-mRNA. They also revealed target clusters of genes, such as autophagy, metabolism, and inflammation, implicated in HF mechanisms, (Shah et al., 2018b).

With the intention to establish a biomarkers panel useful for early detection of HF resulting from MI, Lakhani et al. (2018) found significant upregulation of miR-34a, miR-208b, miR-126, TGFβ-1, TNF-α, IL-6, and MMP-9 and reduced miR-24 and miR-29a levels. A positive association between IL-10 and ejection fraction in MI patients also suggested an important role of IL-10 in predicting HF (Lakhani et al., 2018).

Systems biology analyses of LV remodeling after MI allow molecular comprehensions; for example, miRNA modulation may be used as a marker of HF evolution. Two systems biology strategies were used to define an miRNA mark of LV remodeling in MI. They integrated either multiomics data (proteins and ncRNAs) produced from post-MI plasma or proteomic data generated from a rat model of MI. As a result, several miRNAs were associated with LV remodeling: miR-21-5p, miR-23a-3p, miR-222-3p, miR-17-5p, miR-21-5p, miR-26b-5p, miR-222-3p, miR-335-5p, and miR-375. These outcomes support the use of integrative systems biology analyses for the definition of miRNA marks of HF evolution (Charrier et al., 2019).

LIMITATIONS AND PERSPECTIVES OF THE EPIGENETIC BIOMARKERS

Limitations of the current field include the lack of large multicenter studies to provide convincing evidence for clinical applicability. Rather than a single ncRNA, it is likely that there will be patterns of different ncRNAs and other biomarkers (e.g., protein-based) that, together with machine-learning algorithms, will provide more sensitive and specific diagnostic and prognostic approaches to CVDs. Also, several technical challenges must be overcome before CE-marked ncRNA biomarkers will enter the clinical realm. DNA methylation and histone modifications are epigenetic mechanisms that have been reported to be sources of potential biomarkers useful in clinical practice. However, each CVD is regulated by multiple epigenetic pathways, and different CVDs are regulated by the same epigenetic mechanism, most of which are still under study. For example, hypermethylation of H3K79 (Rodriguez-Iturbe, 2006; Duarte et al., 2012) and ACE2 promoter (Fan et al., 2017) in hypertensive patients has been described. Moreover, H3K4 and H3K9 were also hypermethylated in both mouse models of hypertension (Pojoga et al., 2011) and HF (Angrisano et al., 2014). This makes it difficult to select and implement a set of biomarkers for a particular CVD. Another potential problem is the quality of the samples, especially those obtained from collections in the pathology department. These samples are usually preserved in formaldehyde and paraffin, which highly degrades DNA. The stability, size, and integrity of a sample depend on the duration of fixation and storage (Kristensen et al., 2009). Thus, assessment of the quality of DNA is fundamental. However, the DNA methylation analysis can be performed successfully using polymerase chain reaction (PCR) methods with small amplicons in old samples (Tournier

et al., 2012; Wong et al., 2014). In other cases, it is important to carefully adjust the protocol. It is also important to consider that frozen and paraffin-preserved samples may have different results, and they should not be compared without appropriate correction (García-Giménez et al., 2017).

Among the epigenetic biomarkers, miRNAs are the most promising, and numerous studies have been carried out in the last few years. The relatively easy detection and accessibility to samples in fluids, such as blood, urine, or saliva, make them very attractive. However, a few issues should be solved before their implementation in the clinical practice. The main problem is that miRNAs usually target multiple mRNAs from different genes, and one gene can be targeted by several miRNAs. This complex network should be deeply investigated before determining the use of a specific miRNA as a biomarker for the diagnosis or treatment of a particular disease (Akhtar et al., 2016). Regarding sample preparation, it is highly recommended to use plasma instead of whole blood, because if it is hemolyzed, the circulating miRNA content can be altered. Increasing the centrifugation time is also important in order to reduce platelet contamination (de Gonzalo-Calvo et al., 2017; García-Giménez et al., 2017).

Recently, great advances have been made to implement the new technology in the detection of new epigenetic biomarkers. However, a few concerns should be alleviated before their clinical implementation. Studies with big cohorts in different independent laboratories, using the same experimental design, sample preparation, methodology, and disease specifications, are necessary. Small patient cohorts should be considered as pilot studies before the validation of results in bigger sample analysis. The method of detection should be standardized for clinical application, and the clinical trials have to be randomized and prospective. It is also important to compare the new biomarkers with the classical biomarkers in order to validate them and determine their usefulness. The sensitivity and specificity for a certain disease also have to be determined for each biomarker (Engelhardt, 2012; García-Giménez et al., 2017). Regarding the method of DNA methylation detection, the luminometric methylation assay and the methylation analysis of CpG islands in repeatable elements (LINE-1) are widely used. Although there is a certain correlation with the measurements obtained with both methods, the comparison is not recommended, since a consistent bias between the results has been described (Knothe et al., 2016). Interestingly, a large multicenter study comparing DNA methylation assays compatible with routine clinical use has been performed. According to the authors, good agreement was observed between DNA methylation assays, which can be implemented in large-scale validation studies, development of new biomarkers, and clinical diagnostics (BLUEPRINT Consortium, 2016). The most used system to detect miRNAs is quantitative PCR, being the normalization protocol critical. Most laboratories use housekeeping genes or miRNAs as normalizers, changing their expression levels within serums. Another approach employs identical volumes of serum for all samples, generating different amounts of total RNA (Chen et al., 2008; Wang et al., 2009; Rockenbach et al., 2012). Both approaches include spike-in normalization, which consists of adding RNA of known sequence and quantity to calibrate measurements. However, spike-in normalization does not consider internal variation in circulating miRNA between different individuals. Thus, a combination of both methods should always be performed to guarantee results reliability (van Empel et al., 2012). Polymerase chain reaction technology has to be performed with rigorous controls to avoid artifacts in the amplification step. To overcome this problem, digital PCR based on the amplification of one single molecule per reaction constitutes a valuable option (Hindson et al., 2013). Another attractive alternative for accurate measuring RNAs is the direct nucleic acid sequencing, although it is still expensive when considering large screening analysis (Kozomara and Griffiths-Jones, 2011). Finally, it is also important to understand the processes controlling miRNAs release and stability. The correlation between circulating and tissue miRNAs is not clear, and several studies indicate that miRNA levels in blood are not a reflection of changes in the tissue of origin. The reason is that miRNAs can also be produced by immune cells (Zheng et al., 2018).

CONCLUDING REMARKS

Over the past few years, a great amount of research has focused on epigenetics and its dynamic cross-talk with genetics. Unveiling a personalized epigenetic pattern can provide a large amount of information on epigenetic machinery that could be employed to tailor diagnosis and therapeutic strategies in CVDs. Recent advances in technology and data analysis have made it possible to create detailed epigenetic maps, which may represent a new tool in the clinical practice to discern cardiovascular risk beyond traditional risk determinants. Epigenetic information can also help in predicting individual drug responses. Importantly, epigenetic biomarkers are gaining ground in the scientific community as tools for the diagnosis and prognosis of CVDs. However, discrepancies in specific diagnostic biomarkers make replication of the current results in independent laboratories, with multiple research centers and a big sample size, mandatory. All of this will lead to a standardized clinical application in the near future.

AUTHOR CONTRIBUTIONS

CS-B and AB-G conceived the idea and wrote the manuscript with support from CG-M. CG-M performed the drawings and structure of the figures. All authors contributed to manuscript revision, read and approved the submitted version.

FUNDING

This work was supported by grants from the Spanish Ministry of Economy and Competitiveness-MINECO (SAF2017-84324-C2-1-R), the Instituto de Salud Carlos III (PIC18/0014, PI18/00256), the Red de Terapia Celular–TerCel (RD16/0011/0006) and the CIBER Cardiovascular (CB16/11/00403) projects, as part of the Plan Nacional de I+D+I, and it was co-funded by ISCIII-Sudirección General de Evaluación y el Fondo Europeo de Desarrollo Regional (FEDER). This work was also funded by the Fundació La MARATÓ de TV3 (201516-10, 201502-20), the Generalitat de Catalunya (SGR2017 00483, SLT002/16/00234), the CERCA Programme/Generalitat de Catalunya, and "la Caixa" Banking Foundation.

ACKNOWLEDGMENTS

We apologize to all authors whose work could not be mentioned because of space limitations or inadvertent omissions. We are greatly grateful to Sonia V Forcales for her comments and discussion on epigenetic regulation.

REFERENCES

1. Adachi, T., Nakanishi, M., Otsuka, Y., Nishimura, K., Hirokawa, G., Goto, Y., et al. (2010). Plasma microRNA 499 as a biomarker of acute myocardial infarction. *Clin. Chem.* 56, 1183–1185. doi: 10.1373/clinchem.2010.144121
2. Ai, J., Zhang, R., Li, Y., Pu, J., Lu, Y., Jiao, J., et al. (2010). Circulating microRNA-1 as a potential novel biomarker for acute myocardial infarction. *Biochem. Biophys. Res. Commun.* 391, 73–77. doi: 10.1016/j.bbrc.2009.11.005
3. Akat, K. M., Moore-McGriff, D., Morozov, P., Brown, M., Gogakos, T., Correa Da Rosa, J., et al. (2014). Comparative RNA-sequencing analysis of myocardial and circulating small RNAs in human heart failure and their utility as biomarkers. *Proc. Natl. Acad. Sci. U. S. A* 111, 11151–11156. doi: 10.1073/pnas.1401724111
4. Akhtar, M. M., Micolucci, L., Islam, M. S., Olivieri, F., and Procopio, A. D. (2016). Bioinformatic tools for microRNA dissection. *Nucleic Acids Res.* 44, 24–44. doi: 10.1093/nar/gkv1221
5. Alavi-Moghaddam, M., Chehrazi, M., Alipoor, S. D., Mohammadi, M., Baratloo, A., Mahjoub, M. P., et al. (2018). A preliminary study of microRNA-208b after acute myocardial infarction: impact on 6-month survival. *Dis. Markers* 2018, 2410451–7. doi: 10.1155/2018/2410451
6. Alikhani-Koopaei, R., Fouladkou, F., Frey, F. J., and Frey, B. M. (2004). Epigenetic regulation of 11 beta-hydroxysteroid dehydrogenase type 2 expression. *J. Clin. Investig.* 114, 1146–1157. doi: 10.1172/JCI21647
7. Angrisano, T., Schiattarella, G. G., Keller, S., Pironti, G., Florio, E., Magliulo, F., et al. (2014). Epigenetic switch at atp2a2 and myh7 gene promoters in pressure overload-induced heart failure. *PLoS One* 9, e106024. doi: 10.1371/journal.pone.0106024

8. Authors/Task Force members, Windecker, S., Kolh, P., Alfonso, F., Collet, J.-P., Cremer, J., et al. (2014). 2014 ESC/EACTS guidelines on myocardial revascularization: the task force on myocardial revascularization of the European Society of Cardiology (ESC) and the European Association for Cardio-Thoracic Surgery (EACTS) developed with the special contribution of the European Association of Percutaneous Cardiovascular Interventions (EAPCI). *Eur. Heart J.* 35, 2541–2619. doi: 10.1093/eurheartj/ehu278
9. Babuin, L., and Jaffe, A. S. (2005). Troponin: the biomarker of choice for the detection of cardiac injury. *CMAJ* 173, 1191–1202. doi: 10.1503/cmaj/051291
10. Baccarelli, A., Rienstra, M., and Benjamin, E. J. (2010). Cardiovascular epigenetics: basic concepts and results from animal and human studies. *Circ. Cardiovasc. Genet.* 3, 567–573. doi: 10.1161/CIRCGENETICS.110.958744
11. Baptista, R., Marques, C., Catarino, S., Enguita, F. J., Costa, M. C., Matafome, P., et al. (2018). MicroRNA-424(322) as a new marker of disease progression in pulmonary arterial hypertension and its role in right ventricular hypertrophy by targeting SMURF1. *Cardiovasc. Res.* 114, 53–64. doi: 10.1093/cvr/cvx187
12. Bartel, D. P. (2009). MicroRNAs: target recognition and regulatory functions. *Cell* 136, 215–233. doi: 10.1016/j.cell.2009.01.002
13. Bauters, C., Kumarswamy, R., Holzmann, A., Bretthauer, J., Anker, S. D., Pinet, F., et al. (2013). Circulating miR-133a and miR-423-5p fail as biomarkers for left ventricular remodeling after myocardial infarction. *Int. J. Cardiol.* 168, 1837–1840. doi: 10.1016/j.ijcard.2012.12.074
14. Bayés-Genis, A., Lanfear, D. E., de Ronde, M. W. J., Lupón, J., Leenders, J. J., Liu, Z., et al. (2018). Prognostic value of circulating microRNAs on heart failure–related morbidity and mortality in two large diverse cohorts of general heart failure patients. *Eur. J. Heart Fail.* 20, 67–75. doi: 10.1002/ejhf.984
15. Beaumont, J., López, B., Ravassa, S., Hermida, N., José, G. S., Gallego, I., et

al. (2017). MicroRNA-19b is a potential biomarker of increased myocardial collagen cross-linking in patients with aortic stenosis and heart failure. *Sci. Rep.* 7, 40696. doi: 10.1038/srep40696

16. Beekering, M., Nederstigt, C., Suchiman, H. E. D., Kremer, D., van der Breggen, R., Lakenberg, N., et al. (2010). Genome-wide association study (GWAS)–identified disease risk alleles do not compromise human longevity. *Proc. Natl. Acad. Sci. U. S. A* 107, 18046–18049. doi: 10.1073/pnas.1003540107

17. Beg, F., Wang, R., Saeed, Z., Devaraj, S., Masoor, K., and Nakshatri, H. (2017). Inflammation-associated microRNA changes in circulating exosomes of heart failure patients. *BMC Res. Notes* 10, 751. doi: 10.1186/s13104-017-3090-y

18. Bekkering, S., van den Munckhof, I., Nielen, T., Lamfers, E., Dinarello, C., Rutten, J., et al. (2016). Innate immune cell activation and epigenetic remodeling in symptomatic and asymptomatic atherosclerosis in humans *in vivo*. *Atherosclerosis* 254, 228–236. doi: 10.1016/j.atherosclerosis.2016.10.019

19. Białek, S., Górko, D., Zajkowska, A., Kołtowski, Ł., Grabowski, M., Stachurska, A., et al. (2015). Release kinetics of circulating miRNA-208a in the early phase of myocardial infarction. *Kardiologia Polska* 73, 613–619. doi: 10.5603/KP.a2015.0067

20. Bildirici, A. E., Arslan, S., Özbilüm Şahin, N., Berkan, Ö., Beton, O., and Yilmaz, M. B. (2018). MicroRNA-221/222 expression in atherosclerotic coronary artery plaque versus internal mammarian artery and in peripheral blood samples. *Biomarkers* 23, 670–675. doi: 10.1080/1354750X.2018.1474260 BLUEPRINT Consortium. (2016). Quantitative comparison of DNA methylation assays for biomarker development and clinical applications. *Nat. Biotechnol.* 34, 726–737. doi: 10.1038/nbt.3605

21. Bogdarina, I., Welham, S., King, P. J., Burns, S. P., and Clark, A. J. L. (2007). Epigenetic modification of the renin–angiotensin system in the fetal programming of hypertension. *Circ. Res.* 100, 520–526. doi: 10.1161/01.RES.0000258855.60637.58

22. Bye, A., Røsjø, H., Nauman, J., Silva, G. J. J., Follestad, T., Omland, T., et al. (2016). Circulating microRNAs predict future fatal myocardial infarction in healthy individuals—the HUNT study. *J. Mol. Cell Cardiol.* 97, 162–168. doi: 10.1016/j.yjmcc.2016.05.009

23. Cakmak, H. A., Coskunpinar, E., Ikitimur, B., Barman, H. A., Karadag, B., Tiryakioglu, N. O., et al. (2015). The prognostic value of circulating microRNAs in heart failure: preliminary results from a genome-wide expression study. *J. Cardiovasc. Med. (Hagerstown)* 16, 431–437. doi: 10.2459/JCM.0000000000000233

24. Cao, J., and Yan, Q. (2012). Histone ubiquitination and deubiquitination in transcription, DNA damage response, and cancer. *Front. Oncol.* 2, 26. doi: 10.3389/fonc.2012.00026

25. Charrier, H., Cuvelliez, M., Dubois-Deruy, E., Mulder, P., Richard, V., Bauters, C., et al. (2019). Integrative system biology analyses identify seven microRNAs to predict heart failure. *Noncoding RNA* 5, E22–E30. doi: 10.3390/ncrna5010022

26. Chelbi, S. T., Mondon, F., Jammes, H., Buffat, C., Mignot, T.-M., Tost, J., et al. (2007). Expressional and epigenetic alterations of placental serine protease inhibitors: SERPINA3 is a potential marker of preeclampsia. *Hypertension* 49, 76–83. doi: 10.1161/01.HYP.0000250831.52876.cb

27. Chen, F., Yang, J., Li, Y., and Wang, H. (2018a). Circulating microRNAs as novel biomarkers for heart failure. *Hellenic J. Cardiol.* 59, 209–214. doi: 10.1016/j.hjc.2017.10.002

28. Chen, J., Xu, L., Hu, Q., Yang, S., Zhang, B., and Jiang, H. (2015a). MiR-17-5p as circulating biomarkers for the severity of coronary atherosclerosis in coronary artery disease. *Int. J. Cardiol.* 197, 123–124. doi: 10.1016/j.ijcard.2015.06.037

29. Chen, M.-C., Chang, T.-H., Chang, J.-P., Huang, H.-D., Ho, W.-C., Lin, Y.-S., et al. (2016). Circulating miR-148b-3p and miR-409-3p as biomarkers for heart failure in patients with mitral regurgitation. *Int. J. Cardiol.* 222, 148–154. doi: 10.1016/j.ijcard.2016.07.179

30. Chen, S., Chen, R., Zhang, T., Lin, S., Chen, Z., Zhao, B., et al. (2018b). Relationship of cardiovascular disease risk factors and noncoding RNAs with hypertension: a case-control study. *BMC Cardiovasc. Disord.* 18, 58. doi: 10.1186/s12872-018-0795-3

31. Chen, W., and Li, S. (2017). Circulating microRNA as a novel biomarker for pulmonary arterial hypertension due to congenital heart disease. *Pediatr. Cardiol.* 38, 86–94. doi: 10.1007/s00246-016-1487-3

32. Chen, X., Ba, Y., Ma, L., Cai, X., Yin, Y., Wang, K., et al. (2008). Characterization of microRNAs in serum: a novel class of biomarkers for diagnosis of cancer and other diseases. *Cell Res.* 18, 997–1006. doi: 10.1038/cr.2008.282

33. Chen, X., Zhang, L., Su, T., Li, H., Huang, Q., Wu, D., et al. (2015b). Kinetics of plasma microRNA-499 expression in acute myocardial infarction. *J. Thorac. Dis.* 7, 890–896. doi: 10.3978/j.issn.2072-1439.2014.11.32

34. Cheng, C., Wang, Q., You, W., Chen, M., and Xia, J. (2014). MiRNAs as biomarkers of myocardial infarction: a meta-analysis. *PLoS ONE* 9, e88566. doi: 10.1371/ journal.pone.0088566

35. Cho, H.-M., Lee, H.-A., Kim, H. Y., Han, H. S., and Kim, I. K. (2011). Expression of Na+-K+ -2Cl- cotransporter 1 is epigenetically regulated during postnatal development of hypertension. *Am. J. Hypertens.* 24, 1286–1293. doi: 10.1038/ ajh.2011.136

36. Choi, J.-H., Nam, K.-H., Kim, J., Baek, M. W., Park, J.-E., Park, H.-Y., et al. (2005). Trichostatin A exacerbates atherosclerosis in low density lipoprotein receptor- deficient mice. *Arteriosclerosis, Thrombosis, and Vascular Biol.* 25, 2404–2409. doi: 10.1161/01.ATV.0000184758.07257.88

37. Choi, S. Y., Yun, J., Lee, O. J., Han, H. S., Yeo, M. K., Lee, M. A., et al. (2013). MicroRNA expression profiles in placenta with severe preeclampsia using a PNA-based microarray. *Placenta* 34, 799–804. doi: 10.1016/j.placenta.2013.06.006

38. Cortez-Dias, N., Costa, M. C., Carrilho-Ferreira, P., Silva, D., Jorge, C., Calisto, C., et al. (2016). Circulating miR-122-5p/miR-133b ratio is a specific early prognostic biomarker in acute myocardial infarction. *Circ. J.* 80, 2183–2191. doi: 10.1253/circj.CJ-16-0568

39. Coskunpinar, E., Cakmak, H. A., Kalkan, A. K., Tiryakioglu, N. O., Erturk, M., and Ongen, Z. (2016). Circulating miR-221-3p as a novel marker for early prediction of acute myocardial infarction. *Gene* 591, 90–96. doi: 10.1016/j.gene.2016.06.059

40. Costantino, S., Libby, P., Kishore, R., Tardif, J.-C., El-Osta, A., and Paneni, F. (2018). Epigenetics and precision medicine in cardiovascular patients: from basic concepts to the clinical arena. *Eur. Heart J.* 39, 4150–4158. doi: 10.1093/eurheartj/ehx568

41. D'Alessandra, Y., Devanna, P., Limana, F., Straino, S., Di Carlo, A., Brambilla, P. G., et al. (2010). Circulating microRNAs are new and sensitive biomarkers of myocardial infarction. *Eur. Heart J.* 31, 2765–2773. doi: 10.1093/eurheartj/ehq167

42. Dasgupta, C., Chen, M., Zhang, H., Yang, S., and Zhang, L. (2012). Chronic hypoxia during gestation causes epigenetic repression of the estrogen receptor-α gene in ovine uterine arteries *via* heightened promoter methylation. *Hypertension* 60, 697–704. doi: 10.1161/HYPERTENSIONAHA.112.198242

43. de Gonzalo-Calvo, D., Cediel, G., Bär, C., Núñez, J., Revuelta-Lopez, E., Gavara, J., et al. (2018). Circulating miR-1254 predicts ventricular remodeling in patients with ST-segment-elevation myocardial infarction: a cardiovascular magnetic resonance study. *Sci. Rep.* 8, 15115. doi: 10.1038/s41598-018-33491-y

44. de Gonzalo-Calvo, D., Cenarro, A., Civeira, F., and Llorente-Cortés, V. (2016). microRNA expression profile in human coronary smooth muscle cell–derived microparticles is a source of biomarkers. *Clin. Investig. Arterioscler.* 28, 167–177. doi: 10.1016/j.arteri.2016.05.005

45. de Gonzalo-Calvo, D., Iglesias-Gutiérrez, E., and Llorente-Cortés, V. (2017). Biomarcadores epigenéticos y enfermedad cardiovascular: los microARN circulantes. *Rev. Española Cardiol.* 70, 763–769. doi: 10.1016/j.recesp.2017.02.027

46. De Rosa, S., Eposito, F., Carella, C., Strangio, A., Ammirati, G., Sabatino, J., et al. (2018). Transcoronary concentration gradients of circulating microRNAs in heart failure. *Eur. J. Heart Fail.* 20, 1000–1010. doi: 10.1002/ejhf.1119

47. Deddens, J. C., Vrijsen, K. R., Colijn, J. M., Oerlemans, M. I., Metz, C. H. G., van der Vlist, E. J., et al. (2016). Circulating extracellular vesicles contain miRNAs and are released as early biomarkers for cardiac injury. *J. Cardiovasc Transl.* 9, 291–301. doi: 10.1007/s12265-016-9705-1

48. Devaux, Y., Vausort, M., Goretti, E., Nazarov, P. V., Azuaje, F., Gilson, G., et al. (2012). Use of circulating microRNAs to diagnose acute myocardial infarction. *Clin. Chem.* 58, 559–567. doi: 10.1373/clinchem.2011.173823

49. Devaux, Y., Vausort, M., McCann, G. P., Zangrando, J., Kelly, D., Razvi, N., et al. (2013). MicroRNA-150: a novel marker of left ventricular remodeling after acute myocardial infarction. *Circ. Cardiovasc. Genet.* 6, 290–298. doi: 10.1161/CIRCGENETICS.113.000077

50. Divakaran, V., and Mann, D. L. (2008). The emerging role of microRNAs in cardiac remodeling and heart failure. *Circ. Res.* 103, 1072–1083. doi: 10.1161/CIRCRESAHA.108.183087

51. Dong, Y.-M., Liu, X.-X., Wei, G.-Q., Da, Y.-N., Cha, L., and Ma, C.-S. (2015). Prediction of long-term outcome after acute myocardial infarction using circulating miR-145. *Scand. J. Clin. Lab. Invest.* 75, 85–91. doi: 10.3109/00365513.2014.981855

52. Duarte, J. D., Zineh, I., Burkley, B., Gong, Y., Langaee, T. Y., Turner, S. T., et al. (2012). Effects of genetic variation in H3K79 methylation regulatory genes on clinical blood pressure and blood pressure response to hydrochlorothiazide. *J. Transl. Med.* 10, 56. doi: 10.1186/1479-5876-10-56

53. Dubois-Deruy, E., Cuvelliez, M., Fiedler, J., Charrier, H., Mulder, P., Hebbar,

E., et al. (2017). MicroRNAs regulating superoxide dismutase 2 are new circulating biomarkers of heart failure. *Sci. Rep.* 7, 14747. doi: 10.1038/s41598-017-15011-6 Eitel, I., Adams, V., Dieterich, P., Fuernau, G., de Waha, S., Desch, S., et al. (2012). Relation of circulating MicroRNA-133a concentrations with myocardial damage and clinical prognosis in ST-elevation myocardial infarction. *Am. Heart J.* 164, 706–714. doi: 10.1016/j.ahj.2012.08.004

54. Ek, W. E., Hedman, Å. K., Enroth, S., Morris, A. P., Lindgren, C. M., Mahajan, A., et al. (2016). Genome-wide DNA methylation study identifies genes associated with the cardiovascular biomarker GDF-15. *Hum. Mol. Genet.* 25, 817–827. doi: 10.1093/hmg/ddv511

55. Ellis, K. L., Cameron, V. A., Troughton, R. W., Frampton, C. M., Ellmers, L. J., and Richards, A. M. (2013). Circulating microRNAs as candidate markers to distinguish heart failure in breathless patients. *Eur. J. Heart Fail.* 15, 1138–1147. doi: 10.1093/eurjhf/hft078

56. Endo, K., Naito, Y., Ji, X., Nakanishi, M., Noguchi, T., Goto, Y., et al. (2013). MicroRNA 210 as a biomarker for congestive heart failure. *Biol. Pharm. Bull.* 36, 48–54. doi: 10.1248/bpb.b12-00578

57. Engelhardt, S. (2012). Small RNA biomarkers come of age. *J. Am. Coll. Cardiol.* 60, 300–303. doi: 10.1016/j.jacc.2012.04.018

58. Eryılmaz, U., Akgullu, C., Beser, N., Yıldız, Ö., Kurt Ömürlü, İ., and Bozdogan, B. (2016). Circulating microRNAs in patients with ST-elevation myocardial infarction. *Anatol. JCardiol* 16, 392–396. doi: 10.5152/AnatolJCardiol.2015.6603 Evans, S., and Mann, D. L. (2013). Circulating p53-responsive microRNAs as predictive biomarkers in heart failure after acute myocardial infarction: the long and arduous road from scientific discovery to clinical utility. *Circ. Res.* 113, 242–244. doi: 10.1161/CIRCRESAHA.113.301951

59. Fagard, R. H. (2006). Exercise is good for your blood pressure: effects of endurance training and resistance training. *Clin. Exp. Pharmacol. Physiol.* 33, 853–856. doi: 10.1111/j.1440-1681.2006.04453.x

60. Fan, R., Mao, S.-Q., Gu, T.-L., Zhong, F.-D., Gong, M.-L., Hao, L.-M., et al. (2017).

61. Preliminary analysis of the association between methylation of the ACE2 promoter and essential hypertension. *Mol. Med. Rep.* 15, 3905–3911. doi: 10.3892/mmr.2017.6460

62. FDA-NIH Biomarker Working Group. (2016). BEST (Biomarkers, EndpointS, and other Tools) Resource.

63. Feng, G., Yan, Z., Li, C., and Hou, Y. (2016). microRNA-208a in an early stage myocardial infarction rat model and the effect on cAMP-PKA signaling pathway. *Mol. Med. Rep.* 14, 1631–1635. doi: 10.3892/mmr.2016.5402

64. Findeisen, H. M., Gizard, F., Zhao, Y., Qing, H., Heywood, E. B., Jones, K. L., et al. (2011). Epigenetic regulation of vascular smooth muscle cell proliferation and neointima formation by histone deacetylase inhibition. *Arteriosclerosis, Thrombosis, and Vascular Biol.* 31, 851–860. doi: 10.1161/ATVBAHA.110.221952

65. Fiorito, G., Guarrera, S., Valle, C., Ricceri, F., Russo, A., Grioni, S., et al. (2014). B-vitamins intake, DNA-methylation of one carbon metabolism and homocysteine pathway genes and myocardial infarction risk: the EPICOR study. *Nutr. Metab. Cardiovasc. Dis.* 24, 483–488. doi: 10.1016/j.numecd.2013.10.026 Fraga, M. F., Ballestar, E., Paz, M. F., Ropero, S., Setien, F., Ballestar, M. L., et al. (2005). Epigenetic differences arise during the lifetime of monozygotic twins. *Proc. Natl. Acad. Sci. U. S. A* 102, 10604–10609. doi: 10.1073/pnas.0500398102

66. Franceschini, N., and Le, T. H. (2014). Genetics of hypertension: discoveries from the bench to human populations. *Am. J. Physiol. Renal Physiol.* 306, F1–F11. doi: 10.1152/ajprenal.00334.2013

67. Friso, S., Pizzolo, F., Choi, S.-W., Guarini, P., Castagna, A., Ravagnani, V., et al. (2008). Epigenetic control of 11 beta-hydroxysteroid dehydrogenase 2 gene promoter is related to human hypertension. *Atherosclerosis* 199, 323–327. doi: 10.1016/j.atherosclerosis.2007.11.029

68. Gao, J., Yang, S., Wang, K., Zhong, Q., Ma, A., and Pan, X. (2019). Plasma miR-126 and miR-143 as potential novel biomarkers for cerebral atherosclerosis. *J. Stroke Cerebrovasc. Dis.* 28, 38–43. doi: 10.1016/j.jstrokecerebrovasdis.2018.09.008

69. García-Giménez, J. L., Mena-Mollá, S., Beltrán-García, J., and Sanchis-Gomar, F. (2017). Challenges in the analysis of epigenetic biomarkers in clinical samples. *Clin. Chem. Lab. Med.* 55, 1474–1477. doi: 10.1515/cclm-2016-1162

70. Gholikhani-Darbroud, R., Khaki-Khatibi, F., Mansouri, F., Hajahmadipoorrafsanjani, M., and Ghojazadeh, M. (2017). Decreased circulatory microRNA-4478 as a specific biomarker for diagnosing nonn-ST-segment elevation myocardial infarction (NSTEMI) and its association with soluble leptin receptor. *Bratisl. Lek. Listy* 118, 684–690. doi: 10.4149/BLL_2017_129

71. Glezeva, N., Moran, B., Collier, P., Moravec, C. S., Phelan, D., Donnellan, E.,

et al. (2019). Targeted DNA methylation profiling of human cardiac tissue reveals novel epigenetic traits and gene deregulation across different heart failure patient subtypes. *Circ. Heart Fail.* 12, e005765. doi: 10.1161/CIRCHEARTFAILURE.118.005765

72. Goldbergova, M. P., Lipkova, J., Fedorko, J., Sevcikova, J., Parenica, J., Spinar, J., et al. (2018). MicroRNAs in pathophysiology of acute myocardial infarction and cardiogenic shock. *Bratisl. Lek. Listy* 119, 341–347. doi: 10.4149/BLL_2018_064

73. Goldraich, L. A., Martinelli, N. C., Matte, U., Cohen, C., Andrades, M., Pimentel, M., et al. (2014). Transcoronary gradient of plasma microRNA 423-5p in heart failure: evidence of altered myocardial expression. *Biomarkers* 19, 135–141. doi: 10.3109/1354750X.2013.870605

74. Gorski, P. A., Jang, S. P., Jeong, D., Lee, A., Lee, P., Oh, J. G., et al. (2019). Role of SIRT1 in modulating acetylation of the sarco-endoplasmic reticulum Ca^{2+}-ATPase in heart failure. *Circ. Res.* 124, e63–e80. doi: 10.1161/CIRCRESAHA.118.313865

75. Goyal, R., Goyal, D., Leitzke, A., Gheorghe, C. P., and Longo, L. D. (2010). Brain renin–angiotensin system: fetal epigenetic programming by maternal protein restriction during pregnancy. *Reprod. Sci.* 17, 227–238. doi: 10.1177/1933719109351935

76. Grabmaier, U., Clauss, S., Gross, L., Klier, I., Franz, W. M., Steinbeck, G., et al. (2017). Diagnostic and prognostic value of miR-1 and miR-29b on adverse ventricular remodeling after acute myocardial infarction—the SITAGRAMI-miR analysis. *Int. J. Cardiol.* 244, 30–36. doi: 10.1016/j.ijcard.2017.06.054

77. Greißel, A., Culmes, M., Burgkart, R., Zimmermann, A., Eckstein, H.-H., Zernecke, A., et al. (2016). Histone acetylation and methylation significantly change with severity of atherosclerosis in human carotid plaques. *Cardiovasc. Pathol.* 25, 79–86. doi: 10.1016/j.carpath.2015.11.001

78. Guarrera, S., Fiorito, G., Onland-Moret, N. C., Russo, A., Agnoli, C., Allione, A., et al. (2015). Gene-specific DNA methylation profiles and LINE-1 hypomethylation are associated with myocardial infarction risk. *Clin. Epigenet.* 7, 133. doi: 10.1186/s13148-015-0164-3

79. Gunel, T., Hosseini, M. K., Gumusoglu, E., Kisakesen, H. I., Benian, A., and Aydinli, K. (2017). Expression profiling of maternal plasma and placenta microRNAs in preeclamptic pregnancies by microarray technology. *Placenta* 52, 77–85. doi: 10.1016/j.placenta.2017.02.019

80. Guo, M., Luo, J., Zhao, J., Shang, D., Lv, Q., and Zang, P. (2018). Combined use of circulating miR-133a and NT-proBNP improves heart failure diagnostic accuracy in elderly patients. *Med. Sci. Monit.* 24, 8840–8848. doi: 10.12659/MSM.911632

81. Guo, M.-L., Guo, L.-L., and Weng, Y.-Q. (2017). Implication of peripheral blood miRNA-124 in predicting acute myocardial infarction. *Eur. Rev. Med. Pharmacol. Sci.* 21, 1054–1059.

82. Haas, J., Frese, K. S., Park, Y. J., Keller, A., Vogel, B., Lindroth, A. M., et al. (2013). Alterations in cardiac DNA methylation in human dilated cardiomyopathy. *EMBO Mol. Med.* 5, 413–429. doi: 10.1002/emmm.201201553

83. Han, L., Zhao, Y., Luo, Q. Q., Liu, X. X., Lu, S. S., and Zou, L. (2017). The significance of miR-145 in the prediction of preeclampsia. *Bratisl. Lek. Listy* 118, 523–528. doi: 10.4149/BLL_2017_101

84. Han, Z., Zhang, L., Yuan, L., Liu, X., Chen, X., Ye, X., et al. (2015). Change of plasma microRNA-208 level in acute myocardial infarction patients and its clinical significance. *Ann. Transl. Med.* 3, 307. doi: 10.3978/j.issn.2305-5839.2015.10.25

85. Hao, X.-Z., and Fan, H.-M. (2017). Identifiation of miRNAs as atherosclerosis biomarkers and functional role of miR-126 in atherosclerosis progression through MAPK signalling pathway. *Eur. Rev. Med. Pharmacol. Sci.* 21, 2725–2733. He, F., Lv, P., Zhao, X., Wang, X., Ma, X., Meng, W., et al. (2014). Predictive value of circulating miR-328 and miR-134 for acute myocardial infarction. *Mol. Cell Biochem* 394, 137–144. doi: 10.1007/s11010-014-2089-0

86. He, X., Ji, J., Wang, T., Wang, M.-B., and Chen, X.-L. (2017). Upregulation of circulating miR-195-3p in heart failure. *Cardiology* 138, 107–114. doi: 10.1159/000476029

87. Hindson, C. M., Chevillet, J. R., Briggs, H. A., Gallichotte, E. N., Ruf, I. K., Hindson, B. J., et al. (2013). Absolute quantification by droplet digital PCR versus analog real-time PCR. *Nat. Methods* 10, 1003–1005. doi: 10.1038/nmeth.2633

88. Hoareau-Aveilla, C., and Meggetto, F. (2017). Crosstalk between microRNA and DNA methylation offers potential biomarkers and targeted therapies in ALK-positive lymphomas. *Cancers (Basel)* 9, E100–E114. doi: 10.3390/cancers9080100

89. Hohl, M., Wagner, M., Reil, J.-C., Müller, S.-A., Tauchnitz, M., Zimmer, A. M., et al. (2013). HDAC4 controls histone methylation in response to elevated cardiac load. *J. Clin. Invest.* 123, 1359–1370. doi: 10.1172/JCI61084

90. Hromadnikova, I., Kotlabova, K., Ondrackova, M., Pirkova, P., Kestlerova, A., Novotna, V., et al. (2015). Expression profile of C19MC microRNAs in placental tissue in pregnancy-related complications. *DNA Cell Biol.* 34, 437–457. doi: 10.1089/dna.2014.2687

91. Hsu, A., Chen, S.-J., Chang, Y.-S., Chen, H.-C., and Chu, P.-H. (2014). Systemic approach to identify serum microRNAs as potential biomarkers for acute myocardial infarction. *Biomed. Res. Int.* 2014, 418628–418613. doi: 10.1155/2014/418628

92. Huang, L., Li, L., Chen, X., Zhang, H., and Shi, Z. (2016a). MiR-103a targeting Piezo1 is involved in acute myocardial infarction through regulating endothelium function. *Cardiol. J.* 23, 556–562. doi: 10.5603/CJ.a2016.0056

93. Huang, Y., Chen, J., Zhou, Y., Yu, X., Huang, C., Li, J., et al. (2016b). Circulating miR-30 is related to carotid artery atherosclerosis. *Clin. Exp. Hypertens.* 38, 489–494. doi: 10.3109/10641963.2016.1163370

94. Huang, Y., Tang, S., Ji-yan, C., Huang, C., Li, J., Cai, A.-P., et al. (2017a). Circulating miR-92a expression level in patients with essential hypertension: a potential marker of atherosclerosis. *J. Hum. Hypertens.* 31, 200–205. doi: 10.1038/jhh.2016.66

95. Huang, Y.-Q., Huang, C., Chen, J.-Y., Li, J., and Feng, Y.-Q. (2017b). Plasma expression level of miRNA let-7 is positively correlated with carotid intima-media thickness in patients with essential hypertension. *J. Hum. Hypertens.* 31, 843–847. doi: 10.1038/jhh.2017.52

96. Huang, Y.-Q., Li, J., Huang, C., and Feng, Y.-Q. (2018). Plasma microRNA-29c levels are associated with carotid intima-media thickness and is a potential biomarker for the early detection of atherosclerosis. *Cell. Physiol. Biochem.* 50, 452–459. doi: 10.1159/000494158

97. Huo, K.-G., Richer, C., Berillo, O., Mahjoub, N., Fraulob-Aquino, J. C., Barhoumi, T., et al. (2019). miR-431-5p knockdown protects against angiotensin II–induced hypertension and vascular injury. *Hypertension* 73, 1007–1017. doi: 10.1161/ HYPERTENSIONAHA.119.12619

98. Iorio, M. V., Piovan, C., and Croce, C. M. (2010). Interplay between microRNAs and the epigenetic machinery: an intricate network. *Biochim. Biophys. Acta* 1799, 694–701. doi: 10.1016/j.bbagrm.2010.05.005

99. Irmak, M. K., and Sizlan, A. (2006). Essential hypertension seems to result from melatonin-induced epigenetic modifications in area postrema. *Med. Hypotheses* 66, 1000–1007. doi: 10.1016/j.mehy.2005.10.016

100. Jaenisch, R., and Bird, A. (2003). Epigenetic regulation of gene expression: how the genome integrates intrinsic and environmental signals. *Nat. Genet.* 33 Suppl, 245–254. doi: 10.1038/ng1089

101. Jaffe, A. S., Babuin, L., and Apple, F. S. (2006). Biomarkers in acute cardiac disease: the present and the future. *J. Am. Coll. Cardiol.* 48, 1–11. doi: 10.1016/j. jacc.2006.02.056

102. Jairajpuri, D. S., Malalla, Z. H., Mahmood, N., and Almawi, W. Y. (2017). Circulating microRNA expression as predictor of preeclampsia and its severity. *Gene* 627, 543–548. doi: 10.1016/j.gene.2017.07.010

103. Jeong, H. S., Kim, J.-Y., Lee, S. H., Hwang, J., Shin, J. W., Song, K. S., et al. (2017). Synergy of circulating miR-212 with markers for cardiovascular risks to enhance estimation of atherosclerosis presence. *PLoS One* 12, e0177809. doi: 10.1371/journal.pone.0177809

104. Ji, X., Takahashi, R., Hiura, Y., Hirokawa, G., Fukushima, Y., and Iwai, N. (2009). Plasma miR-208 as a biomarker of myocardial injury. *Clin. Chem.* 55, 1944–1949. doi: 10.1373/clinchem.2009.125310

105. Jia, K., Shi, P., Han, X., Chen, T., Tang, H., and Wang, J. (2016). Diagnostic value of miR-30d-5p and miR-125b-5p in acute myocardial infarction. *Mol. Med. Rep.* 14, 184–194. doi: 10.3892/mmr.2016.5246

106. Jiang, D., Sun, M., You, L., Lu, K., Gao, L., Hu, C., et al. (2019). DNA methylation and hydroxymethylation are associated with the degree of coronary atherosclerosis in elderly patients with coronary heart disease. *Life Sci.* 224, 241–248. doi: 10.1016/j.lfs.2019.03.021

107. Jiang, F., Li, J., Wu, G., Miao, Z., Lu, L., Ren, G., et al. (2015). Upregulation of microRNA-335 and microRNA-584 contributes to the pathogenesis of severe preeclampsia through downregulation of endothelial nitric oxide synthase. *Mol. Med. Rep.* 12, 5383–5390. doi: 10.3892/mmr.2015.4018

108. Jiang, Y.-Z., Jiménez, J. M., Ou, K., McCormick, M. E., Zhang, L.-D., and Davies, P. F. (2014). Hemodynamic disturbed flow induces differential DNA methylation of endothelial Kruppel-like factor 4 promoter *in vitro* and *in vivo*. *Circ. Res.* 115, 32–43. doi: 10.1161/CIRCRESAHA.115.303883

109. Jiang, Y.-Z., Manduchi, E., Stoeckert, C. J., and Davies, P. F. (2015). Arterial endothelial methylome: differential DNA methylation in athero-susceptible disturbed flow regions *in vivo*. *BMC Genomics* 16, 506. doi: 10.1186/ s12864-015-1656-4

110. Jin, P., Gu, W., Lai, Y., Zheng, W., Zhou, Q., and Wu, X. (2017). The circulating microRNA-206 level predicts the severity of pulmonary hypertension in patients with left heart diseases. *Cell. Physiol. Biochem.* 41, 2150–2160. doi: 10.1159/000475569 Jo, B.-S., Koh, I.-U., Bae, J.-B., Yu, H.-Y., Jeon, E.-S., Lee, H.-Y., et al. (2016).

111. Methylome analysis reveals alterations in DNA methylation in the regulatory regions of left ventricle development genes in human dilated cardiomyopathy. *Genomics* 108, 84–92. doi: 10.1016/j.ygeno.2016.07.001

112. Kanuri, S. H., Ipe, J., Kassab, K., Gao, H., Liu, Y., Skaar, T. C., et al. (2018). Next generation MicroRNA sequencing to identify coronary artery disease patients at risk of recurrent myocardial infarction. *Atherosclerosis* 278, 232–239. doi: 10.1016/j.atherosclerosis.2018.09.021

113. Kato, N., Loh, M., Takeuchi, F., Verweij, N., Wang, X., Zhang, W., et al. (2015). Trans-ancestry genome-wide association study identifies 12 genetic loci influencing blood pressure and implicates a role for DNA methylation. *Nat. Genet.* 47, 1282–1293. doi: 10.1038/ng.3405

114. Khatibzadeh, S., Farzadfar, F., Oliver, J., Ezzati, M., and Moran, A. (2013). Worldwide risk factors for heart failure: a systematic review and pooled analysis. *Int. J. Cardiol.* 168, 1186–1194. doi: 10.1016/j.ijcard.2012.11.065

115. Kim, H. J., Kim, S. Y., Lim, J. H., Kwak, D. W., Park, S. Y., and Ryu, H. M. (2015). Quantification and application of potential epigenetic markers in maternal plasma of pregnancies with hypertensive disorders. *IJMS* 16, 29875–29888. doi: 10.3390/ijms161226201

116. Kim, S. H., Kim, G. J., Umemura, T., Lee, S. G., and Cho, K. J. (2017). Aberrant expression of plasma microRNA-33a in an atherosclerosis-risk group. *Mol. Biol. Rep.* 44, 79–88. doi: 10.1007/s11033-016-4082-z

117. Klenke, S., Eul, S., Peters, J., Neumann, T., Adamzik, M., and Frey, U. H. (2018). Circulating miR-192 is a prognostic marker in patients with ischemic cardiomyopathy. *Future Cardiol.* 14, 283–289. doi: 10.2217/fca-2017-0108

118. Knothe, C., Shiratori, H., Resch, E., Ultsch, A., Geisslinger, G., Doehring, A., et al. (2016). Disagreement between two common biomarkers of global DNA methylation. *Clin. Epigenet.* 8, 60–17. doi: 10.1186/s13148-016-0227-0

119. Koczor, C. A., Lee, E. K., Torres, R. A., Boyd, A., Vega, J. D., Uppal, K., et al. (2013). Detection of differentially methylated gene promoters in failing and nonfailing human left ventricle myocardium using computation analysis. *Physiol. Genomics* 45, 597–605. doi: 10.1152/physiolgenomics.00013.2013

120. Kontaraki, J. E., Marketou, M. E., Zacharis, E. A., Parthenakis, F. I., and Vardas, P. E. (2014). MicroRNA-9 and microRNA-126 expression levels in patients with essential hypertension: potential markers of target-organ damage. *J. Am. Soc. Hypertens.* 8, 368–375. doi: 10.1016/j.jash.2014.03.324

121. Kouzarides, T. (2007). Chromatin modifications and their function. *Cell* 128, 693– 705. doi: 10.1016/j.cell.2007.02.005

122. Kozomara, A., and Griffiths-Jones, S. (2011). miRBase: integrating microRNA annotation and deep-sequencing data. *Nucleic Acids Res.* 39, D152–D157. doi: 10.1093/nar/gkq1027

123. Krishnan, R., Mani, P., Sivakumar, P., Gopinath, V., and Sekar, D. (2017). Expression and methylation of circulating microRNA-510 in essential hypertension. *Hypertens. Res.* 40, 361–363. doi: 10.1038/hr.2016.147

124. Kristensen, L. S., Wojdacz, T. K., Thestrup, B. B., Wiuf, C., Hager, H., and Hansen, L. L. (2009). Quality assessment of DNA derived from up to 30 years old formalin fixed paraffin embedded (FFPE) tissue for PCR-based methylation analysis using SMART-MSP and MS-HRM. *BMC Cancer* 9, 453. doi: 10.1186/1471-2407-9-453

125. Kulkarni, A., Chavan-Gautam, P., Mehendale, S., Yadav, H., and Joshi, S. (2011). Global DNA methylation patterns in placenta and its association with maternal hypertension in pre-eclampsia. *DNA Cell Biol.* 30, 79–84. doi: 10.1089/ dna.2010.1084

126. Kumar, A., Kumar, S., Vikram, A., Hoffman, T. A., Naqvi, A., Lewarchik, C. M., et al. (2013). Histone and DNA methylation–mediated epigenetic downregulation of endothelial Kruppel-like factor 2 by low-density lipoprotein cholesterol. *Arteriosclerosis, Thrombosis, and Vascular Biol.* 33, 1936–1942. doi: 10.1161/ATVBAHA.113.301765

127. Kumarswamy, R., Anker, S. D., and Thum, T. (2010). MicroRNAs as circulating biomarkers for heart failure: questions about MiR-423-5p. *Circ. Res.* 106, e8– author reply e9. doi: 10.1161/CIRCRESAHA.110.220616

128. Kuosmanen, S. M., Hartikainen, J., Hippeläinen, M., Kokki, H., Levonen, A.-L., and Tavi, P. (2015). MicroRNA profiling of pericardial fluid samples from patients with heart failure. *PLoS One* 10, e0119646. doi: 10.1371/journal.pone.0119646

129. Laganà, A. S., Vitale, S. G., Sapia, F., Valenti, G., Corrado, F., Padula, F., et al. (2018). miRNA expression for early diagnosis of preeclampsia onset: hope or hype? *J. Matern. Fetal. Neonatal. Med.* 31, 817–821. doi: 10.1080/14767058.2017.1296426

130. Lai, K.-B., Sanderson, J. E., Izzat, M. B., and Yu, C.-M. (2015). Micro-RNA and mRNA myocardial tissue expression in biopsy specimen from patients

with heart failure. *Int. J. Cardiol.* 199, 79–83. doi: 10.1016/j.ijcard.2015.07.043

131. Lakhani, H. V., Khanal, T., Gabi, A., Yousef, G., Alam, M. B., Sharma, D., et al. (2018). Developing a panel of biomarkers and miRNA in patients with myocardial infarction for early intervention strategies of heart failure in West Virginian population. *PLoS One* 13, e0205329. doi: 10.1371/journal.pone.0205329

132. Lee, H.-A., Baek, I., Seok, Y. M., Yang, E., Cho, H.-M., Lee, D.-Y., et al. (2010). Promoter hypomethylation upregulates Na⁺-K⁺-2Cl⁻ cotransporter 1 in spontaneously hypertensive rats. *Biochem. Biophys. Res. Commun.* 396, 252–257. doi: 10.1016/j.bbrc.2010.04.074

133. Li, B., Feng, Z.-H., Sun, H., Zhao, Z.-H., Yang, S.-B., and Yang, P. (2017a). The blood genome-wide DNA methylation analysis reveals novel epigenetic changes in human heart failure. *Eur. Rev. Med. Pharmacol. Sci.* 21, 1828–1836.

134. Li, G., Song, Y., Li, Y.-D., Jie, L.-J., Wu, W.-Y., Li, J.-Z., et al. (2018a). Circulating miRNA-302 family members as potential biomarkers for the diagnosis of acute heart failure. *Biomark. Med* 12, 871–880. doi: 10.2217/bmm-2018-0132

135. Li, H., Fan, J., Yin, Z., Wang, F., Chen, C., and Wang, D. W. (2016). Identification of cardiac-related circulating microRNA profile in human chronic heart failure. *Oncotarget* 7, 33–45. doi: 10.18632/oncotarget.6631

136. Li, K., Chen, Z., Qin, Y., and Wei, Y. (2018b). MiR-664a-3p expression in patients with obstructive sleep apnea: a potential marker of atherosclerosis. *Medicine (Baltimore)* 97, e9813. doi: 10.1097/MD.0000000000009813

137. Li, L., Li, S., Wu, M., Chi, C., Hu, D., Cui, Y., et al. (2019). Early diagnostic value of circulating microRNAs in patients with suspected acute myocardial infarction. *J. Cell Physiol.* 234, 13649–13658. doi: 10.1002/jcp.28045

138. Li, L.-M., Cai, W.-B., Ye, Q., Liu, J.-M., Li, X., and Liao, X.-X. (2014a). Comparison of plasma microRNA-1 and cardiac troponin T in early diagnosis of patients with acute myocardial infarction. *World. J. Emerg. Med.* 5, 182–186. doi: 10.5847/wjem.j.issn.1920-8642.2014.03.004

139. Li, S., Guo, L. Z., Kim, M. H., Han, J.-Y., and Serebruany, V. (2017b). Platelet microRNA for predicting acute myocardial infarction. *J. Thromb. Thrombolysis* 44, 556–564. doi: 10.1007/s11239-017-1537-6

140. Li, T., Cao, H., Zhuang, J., Wan, J., Guan, M., Yu, B., et al. (2011). Identification of miR-130a, miR-27b and miR-210 as serum biomarkers for atherosclerosis obliterans. *Clin. Chim. Acta* 412, 66–70. doi: 10.1016/j.cca.2010.09.029

141. Li, Y., Du, W., Zhao, R., Hu, J., Li, H., Han, R., et al. (2017c). New insights into epigenetic modifications in heart failure. *Front. Biosci. (Landmark Ed)* 22, 230–247. doi: 10.2741/4483

142. Li, Y.-Q., Zhang, M.-F., Wen, H.-Y., Hu, C.-L., Liu, R., Wei, H.-Y., et al. (2013). Comparing the diagnostic values of circulating microRNAs and cardiac troponin T in patients with acute myocardial infarction. *Clinics (Sao Paulo)* 68, 75–80. doi: 10.6061/clinics/2013(01)OA12

143. Li, Z., Lu, J., Luo, Y., Li, S., and Chen, M. (2014b). High association between human circulating microRNA-497 and acute myocardial infarction. *Sci. World J.* 2014, 931845–931847. doi: 10.1155/2014/931845

144. Liang, J., Bai, S., Su, L., Li, C., Wu, J., Xia, Z., et al. (2015). A subset of circulating microRNAs is expressed differently in patients with myocardial infarction. *Mol. Med. Rep.* 12, 243–247. doi: 10.3892/mmr.2015.3422

145. Lin, X., Zhang, S., and Huo, Z. (2019). Serum circulating miR-150 is a predictor of post-acute myocardial infarction heart failure. *Int. Heart J.* 60, 280–286. doi: 10.1536/ihj.18-306

146. Liu, G., Niu, X., Meng, X., and Zhang, Z. (2018a). Sensitive miRNA markers for the detection and management of NSTEMI acute myocardial infarction patients. *J. Thorac. Dis.* 10, 3206–3215. doi: 10.21037/jtd.2018.05.141

147. Liu, W., Zheng, J., Dong, J., Bai, R., Song, D., Ma, X., et al. (2018b). Association of miR-197-5p, a circulating biomarker for heart failure, with myocardial fibrosis and adverse cardiovascular events among patients with stage C or D heart failure. *Cardiology* 141, 212–225. doi: 10.1159/000493419

148. Liu, X., Dong, Y., Chen, S., Zhang, G., Zhang, M., Gong, Y., et al. (2015a). Circulating microRNA-146a and microRNA-21 predict left ventricular remodeling after ST-elevation myocardial infarction. *Cardiology* 132, 233–241. doi: 10.1159/000437090

149. Liu, X., Fan, Z., Zhao, T., Cao, W., Zhang, L., Li, H., et al. (2015b). Plasma miR-1, miR-208, miR-499 as potential predictive biomarkers for acute myocardial infarction: an independent study of Han population. *Exp. Gerontol.* 72, 230–238. doi: 10.1016/j.exger.2015.10.011

150. Liu, X., Meng, H., Jiang, C., Yang, S., Cui, F., and Yang, P. (2016). Differential microRNA Expression and regulation in the rat model of post-infarction heart failure. *PLoS One* 11, e0160920. doi: 10.1371/journal.pone.0160920

151. Liu, X., Yuan, L., Chen, F., Zhang, L., Chen, X., Yang, C., et al. (2017). Circulating miR-208b: a potentially sensitive and reliable biomarker for the diagnosis and prognosis of acute myocardial infarction. *Clin. Lab.* 63, 101–109. doi: 10.7754/Clin.Lab.2016.160632

152. Liu, Y., Liu, P., Yang, C., Cowley, A. W., and Liang, M. (2014). Base-resolution maps of 5-methylcytosine and 5-hydroxymethylcytosine in Dahl S rats: effect of salt and genomic sequence. *Hypertension* 63, 827–838. doi: 10.1161/HYPERTENSIONAHA.113.02637

153. Long, G., Wang, F., Duan, Q., Chen, F., Yang, S., Gong, W., et al. (2012a). Human circulating microRNA-1 and microRNA-126 as potential novel indicators for acute myocardial infarction. *Int. J. Biol. Sci.* 8, 811–818. doi: 10.7150/ijbs.4439 Long, G., Wang, F., Duan, Q., Yang, S., Chen, F., Gong, W., et al. (2012b). Circulating miR-30a, miR-195 and let-7b associated with acute myocardial infarction. *PLoS One* 7, e50926. doi: 10.1371/journal.pone.0050926

154. Luque, A., Farwati, A., Krupinski, J., and Aran, J. M. (2018). Association between low levels of serum miR-638 and atherosclerotic plaque vulnerability in patients with high-grade carotid stenosis. *J. Neurosurg.* 131, 1–8. doi: 10.3171/2018.2.JNS171899

155. Lv, P., Zhou, M., He, J., Meng, W., Ma, X., Dong, S., et al. (2014). Circulating miR-208b and miR-34a are associated with left ventricular remodeling after acute myocardial infarction. *IJMS* 15, 5774–5788. doi: 10.3390/ijms15045774

156. Ma, S.-C., Zhang, H.-P., Kong, F.-Q., Zhang, H., Yang, C., He, Y.-Y., et al. (2016). Integration of gene expression and DNA methylation profiles provides a molecular subtype for risk assessment in atherosclerosis. *Mol. Med. Rep.* 13, 4791–4799. doi: 10.3892/mmr.2016.5120

157. Maciejak, A., Kiliszek, M., Opolski, G., Segiet, A., Matlak, K., Dobrzycki, S., et al. (2016). miR-22-5p revealed as a potential biomarker involved in the acute phase of myocardial infarction via profiling of circulating microRNAs. *Mol. Med. Rep.* 14, 2867–2875. doi: 10.3892/mmr.2016.5566

158. Maciejak, A., Kostarska-Srokosz, E., Gierlak, W., Dluzniewski, M., Kuch, M., Marchel, M., et al. (2018). Circulating miR-30a-5p as a prognostic biomarker of left ventricular dysfunction after acute myocardial infarction. *Sci. Rep.* 8, 9883. doi: 10.1038/s41598-018-28118-1

159. Magenta, A., Sileno, S., D'Agostino, M., Persiani, F., Beji, S., Paolini, A., et al. (2018). Atherosclerotic plaque instability in carotid arteries: miR-200c as a promising biomarker. *Clin. Sci.* 132, 2423–2436. doi: 10.1042/CS20180684

160. Majchrzak-Celińska, A., Kosicka, K., Paczkowska, J., Główka, F. K., Bręborowicz, G. H., Krzyścin, M., et al. (2017). HSD11B2, RUNX3, and LINE-1 methylation in placental DNA of hypertensive disorders of pregnancy patients. *Reprod. Sci.* 24, 1520–1531. doi: 10.1177/1933719117692043

161. Mao, Z., Wu, F., and Shan, Y. (2018). Identification of key genes and miRNAs associated with carotid atherosclerosis based on mRNA-seq data. *Medicine (Baltimore)* 97, e9832. doi: 10.1097/MD.0000000000009832

162. Marketou, M. E., Kontaraki, J. E., Maragkoudakis, S., Patrianakos, A., Konstantinou, J., Nakou, H., et al. (2018). MicroRNAs in peripheral mononuclear cells as potential biomarkers in hypertensive patients with heart failure with preserved ejection fraction. *Am. J. Hypertens.* 31, 651–657. doi: 10.1093/ajh/hpy035

163. Masson, S., Batkai, S., Beermann, J., Bär, C., Pfanne, A., Thum, S., et al. (2018). Circulating microRNA-132 levels improve risk prediction for heart failure hospitalization in patients with chronic heart failure. *Eur. J. Heart Fail.* 20, 78–85. doi: 10.1002/ejhf.961

164. Matsumoto, S., Sakata, Y., Suna, S., Nakatani, D., Usami, M., Hara, M., et al. (2013). Circulating p53-responsive microRNAs are predictive indicators of heart failure after acute myocardial infarction. *Circ. Res.* 113, 322–326. doi: 10.1161/CIRCRESAHA.113.301209

165. Meder, B., Haas, J., Sedaghat-Hamedani, F., Kayvanpour, E., Frese, K., Lai, A., et al. (2017). Epigenome-wide association study identifies cardiac gene patterning and a novel class of biomarkers for heart failure. *Circulation* 136, 1528–1544. doi: 10.1161/CIRCULATIONAHA.117.027355

166. Mei, Z., Huang, B., Mo, Y., and Fan, J. (2017). An exploratory study into the role of miR-204-5p in pregnancy-induced hypertension. *Exp Ther Med* 13, 1711–1718. doi: 10.3892/etm.2017.4212

167. Miyamoto, S., Kawamura, T., Morimoto, T., Ono, K., Wada, H., Kawase, Y., et al. (2006). Histone acetyltransferase activity of p300 is required for the promotion of left ventricular remodeling after myocardial infarction in adult mice in vivo. *Circulation* 113, 679–690. doi: 10.1161/CIRCULATIONAHA.105.585182

168. Moutinho, C., and Esteller, M. (2017). MicroRNAs and epigenetics. *Adv. Cancer Res.* 135, 189–220. doi: 10.1016/bs.acr.2017.06.003

169. Movassagh, M., Choy, M.-K., Knowles, D. A., Cordeddu, L., Haider, S., Down, T., et al. (2011). Distinct epigenomic features in end-stage failing human hearts. *Circulation* 124, 2411–2422. doi: 10.1161/CIRCULATIONAHA.111.040071

170. Mu, S., Shimosawa, T., Ogura, S., Wang, H., Uetake, Y., Kawakami-Mori, F., et al. (2011). Epigenetic modulation of the renal β-adrenergic-WNK4 pathway in salt-sensitive hypertension. *Nat. Med.* 17, 573–580. doi: 10.1038/nm.2337

171. Nagata, S., Marunouchi, T., and Tanonaka, K. (2019). Histone deacetylase inhibitor SAHA treatment prevents the development of heart failure after myocardial infarction *via an* induction of heat-shock proteins in rats. *Biol. Pharm. Bull.* 42, 453–461. doi: 10.1248/bpb.b18-00785

172. Nakatochi, M., Ichihara, S., Yamamoto, K., Naruse, K., Yokota, S., Asano, H., et al. (2017). Epigenome-wide association of myocardial infarction with DNA methylation sites at loci related to cardiovascular disease. *Clin. Epigenet.* 9, 54. doi: 10.1186/s13148-017-0353-3

173. Nishiguchi, T., Imanishi, T., and Akasaka, T. (2015). MicroRNAs and cardiovascular diseases. *Biomed. Res. Int.* 2015, 682857. doi: 10.1155/2015/682857

174. Noack, F., Ribbat-Idel, J., Thorns, C., Chiriac, A., Axt-Fliedner, R., Diedrich, K., et al. (2011). miRNA expression profiling in formalin-fixed and paraffin-embedded placental tissue samples from pregnancies with severe preeclampsia. *J. Perinat. Med.* 39, 267–271. doi: 10.1515/jpm.2011.012

175. Nuyt, A. M., and Alexander, B. T. (2009). Developmental programming and hypertension. *Curr. Opin. Nephrol. Hypertens.* 18, 144–152. doi: 10.1097/MNH.0b013e328326092c

176. O'Sullivan, J. F., Neylon, A., McGorrian, C., and Blake, G. J. (2016). miRNA-93-5p and other miRNAs as predictors of coronary artery disease and STEMI. *Int. J. Cardiol.* 224, 310–316. doi: 10.1016/j.ijcard.2016.09.016

177. Olivieri, F., Antonicelli, R., Lorenzi, M., D'Alessandra, Y., Lazzarini, R., Santini, G., et al. (2013). Diagnostic potential of circulating miR-499-5p in elderly patients with acute non ST-elevation myocardial infarction. *Int. J. Cardiol.* 167, 531–536. doi: 10.1016/j.ijcard.2012.01.075

178. Ovchinnikova, E. S., Schmitter, D., Vegter, E. L., ter, J. M., Valente, M. A. E., Liu, L. C. Y., et al. (2016). Signature of circulating microRNAs in patients with acute heart failure. *Eur. J. Heart Fail.* 18, 414–423. doi: 10.1002/ejhf.332

179. Panico, C., and Condorelli, G. (2018). microRNA-132: a new biomarker of heart failure at last? *Eur. J. Heart Fail.* 20, 86–88. doi: 10.1002/ejhf.1044

180. Parahuleva, M. S., Euler, G., Mardini, A., Parviz, B., Schieffer, B., Schulz, R., et al. (2017). Identification of microRNAs as potential cellular monocytic biomarkers in the early phase of myocardial infarction: a pilot study. *Sci. Rep.* 7, 15974. doi: 10.1038/s41598-017-16263-y

181. Parthenakis, F., Marketou, M., Kontaraki, J., Patrianakos, A., Nakou, H., Touloupaki, M., et al. (2017). Low levels of microRNA-21 are a marker of reduced arterial stiffness in well-controlled hypertension. *J. Clin. Hypertens. (Greenwich)* 19, 235–240. doi: 10.1111/jch.12900

182. Peng, L., Chun-guang, Q., Bei-fang, L., Xue-zhi, D., Zi-hao, W., Yun-fu, L., et al. (2014). Clinical impact of circulating miR-133, miR-1291 and miR-663b in plasma of patients with acute myocardial infarction. *Diagn. Pathol.* 9, 89. doi: 10.1186/1746-1596-9-89

183. Pereira-da-Silva, T., Coutinho Cruz, M., Carrusca, C., Cruz Ferreira, R., Napoleão, P., and Mota Carmo, M. (2018). Circulating microRNA profiles in different arterial territories of stable atherosclerotic disease: a systematic review. *Am J Cardiovasc Dis* 8, 1–13.

184. Pojoga, L. H., Williams, J. S., Yao, T. M., Kumar, A., Raffetto, J. D., do Nascimento, G. R. A., et al. (2011). Histone demethylase LSD1 deficiency during high-salt diet is associated with enhanced vascular contraction, altered NO-cGMP relaxation pathway, and hypertension. *AJP: Heart Circ. Physiol.* 301, H1862–H1871. doi: 10.1152/ajpheart.00513.2011

185. Qipshidze Kelm, N., Piell, K. M., Wang, E., and Cole, M. P. (2018). MicroRNAs as predictive biomarkers for myocardial injury in aged mice following myocardial infarction. *J. Cell Physiol.* 233, 5214–5221. doi: 10.1002/jcp.26283

186. Qiu, X.-K., and Ma, J. (2018). Alteration in microRNA-155 level correspond to severity of coronary heart disease. *Scand. J. Clin. Lab. Invest.* 78, 219–223. doi: 10.1080/00365513.2018.1435904

187. Rask-Andersen, M., Martinsson, D., Ahsan, M., Enroth, S., Ek, W. E., Gyllensten, U., et al. (2016). Epigenome-wide association study reveals differential DNA methylation in individuals with a history of myocardial infarction. *Hum. Mol. Genet.* 25, 4739–4748. doi: 10.1093/hmg/ddw302

188. Rau, C. D., and Vondriska, T. M. (2017). DNA methylation and human heart failure: mechanisms or prognostics. *Circulation* 136, 1545–1547. doi: 10.1161/CIRCULATIONAHA.117.029840

189. Reed, G. W., Rossi, J. E., and Cannon, C. P. (2017). Acute myocardial infarction. *Lancet* 389, 197–210. doi: 10.1016/S0140-6736(16)30677-8

190. Rezaei, M., Eskandari, F., Mohammadpour-Gharehbagh, A., Harati-Sadegh, M., Teimoori, B., and Salimi, S. (2018). Hypomethylation of the miRNA-34a gene promoter is associated with severe preeclampsia. *Clin. Exp. Hypertens.* 41, 1–5. doi: 10.1080/10641963.2018.1451534

191. Rivière, G., Lienhard, D., Andrieu, T., Vieau, D., Frey, B. M., and Frey, F. J. (2011). Epigenetic regulation of somatic angiotensin-converting enzyme by DNA methylation and histone acetylation. *Epigenetics* 6, 478–489. doi: 10.4161/ epi.6.4.14961

192. Rockenbach, G., De Melo Neto, A. J., Barcellos, N. T., and Wolff, F. H. (2012). Ethnic differences in viral dominance patterns in patients with hepatitis B virus and hepatitis C virus dual infection. *Hepatology* 55, 1640–author reply 1640. doi: 10.1002/hep.24533

193. Rodriguez-Iturbe, B. (2006). Arteriolar remodeling in essential hypertension: are connective tissue growth factor and transforming growth factor involved? *Kidney Int.* 69, 1104–1105. doi: 10.1038/sj.ki.5000222

194. Rossetto, D., Avvakumov, N., and Côté, J. (2012). Histone phosphorylation: a chromatin modification involved in diverse nuclear events. *Epigenetics* 7, 1098–1108. doi: 10.4161/epi.21975

195. Sabia, C., Picascia, A., Grimaldi, V., Amarelli, C., Maiello, C., and Napoli, C. (2017). The epigenetic promise to improve prognosis of heart failure and heart transplantation. *Transplant. Rev. (Orlando)* 31, 249–256. doi: 10.1016/j. trre.2017.08.004

196. Sano, M., Minamino, T., Toko, H., Miyauchi, H., Orimo, M., Qin, Y., et al. (2007). p53-Induced inhibition of Hif-1 causes cardiac dysfunction during pressure overload. *Nature* 446, 444–448. doi: 10.1038/nature05602

197. Sato, F., Tsuchiya, S., Meltzer, S. J., and Shimizu, K. (2011). MicroRNAs and epigenetics. *FEBS J.* 278, 1598–1609. doi: 10.1111/j.1742-4658.2011.08089.x

198. Schulte, C., Westermann, D., Blankenberg, S., and Zeller, T. (2015). Diagnostic and prognostic value of circulating microRNAs in heart failure with preserved and reduced ejection fraction. *WJC* 7, 843–860. doi: 10.4330/wjc.v7.i12.843

199. Scrutinio, D., Conserva, F., Passantino, A., Iacoviello, M., Lagioia, R., and Gesualdo, L. (2017). Circulating microRNA-150-5p as a novel biomarker for advanced heart failure: a genome-wide prospective study. *J. Heart Lung Transplant.* 36, 616–624. doi: 10.1016/j.healun.2017.02.008

200. Sekar, D., Shilpa, B. R., and Das, A. J. (2017). Relevance of microRNA 21 in different types of hypertension. *Curr. Hypertens. Rep.* 19, 57. doi: 10.1007/ s11906-017-0752-z

201. Seronde, M.-F., Vausort, M., Gayat, E., Goretti, E., Ng, L. L., Squire, I. B., et al. (2015). Circulating microRNAs and outcome in patients with acute heart failure. *PLoS One* 10, e0142237. doi: 10.1371/journal.pone.0142237

202. Shah, R. V., Rong, J., Larson, M. G., Yeri, A., Ziegler, O., Tanriverdi, K., et al. (2018a). Associations of circulating extracellular RNAs with myocardial remodeling and heart failure. *JAMA Cardiol.* 3, 871–876. doi: 10.1001/ jamacardio.2018.2371

203. Shah, R., Ziegler, O., Yeri, A., Liu, X., Murthy, V., Rabideau, D., et al. (2018b). MicroRNAs associated with reverse left ventricular remodeling in humans identify pathways of heart failure progression. *Circ. Heart Fail.* 11, e004278. doi: 10.1161/CIRCHEARTFAILURE.117.004278

204. Shi, B., Guo, Y., Wang, J., and Gao, W. (2010). Altered expression of microRNAs in the myocardium of rats with acute myocardial infarction. *BMC Cardiovasc. Disord.* 10, 11. doi: 10.1186/1471-2261-10-11

205. Singh, K., Williams, J., Brown, J., Wang, E. T., Lee, B., Gonzalez, T. L., et al. (2017). Up-regulation of microRNA-202-3p in first trimester placenta of pregnancies destined to develop severe preeclampsia, a pilot study. *Pregnancy Hypertens.* 10, 7–9. doi: 10.1016/j.preghy.2017.04.002

206. Small, E. M., and Olson, E. N. (2011). Pervasive roles of microRNAs in cardiovascular biology. *Nature* 469, 336–342. doi: 10.1038/nature09783

207. Smolarek, I., Wyszko, E., Barciszewska, A. M., Nowak, S., Gawronska, I., Jablecka, A., et al. (2010). Global DNA methylation changes in blood of patients with essential hypertension. *Med. Sci. Monit.* 16, CR149–CR155.

208. Strimbu, K., and Tavel, J. A. (2010). What are biomarkers? *Curr. Opin. HIV AIDS* 5, 463–466. doi: 10.1097/COH.0b013e32833ed177

209. Su, M., Wang, J., Wang, C., Wang, X., Dong, W., Qiu, W., et al. (2015). MicroRNA-221 inhibits autophagy and promotes heart failure by modulating the p27/CDK2/ mTOR axis. *Cell Death Differ.* 22, 986–999. doi: 10.1038/ cdd.2014.187

210. Sun, T., Dong, Y.-H., Du, W., Shi, C.-Y., Wang, K., Tariq, M.-A., et al. (2017). The role of MicroRNAs in myocardial infarction: from molecular mechanism to clinical application. *IJMS* 18, 745. doi: 10.3390/ijms18040745

211. Sygitowicz, G., Tomaniak, M., Błaszczyk, O., Kołtowski, Ł., Filipiak, K. J., and Sitkiewicz, D. (2015). Circulating microribonucleic acids miR-1, miR-21 and miR-208a in patients with symptomatic heart failure: preliminary results. *Arch. Cardiovasc. Dis.* 108, 634–642. doi: 10.1016/j.acvd.2015.07.003

212. Talens, R. P., Jukema, J. W., Trompet, S., Kremer, D., Westendorp, R. G. J., Lumey, L. H., et al. (2012). Hypermethylation at loci sensitive to the prenatal environment is associated with increased incidence of myocardial infarction. *Int. J. Epidemiol.* 41, 106–115. doi: 10.1093/ije/dyr153

213. Thomas, H., Diamond, J., Vieco, A., Chaudhuri, S., Shinnar, E., Cromer,

S., et al. (2018). Global atlas of cardiovascular disease 2000–2016: the path to prevention and control. *Glob. Heart* 13, 143–163. doi: 10.1016/j. gheart.2018.09.511

214. Tijsen, A. J., Creemers, E. E., Moerland, P. D., de Windt, L. J., van der Wal, A. C., Kok, W. E., et al. (2010). MiR423-5p as a circulating biomarker for heart failure. *Circ. Res.* 106, 1035–1039. doi: 10.1161/CIRCRESAHA.110.218297

215. Tournier, B., Chapusot, C., Courcet, E., Martin, L., Lepage, C., Faivre, J., et al. (2012). Why do results conflict regarding the prognostic value of the methylation status in colon cancers? The role of the preservation method. *BMC Cancer* 12, 12–12. doi: 10.1186/1471-2407-12-12

216. Ura, B., Feriotto, G., Monasta, L., Bilel, S., Zweyer, M., and Celeghini, C. (2014). Potential role of circulating microRNAs as early markers of preeclampsia. *Taiwan J. Obstet. Gynecol.* 53, 232–234. doi: 10.1016/j.tjog.2014.03.001

217. Valencia-Morales, M. D. P., Zaina, S., Heyn, H., Carmona, F. J., Varol, N., Sayols, S., et al. (2015). The DNA methylation drift of the atherosclerotic aorta increases with lesion progression. *BMC Med. Genomics* 8, 7. doi: 10.1186/s12920-015-0085-1

218. van Boven, N., Akkerhuis, K. M., Anroedh, S. S., Rizopoulos, D., Pinto, Y., Battes, L. C., et al. (2017). Serially measured circulating miR-22-3p is a biomarker for adverse clinical outcome in patients with chronic heart failure: the Bio-SHiFT study. *Int. J. Cardiol.* 235, 124–132. doi: 10.1016/j. ijcard.2017.02.078

219. van Empel, V. P. M., de Windt, L. J., and da Costa Martins, P. A. (2012). Circulating miRNAs: reflecting or affecting cardiovascular disease? *Curr. Hypertens. Rep.* 14, 498–509. doi: 10.1007/s11906-012-0310-7

220. Vegter, E. L., Ovchinnikova, E. S., van Veldhuisen, D. J., Jaarsma, T., Berezikov, E., van der Meer, P., et al. (2017). Low circulating microRNA levels in heart failure patients are associated with atherosclerotic disease and cardiovascular-related rehospitalizations. *Clin. Res. Cardiol.* 106, 598–609. doi: 10.1007/s00392-017-1096-z

221. Vegter, E. L., Schmitter, D., Hagemeijer, Y., Ovchinnikova, E. S., van der Harst, P., Teerlink, J. R., et al. (2016). Use of biomarkers to establish potential role and function of circulating microRNAs in acute heart failure. *Int. J. Cardiol.* 224, 231–239. doi: 10.1016/j.ijcard.2016.09.010

222. Vogel, B., Keller, A., Frese, K. S., Leidinger, P., Sedaghat-Hamedani, F., Kayvanpour, E., et al. (2013). Multivariate miRNA signatures as biomarkers for non-ischaemic systolic heart failure. *Eur. Heart J.* 34, 2812–2822. doi: 10.1093/ eurheartj/eht256

223. Wang, C., Xu, G., Wen, Q., Peng, X., Chen, H., Zhang, J., et al. (2019a). CBS promoter hypermethylation increases the risk of hypertension and stroke. *Clinics (Sao Paulo)* 74, e630. doi: 10.6061/clinics/2019/e630

224. Wang, F., Demura, M., Cheng, Y., Zhu, A., Karashima, S., Yoneda, T., et al. (2014a). Dynamic CCAAT/enhancer binding protein-associated changes of DNA methylation in the angiotensinogen gene. *Hypertension* 63, 281–288. doi: 10.1161/HYPERTENSIONAHA.113.02303

225. Wang, F., Long, G., Zhao, C., Li, H., Chaugai, S., Wang, Y., et al. (2013a). Plasma microRNA-133a is a new marker for both acute myocardial infarction and underlying coronary artery stenosis. *J. Transl. Med.* 11, 222. doi: 10.1186/1479-5876-11-222

226. Wang, F., Long, G., Zhao, C., Li, H., Chaugai, S., Wang, Y., et al. (2014b). Atherosclerosis-related circulating miRNAs as novel and sensitive predictors for acute myocardial infarction. *PLoS One* 9, e105734. doi: 10.1371/journal. pone.0105734

227. Wang, F., Ma, Y., Wang, H., and Qin, H. (2017a). Reciprocal regulation between microRNAs and epigenetic machinery in colorectal cancer. *Oncol Lett.* 13, 1048–1057. doi: 10.3892/ol.2017.5593

228. Wang, H., Naghavi, M., Allen, C., Barber, R. M., Bhutta, Z. A., Carter, A., et al. (2016a). Articles Global, regional, and national life expectancy, all-cause mortality, and cause-specific mortality for 249 causes of death, 1980–2015: a systematic analysis for the Global Burden of Disease Study 2015. *Lancet* 388, 1459–1544. doi: 10.1016/S0140-6736(16)31012-1

229. Wang, K., Zhang, S., Marzolf, B., Troisch, P., Brightman, A., Hu, Z., et al. (2009). Circulating microRNAs, potential biomarkers for drug-induced liver injury. *Proc. Natl. Acad. Sci. U. S. A* 106, 4402–4407. doi: 10.1073/pnas.0813371106

230. Wang, K.-J., Zhao, X., Liu, Y.-Z., Zeng, Q.-T., Mao, X.-B., Li, S.-N., et al. (2016b). Circulating MiR-19b-3p, MiR-134-5p and MiR-186-5p are promising novel biomarkers for early diagnosis of acute myocardial infarction. *Cell. Physiol. Biochem.* 38, 1015–1029. doi: 10.1159/000443053

231. Wang, L., Liu, J., Xu, B., Liu, Y.-L., and Liu, Z. (2018a). Reduced exosome miR-425 and miR-744 in the plasma represents the progression of fibrosis and heart failure. *Kaohsiung J. Med. Sci.* 34, 626–633. doi: 10.1016/j.kjms.2018.05.008

232. Wang, P., Shen, C., Diao, L., Yang, Z., Fan, F., Wang, C., et al. (2015). Aberrant

hypermethylation of aldehyde dehydrogenase 2 promoter upstream sequence in rats with experimental myocardial infarction. *Biomed. Res. Int.* 2015, 503692–503613. doi: 10.1155/2015/503692

233. Wang, X., Falkner, B., Zhu, H., Shi, H., Su, S., Xu, X., et al. (2013b). A genome-wide methylation study on essential hypertension in young African American males. *PLoS One* 8, e53938. doi: 10.1371/journal.pone.0053938

234. Wang, Y., Chang, W., Zhang, Y., Zhang, L., Ding, H., Qi, H., et al. (2019b). Circulating miR-22-5p and miR-122-5p are promising novel biomarkers for diagnosis of acute myocardial infarction. *J. Cell Physiol.* 234, 4778–4786. doi: 10.1002/jcp.27274

235. Wang, Y., Yan, L., Zhang, Z., Prado, E., Fu, L., Xu, X., et al. (2018b). Epigenetic regulation and its therapeutic potential in pulmonary hypertension. *Front. Pharmacol.* 9, 241. doi: 10.3389/fphar.2018.00241

236. Wang, Y.-L., and Yu, W. (2018). Association of circulating microRNA-122 with presence and severity of atherosclerotic lesions. *PeerJ* 6, e5218. doi: 10.7717/peerj.5218

237. Wang, Z.-H., Sun, X.-Y., Li, C.-L., Sun, Y.-M., Li, J., Wang, L.-F., et al. (2017b). miRNA-21 expression in the serum of elderly patients with acute myocardial infarction. *Med. Sci. Monit.* 23, 5728–5734. doi: 10.12659/MSM.904933

238. Ward, J. A., Esa, N., Pidikiti, R., Freedman, J. E., Keaney, J. F., Tanriverdi, K., et al. (2013). Circulating cell and plasma microRNA profiles differ between non-ST-segment and ST-segment-elevation myocardial infarction. *Fam. Med. Med. Sci. Res.* 2, 108. doi: 10.4172/2327-4972.1000108

239. Watson, C. J., Gupta, S. K., O'Connell, E., Thum, S., Glezeva, N., Fendrich, J., et al. (2015). MicroRNA signatures differentiate preserved from reduced ejection fraction heart failure. *Eur. J. Heart Fail.* 17, 405–415. doi: 10.1002/ejhf.244

240. Wei, L., Zhao, S., Wang, G., Zhang, S., Luo, W., Qin, Z., et al. (2018). SMAD7 methylation as a novel marker in atherosclerosis. *Biochem. Biophys. Res. Commun.* 496, 700–705. doi: 10.1016/j.bbrc.2018.01.121

241. Wei, X. J., Han, M., Yang, F. Y., Wei, G. C., Liang, Z. G., Yao, H., et al. (2015). Biological significance of miR-126 expression in atrial fibrillation and heart failure. *Braz. J. Med. Biol. Res.* 48, 983–989. doi: 10.1590/1414-431x20154590

242. Wierda, R. J., Rietveld, I. M., van Eggermond, M. C. J. A., Belien, J. A. M., van Zwet, E. W., Lindeman, J. H. N., et al. (2015). Global histone H3 lysine 27 triple methylation levels are reduced in vessels with advanced atherosclerotic plaques. *Life Sci.* 129, 3–9. doi: 10.1016/j.lfs.2014.10.010

243. Wissler, R. W. (1991). Update on the pathogenesis of atherosclerosis. *Am. J. Med.* 91, 3S–9S. doi: 10.1016/0002-9343(91)90050-8

244. Wong, L. L., Armugam, A., Sepramaniam, S., Karolina, D. S., Lim, K. Y., Lim, J. Y., et al. (2015). Circulating microRNAs in heart failure with reduced and preserved left ventricular ejection fraction. *Eur. J. Heart Fail.* 17, 393–404. doi: 10.1002/ejhf.223

245. Wong, L. L., Rademaker, M. T., Saw, E. L., Lew, K. S., Ellmers, L. J., Charles, C. J., et al. (2017). Identification of novel microRNAs in the sheep heart and their regulation in heart failure. *Sci. Rep.* 7, 8250. doi: 10.1038/s41598-017-08574-x

246. Wong, S. Q., Li, J., Tan, A. Y.-C., Vedururu, R., Pang, J.-M. B., Do, H., et al. (2014). Sequence artefacts in a prospective series of formalin-fixed tumours tested for mutations in hotspot regions by massively parallel sequencing. *BMC Med. Genomics* 7, 23–10. doi: 10.1186/1755-8794-7-23

247. Wu, K., Zhao, Q., Li, Z., Li, N., Xiao, Q., Li, X., et al. (2018a). Bioinformatic screening for key miRNAs and genes associated with myocardial infarction. *FEBS Open Bio.* 8, 897–913. doi: 10.1002/2211-5463.12423

248. Wu, T., Chen, Y., Du, Y., Tao, J., Li, W., Zhou, Z., et al. (2018b). Circulating exosomal miR-92b-5p is a promising diagnostic biomarker of heart failure with reduced ejection fraction patients hospitalized for acute heart failure. *J. Thorac. Dis.* 10, 6211–6220. doi: 10.21037/jtd.2018.10.52

249. Wu, T., Chen, Y., Du, Y., Tao, J., Zhou, Z., and Yang, Z. (2018c). Serum exosomal MiR-92b-5p as a potential biomarker for acute heart failure caused by dilated cardiomyopathy. *Cell. Physiol. Biochem.* 46, 1939–1950. doi: 10.1159/000489383 Xiao, J., Gao, R., Bei, Y., Zhou, Q., Zhou, Y., Zhang, H., et al. (2017). Circulating miR-30d predicts survival in patients with acute heart failure. *Cell. Physiol. Biochem.* 41, 865–874. doi: 10.1159/000459899

250. Xiao, J., Shen, B., Li, J., Lv, D., Zhao, Y., Wang, F., et al. (2014). Serum microRNA-499 and microRNA-208a as biomarkers of acute myocardial infarction. *Int. J. Clin. Exp. Med.* 7, 136–141.

251. Xu, M., Li, J., Chen, X., Han, L., Li, L., and Liu, Y. (2019). MTHFD1 promoter hypermethylation increases the risk of hypertension. *Clin. Exp. Hypertens.* 41, 422–427. doi: 10.1080/10641963.2018.1501057

252. Xu, P., Zhao, Y., Liu, M., Wang, Y., Wang, H., Li, Y.-X., et al. (2014). Variations of microRNAs in human placentas and plasma from preeclamptic pregnancy. *Hypertension* 63, 1276–1284. doi: 10.1161/HYPERTENSIONAHA.113.02647

253. Xu, S., Pelisek, J., and Jin, Z. G. (2018). Atherosclerosis is an epigenetic disease. *Trends Endocrinol. Metab.* 29, 739–742. doi: 10.1016/j.tem.2018.04.007

254. Xue, S., Liu, D., Zhu, W., Su, Z., Zhang, L., Zhou, C., et al. (2019). Circulating MiR- 17-5p, MiR-126-5p and MiR-145-3p are novel biomarkers for diagnosis of acute myocardial infarction. *Front. Physiol.* 10, 123. doi: 10.3389/ fphys.2019.00123

255. Yamada, Y., Nishida, T., Horibe, H., Oguri, M., Kato, K., and Sawabe, M. (2014). Identification of hypo- and hypermethylated genes related to atherosclerosis by a genome-wide analysis of DNA methylation. *Int. J. Mol. Med.* 33, 1355– 1363. doi: 10.3892/ijmm.2014.1692

256. Yan, Y., Song, X., Li, Z., Zhang, J., Ren, J., Wu, J., et al. (2017). Elevated levels of granzyme B correlated with miR-874-3p downregulation in patients with acute myocardial infarction. *Biomark. Med.* 11, 761–767. doi: 10.2217/ bmm-2017-0144

257. Yang, G., Weng, X., Zhao, Y., Zhang, X., Hu, Y., Dai, X., et al. (2017a). The histone H3K9 methyltransferase SUV39H links SIRT1 repression to myocardial infarction. *Nat. Commun.* 8, 14941. doi: 10.1038/ncomms14941

258. Yang, Q., Jia, C., Wang, P., Xiong, M., Cui, J., Li, L., et al. (2014). MicroRNA-505 identified from patients with essential hypertension impairs endothelial cell migration and tube formation. *Int. J. Cardiol.* 177, 925–934. doi: 10.1016/j. ijcard.2014.09.204

259. Yang, Q., Lu, J., Wang, S., Li, H., Ge, Q., and Lu, Z. (2011). Application of next-generation sequencing technology to profile the circulating microRNAs in the serum of preeclampsia versus normal pregnant women. *Clin. Chim. Acta* 412, 2167–2173. doi: 10.1016/j.cca.2011.07.029

260. Yang, S.-Y., Wang, Y.-Q., Gao, H.-M., Wang, B., and He, Q. (2016a). The clinical value of circulating miR-99a in plasma of patients with acute myocardial infarction. *Eur. Rev. Med. Pharmacol. Sci.* 20, 5193–5197.

261. Yang, V. K., Loughran, K. A., Meola, D. M., Juhr, C. M., Thane, K. E., Davis, A. M., et al. (2017b). Circulating exosome microRNA associated with heart failure secondary to myxomatous mitral valve disease in a naturally occurring canine model. *J. Extracell Vesicles* 6, 1350088. doi: 10.1080/20013078.2017.1350088

262. Yang, W., Wang, A., Zhao, C., Li, Q., Pan, Z., Han, X., et al. (2016b). miR-125b enhances IL-8 production in early-onset severe preeclampsia by targeting sphingosine-1-phosphate lyase 1. *PLoS One* 11, e0166940. doi: 10.1371/ journal. pone.0166940

263. Yao, X.-L., Lu, X.-L., Yan, C.-Y., Wan, Q.-L., Cheng, G.-C., and Li, Y.-M. (2015). Circulating miR-122-5p as a potential novel biomarker for diagnosis of acute myocardial infarction. *Int. J. Clin. Exp. Pathol.* 8, 16014–16019.

264. Yilmaz, S. G., Isbir, S., Kunt, A. T., and Isbir, T. (2018). Circulating microRNAs as novel biomarkers for atherosclerosis. *In Vivo* 32, 561–565. doi: 10.21873/ invivo.11276

265. Yuan, L., Liu, X., Chen, F., Zhang, L., Chen, X., Huang, Q., et al. (2016). Diagnostic and prognostic value of circulating microRNA-133a in patients with acute myocardial infarction. *Clin. Lab.* 62, 1233–1241. doi: 10.7754/Clin. Lab.2015.151023

266. Zampetaki, A., Zeng, L., Margariti, A., Xiao, Q., Li, H., Zhang, Z., et al. (2010). Histone deacetylase 3 is critical in endothelial survival and atherosclerosis development in response to disturbed flow. *Circulation* 121, 132–142. doi: 10.1161/CIRCULATIONAHA.109.890491

267. Zhang, C., Li, Q., Ren, N., Li, C., Wang, X., Xie, M., et al. (2015a). Placental miR- 106a~363 cluster is dysregulated in preeclamptic placenta. *Placenta* 36, 250– 252. doi: 10.1016/j.placenta.2014.11.020

268. Zhang, D., Yu, Z.-Y., Cruz, P., Kong, Q., Li, S., and Kone, B. C. (2009). Epigenetics and the control of epithelial sodium channel expression in collecting duct. *Kidney Int.* 75, 260–267. doi: 10.1038/ki.2008.475

269. Zhang, J., Li, Y., and Zhao, Q. (2018a). Circulating miR-23b as a novel biomarker for early risk stratification after ST-elevation myocardial infarction. *Med. Sci. Monit.* 24, 1517–1523. doi: 10.12659/MSM.908060

270. Zhang, J., Xing, Q., Zhou, X., Li, J., Li, Y., Zhang, L., et al. (2017a). Circulating miRNA-21 is a promising biomarker for heart failure. *Mol. Med. Rep.* 16, 7766– 7774. doi: 10.3892/mmr.2017.7575

271. Zhang, L. X., Du, J., Zhao, Y. T., Wang, J., Zhang, S., Dubielecka, P. M., et al. (2018b). Transgenic overexpression of active HDAC4 in the heart attenuates cardiac function and exacerbates remodeling in infarcted myocardium. *J. Appl. Physiol.* 125, 1968–1978. doi: 10.1152/japplphysiol.00006.2018

272. Zhang, L., Chen, X., Su, T., Li, H., Huang, Q., Wu, D., et al. (2015b). Circulating miR-499 are novel and sensitive biomarker of acute myocardial infarction. *J. Thorac. Dis.* 7, 303–308. doi: 10.3978/j.issn.2072-1439.2015.02.05

273. Zhang, L.-N., Liu, P.-P., Wang, L., Yuan, F., Xu, L., Xin, Y., et al. (2013a). Lower ADD1 gene promoter DNA methylation increases the risk of essential hypertension. *PLoS ONE* 8, e63455. doi: 10.1371/journal.pone.0063455

274. Zhang, M., Cheng, Y.-J., Sara, J. D., Liu, L.-J., Liu, L.-P., Zhao, X., et al. (2017b). Circulating microRNA-145 is associated with acute myocardial infarction and heart failure. *Chin. Med. J.* 130, 51–56. doi: 10.4103/0366-6999.196573

275. Zhang, R., Lan, C., Pei, H., Duan, G., Huang, L., and Li, L. (2015c). Expression of circulating miR-486 and miR-150 in patients with acute myocardial infarction. *BMC Cardiovasc. Disord.* 15, 51. doi: 10.1186/s12872-015-0042-0

276. Zhang, R., Niu, H., Ban, T., Xu, L., Li, Y., Wang, N., et al. (2013b). Elevated plasma microRNA-1 predicts heart failure after acute myocardial infarction. *Int. J. Cardiol.* 166, 259–260. doi: 10.1016/j.ijcard.2012.09.108

277. Zhang, W.-Q., and Xie, B.-Q. (2017). A meta-analysis of the relations between blood microRNA-208b detection and acute myocardial infarction. *Eur. Rev. Med. Pharmacol. Sci.* 21, 848–854.

278. Zhang, X., Wang, X., Wu, J., Peng, J., Deng, X., Shen, Y., et al. (2018c). The diagnostic values of circulating miRNAs for hypertension and bioinformatics analysis. *Biosci. Rep.* 38, BSR20180525. doi: 10.1042/ BSR20180525

279. Zhang, Y., Cheng, J., Chen, F., Wu, C., Zhang, J., Ren, X., et al. (2017c). Circulating endothelial microparticles and miR-92a in acute myocardial infarction. *Biosci. Rep.* 37, BSR20170047. doi: 10.1042/BSR20170047

280. Zhang, Y., Liu, Y.-J., Liu, T., Zhang, H., and Yang, S.-J. (2016). Plasma microRNA-21 is a potential diagnostic biomarker of acute myocardial infarction. *Eur. Rev. Med. Pharmacol. Sci.* 20, 323–329.

281. Zhao, D.-S., Chen, Y., Jiang, H., Lu, J.-P., Zhang, G., Geng, J., et al. (2013). Serum miR-210 and miR-30a expressions tend to revert to fetal levels in Chinese adult patients with chronic heart failure. *Cardiovasc. Pathol.* 22, 444– 450. doi: 10.1016/j.carpath.2013.04.001

282. Zhao, L., Chen, C.-N., Hajji, N., Oliver, E., Cotroneo, E., Wharton, J., et al. (2012). Histone deacetylation inhibition in pulmonary hypertension: therapeutic potential of valproic acid and suberoylanilide hydroxamic acid. *Circulation* 126, 455–467. doi: 10.1161/CIRCULATIONAHA.112.103176

283. Zheng, B., Xi, Z., Liu, R., Yin, W., Sui, Z., Ren, B., et al. (2018). The function of microRNAs in B-cell development, lymphoma, and their potential in clinical practice. *Front. Immunol.* 9, 936. doi: 10.3389/fimmu.2018.00936

284. Zhong, J., He, Y., Chen, W., Shui, X., Chen, C., and Lei, W. (2014). Circulating microRNA19a as a potential novel biomarker for diagnosis of acute myocardial infarction. *IJMS* 15, 20355–20364. doi: 10.3390/ijms151120355

285. Zhu, J., Yao, K., Wang, Q., Guo, J., Shi, H., Ma, L., et al. (2016). Circulating miR-181a as a potential novel biomarker for diagnosis of acute myocardial infarction. *Cell. Physiol. Biochem.* 40, 1591–1602. doi: 10.1159/000453209

286. Zhu, L., Liu, F., Xie, H., and Feng, J. (2018). Diagnostic performance of microRNA- 133a in acute myocardial infarction: a meta-analysis. *Cardiol. J.* 25, 260–267. doi: 10.5603/CJ.a2017.0126

287. Zhu, X.-M., Han, T., Sargent, I. L., Yin, G.-W., and Yao, Y.-Q. (2009). Differential expression profile of microRNAs in human placentas from preeclamptic pregnancies vs normal pregnancies. *Am. J. Obstet. Gynecol.* 200, 661.e1–661.e7. doi: 10.1016/j.ajog.2008.12.045

Permissions

The contributors of this book come from diverse backgrounds, making this book a truly international effort. This book will bring forth new frontiers with its revolutionizing research information and detailed analysis of the nascent developments around the world.

We would like to thank all the contributing authors for lending their expertise to make the book truly unique. They have played a crucial role in the development of this book. Without their invaluable contributions this book wouldn't have been possible. They have made vital efforts to compile up to date information on the varied aspects of this subject to make this book a valuable addition to the collection of many professionals and students.

This book was conceptualized with the vision of imparting up-to-date information and advanced data in this field. To ensure the same, a matchless editorial board was set up. Every individual on the board went through rigorous rounds of assessment to prove their worth. After which they invested a large part of their time researching and compiling the most relevant data for our readers.

The editorial board has been involved in producing this book since its inception. They have spent rigorous hours researching and exploring the diverse topics which have resulted in the successful publishing of this book. They have passed on their knowledge of decades through this book. To expedite this challenging task, the publisher supported the team at every step. A small team of assistant editors was also appointed to further simplify the editing procedure and attain best results for the readers.

Apart from the editorial board, the designing team has also invested a significant amount of their time in understanding the subject and creating the most relevant covers. They scrutinized every image to scout for the most suitable representation of the subject and create an appropriate cover for the book.

The publishing team has been an ardent support to the editorial, designing and production team. Their endless efforts to recruit the best for this project, has resulted in the accomplishment of this book. They are a veteran in the field of academics and their pool of knowledge is as vast as their experience in printing. Their expertise and guidance has proved useful at every step. Their uncompromising quality standards have made this book an exceptional effort. Their encouragement from time to time has been an inspiration for everyone.

The publisher and the editorial board hope that this book will prove to be a valuable piece of knowledge for researchers, students, practitioners and scholars across the globe.

List of Contributors

Yi Zhang, Zhihui Zhao, Qing Zhao, Lu Yan, Xin Li, Anqi Duan, Chenhong An, Xiuping Ma, Changming Xiong, Qin Luo and Zhihong Liu
Center for Pulmonary Vascular Diseases, Fuwai Hospital, National Center for Cardiovascular Diseases, Chinese Academy of Medical Sciences and Peking Union Medical College, Beijing, China

Qi Jin
Center for Pulmonary Vascular Diseases, Fuwai Hospital, National Center for Cardiovascular Diseases, Chinese Academy of Medical Sciences and Peking Union Medical College, Beijing, China
Department of Cardiology, Shanghai Institute of Cardiovascular Diseases, Zhongshan Hospital, Fudan University, Shanghai, China

Xue Yu
Center for Pulmonary Vascular Diseases, Fuwai Hospital, National Center for Cardiovascular Diseases, Chinese Academy of Medical Sciences and Peking Union Medical College, Beijing, China
Department of Cardiology, Qingdao Municipal Hospital, Qingdao, China

Jiaquan Chen, Qihong Ni, Xiangjiang Guo, Guanhua Xue and Shuofei Yang
Department of Vascular Surgery, Renji Hospital, School of Medicine, Shanghai Jiaotong University, Shanghai, China

Yongsheng Xiao
Department of Vascular Surgery, Tianjin 4th Centre Hospital, The Fourth Central Hospital Affiliated to Nankai University, The Fourth Center Clinical College of Tianjin Medical University, Tianjin, China

Yuanfeng Du
Department of Neurosurgery, School of Medicine, Affiliated Hangzhou First People's Hospital, Zhejiang University, Hangzhou, China

Xupin Xie
Department of Vascular Surgery, School of Medicine, Affiliated Hangzhou First People's Hospital, Zhejiang University, Hangzhou, China

Guangyao Zhai, Jianlong Wang, Yuyang Liu and Yujie Zhou
Beijing Anzhen Hospital, Capital Medical University, Beijing, China

Rebecca Angoff and Connie W. Tsao
Cardiovascular Division, Department of Medicine, Beth Israel Deaconess Medical Center, Boston, MA, United States

Ramya C. Mosarla
Division of Cardiology, Department of Medicine, New York University Langone Health, New York, NY, United States

D. Elizabeth Le, Sanjiv Kaul and Diana Rinkevich
Knight Cardiovascular Institute, Oregon Health and Science University, Portland, OR, United States

Manuel García-Jaramillo
Nutrition Program, School of Biological and Population Health Sciences, Oregon State University, Corvallis, OR, United States
Linus Pauling Institute, Oregon State University, Corvallis, OR, United States
Helfgott Research Institute, National University of Natural Medicine, Portland, OR, United States

Donald B. Jump
Nutrition Program, School of Biological and Population Health Sciences, Oregon State University, Corvallis, OR, United States
Linus Pauling Institute, Oregon State University, Corvallis, OR, United States

Gerd Bobe
Linus Pauling Institute, Oregon State University, Corvallis, OR, United States
Department of Animal and Rangeland Sciences, Oregon State University, Corvallis, OR, United States

Armando Alcazar Magana, Ashish Vaswani and Claudia S. Maier
Linus Pauling Institute, Oregon State University, Corvallis, OR, United States
Department of Chemistry, Oregon State University, Corvallis, OR, United States

Jessica Minnier
Department of Biostatistics and Knight Cancer Institute, Oregon Health and Science University, Portland, OR, United States

Nabil J. Alkayed
Knight Cardiovascular Institute, Oregon Health and Science University, Portland, OR, United States
Department of Anesthesiology and Perioperative Medicine, Oregon Health and Science University, Portland, OR, United States

Koki Mise, Mariko Imamura, Satoshi Yamaguchi, Mayu Watanabe, Chigusa Higuchi, Atsuko Nakatsuka, Jun Eguchi and Jun Wada
Department of Nephrology, Rheumatology, Endocrinology and Metabolism, Okayama University Graduate School of Medicine, Dentistry and Pharmaceutical Sciences, Okayama, Japan

Akihiro Katayama
Diabetes Center, Okayama University Hospital, Okayama, Japan

Satoshi Miyamoto, Michihiro Yoshida and Kenichi Shikata
Center for Innovative Clinical Medicine, Okayama University Hospital, Okayama, Japan

Haruhito A. Uchida
Department of Chronic Kidney Disease and Cardiovascular Disease, Okayama University Graduate School of Medicine, Dentistry and Pharmaceutical Sciences, Okayama, Japan

Kazuyuki Hida
Department of Diabetology and Metabolism, National Hospital Organization Okayama Medical Center, Okayama, Japan

Tatsuaki Nakato, Atsuhito Tone and Sanae Teshigawara
Okayama Saiseikai General Hospital, Okayama, Japan

Takashi Matsuoka, Shinji Kamei and Kazutoshi Murakami
Kurashiki Central Hospital, Kurashiki, Japan

Ikki Shimizu
The Sakakibara Heart Institute of Okayama, Okayama, Japan

Katsuhiro Miyashita
Japanese Red Cross Okayama Hospital, Okayama, Japan

Shinichiro Ando
Okayama City General Medical Center, Okayama, Japan

Tomokazu Nunoue
Nunoue Clinic, Tsuyama, Japan

Masao Yamada
GlycoTechnica Ltd., Yokohama, Japan

Eva Janssen, J. Wouter Jukema, Saskia L. M. A. Beeres, Martin J. Schalij and Laurens F. Tops
Department of Cardiology, Leiden University Medical Center, Leiden, Netherlands

Ahmed Zaky, Iram Zafar, Juan Xavier Masjoan-Juncos, Maroof Husain, Nithya Mariappan, Michael A. Frölich, Shama Ahmad and Aftab Ahmad
Department of Anesthesiology and Perioperative Medicine, University of Alabama at Birmingham, Birmingham, AL, United States

Charity J. Morgan
Department of Biostatistics, University of Alabama at Birmingham, Birmingham, AL, United States

Tariq Hamid
Division of Cardiovascular Disease, Department of Medicine, University of Alabama at Birmingham, Birmingham, AL, United States

Jin Sug Kim, Yang Gyun Kim, Ju-Young Moon, Sang-Ho Lee, Hyeon Seok Hwang and Kyung Hwan Jeong
Division of Nephrology, Department of Internal Medicine, Kyung Hee University, Seoul, South Korea

Dong-Young Lee
Division of Nephrology, Department of Internal Medicine, Veterans Health Service Medical Center, Seoul, South Korea

Shin Young Ahn and Gang-Jee Ko
Division of Nephrology, Department of Internal Medicine, Korea University College of Medicine, Seoul, South Korea

Qin-Hua Zhao, Su-Gang Gong, Rong Jiang, Ci-Jun Luo, Hong-Ling Qiu and Jin-Ming Liu
Department of Pulmonary Circulation, Shanghai Pulmonary Hospital, Tongji University School of Medicine, Shanghai, China

Lan Wang and Rui Zhang
Department of Pulmonary Circulation, Shanghai Pulmonary Hospital, Tongji University School of Medicine, Shanghai, China

Chao Li
Tongji University School of Medicine, Shanghai, China

Ge-Fei Chen
Department of Biosciences and Nutrition, Karolinska Institutet, Stockholm, Sweden

Xiao Ma, Changhua Mo, Liangzhao Huang, Peidong Cao, Louyi Shen and Chun Gui
Department of Cardiology, First Affiliated Hospital of Guangxi Medical University, Nanning, China

Chaojun Yang, Zhixing Fan, Jing Zhang and Jun Yang
Central Laboratory, Department of Cardiology, The First College of Clinical Medical Science, China Three Gorges University and Yichang Central People's Hospital, Yichang, China

Jinchun Wu
Department of Cardiology, Qinghai Provincial People's Hospital, Xining, China

Wei Zhang
Department of Cardiology, Renmin Hospital of Wuhan University, Wuhan, China

Jian Yang
Department of Cardiology, The People's Hospital of Three Gorges University and The First People' s Hospital of Yichang, Yichang, China

Yifan, Shi Jianfeng and Pu Jun
State Key Laboratory for Oncogenes and Related Genes, Division of Cardiology, Renji Hospital, School of Medicine, Shanghai Jiao Tong University, Shanghai Cancer Institute, Shanghai, China

Dae Kyu Kim
Department of Medicine, Graduate School, Kyung Hee University, Seoul, South Korea

Yu Ho Lee and So-Young Lee
Division of Nephrology, Department of Internal Medicine, CHA Bundang Medical Center, CHA University, Seongnam, South Korea

Muzheng Li, Zhijian Wu, Ilyas Tudahun, Na Liu, Qiuzhen Lin, Yingmin Wang, Mingxian Chen, Yaqin Chen, Nenghua Qi, Qingyi Zhu, Jianjun Tang and Qiming Liu
Department of Cardiovascular Medicine, The Second Xiangya Hospital of Central South University, Changsha, China

Jiang Liu
Department of Cardiovascular Surgery, The Second Xiangya Hospital of Central South University, Changsha, China

JunLi Li
Department of Radiology, The Second Xiangya Hospital of Central South University, Changsha, China

Wei Li
Department of Cardiology, Huaihua Hospital of Traditional Chinese Medicine, Huaihua, China

Xing Liu, Qian Chen, Yuanyuan Zhang and Long Peng
Department of Cardiovascular Medicine, The Third Affiliated Hospital, Sun Yat-sen University, Guangzhou, China

Shiyue Xu
Department of Hypertension and Vascular Disease, The First Affiliated Hospital, Sun Yat-sen University, Guangzhou, China

Ying Li
Department of Dermatology, Guangzhou Eighth People's Hospital, Guangzhou Medical University, Guangzhou, China

Shinichiro Niizuma
Department of Cardiology, Nihon University Hospital, Tokyo, Japan

Yoshitaka Iwanaga and Shunichi Miyazaki
Division of Cardiology, Kindai University Faculty of Medicine, Osakasayama, Japan

Takaharu Yahata
Department of Cardiology, Yokohama Chuo Hospital, Yokohama, Japan

Carolina Soler-Botija and Carolina Gálvez-Montón
Heart Failure and Cardiac Regeneration (ICREC) Research Program, Health Science Research Institute Germans Trias i Pujol (IGTP), Badalona, Spain
CIBERCV, Instituto de Salud Carlos III, Madrid, Spain

Antoni Bayés-Genís
Heart Failure and Cardiac Regeneration (ICREC) Research Program, Health Science Research Institute Germans Trias i Pujol (IGTP), Badalona, Spain
CIBERCV, Instituto de Salud Carlos III, Madrid, Spain
Cardiology Service, HUGTiP, Badalona, Spain
Department of Medicine, Barcelona Autonomous University (UAB), Badalona, Spain

Index